Molecular Allergy Diagnostics

Jörg Kleine-Tebbe • Thilo Jakob
Editors

Molecular Allergy Diagnostics

Innovation for a Better Patient Management

Foreword 1 by Robert G. Hamilton
Foreword 2 by Stefan Vieths

Springer

Editors
Jörg Kleine-Tebbe, MD
Professor of Dermatology and Allergology
Allergy and Asthma Center Westend
Outpatient Clinic Hanf
Ackermann and Kleine-Tebbe
Berlin
Germany

Thilo Jakob, MD
Professor of Dermatology and Allergology
Chairman of the Department of
Dermatology and Allergology
University Medical Center Gießen and
Marburg, Campus Gießen
Justus Liebig University Gießen
Gießen
Germany

ISBN 978-3-319-42498-9 ISBN 978-3-319-42499-6 (eBook)
DOI 10.1007/978-3-319-42499-6

Library of Congress Control Number: 2016963214

The editors gratefully thank Thermo Fisher Scientific, Phadia AB, Uppsala, Sweden, for the educational grant provided supporting English translation and language revision.
Based partially on the German language edition: Molekulare Allergiediagnostik by Jörg Kleine-Tebbe, Thilo Jakob.

Printed on acid-free paper

This Springer imprint is published by Springer Nature
The registered company is Springer International Publishing AG
The registered company address is: Gewerbestrasse 11, 6330 Cham, Switzerland

Foreword 1

Since 1967, when immunoglobulin E (IgE) was identified as the reagin in the blood that could transfer allergic sensitization, allergists have been striving to achieve increasingly "allergen-specific" diagnoses to help their patients with more targeted management strategies. In the USA in particular, complex allergen extracts have been almost exclusively used in both, in vivo (skin test and provocation testing) and in vitro (serological IgE antibody) assays. Of the 1269 extracts used in vivo for diagnosis in the USA, only 19 have limited "standardization." Thus, the remaining 1250 extracts have no defined potency, no known composition, and no documented stability. Importantly, 45 % of extracts used in skin testing have no peer-reviewed literature documenting their efficacy and may be deleted from use in the USA. Moreover, extracts cannot readily differentiate between primary sensitization and immunological cross-reactivity, and they cannot predict risk or identify a prognostically significant sensitization. Despite these serious limitations, these crude extracts are being exclusively used in allergy diagnosis throughout North America because they are grandfathered by regulatory agencies, relatively easy to prepare, and are thought to contain the most comprehensive profile of allergens of clinical relevance achievable for that specificity.

The increasing availability of clinically relevant allergenic molecules has begun to change the manner in which allergy diagnosis is performed. The age of "molecular allergology" has brought with it the promise of enhanced specificity and increased predictability for serious allergic reactions. Much of the innovative science related to allergenic molecules has emerged from basic and clinical studies performed in Europe. Thus, it is fitting that this excellent, comprehensive, practical text entitled *Molecular Allergy Diagnostics* has been edited by our German colleagues Drs. Kleine-Tebbe and Jakob. They have succeeded in obtaining authoritative and well-referenced reviews from the most experienced and knowledgeable authors from all over the world on topics relating to the allergenic plant and animal protein families and cross-reactive allergens due to their structure similarity. Despite the expanding repertoire of allergenic molecules available for serological dissection of the patient's IgE antibody sensitization profile, the North American allergist has been slow to adopt most of the available molecular allergen-specific IgE analyses into their routine diagnostic algorithm. The exceptions are peanut (Ara h 1, 2, 3, 8, and 9) and hazelnut (Cor a 1, 8, 9, and 14) where distinction can be made between cross-reactive and primary sensitization and in some cases relative risk for serious allergic reactions.

Drs. Kleine-Tebbe and Jakob and the contributing authors of *Molecular Allergy Diagnostics* are to be commended for their hard work and insightful preparation of this practical guide. This text serves as a unique, comprehensive, and simplified guidance with practical applications of the clinically important molecular allergen families as they are increasingly applied to the mainstream diagnostic algorithm for human allergic disease. For North American allergists who will probably not see recombinant molecular allergens used in skin testing or therapy, this textbook serves as a well-written primer on the topic of molecular allergen families available in IgE antibody serology and how they can enhance the accuracy (analytical and subsequently diagnostic sensitivity and specificity) of allergic diagnosis. This textbook also serves as a comprehensive compendium of the current science related to the application of allergen molecules in the diagnosis of the allergic patient. It is a must read for clinicians, clinical and research laboratory personnel, and governmental regulators who are involved in the use, interpretation, or regulation of allergen reagents and IgE antibody measurement used in allergy diagnosis. Finally, the lay public who suffer from allergic disease will enjoy reading this well-organized text while also gaining a clearer understanding of how diagnostic molecular allergens can simplify the complexity of their disease.

Robert G. Hamilton, Ph.D., D.ABMLI
Professor of Medicine and Pathology
Johns Hopkins University School of Medicine, and
Director of the Johns Hopkins Dermatology, Allergy and
Clinical Immunology Reference Laboratory,
Baltimore, MD, USA

Foreword 2

The term "molecular allergology" refers to the use of allergen molecules or particular fragments, such as peptides or carbohydrate chains for the diagnosis and allergen-specific immunotherapy of allergic diseases. The focus of this book is a clear and practice-oriented introduction to this complex topic.

The first allergens, from house dust mite and birch pollen, were cloned in the late 1980s, becoming available as highly purified recombinant proteins for molecular allergy research. The enormous potential for basic and clinical research was quickly recognized. Since then, more than 1000 allergen sequences have been identified. The availability of molecular allergens has caused a quantum leap in the field of allergy and offers great potential for the diagnosis and treatment of allergic diseases. The following areas of application are particularly worthy of note:

- Molecular-level studies on the mechanisms of type-I allergies (IgE-mediated immediate-type hypersensitivity reactions)
- Analysis of the B- and T-cell epitopes of allergens, with the goal of optimizing allergen-specific immunotherapy (AIT)
- Study on the mode of action of AIT
- Differentiation between clinically important and less relevant allergens from an allergen source or from comparable allergen families of different allergen sources
- Development of innovative immunotherapeutics of precisely defined composition and dosage
- Potential for the development of personalized mixtures of recombinant allergens for immunotherapy

Molecular diagnostics using single allergens is without doubt the area of application that has seen the greatest development and has already found its way into many areas of clinical routine. For allergists not primarily involved in research or molecular diagnostics, the multitude of publications on the topic can be confusing: What are the clinical consequences, e.g., of IgE binding to strongly cross-reactive minor allergens vs. species-specific major allergens from pollen? Which treatment recommendations for AIT can be derived from this? Should IgE responses to cross-reactive carbohydrate epitopes be classified as clinically irrelevant? Are all patients with IgE to the major allergen Ara h 2 from peanut at significant risk of anaphylaxis? Are these patients at high risk of reacting to trace quantities of peanut? Is the evidence solid enough to form the basis for recommendations for routine clinical practice?

This work addresses these questions by elaborating the background of molecular allergology in an easily comprehensible manner, hopefully without succumbing to the temptation to over-interpret the often exciting science uncovered in this still-evolving field. The authors, many of them well-known allergy researchers in German-speaking countries, have attempted to impart the interdisciplinary fundamentals in a clear and concise manner.

The boundaries of serological IgE diagnostics using single allergens are also clearly defined: Each IgE test represents a detection of sensitization, equivalent to an increased predisposition to allergies, not an actual allergy test. The use of allergen components changes nothing in this regard; the guidelines and basic principles of allergy diagnostics continue to remain valid.

With this book, the editors have succeeded in making the field of molecular allergy diagnostics accessible to a wide readership, thereby smoothing the way to an increased application in clinical practice.

Stefan Vieths, PhD
Vice President of the Paul-Ehrlich-Institut, and
Deputy Research Manager of the Allergology Unit,
Federal Institute for Vaccines and Biomedicines,
Langen, Germany

Preface

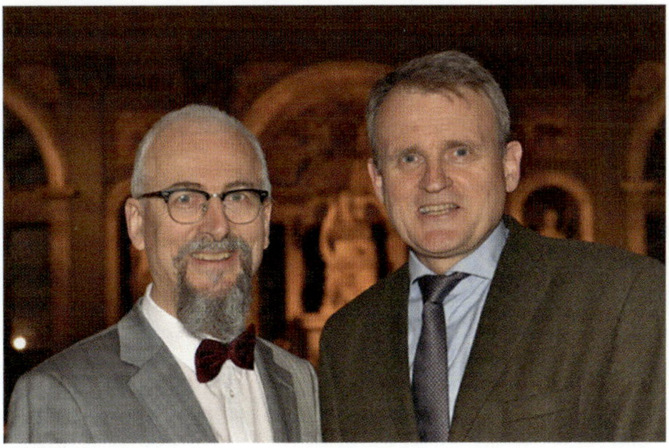

Molecular Allergology: From Research Topic to Innovative Allergy Diagnosis

Allergology—the recognition and treatment of allergic diseases—is regarded as an interdisciplinary field. Indeed, physicians with various organ specialties (i.e., dermatology, ENT, pediatrics, pulmonology) take care of allergic patients in Germany. In other countries, physicians practice as full specialists of allergy and clinical immunology. Immediate-type allergic reactions can affect multiple organs and all age groups. A multidisciplinary conceptual and detailed approach is key to understanding patterns of allergic responses and sequelae. The "scientific method," medical detective work, and clinical experience go hand in hand here. Successfully practiced allergology always considers the whole person, seeks individual solutions, and requires narrative-based medicine.

Rapid advances in modern allergy research have set this medically diverse specialty on a new course. With purified and synthetically produced (recombinant) allergens, basic and clinical research have gained important reagents with which new areas of allergology can be explored and old problems surprisingly easily solved.

This work on molecular allergology summarizes the most important developments of recent years. The first section presents examples of various allergic plant protein families and structurally related allergens, such as the Bet v 1 homologs/PR-10-like proteins, profilins, polcalcins, lipid transfer proteins, and storage proteins. This is followed by an introduction to animal allergens from the lipocalin, albumin, and Ca^{++}-binding protein families. Thus, the biological definition of important allergen sources (e.g., pollen, mites, mammals, molds, and foods) is expanded to a molecular dimension. It is, in fact, the actual allergic constituents that really matter!

The second section deals with methods of immunoglobulin E (IgE) determination to identify specific allergenic triggers: single determinations using singleplex or allergen screening using multiplex assays. Which type of diagnostician are you? Hunter or gatherer? Single allergens primarily improve the accuracy of IgE determinations, the test variants of which will be discussed in detail. The basic diagnostic rules remain unchanged: Positive IgE tests are only relevant in the case of corresponding symptoms. Thus, the individual patient history, quantifiable challenge tests, and astute interpretation retain their central importance in allergy diagnostics. Ultimately, it is the physician who determines the clinical relevance of allergy findings, not the test. The third section is devoted to molecular allergy diagnostics in routine clinical practice. How does one interpret symptoms conclusively and identify reaction patterns correctly? How can one effectively enhance the accuracy of allergy diagnostics? Molecular allergology opens up new avenues—it begins when one "thinks molecular" and makes use of the testing options which have recently become available. The benefits and boundaries of molecular allergy diagnostics are discussed using the gamut of common allergen sources as a basis. The final section looks ahead to future applications of molecular allergology, such as the development of recombinant allergy vaccines and hypoallergenic foods.

Molecular allergology is an exciting and rapidly developing field that has evolved from fragmented foci of research to an essential body of knowledge—particularly in relation to diagnostic questions in clinical allergology. It is our hope that, with this book, the authors will succeed in stimulating the reader's enthusiasm for this still-evolving discipline and provide possibilities for its implementation in clinical routine. Well-targeted, specific allergy diagnostics will, hopefully, augment the counseling and treatment of allergic patients in the future.

Berlin/Gießen, Germany
January 2017

Jörg Kleine-Tebbe
Thilo Jakob

Acknowledgments

First and foremost, we would like to extend our sincere thanks to the coauthors, co-contributors, and reviewers, all of whom are scientists active in the field of research. Their detailed knowledge, enthusiasm, and publishing experience were crucial to this team project. The goal of publishing the most comprehensive text book on molecular allergology worldwide available was only made possible by the authors' many years of experience in their specific fields. Truthfully, much of the content of this book has evolved over a number of years: most chapters have already been published at an earlier stage in the *Allergo Journal International* and have been revised, updated, and expanded for this book. Particular thanks are due to Marion Weber, Sebastian Lux, and Markus Seidl at Urban & Vogel Publishers/Springer Medicine for their unwavering support and careful stewardship of the article series "In Focus: Molecular Allergology," which later became the blueprint for a German book, released in 2015 by Springer Medicine, and eventually evolved into this book.

In this time of increasingly rapid global information exchange, international knowledge networks assume great importance. It is only by virtue of long-standing contact with visionary allergists and world-class European scientists—such as Rudolf Valenta, the founder of molecular allergology; Adriano Mari, the originator of Allergome, the largest allergen database worldwide; Jonas Lidholm, a molecular biologist highly productive in research and development in industry; Paolo M. Matricardi, a dedicated scientist with a creative view of future opportunities applying molecular allergology, Ronald van Ree, with his multinational, ground-breaking research projects; and many others—that the editors and authors were in a position to flow with the rapid pace of this young discipline. On behalf of ourselves and all the coauthors, we would like to express our sincere thanks to Caroline Beyer, Christopher Richardson, Christine Schäfer, and Stefan Schülke for professional translations; Steve Love for his meticulous style corrections; Jan Bernhisel-Broadbent, Kenneth Broadbent, Robert K. Bush, David B. K. Golden, Marianne van Hage, Robert G. Hamilton, David A. Levy, Greg Plunkett, Sarbjit S. Saini, Wayne Thomas, Anna Nowak-Wegrzyn, and Robert A. Wood, for their excellent comments and final editorial assistance; and last but not least to all pioneers and enthusiasts of modern molecular allergology.

We, the editors, would also like to take this opportunity to thank our mentors and colleagues of many years' standing, both here and abroad, who have been instrumental in supporting our professional passion for clinical and, more particularly, molecular allergology with their specialized expertise. Particular and special thanks go to our academic teachers, mentors and friends Ivan M Roith, London, Mark C. Udey and Steven I. Katz, Bethesda, Johannes Ring and Heidrun Behrendt, Munich, and Lena Bruckner-Tuderman, Freiburg (T.J.) as well as Gert Kunkel, Berlin, Susan M. MacDonald, Robert G. Hamilton, Donald W. MacGlashan Jr., Lawrence M. Lichtenstein, Shau-Ku Huang, David G. Marsh†, Baltimore, and Uwe-Frithjof Haustein, Leipzig (J.K-T.) as well as our colleagues and staff at our past and present affiliations. Thanks to regular expert and collegial exchanges with them, many important aspects relating to the theoretical understanding of and practical approach to molecular allergology have found their way into this book.

Every book project comes at a price—the time and effort devoted on a professional level often means shortfalls elsewhere. We are extremely grateful, therefore, to our families, in particular our wives, Uta Bella Zielke (Berlin) and Virginia Jakob (Wetzlar), for their patience and support. Our thanks also go to the staff at Springer Nature, particularly Juliette R. Kleemann for the realization of the English version of this work and continuous support throughout the project.

Finally, special thanks are due to Rahul Kumar Sharma for his professional copyediting of the manuscript and Muthu Pradeep Kumar for coordinating production of the book, as well as Stephanie Hofmaier for her meticulous correction and Wolf-Meinhard Becker for his careful preparation of an excellent index. With their enthusiasm and commitment, they all contributed substantially to making it possible to produce this book with high quality.

Jörg Kleine-Tebbe
Thilo Jakob

Contents

Part III Marker Allergens

Contributors

Barbara K. Ballmer-Weber, MD, Prof. Center of Dermatology and Allergology, Kantonsspital Luzern, Lucerne, Switzerland

Department of Dermatology, University Hospital Zürich, Zurich, Switzerland

Kirsten Beyer, MD, Prof. Department of Pediatric Pneumology and Immunology, Charité-Universitätsmedizin, Berlin, Germany

Tilo Biedermann, MD, Prof. Department of Dermatology and Allergology, Technical University of Munich, Munich, Germany

Simon Blank, PhD Center of Allergy and Environment (ZAUM), Technical University of Munich and Helmholtz Center Munich, Munich, Germany

Heimo Breiteneder, PhD, Prof. Department of Pathophysiology and Allergy Research, Center for Pathophysiology, Infectiology and Immunology, Medical University of Vienna, Vienna, Austria

Peter S. Creticos, MD, Prof. Johns Hopkins University School of Medicine, Division of Allergy and Clinical Immunology, Baltimore, MD, USA

Creticos Research Group, LLC, Crownsville, MD, USA

Janet M. Davies, PhD, Prof. Centre for Children's Health Research, Institute of Health and Biomedical Innovation, Queensland University of Technology, South Brisbane, QLD, Australia

Fatima Ferreira, PhD, Prof. Department of Molecular Biology, University of Salzburg, Salzburg, Austria

Jörg Fischer, MD Department of Dermatology, University Hospital Tübingen, Tübingen, Germany

Peter Forstenlechner, PhD Phadia – Thermo Fisher Scientific, Wien, Austria

Gabriele Gadermaier, PhD, Prof. Department of Molecular Biology, University of Salzburg, Salzburg, Austria

Katharina Gangl, MD Department of Otorhinolaryngology, Medical University of Vienna, Vienna, Austria

Richard E. Goodman, PhD, Prof. Department of Food Science & Technology, University of Nebraska, Lincoln, NE, USA

Dietrich Häfner, PhD Allergopharma GmbH and Co. KG, Reinbek, Germany

Robert G. Hamilton, PhD, Prof. Department of Medicine, Johns Hopkins University School of Medicine, Baltimore, MD, USA

Johns Hopkins Dermatology, Allergy and Clinical Immunology Reference Laboratory, Baltimore, MD, USA

Johns Hopkins Asthma and Allergy Center, Baltimore, MD, USA

Michael Hauser, PhD Department of Molecular Biology, University of Salzburg, Salzburg, Austria

Thomas Hawranek, MD Department of Dermatology, Paracelsus Private Medical University Salzburg, Salzburg, Austria

Wolfgang Hemmer, PhD, Assoc Prof. FAZ – Floridsdorf Allergy Center, Vienna, Austria

Christiane Hilger, PhD Allergology – Immunology – Inflammation Research Unit, Department of Infection and Immunity, Luxembourg Institute of Health, Esch-sur-Alzette, Luxembourg

Heidi Hofer, PhD Department of Molecular Biology, University of Salzburg, Salzburg, Austria

Karin Hoffmann-Sommergruber, PhD, Prof. Department of Pathophysiology and Allergy Research, Medical University of Vienna, Vienna, Austria

Silke C. Hofmann, MD Center for Dermatology, Allergy and Dermatosurgery, HELIOS University Hospital Wuppertal, University Witten/Herdecke, Wuppertal, Germany

Johannes Huss-Marp, MD, MBA, Assoc Prof. Therapeutic Area Dermatology, AbbVie Deutschland GmbH & Co KG, Wiesbaden, Germany

Thilo Jakob, MD, Prof. Department of Dermatology and Allergology, University Medical Center Giessen (UKGM), Justus-Liebig-University, Giessen, Germany

Uta Jappe, MD, Prof. Division of Clinical and Molecular Allergology, Research Center Borstel, Airway Research Center North (ARCN), Member of the German Center for Lung Research (DZL), Borstel, Germany

Interdisciplinary Allergy Unit, Department of Pneumology, University Medical Center, University of Lübeck, Lubeck, Germany

Sandip D. Kamath, PhD Molecular Allergy Research Laboratory, Centre for Biodiscovery and Molecular Development of Therapeutics, Australian Institute of Tropical Health and Medicine, James Cook University, Townsville, QLD, Australia

Sabine Kespohl, PhD Institute for Prevention and Occupational Medicine of the German Social Accident Insurance, Institute of the Ruhr-Universität Bochum (IPA), Bochum, Germany

Jörg Kleine-Tebbe, MD, Prof. Allergy and Asthma Center Westend, Outpatient Clinic Hanf, Ackermann and Kleine-Tebbe, Berlin, Germany

Annette Kuehn, PhD Allergology – Immunology – Inflammation Research Unit, Department of Infection and Immunity, Luxembourg Institute of Health, Esch-sur-Alzette, Luxembourg

Skadi Kull, PhD Clinical and Molecular Allergology, Research Center Borstel, Leibniz-Center for Medicine and Biosciences, Borstel, Germany

Lars Lange, MD, Assoc Prof. St. Marien Hospital, Bonn, Germany

Department of Pediatrics, St. Marien-Hospital, Bonn, Germany

Andreas L. Lopata, PhD, Prof. Molecular Allergy Research Laboratory, Centre for Biodiscovery and Molecular Development of Therapeutics, Australian Institute of Tropical Health and Medicine, James Cook University, Townsville, QLD, Australia

Vera Mahler, MD, Prof. Paul-Ehrlich-Institute, Allergy Department, Federal Institute for Vaccines and Biomedicines, Langen, Germany

Paolo M. Matricardi, MD, Assoc Prof. Molecular Allergology and Immunomodulation Working Group, Department of Pediatric Pneumology and Immunology, Charité-Universitätsmedizin, Berlin, Germany

Martine Morisset, MD Immunology Allergology Unit, Centre Hospitalier de Luxembourg, Luxembourg, Luxembourg

Andreas Nandy, PhD Business Unit Allergy, Research & Development, Allergopharma GmbH and Co. KG, Reinbek, Germany

Verena Niederberger, MD, Prof. Department of Otorhinolaryngology, Medical University of Vienna, Vienna, Austria

Markus Ollert, MD, Prof. Department of Infection and Immunity, Luxembourg Institute of Health (LIH), Esch-sur-Alzette, Luxembourg

Odense Research Center for Anaphylaxis (ORCA), Department of Dermatology and Allergy Center, Odense University Hospital, University of Southern Denmark, Odense C, Denmark

Arnd Petersen, PhD Research Center Borstel, Borstel, Germany

Thomas Platts-Mills, MD, PhD, Prof. Division of Allergy, Asthma, & Immunology, Department of Medicine, University of Virginia Health System, Charlottesville, VA, USA

Anna Pomés, PhD Basic Research Department, Indoor Biotechnologies, Inc, Charlottesville, VA, USA

Christian Radauer, PhD, Prof. Department of Pathophysiology and Allergy Research, Center for Pathophysiology, Infectiology and Immunology, Medical University of Vienna, Vienna, Austria

Monika Raulf, PhD, Prof. Center Allergology/Immunology, Institute for Prevention and Occupational Medicine of the German Social Accident Insurance, Institute of the Ruhr-Universität Bochum, Bochum, Germany

Imke Reese, Dr. oec troph. Nutrition Counseling and Therapy with Special Focus on Allergology, Munich, Germany

Hans-Peter Rihs, PhD Institute for Prevention and Occupational Medicine of the German Social Accident Insurance, Institute of the Ruhr-University Bochum (IPA), Bochum, Germany

Stephan Scheurer, PhD, Assoc Prof. Paul-Ehrlich-Institut, Federal Institute for Vaccines and Biomedicines, Langen, Germany

Edzard Spillner, PhD, Prof. Immunological Engineering, Department of Engineering, Aarhus University, Aarhus, Denmark

Teresa Stemeseder Department of Molecular Biology, University of Salzburg, Salzburg, Austria

Ines Swoboda, PhD, Prof. Molecular Biotechnology Section, FH Campus Wien, University of Applied Sciences, Vienna, Austria

Anubha Tripathi, MD Division of Allergy, Asthma, & Immunology, Department of Medicine, University of Virginia Health System, Charlottesville, VA, USA

Rudolf Valenta, MD, Prof. Center for Pathophysiology, Infectiology and Immunology, Medical University of Vienna, Vienna, Austria

Marianne van Hage, MD, Prof. Immunology and Allergy Unit, Department of Medicine Solna, Karolinska Institutet and Karolinska University Hospital, Stockholm, Sweden

Stefan Vieths, PhD, Prof. Paul-Ehrlich-Institute, Management, Federal Institute for Vaccines and Biomedicines, Langen, Germany

Susanne Vrtala, PhD, Prof. Department of Pathophysiology and Allergy Research, Center for Pathophysiology, Infectiology and Immunology, Medical University of Vienna, Vienna, Austria

Michael Wallner, PhD Department of Molecular Biology, University of Salzburg, Salzburg, Austria

Part I

Protein Families and Relationships

Introduction to Molecular Allergology: Protein Families, Databases, and Potential Benefits

1

J. Kleine-Tebbe, M. Ollert, C. Radauer, and T. Jakob

This contribution is based on a publication that appeared in the *Allergo Journal* in 2010 (Kleine-Tebbe J, Ollert M, Jakob T: Molekulare Allergologie: Nomenklatur, Proteinfamilien, Datenbanken und potenzieller Nutzen. Allergo J 2010; 19: 390–394) and which has been updated, expanded, and translated into English as a chapter for this book.
The authors gratefully thank Dr. Steve Love, PhD, Laguna Niguel, CA, USA, for reading the manuscript, helpful suggestions, and editorial assistance with the English translation.

J. Kleine-Tebbe, MD, Prof. (✉)
Allergy & Asthma Center Westend, Outpatient Clinic Hanf, Ackermann & Kleine-Tebbe, Berlin, Germany
e-mail: kleine-tebbe@allergie-experten.de

M. Ollert, MD, Prof.
Department of Infection and Immunity, Luxembourg Institute of Health (LIH), Esch-sur-Alzette, Luxembourg

Odense Research Center for Anaphylaxis (ORCA), Department of Dermatology and Allergy Center, Odense University Hospital, University of Southern Denmark, Odense C, Denmark
e-mail: markus.ollert@lih.lu; markus.ollert@rsyd.dk; Web: http://www.lih.lu; http://www.anafylaksi.net/

C. Radauer, PhD, Prof.
Department of Pathophysiology and Allergy Research, Center for Pathophysiology, Infectiology and Immunology, Medical University of Vienna, Vienna, Austria
e-mail: christian.radauer@meduniwien.ac.at

T. Jakob, MD, Prof.
Department of Dermatology and Allergology, University Medical Center Giessen (UKGM), Justus-Liebig-University, Giessen, Germany
e-mail: thilo.jakob@derma.med.uni-giessen.de

J. Kleine-Tebbe, T. Jakob (eds.), *Molecular Allergy Diagnostics*,
DOI 10.1007/978-3-319-42499-6_1

1.1 The Era of Molecular Allergology

Thanks to advances in methods of protein biochemistry and molecular biology, the past 30 years have seen the identification of the most important allergens that induce IgE-mediated immediate-type reactions and atopic conditions. The study of allergens (the main focus of which was previously the biological relatedness of allergy sources, e.g., plant, mite, and mammalian species) was thus mounting a molecular dimension and new terminology (▶ brief glossary). Modern allergen research is providing the foundation for improved allergy diagnostics and therapy which complements and/or replaces our previous allergological methodology (for review, see also Matricardi et al. 2016).

Molecular Allergology: A Brief Glossary (modified from Kleine-Tebbe et al 2010)

Allergen (also single allergen or allergen component)	A molecule (protein, e.g., major allergen Bet v 1 from birch pollen, in rare cases carbohydrate moieties) that may induce an allergic immune response
Allergen extract	Mixture of allergenic and nonallergenic components extracted from the allergen source (e.g., birch pollen)
Allergen nomenclature	International agreement on the designation (naming) of allergens
Allergen source	Biological species that produces (single) allergens and releases them into the environment
CRD	Component-resolved diagnostics (allergy diagnostic procedures with single allergens)
Epitope	Binding site for antibodies
Isoallergen	Variant form of an allergen with similar amino acid sequence (>67 % identity score)
Linear epitope	Peptide sequence that may be bound by an antibody or a T cell receptor
Conformational epitope	Discontinuous, structure-dependent binding site for antibodies
Cross-reaction	Immunological response caused by structural similarity and involving molecules not responsible for the original sensitization
Major allergen	An allergen that binds IgE in ≥50 % of allergic individuals
Minor allergen	Allergen that binds IgE in <50 % of allergic individuals
Multiplex assay	In vitro diagnostic test with concurrent testing of antibodies (e.g., IgE) to many (single) allergens
Panallergen	An allergen that is ubiquitous or present in many allergen sources, generally highly conserved (i.e., little changed by evolution)

Protein family	Group of proteins related in terms of sequence and structural similarity
Recombinant	Produced by means of genetically modified microorganisms
Recombinant allergen	Allergenic protein frequently produced in *Escherichia coli* that lacks modifications occurring in native allergens (e.g., carbohydrate side chains)
Sequential epitope	Antibody binding site whose basis is a continuous peptide sequence (▶ linear epitope)
Singleplex assay	In vitro diagnostic test (e.g., antibody test) detecting allergy to *a single* allergen
Species specific	Allergen or other characteristic present in only *one* species

1.2 Immediate-Type Allergens and Their Names

As early as the 1980s, a systematic naming convention was proposed for the first purified protein allergens and an allergen nomenclature devised (Marsh et al. 1986). The organization responsible is the Allergen Nomenclature Sub-Committee (▶ www.allergen.org) under the auspices of the International Union of Immunological Societies (IUIS, ▶ www.iuisonline.org) and the World Health Organization (WHO, ▶ www.who.int).

This official nomenclature (Chapman 2004, 2008; King et al. 1995; Radauer et al. 2014) is based on the allergen source, using abbreviations of Linnaean species names and with numbering related to the order of discovery (◉ Table 1.1), for example, Bet v 1 as the major allergen of the silver birch (*Betula verrucosa*). The nomenclature also incorporates isoallergens and allergen variants, allergen-coding genes, mRNA and cDNA, as well as allergenic peptides of recombinant or synthetic

Table 1.1 Allergen nomenclature: names of allergens illustrated with reference to rBet v 1.0102, a major allergen of the silver birch (*Betula verrucosa*)

Abbreviation	Full term	Explanatory notes
n	Natural	Obtained from the allergen source (= purified)
r	Recombinant	Produced in microorganisms such as bacteria
Bet	*Betula*	The first 3–4 letters of the genus name
v	*verrucosa*	The first 1–2 letters of the species name
1	Allergen number	Indicates order in which allergens were first reported
.01	Isoallergen number	Different sequences of an allergen with >67 % sequence identity are termed isoallergens
02	Variant number	Different sequences of an allergen with >90 % sequence identity are termed variants

origin, in both their original and modified forms. Data on new allergens or related molecules are examined carefully before the name is included in the official list of allergens (▶ www.allergen.org).

1.3 Sequence and Structure: From T Cell to Antibody (B Cell) Epitopes

As with other proteins, each allergen (including its natural variants) is coded for by corresponding genes.

By means of its physicochemical properties, the resulting amino acid sequence (primary structure) gives rise to folding and the spatial arrangement of the polypeptide chain in regular structural elements (◉ Fig. 1.1): examples are α-helix, β-sheet, and β-turn (secondary structure). The overall arrangement of the secondary structure elements determines a protein's three-dimensional structure (tertiary structure). Additionally, several polypeptide chains can combine to form larger complexes (quaternary structure). Practically, allergen molecules or their fragments correspond to the general structural hierarchy of proteins.

Structural Hierarchy of Proteins: From Peptide to Protein Complex

- *Primary structure:* amino acid sequence, linear peptide
- *Secondary structure:* folding of the polypeptide chain into regular structural elements (e.g., α-helix, β-sheet)
- *Tertiary structure:* three-dimensional structure of a polypeptide chain
- *Quaternary structure:* complex consisting of several (identical or different) polypeptide chains (= subunits), e.g., Ara h 1 trimer

Whereas T cells recognize only short linear peptides (linear peptide epitopes) following their processing by antigen-presenting cells, antibodies primarily bind *conformational epitopes*. These are formed by several single amino acids or short peptides that are located at noncontiguous sites in the amino acid sequence and arranged at adjacent positions on the protein surface (only if the protein is correctly folded). Thus, they are alternatively designated *discontinuous epitopes* (◉ Fig. 1.1e, f).

1.4 Protein Families and Relatedness of Type I Allergens

Similar proteins are assigned to families based on their amino acid sequences. Evolutionarily related protein families, whose members exhibit similar three-dimensional structures, are grouped into superfamilies (◉ Fig. 1.2). While it can be assumed that two proteins with a sequence identity of as low as 25 % are evolutionarily related, cross-reactivity generally requires a sequence identity of >50 %.

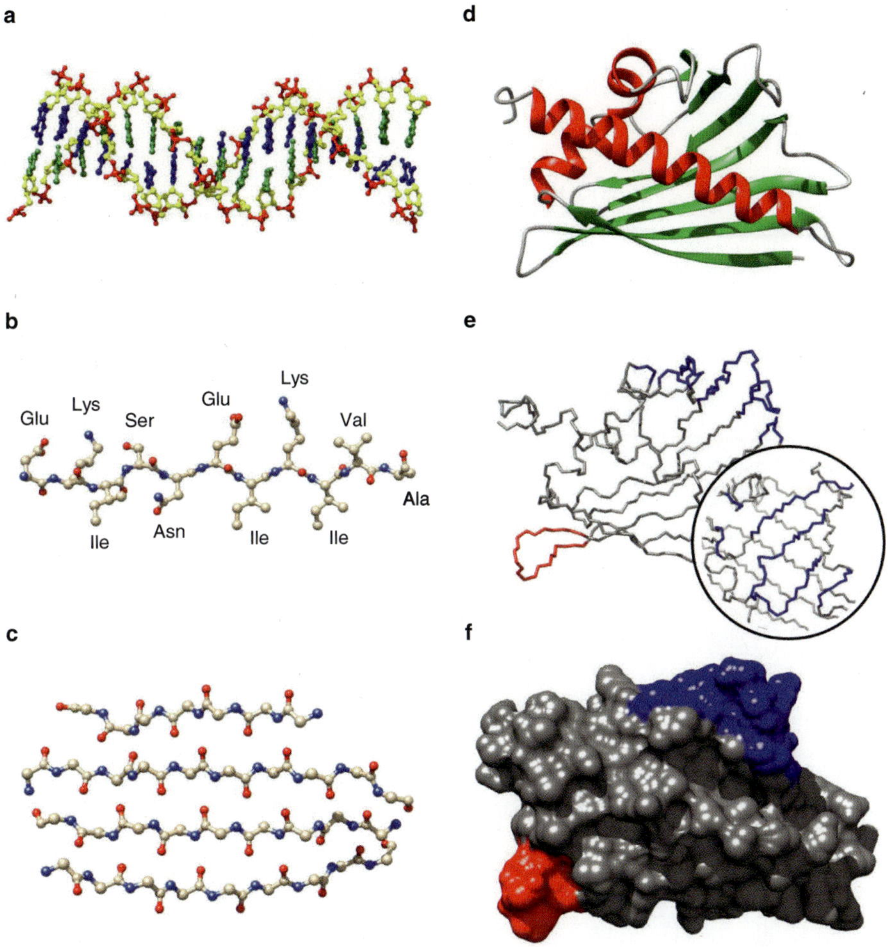

Fig. 1.1 From gene to epitope. (**a**) Structure of the DNA double helix (*red*: phosphate, *yellow*: deoxyribose, *green* and *blue*: bases). (**b**) Primary structure of a polypeptide chain. (**c**) Regular folding of the polypeptide chain in a secondary structure, using the β-sheet of Bet v 1 as an example. The molecules in **b** and **c** are colored by type of atom (*gray*: carbon, *red*: oxygen, *blue*: nitrogen). (**d–f**) Tertiary structure of Bet v 1: **d** Ribbon diagram illustrating secondary structure elements (*red* α-helix, *green*: β-sheet). (**e**) Polypeptide chain (without side chains) with two possible epitopes (*red*: linear epitope, *blue*: conformational epitope with top view circled). (**f**) Surface of Bet v 1 highlighting the same epitopes as in **e**

Proteins with this degree of similarity have many identical surface patches that may act as potential epitopes for cross-reactive antibodies.

Apparently, a mere fraction of known protein families include potential immediate-type allergens (Breiteneder 2009; Breiteneder and Radauer 2004; Radauer et al. 2008). It should also be emphasized that, even within protein families containing allergens, most proteins are not allergenic. The factors predisposing a

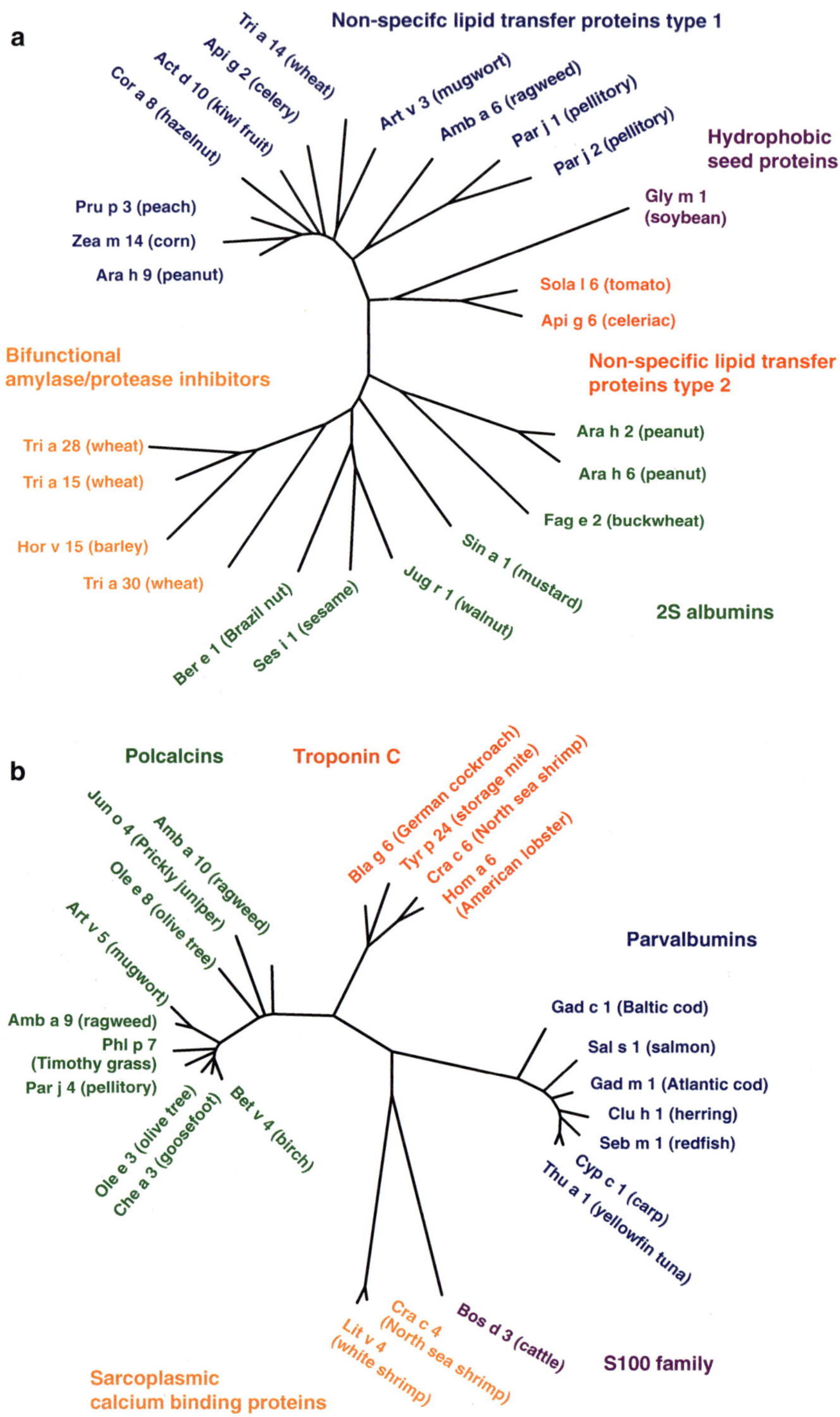

Fig. 1.2 Evolutionary relatedness within allergen superfamilies using the examples of (**a**) the prolamin superfamily and (**b**) the EF-hand superfamily. Protein families defined by sequence similarity (highlighted in *color*) are grouped into superfamilies on the basis of structural similarity

protein to be an allergen are still a matter of active research (Poulsen 2009) and, to date, known only for certain proteins. Among these factors are the following:

- Occurrence, opportunities for exposure
- Physicochemical properties, such as solubility in water, and extractability (mainly with inhalant allergens) or stability (mainly with food allergens)
- Proportion of total protein in a species, organism, or allergen source
- Proteolytic activity, resulting in easier penetration of epithelium (group 1 allergens of the house-dust mite, e.g., Der p 1, Der f 1) (Kauffman et al. 2006)
- Binding to receptors of dendritic cells (group 2 allergens of the house-dust mite, e.g., Der p 2, Der f 2; peanut allergen Ara h 1) and structural mimicry with other danger signals (Karp 2010)

There is, in fact, no single reason why a protein becomes an allergen. This must be clarified separately for each allergen. The answers will help to broaden our understanding of the interaction between foreign proteins and the human body, as well as the cause of hypersensitivity.

In regard to proteins that also occur in humans, the degree of evolutionary relatedness – expressed as sequence identity/similarity – is probably the crucial factor leading either to tolerance (where relatedness is close) or the possibility of type I allergy (where proteins are distantly related). Likewise, cross-reactions between allergens not present in humans can be predicted on the basis of their evolutionary relatedness (percent sequence identity) and resulting structural similarity (Jenkins et al. 2007).

1.5 Databases for Clinical Practice and Research

Extensive databases of allergens and their protein families now exist (◉ Table 1.2) (Sircar et al. 2014).

The official source of allergen designations is the database of the WHO/IUIS Allergen Nomenclature Sub-Committee (www.allergen.org). Researchers who describe new allergens are required to submit the key data to this body prior to their publication, upon which they receive an official name for the allergen; this name should, thereafter, be used consistently in the literature (with referencing if necessary). As well as the names and sources of allergens, this database also contains data on allergenicity provided at the time of submission, the citation of the first description, and links to other databases (DNA sequence, protein sequence, protein structure).

The largest database of protein allergens at present was established and is maintained by Adriano Mari, a clinical allergist and research scientist from Rome, Italy (▶ www.allergome.org; Mari and Scala 2006). It offers free public access for searches of all allergens identified to date. Additionally, it contains information on allergenic molecules; potential variants and modifications; links to databases of sequences, structures, and taxonomy; allergen sources with illustrations; and epidemiologic statistics.

Table 1.2 Important allergen databases and their areas of application

Name	Internet Address	Data included	Search tools	Target groups	Remarks
IUIS Allergen Nomenclature Database	www.allergen.org	Allergen names, biochemical designations, allergen source, isoallergens, literature (first description), links to external databases (sequence, structure)	Search by allergen names and source	Clinicians, scientists, industry	Official reference for allergen names and corresponding sequences
Allergome	www.allergome.org	Allergen names, biochemical functions, isoallergens, allergen source, type of exposure, diagnostic reagents, links to sequences and structures, sequence homologies, cross-reactive allergens, allergenic properties and epidemiology, extensive bibliography grouped by subject area	Text search in all database fields, sequence comparison, sophisticated literature search	Clinicians, scientists, industry	Extensive collection of data on allergens, obtained from other databases and the literature. All allergens with published data are included, without filtering by relevance
AllergenOnline	www.allergenonline.org	Allergen names, type (inhalant, food, etc.) and source, sequence, selected literature	Text search, different methods of sequence comparison	Scientists, industry	List of allergens reviewed by panel of experts, provision of a reliable database with relevant allergen sequences
Structural Database of Allergenic Proteins (SDAP)	https://fermi.utmb.edu	Allergen names and source, protein family, selected literature, links to sequences, and structures	Sequence comparison, peptide comparison, links to external servers (e.g., BLAST)	Scientists, industry	Allergen sequence database with collection of bioinformatics tools; emphasis on allergen structures and epitopes
AllFam	www.meduniwien.ac.at/allfam/	Allergen names with links to IUIS database and AllergenOnline, type of exposure, abstracts on protein families with selected literature	List of members of allergen families (filtered by source and exposure), text search by protein family	Clinicians, scientists, industry	Classification of allergens by protein family

Each allergen record in the www.allergome.org database includes an extensive list of references arranged by subject area:

- Biochemistry/structure/function
- Molecular biology
- Immunochemistry and allergenicity
- Immune mechanism and genetics
- Detection
- Epidemiology
- Diagnosis
- Immunotherapy
- Experimental models
- Reviews

Further online instruments – whose use is in some cases restricted to active collaborators – continuously enhance the value of this database, as does its comprehensive maintenance. Because Allergome's objective is, insofar as possible, a full analysis of the allergological literature, this database also includes allergens without an official designation and a listing in www.allergen.org.

The AllergenOnline database (▶ www.allergenonline.org) is maintained by the Food Allergy Research and Resource Program (FARRP) at the University of Nebraska-Lincoln, Lincoln, NB. It provides a list of allergen sequences that can be searched using various bioinformatics tools. Users can compare a protein sequence with the database and, thus, search for similar allergen sequences. The list of allergens included in AllergenOnline is reviewed by an international panel of experts and updated annually. One application is risk assessment of genetically modified foods. It is crucial, in order to minimize the risk of allergic reactions, that the sequences of the newly introduced genes have no similarity to known allergens.

The Structural Database of Allergenic Proteins (SDAP) is operated by the Department of Biochemistry and Molecular Biology at the University of Texas, Galveston, Texas (▶ https://fermi.utmb.edu). It gathers data on allergen sequences, structures, epitopes, and protein families from both the IUIS allergen database and the literature. A particular strength of the SDAP is the extensive repertoire of bioinformatics tools with which investigators can compare their own sequences to the database.

For protein families that contain structurally related allergens, a valuable website (AllFam) has been created in Vienna (▶ www.meduniwien.ac.at/allfam/). It draws upon existing databases of allergens (www.allergome.org; www.allergen.org) and protein families (http://pfam.xfam.org), informs users about the properties of a given allergen family or superfamily, and lists the allergens within each family with links to allergenonline.com and allergen.org.

1.6 Potential Use of Single Allergens

1.6.1 Quantification of Allergens in Extracts

Recombinant allergens and corresponding (monoclonal) antibodies are potentially suitable for immunoassays of the allergen content of extracts. The reagents required for assays to test for major allergens, such as the major birch pollen allergen Bet v 1 and the major grass pollen allergen Phl p 5a, have already been identified in an EU-funded research project (CREATE; van Ree et al. 2008). They were then individually reviewed by the Biological Standardization Program (BSP090) of the European Directorate for the Quality of Medicines & HealthCare (EDQM) and, in an interlaboratory trial, tested as to their likely reliability (Vieths et al. 2012). The recombinant major allergens Bet v 1 (▶ https://crs.edqm.eu/db/4DCGI/View=Y0001565) and Phl p 5a (▶ https://crs.edqm.eu/db/4DCGI/View=Y0001566) have, since 2012, been used by the European Pharmacopoeia (Ph. Eur.) as biological reference products (BRPs). Now that the corresponding antibody pairs have also been officially accepted by the EDQM, robust testing methods will be available for the first time, allowing for the reliable testing and subsequent labeling of major allergens in complex allergen extracts – a "Holy Grail" of allergists for a long time.

Benefits of Molecular Allergology in Routine Clinical Practice (for review see also Matricardi et al. 2016)

- Advantages of using single allergens for extract standardization:
  - Facilitates quality management in the production of allergen extracts
  - Greater comparability of allergen extracts for diagnostics and immunotherapy
  - Greater safety because of improved batch conformity of allergen products
- Differential diagnostic procedures where allergen components are used, allowing the following:
  - Greater analytical and (if applicable) diagnostic sensitivity of in vitro tests
  - Improved analytical specificity and selectivity for associating allergens with risks
  - Identification of species-specific allergens (detection of true sensitization as opposed to cross-sensitization)
  - Identification of (pan-)allergens as the cause of cross-reactions
- Advantages of multiplex methods (multiple analytes in one assay run) in allergy diagnostics (e.g., using microchips for IgE detection):
  - IgE-mediated sensitization essentially ruled out where a result is negative

- Effective assessment of complex sensitization patterns in polyvalent allergy
- Comprehensive screening if etiology of IgE-mediated anaphylactic reaction is unknown

• Potential use of recombinant single allergens in specific immunotherapy

1.6.2 Molecular Epidemiology

Historical data on the frequency of allergic sensitization are based primarily on IgE diagnostics with allergen extracts (Haftenberger et al. 2013). Their complex composition – a mixture of species-specific (major) allergens, cross-reactive panallergens, and cross-reactive minor allergens – makes it difficult to clearly assign prevalence to the relevant allergy sources (Schmitz et al. 2013). Systematic investigations into regional sensitization profiles by means of single allergens (Barber et al. 2008) therefore have huge potential for mapping of regional (inhalant) allergen load, lifestyle factors and dietary habits, and the consequent impact on atopic individuals.

Longitudinal studies are suitable (based on the sequence of new sensitizations) for clarifying the relevance of single allergens in the allergic immune response at relevant exposure levels. For example, in the majority of the children in the Berlin MAS birth cohort, Phl p 1, a major allergen of Timothy grass pollen and a member of the group 1 grass allergen family, was the first allergen for which specific IgE was detected. This sensitization predated by years the onset of clinical symptoms (Hatzler et al. 2012).

1.6.3 Diagnostics with Single Allergens

The increasing availability of known and commercially available allergen molecules opens up new diagnostic possibilities for testing specific IgE antibodies (examples, no complete listing):

- www.phadia.com/en/Products/Allergy-testing-products/ImmunoCAP-Molecular-Allergology/
- https://www.healthcare.siemens.com/clinical-specialities/allergy/laboratorian-information
- www.fooke-labs.com/produktbereiche/in-vitro-allergie-diagnostik/index.html *(in German only)*

Purified natural and recombinant allergens can be used as follows:

1. As single test reagents (singleplex method, ▶ Chap. 7)
2. As a combination of multiple allergens in component-resolved diagnostics, such as in a microarray (multiplex method, ▶ Chap. 9) (Scala et al. 2010)

3. Spiked onto extracts (▶ Chap. 8)
4. Combined as extract substitutes (not yet available due to high costs)

The first two options allow molecule-specific diagnosis, whereas the last two variants increase the sensitivity and reliability of the tests.

In general, single allergens used in IgE diagnostics primarily improve the nature of the tests and, to a lesser extent, its clinical interpretation (▶ Sect. 1.7):

- Test sensitivity (= limit of quantitation, LoQ) is enhanced (lower LoQ) by single allergens especially when they are not sufficiently present in the allergen extract or absent altogether.
- The analytical specificity (selectivity), i.e., the ability to identify only a relevant part of the allergen-specific IgE repertoire is enhanced. This is beneficial if IgE sensitization to the single relevant allergen is associated with certain clinical observations (e.g., extent of risk of reaction to food, the severity of a reaction, or the patient's specific condition).
- Certain single allergens function as indicators of serological, IgE-mediated cross-reactions between structurally similar allergens.
- By contrast, some single allergens are regarded as serological, species-specific markers of primary, genuine IgE sensitization to a specific allergen source.

Apart from the second point, these advantages relate solely to testing, i.e., improvement in detection of sensitization – even without knowledge of the patient's clinical symptoms. Molecular allergy diagnostics may allow differentiation of multiple sensitizations by identification of species-specific reactions. It may also uncover cross-sensitizations and previously undetected sensitizations to single allergens that are underrepresented in the extract or are associated with an increased risk of severe reactions, such as to certain food allergens. Enhanced test sensitivity increases the number of positive specific IgE findings, whose clinical relevance is – as this was the case with extract diagnostics – valid only if there are corresponding symptoms present.

Clinical trials will help to define the diagnostic role of single allergens for the development of tolerance and prognosis of food allergies in early childhood, the progression of inhalant allergies, and the transition from monosensitization to polysensitization.

A task force of the interest group on allergy diagnosis (IGAD) within the European Academy of Allergy and Clinical Immunology (EAACI) had recently focussed on a comprehensive and practical compendium on molecular allergology for diagnostic purposes. Due to the common efforts of 65 authors, researchers, and clinicians from 20 countries, coordinated by Paolo M. Matricardi (Berlin, Germany) and his team, a unique *EAACI Molecular Allergology User's Guide* (*MAUG*) was released in June 2016 (Matricardi et al. 2016). This impressive compilation is publicly available through *free access* to a supplement (Matricardi et al. 2016) of the journal *Pediatric Allergy and Immunology (PAI)* (http://onlinelibrary.wiley.com/doi/10.1111/pai.12563/epdf). This publication and our present text book on molecular allergology document the rapid progression of the field from basic research to its integration into clinical practice, a quantum leap in the management of allergic patients.

1.7 Scope and Limits of Interpretation

The rules for allergen extract diagnostics also apply to the interpretation of the findings applying allergen molecules:

- Positive specific IgE corresponds to a sensitization (increased susceptibility to allergy) that is clinically relevant only where there are corresponding symptoms.
- If specific IgE is not detected in the serum, this essentially rules out sensitization – and hence the possibility of allergy but only if the following conditions obtain
  - The total IgE of the serum sample is high enough (>20 kU/l).
  - The allergen is suitable as a reagent, representative, and capable of complete IgE binding.
  - The sensitivity of the IgE testing method is optimized (e.g., detection threshold for specific IgE, 0.1 kU_A/l).

In actual practice, it is the physician, who knows the patient's history and symptoms, which determine the clinical relevance and not the test as such.

A frequent misunderstanding derives from the hope that IgE findings can enhance the prediction of clinical symptoms. This is not intrinsically possible, since specific IgE testing – as the skin prick test or the basophil activation test (BAT) – is primarily a method of demonstrating sensitization. Attempts to improve clinical predictivity with sole reference to single allergens (and without clinical data) often fail. Despite continuing desire to achieve it, improving diagnostic sensitivity and specificity by means of molecular allergology will not be straightforward. More reliable predictions of clinical outcomes, clinical cross-reactions, or even defined IgE threshold levels cannot be made without considerable effort. Moreover, as target parameters, they do not – in the author's view – truly serve to capture the primary utility of molecular allergology.

1.8 Immunotherapy and Single Allergens

Recombinant allergens, produced under conditions of good manufacturing practice (GMP), are promising candidates for allergen-specific immunotherapy (Ferreira et al. 2014; Jutel et al. 2012; Makatsori et al. 2013) (▶ Chap. 22). Because, in the temperate climate zones of the northern hemisphere, birch pollen allergy is largely induced by IgE binding to the major allergen Bet v 1, this allergen has now been developed and tested for allergen-specific immunotherapy (AIT) as an alternative to the well-established pollen extracts. Two candidates have already been in clinical development: a recombinant, non-modified Bet v 1 used in sublingual immunotherapy (Stallergenes-Greer, London, United

Kingdom; ▸ www.stallergenesgreer.com) and a recombinant hypoallergenic folding variant for subcutaneous AIT (Allergopharma, Reinbek, Germany; ▸ www.allergopharma.com) (Meyer et al. 2013). This avenue is not, however, being pursued at present (▸ Chap. 23).

More complex allergen extracts, such as those from grass pollen or house-dust mites, require a greater number of recombinant single allergens in order to represent the individually variable IgE repertoires and to be candidates for AIT. A suitable "cocktail" of essential major allergens of Timothy grass has been successfully tested in a proof-of-concept study for subcutaneous AIT of grass pollen allergy (Jutel et al. 2005). The results were, however, not really superior compared to grass extract-based AIT trials. In addition, the non-modified grass allergens still carried the risk of unwanted, presumably rare anaphylactic reactions after AIT injection. Further clinical developments have therefore been put on hold.

Owing to the strict requirements of the European Medicines Agency (EMA), it is unlikely that any products derived from recombinant allergens will become available for AIT in the years ahead. New products based on recombinant molecules have to achieve market access through a centralized authorization procedure of the EMA. Limited advantages in efficacy, costs, and no previous experience with the competent authorities are the main drawbacks leading to a stop of further clinical developments.

1.9 Molecular Allergology Drives Innovation

Following their identification and official naming, many purified and recombinant protein allergens – triggers of IgE-mediated reactions and diseases – have undergone closer investigation. These studies looked at the following: structure and physiochemical properties, relationship to other allergens, membership in protein families, biological function, occurrence and geographic distribution in allergen sources in the natural environment. This has provided a strong momentum to both basic and clinical research.

The *first section* of this book introduces important protein families and related (structurally similar) allergens: Bet v 1 homologs/PR10 proteins, profilins, polcalcins, lipid transfer proteins, and storage proteins. Their description encompasses both molecular characteristics and any clinical role in allergology, which is at present being elucidated.

Methods of testing for allergen-specific IgE antibodies are described in the *second section*. Both IgE singleplex assays and IgE multiplex assays (i.e., screening) for allergen molecules are already routine diagnostic procedures, to an extent replacing the previously used extracts, and are being gradually refined. The available versions of relevant tests and different assay designs have a direct impact on the accuracy of the outcome. Molecular IgE diagnostics with single allergens improve the nature of these tests and, ideally, the clinical interpretation of the results as well.

The *third section* addresses molecular allergy diagnostics in everyday clinical practice. To this end, clinical research problems are broken down with reference to common allergy sources such as tree, grass or weed pollen, insect venom, peanuts and tree nuts, fish, and house dust mite. It is already possible to critically evaluate the benefits of, and limits to, molecular allergy diagnostics with specific single allergens.

Finally, the development of recombinant allergen vaccines or hypoallergenic foods will eventually lead to clinical applications of molecular allergology. The molecular approach with single allergens is giving valuable impetus to modern allergology, to both laboratory research and improved patient care. These innovations will yield lasting benefits in both basic and clinical allergy research.

Conclusions

Most allergens triggering IgE-mediated immediate-type hypersensitivity reactions and diseases are proteins from selected protein families (www.meduniwien.ac.at/allfam/). Their members occur in various natural allergen sources such as pollen, mites, animal dander and secretions, mold spores, foods, and insect venoms. An international nomenclature for protein allergens and an official list of the approved molecular allergens (www.allergen.org) is regularly updated. Various databases offer additional and detailed information on allergen candidates (www.allergome.com; www.allergenonline.org) and link them to general protein databases.

Molecular allergen research aims to improve

- our understanding of the biological and structural relationship of important allergenic molecules driving IgE-mediated reactions,
- quantitation of allergens in biological products, aiming for improved comparability and quality of diagnostic and therapeutic extract-based reagents,
- geographic mapping of IgE-mediated responses (molecular epidemiology),
- individual routine allergy diagnostics, particularly novel tests for allergen-specific IgE applying single allergenic molecules,
- development of unique materials modified on the molecular level, either for safe use in allergic individuals (e.g. hypoallergenic foods) or for improved modes of allergen-specific immunotherapy.

The fast progress in molecular allergen research enhances our general understanding of IgE-mediated responses, provides new diagnostic tools to work-up IgE-mediated allergic conditions and may lead to novel reagents for the treatment of allergic diseases.

References

Barber D, de la Torre F, Feo F, Florido F, Guardia P, Moreno C, Quiralte J, Lombardero M, Villalba M, Salcedo G, Rodriguez R. Understanding patient sensitization profiles in complex pollen areas: a molecular epidemiological study. Allergy. 2008;63:1550–8.

Breiteneder H. Protein families: implications for allergen nomenclature, standardisation and specific immunotherapy. Arb Paul Ehrlich Inst Bundesinstitut Impfstoffe BiomedArzneim Langen Hess. 2009;96:249–54; discussion 254–246.

Breiteneder H, Radauer C. A classification of plant food allergens. J Allergy Clin Immunol. 2004;113:821–30; quiz 831.

Chapman MD. Allergen nomenclature. Clin Allergy Immunol. 2004;18:51–64.

Chapman MD. Allergen nomenclature. Clin Allergy Immunol. 2008;21:47–58.
Ferreira F, Wolf M, Wallner M. Molecular approach to allergy diagnosis and therapy. Yonsei Med J. 2014;55:839–52.
Haftenberger M, Laussmann D, Ellert U, Kalcklosch M, Langen U, Schlaud M, Schmitz R, Thamm M. Prevalence of sensitisation to aeraoallergens and food allergens: results of the German Health Interview and Examination Survey for Adults (DEGS1). Bundesgesundheitsblatt Gesundheitsforschung Gesundheitsschutz. 2013;56:687–97.
Hatzler L, Panetta V, Lau S, Wagner P, Bergmann RL, Illi S, Bergmann KE, Keil T, Hofmaier S, Rohrbach A, Bauer CP, Forster J, Hoffman U, Zepp F, Schuster A, Wahn U, Matricardi PM. Molecular spreading and predictive value of preclinical IgE response to Phleum pratense in children with hay fever. J Allergy Clin Immunol. 2012;130:894–901.
Jenkins JA, Breiteneder H, Mills EN. Evolutionary distance from human homologs reflects allergenicity of animal food proteins. J Allergy Clin Immunol. 2007;120:1399–405.
Jutel M, Jaeger L, Suck R, Meyer H, Fiebig H, Cromwell O. Allergen-specific immunotherapy with recombinant grass pollen allergens. J Allergy Clin Immunol. 2005;116:608–13.
Jutel M, Solarewicz-Madejek K, Smolinska S. Recombinant allergens: the present and the future. Hum Vaccin Immunother. 2012;8:1534–43.
Karp CL. Guilt by intimate association: what makes an allergen an allergen? J Allergy Clin Immunol. 2010;125:955–60; quiz 961–952.
Kauffman HF, Tamm M, Timmerman JA, Borger P. House dust mite major allergens Der p 1 and Der p 5 activate human airway-derived epithelial cells by protease-dependent and protease-independent mechanisms. Clin Mol Allergy. 2006;4:5.
King TP, Hoffman D, Lowenstein H, Marsh DG, Platts-Mills TA, Thomas W. Allergen nomenclature. Allergy. 1995;50:765–74.
Kleine-Tebbe J, Ollert M, Jakob T. Molekulare Allergologie: Nomenklatur, Proteinfamilien, Datenbanken und potenzieller Nutzen. Allergo J. 2010;19:390–4.
Makatsori M, Pfaar O, Lleonart R, Calderon MA. Recombinant allergen immunotherapy: clinical evidence of efficacy – a review. Curr Allergy Asthma Rep. 2013;13:371–80.
Mari A, Scala E. Allergome: a unifying platform. Arb Paul Ehrlich Inst Bundesamt Sera Impfstoffe Frankf A M. 2006;95:29–39; discussion 39–40.
Marsh DG, Goodfriend L, King TP, Løwenstein H, Platts-Mills TA. Allergen nomenclature. Bull World Health Organ. 1986;64:767–74.
Matricardi PM, Kleine-Tebbe J, Hoffmann HJ, Valenta R, Hilger C, Hofmaier S, Aalberse RC, Agache I, Asero R, Ballmer-Weber B, Barber D, Beyer K, Biedermann T, Biló MB, Blank S, Bohle B, Bosshard PP, Breiteneder H, Brough HA, Caraballo L, Caubet JC, Crameri R, Davies JM, Douladiris N, Ebisawa M, Eigenmann PA, Fernandez-Rivas M, Ferreira F, Gadermaier G, Glatz M, Hamilton RG, Hawranek T, Hellings P, Hoffmann-Sommergruber K, Jakob T, Jappe U, Jutel M, Kamath SD, Knol EF, Korosec P, Kuehn A, Lack G, Lopata AL, Mäkelä M, Morisset M, Niederberger V, Nowak-Wezgrzyn AH, Papadopoulos NG, Pastorello EA, Pauli G, Platts-Mills T, Posa D, Poulsen LK, Raulf M, Sastre J, Scala E, Schmid JM, Schmid-Grendelmeier P, van Hage M, van Ree R, Vieths S, Weber R, Wickman M, Muraro A, Ollert M. EAACI molecular allergology user's guide. Pediatr Allergy Immunol. 2016;27(Suppl23): 1–250.
Meyer W, Narkus A, Salapatek AM, Hafner D. Double-blind, placebo-controlled, dose-ranging study of new recombinant hypoallergenic Bet v 1 in an environmental exposure chamber. Allergy. 2013;68:724–31.
Poulsen LK. What makes an allergen more than an allergen? Clin Exp Allergy. 2009;39:623–5.
Radauer C, Bublin M, Wagner S, Mari A, Breiteneder H. Allergens are distributed into few protein families and possess a restricted number of biochemical functions. J Allergy Clin Immunol. 2008;121:847–52 e847.
Radauer C, Nandy A, Ferreira F, Goodman RE, Larsen JN, Lidholm J, Pomes A, Raulf-Heimsoth M, Rozynek P, Thomas WR, Breiteneder H. Update of the WHO/IUIS Allergen Nomenclature Database based on analysis of allergen sequences. Allergy. 2014;69:413–9.

Scala E, Alessandri C, Bernardi ML, Ferrara R, Palazzo P, Pomponi D, Quaratino D, Rasi C, Zaffiro A, Zennaro D, Mari A. Cross-sectional survey on immunoglobulin E reactivity in 23,077 subjects using an allergenic molecule-based microarray detection system. Clin Exp Allergy. 2010;40:911–21.

Schmitz R, Ellert U, Kalcklosch M, Dahm S, Thamm M. Patterns of sensitization to inhalant and food allergens – findings from the German Health Interview and Examination Survey for Children and Adolescents. Int Arch Allergy Immunol. 2013;162:263–70.

Sircar G, Sarkar D, Bhattacharya SG, Saha S. Allergen databases. Methods Mol Biol. 2014;1184:165–81.

van Ree R, Chapman MD, Ferreira F, Vieths S, Bryan D, Cromwell O, Villalba M, Durham SR, Becker WM, Aalbers M, Andre C, Barber D, CisteroBahima A, Custovic A, Didierlaurent A, Dolman C, Dorpema JW, Di Felice G, Eberhardt F, Fernandez Caldas E, et al. The CREATE project: development of certified reference materials for allergenic products and validation of methods for their quantification. Allergy. 2008;63:310–26.

Vieths S, Barber D, Chapman M, Costanzo A, Daas A, Fiebig H, Hanschmann KM, Hrabina M, Kaul S, Ledesma A, Moingeon P, Reese G, Schorner C, van Ree R, Weber B, Buchheit KH. Establishment of recombinant major allergens Bet v 1 and Phl p 5a as Ph. Eur. reference standards and validation of ELISA methods for their measurement. Results from feasibility studies. Pharmeur Bio Sci Notes. 2012;2012:118–34.

Bet v 1 and its Homologs: Triggers of Tree-Pollen Allergy and Birch Pollen-Associated Cross-Reactions

2

J. Kleine-Tebbe, B.K. Ballmer-Weber, H. Breiteneder, and S. Vieths

2.1 Introduction

The major allergen of birch (*Betula verrucosa*), Bet v 1, is of crucial importance in molecular allergology. First identified as an allergen in 1988, Bet v 1 has attained a key role in both basic and clinical research. Many structurally similar (homologous) molecules in tree pollen from the Fagales order, as well as from plant foods, have been identified as related allergens. From an allergological perspective, Bet v 1 and its homologs are:

The present chapter is based on, and modified from, an article by the authors published in 2010 in *Allergo Journal* (Kleine-Tebbe J, Ballmer-Weber B, Breiteneder H, Vieths S: Bet v 1 und Homologe: Verursacher der Baumpollenallergie und birkenpollenassoziierter Kreuzreaktionen. Allergo J 2010; 19: 462–463).
The authors gratefully thank Dr. Steve Love, PhD, Laguna Niguel, CA, USA, for reading the manuscript, helpful suggestions, and editorial assistance with the English translation.

J. Kleine-Tebbe, MD, Prof. (✉)
Allergy and Asthma Center Westend, Outpatient Clinic Hanf, Ackermann and Kleine-Tebbe, Berlin, Germany
e-mail: kleine-tebbe@allergie-experten.de

B.K. Ballmer-Weber, MD, Prof.
Center of Dermatology and Allergology, Kantonsspital Luzern, Lucerne, Switzerland

Department of Dermatology, University Hospital Zürich, Zurich, Switzerland
e-mail: Barbara.Ballmer@usz.ch

H. Breiteneder, PhD, Prof.
Department of Pathophysiology and Allergy Research, Center for Pathophysiology, Infectiology and Immunology, Medical University of Vienna, Vienna, Austria
e-mail: Heimo.Breiteneder@meduniwien.ac.at

S. Vieths, PhD, Prof.
Paul-Ehrlich-Institute, Federal Institute for Vaccines and Biomedicines, Langen, Germany
e-mail: Stefan.Vieths@pei.de; viest@pei.de

J. Kleine-Tebbe, T. Jakob (eds.), *Molecular Allergy Diagnostics*,
DOI 10.1007/978-3-319-42499-6_2

- Among the most important pollen allergens (in the upper Northern hemisphere, i.e., Northern and Central Europe, Northern Asia, and Northern America)
- Among the most common triggers of pollen-associated food allergies after sensitization to Bet v 1
- Among the most common triggers of food allergies in adolescence and adulthood in areas of strong birch pollen exposure

Thus, both Bet v 1 and its related allergens play an important role in our understanding of cross-reactivity, diagnostics, counseling, and allergen-specific immunotherapy (AIT) in allergy sufferers. The present chapter summarizes the most important facts and discusses in detail the clinical symptoms and patterns of allergic disease caused by Bet v 1 and its homologs. The chapter then goes on to describe the options for molecular diagnostics and their interpretation as the basis for individual counseling and treatment (AIT).

2.2 Biological Facts and Characteristics

2.2.1 Allergen Identification

For detailed information on the Bet v 1 homologous allergenic proteins please consult the database AllFam (http://www.meduniwien.ac.at/allfam/; ▶ Bet v 1)

2.2.2 Family

PR-10 proteins (PR: pathogenesis related)

2.2.3 Bet v 1 and the Bet v 1 Superfamily

The cDNA sequence that codes for the major allergen of birch pollen was discovered in July 1988 and published in 1989 as the first known sequence of a plant allergen (Breiteneder et al. 1989). Bet v 1 lent its name to a superfamily of proteins, the Bet v 1-like superfamily, which currently contains 23,609 members and 4418 species (http://pfam.xfam.org/clan/CL0209). These proteins, which are found in all three domains of life – Archaea (prokaryotic microorganisms with membranes containing branched hydrocarbon chains), Bacteria (prokaryotes with membranes containing unbranched hydrocarbon chains), and Eukaryota (eukaryotic cells and organisms, including Plantae as well as Animalia) – are based on the typical Bet v 1 architecture. This consists of a seven-stranded, antiparallel β-pleated sheet and two short α-helices in a V-shaped arrangement, which, together with a long C-terminal α-helix, form a hydrophobic cavity (which effectively binds lipophilic ligands) (◉ Fig. 2.1) (Gajhede et al. 1996). The Bet v 1 architecture, with its characteristic topology (precise spatial organization of the individual structural elements, such as the β-strands and α-helices), can be traced back to the origins of life on Earth (Radauer et al. 2008).

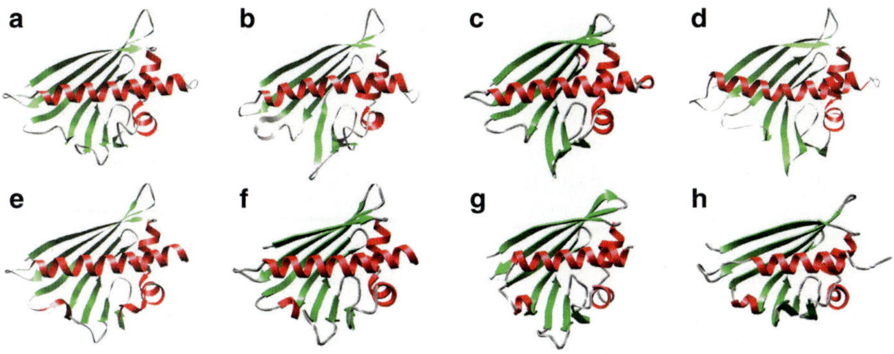

Fig. 2.1 Structures of Bet v 1 homologous allergens: (**a**) Bet v 1 (birch pollen), (**b**) Pru av 1 (cherry), (**c**) Ara h 8 (peanut), (**d**) Gly m 4 (soybean), (**e**) Api g 1 (celery), (**f**) Dau c 1 (carrot), (**g**) Vig r 6 (mung bean), (**h**) Act d 11 (kiwi fruit)

The Bet v 1-like superfamily contains 14 families, one of which bears the name, Bet v 1 family. The Bet v 1 family contains in turn 11 subfamilies (Villalta and Asero 2010). Most allergenic Bet v 1 homologs known today are found in the *PR-10 subfamily*. In addition, two allergens from two further subfamilies (one from each) are also known. Act d 11, a kiwifruit allergen, belongs to the *RRP/MLP subfamily* (RRP/MLP: ripening-related proteins/major latex proteins) and is recognized by IgE in 10% of kiwifruit-allergic individuals (D'Avino et al. 2011). Although the sequence identity between Act d 11 and Bet v 1 is only around 20%, the two allergens are immunologically related by virtue of the 3-dimensional structure of Act d 11 (Chruszcz et al. 2013). Vig r 6 is a mung bean allergen and belongs to the *CSBP subfamily* (CSBP: cytokine-specific binding protein). It is recognized in particular by sera from patients with mung bean sprout allergy but also by around a third of Bet v 1-sensitized individuals, in whom IgE binding can be completely inhibited by Bet v 1 (Guhsl et al. 2014).

2.2.4 Physiological Function of Bet v 1

The capacity of Bet v 1 to bind physiologically important lipophilic ligands has been demonstrated in in vitro systems in the past. These included fatty acids, flavonoids, and a group of plant hormones, the so-called cytokinins (Bublin et al. 2014). Recently it was possible to identify the natural ligand of Bet v 1 as it is found in pollen (Seutter von Loetzen et al. 2014): quercetin-3-O-sophoroside (Q3OS), a glycosylated flavonol. The Bet v 1–Q3OS complex may protect the DNA present in the pollen from damage caused by ultraviolet (UV) light. Bet v 1 is found in high concentrations in the pollen, and flavonoids absorb both UV-A and UV-B. Furthermore, deglycosylated quercetin may deliver an important signal for pollen germination following contact between pollen and stigma. There is also speculation that Q3OS plays a crucial role in allergic sensitization.

2.2.5 Characteristics

- Heat and acid labile
- Numerous structural relatives:
  - Within a species (isoforms)
  - Between different species (homologs)

2.3 Importance of Bet v 1 and Related Allergens

The major birch pollen allergen Bet v 1 induces IgE-mediated sensitization (more than 95 % of IgE binding to birch pollen allergens) and probably the majority of allergic symptoms associated with tree pollen allergy during the spring in Northern and Central Europe, Northern America, and Northern Asia.

2.3.1 Sources of Bet v 1 and its Biological and Allergological Role

No other allergen has been investigated in as much depth as Bet v 1. This applies both to its basic characteristics and to the clinical aspects of the allergic immune response elicited by it. The Allergome database (www.allergome.org) provides a detailed list of links to references on the following Bet v 1-relevant topics on the "Bet v 1" page (Allergen search: ▶ Bet v 1):

- General information
  - Biochemistry, structure, and function of Bet v 1
  - Molecular biology
  - Immunochemistry and allergenicity
  - Immune-mechanisms and genetics
- Measurement/detection of Bet v 1 in the following:
  - Indoor and outdoor environments
  - Allergen sources (extracts), food products, and drugs
  - In the context of allergy diagnostic and immunotherapeutic agents
  - In allergen sources (plant tissues)
  - In the human body (biological distribution)
- Significance and applications of Bet v 1:
  - Epidemiology
  - Diagnosis
  - Allergen-specific immunotherapy
- Experimental models:
  - The allergic immune response (caused by Bet v 1)
  - Foods reactions (caused by Bet v 1 homologs)
  - Inhalant allergies (caused by Bet v 1 and homologs)

  - Skin diseases (caused by Bet v 1 and homologs)
- Overviews, reports, and other sources

The structured links on www.allergome.org are designed to simplify specific searches for relevant information on Bet v 1, relevant sources, and original papers.

2.3.2 Prevalence and Distribution of Sensitization

According to data obtained in the European Community Respiratory Health Survey, the average sensitization rate to birch pollen is 6.4 %, while the highest prevalence rates were found in Northern and Central Europe (up to 22.4 %) (Bousquet et al. 2007). Large-scale screening programs in Germany (KIGGS trial) detected birch pollen-specific IgE in 15 % of children and adolescents aged between 3 and 17 years; rates in the 13- to 17-year age group were 15.7 % for girls and 21.7 % for boys (Schmitz et al. 2013). IgE sensitization to birch pollen was detected in 17.4 % of adults (19–79 years) and in 15.2 %, to Bet v 1 (Haftenberger et al. 2013).

It has been estimated that half of the sensitized subjects developed symptoms of allergic rhinoconjunctivitis or bronchial asthma. Regional differences exist depending on local distribution of allergens and exposure. A Danish study reported the probability of a clinical reaction to birch pollen-related allergenic foods in patients with isolated birch pollen allergy to be 25 %, rising to 50 % in the case of co-sensitization to other pollens. The percentage was significantly higher in reactive versus asymptomatic birch pollen-sensitized adults (Osterballe et al. 2005).

2.3.3 Bet v 1: A Marker Allergen for Tree (Fagales Order) Pollen Sensitization and IgE Cross-Reactivity to Plant-Derived Foods

IgE to Bet v 1 can be considered to be either of the following:

(a) A marker allergen for primary tree pollen sensitization to birch (as well as all other members of the birch and beech families)
(b) A major allergen and indicator for cross-reactivity with a number of related major allergens in other pollen producers (birch and beech families) and plant-derived foods

2.3.3.1 Bet v 1 Cross-Reactive Inhalant Allergens

Pollen from hazel, alder, oak, beech, hornbeam, and chestnut have structurally related allergens (Bet v 1 homologs, ◉ Table 2.1) with common (forming the basis for cross-reactivity) as well as individually variable IgE-binding sites (only discontinuous conformational epitopes).

Table 2.1 List of Bet v 1 homologs (common name of the allergen source in parentheses)

Pollen allergens	Aln g 1 (alder)
	Bet v 1 (birch)
	Car b 1 (hornbeam)
	Cas s 1 (chestnut)
	Cor a 1 (hazel)
	Fag s 1 (beech)
	Que a 1 (oak)
Food allergens	
Pome and stone fruits; tree nuts	Act c 8 (gold kiwi)
	Act d 8 (large-fruited kiwi)
	Cas s 1 (chestnut)
	Cor a 1.04 (hazelnut[a])
	Fra a 1 (strawberry)
	Mal d 1 (apple)
	Pru ar 1 (apricot)
	Pru av 1 (cherry)
	Pru p 1 (peach)
	Pyr c 1 (pear)
	Rub i 1(raspberry)
Vegetables, legumes	Api g 1 (celery[a])
	Ara h 8 (peanut)
	Dau c 1 (carrot[a])
	Gly m 4 (soybean[a])
	Vig r 1 (mung bean)
	Sola l 4 (tomato) (Wangorsch et al. 2014)
Foods for which no Bet v 1 homologs have been identified or officially named as yet	Asparagus, potato, parsley, plum, nectarine, fig, mango, persimmon, jack fruit, walnut, chickpea

[a]Foods containing Bet v 1 homologs that potentially trigger frequent systemic or serious local reactions

2.3.3.2 Bet v 1 Cross-Reactive Food Allergens

Bet v 1 is the most frequent cause of pollen-related food allergies (Ballmer-Weber, Hoffmann-Sommergruber 2011), which are the most frequent type of food allergy in adults in Northern and Central Europe (◉ Table 2.1). The clinical symptoms observed are elicited by Bet v 1-induced IgE, which can then cross-react with a number of Bet v 1-related proteins from plant-derived foods.

The known structures of the Bet v 1 homologs from cherry (Neudecker et al. 2001), celery (Schirmer et al. 2005), carrot (Markovic-Housley et al. 2009), soybean (Berkner et al. 2009; Kleine-Tebbe et al. 2002), and peanut (Hurlburt et al. 2013) demonstrate the strong similarity between the molecular surface conformations of these allergens, thereby explaining their cross-reactivity. The structures of the two allergens that do not belong to the PR-10 subfamily are also known, e.g., that of Act d 11 from kiwi (Chruszcz et al. 2013) and of Vig r 6 from mung bean (Pasternak et al. 2006). The variable IgE epitope patterns, as

Table 2.2 Possible symptoms caused by Bet v 1-induced IgE cross-reactivity

	Symptom complex	Symptoms	Localization
A	Solely oropharyngeal symptoms (frequent)	Itching (including "tingling," "prickling," "tickling")	Labial mucosa, buccal mucosa, palate
		Burning, stinging	Palate, pharynx
		Mild mucosal swelling	Labial mucosa, buccal mucosa, palate, pharynx
B	Additional symptoms in the head area [in isolation or in combination with symptoms in (A)] (rare)	Itching, redness, watering of the eyes	Conjunctiva
		Itching, sneezing, runny nose, nasal congestion	Nose
		Itching	Ears, inner (Eustachian tubes)
		External swelling (angioedema)	Eyelids, lips, cheeks, ears, face
		Internal, pronounced swelling, globus hystericus, difficulty swallowing, hoarseness (sign of vocal cord or laryngeal edema), respiratory distress, stridor	Palate, pharynx, larynx
C	Systemic manifestations (extremely rare)	Itching, redness, wheal formation, swelling	Localized, multifocal, or generalized to the skin
		Nausea, vomiting, abdominal pain, diarrhea	Gastrointestinal tract
		Difficulty breathing and chest pressure or tightness, respiratory distress, wheezing, coughing, possibly productive	Bronchi
		Vertigo (non-otologic), general weakness, syncope, circulatory collapse	Cardiovascular system

described for Bet v 1 in birch pollen-allergic individuals (Gepp et al. 2014), may be responsible for the list of foods not tolerated on an individual basis. The responsible Bet v 1 epitopes are currently being investigated more closely using synthetic allergen epitopes precisely defined on a molecular level (Berkner et al. 2014). This should provide insight into the reasons for the highly individual variability of cross-reactivity. The ultimate goal is to predict serological and, possibly, clinical cross-reactivity to other Bet v 1 homologs by means of Bet v 1 epitope-specific IgE.

The Bet v 1 homologs, often comprising only a fraction of the total protein content of the allergen source, frequently induce not only oropharyngeal symptoms but occasionally systemic and serious (local) reactions in the facial area (Worm et al. 2014) (◉ Table 2.2). However, patients need only avoid those foods that have not been tolerated (Kleine-Tebbe et al. 2010). Even these foods are often unproblematic (approach carefully) in cooked form.

2.4 Diagnosis

Allergy diagnostics for tree pollen allergy and associated food allergies generally consist of the following:

- Patient history (clinical symptoms, course, duration, time, and location of exposure)
- Detection of sensitization (e.g., skin prick test, specific IgE)
- Assessment of sensitization test results in relation to symptoms, possibly confirmed by challenge tests

The following sections discuss first the diagnostic workup of tree pollen allergy, followed by birch pollen (Bet v 1)-associated food allergies. The diagnosis of these two entities usually goes hand in hand, since the cause is the same in both, i.e., Bet v 1-specific IgE, as is the mechanism: IgE cross-reactivity based on structurally similar proteins (Matricardi et al. 2016).

2.4.1 Airway Symptoms Caused by Tree Pollen Allergy

Clinical Presentation and Symptoms

The typical symptoms of tree pollen allergy are present in Central Europe during spring (peaking in April; possible total duration, February to early May) and appear principally related to the mucosa.

- Itching, redness, and watering of the eyes
- Nasal itchiness, sneezing, runny nose and/or nasal congestion
- Possibly also dry cough (particularly during or shortly after physical exertion), difficulty breathing and chest pressure, wheezing, secretion, and respiratory distress as a sign of increased lower airway involvement ("allergic march")

The diagnosis of seasonal allergic rhinoconjunctivitis or allergic bronchial asthma is extremely likely in the case of recurrent, possibly progressive mucosal symptoms that occur during the same season for several consecutive years.

Probing for possible oropharyngeal symptoms following the consumption of raw, relevant plant-derived foods (present in around two thirds of tree pollen-allergic individuals) can confirm, albeit indirectly, the suspicion of birch pollen allergy due to Bet v 1 sensitization.

Detection of Sensitization

Skin prick tests or, in the case of contraindications or unavailability, specific IgE tests with tree pollen extracts are traditionally performed for diagnostic screening in rhinoconjunctivitis with symptoms occurring during the spring.

The Bet v 1 homologs and their strong similarity in pollens from hazel, alder, oak, beech, hornbeam, and chestnut inevitably cause positive reactions to all extracts based on IgE cross-reactivity to the corresponding major allergens Cor a 1, Aln g 1, Que a 1, Fag s 1, Car b 1, and Cas s 1. As the clinical relevance of these tree pollen sensitizations cannot be established from skin prick testing or from the results of IgE specific to the birch and beech families, birch is, for practical purposes, sufficient as a "principal allergen source" for diagnosis.

Due to the botanical relationship between birch, hazel, and alder pollen and the similarity of their major allergens, these pollens are subsumed today in a homologous group. This principle is also recognized in a guideline issued by the European Medicines Agency (EMA) on allergen extract quality. As a result, manufacturers of allergen extracts for AIT have the option to submit studies with birch pollen or combined hazel/alder/birch pollen extracts to document the safety and efficacy of their tree pollen preparations.

Whether potential species-specific sensitization to related trees remains a possibility when other early blooming pollens are excluded in routine diagnostics is not known. Bet v 1 IgE reactivity dominates (>95 % of IgE binding) to such an extent that differential testing of other Fagales pollen preparations rarely yields useful information.

Thus, Bet v 1-specific IgE is well suited as a screening instrument for sensitizations to early blooming species and sometimes increases analytical specificity relative to birch pollen extract (Matricardi et al. 2016). This is because other rarer birch pollen allergens (birch pollen profilin Bet v 2, birch pollen polcalcin Bet v 4, Bet v 6 and 7) in the extract do not obscure identification of IgE reactivity to the major allergens of the birch and beech families.

Additionally, measuring IgE to other Bet v 1-homologous major allergens, e.g., Cor a 1 (hazelnut pollen) or Aln g 1 (alder pollen), confers no additional diagnostic benefit, as Bet v 1 is sufficient to detect or exclude IgE sensitization in suspected early blooming tree pollen allergy.

Whether other birch pollen allergens are required for the specific diagnosis of allergy to early blooming species is questionable for most individuals. In contrast, IgE sensitization and cross-reactivity to the pollen panallergens Bet v 2 and Bet v 4 (▶ Chap. 3) present a diagnostic problem: the analytical specificity of sensitization tests using pollen extracts is generally lost and can only be compensated for by using species-specific marker allergens (for tree, grass, and weed pollen) (▶ Chap. 3).

Practical Tip

If skin prick tests as well as specific IgE tests are ordered as sensitization tests for suspected "spring bloomer" allergy, skin prick testing with birch pollen extract (or mixed hazel/alder/birch extract) should be supplemented by specific IgE to Bet v 1. This increases analytical specificity and yields additional information (see below).

Interpreting Diagnostic Results in Suspected Tree Pollen Allergy

IgE sensitization is only relevant in the presence of corresponding symptoms (seen in around 50 % of sensitized individuals in Central Europe).

Tree pollen allergy sufferers report variable symptoms that are usually confined to the birch pollen season (primarily April in Central Europe) or which extend over several months (February to early May) depending on the flowering period: hazel (Jan/Feb/March), birch (April), beech and oak (April/May). In many cases, however, an initially short period of symptoms in April gradually develops into a longer season in later years. This phenomenon is probably based on higher-avidity antibodies and a Bet v 1-specific IgE repertoire that:

- Grows in complexity
- Recognizes ever more epitopes
- Behaves in an increasingly cross-reactive manner

It is not possible to measure these dynamics with the IgE tests currently available; at best, they are reflected in a relatively high percentage (>10 %, >20 %, occasionally >40 %) of Bet v 1-specific IgE in total IgE.

Thus, the diagnosis of tree pollen allergy should be based on the available clinical information and not on the results of the general sensitization tests rendered positive by Bet v 1 cross-reactivity. It is the symptom history of the tree pollen-allergic individual which is of paramount importance. The majority of affected individuals knows from experience whether they develop allergic symptoms only in April or whether these may appear in the preceding winter months.

It is probably irrelevant to the efficacy and safety of AIT with a tree pollen extract whether the patient is treated with a 100 % birch pollen or with a combined hazel/alder/birch pollen extract, as long as the content of Bet v 1-homologous major allergens is equivalent to the amount of Bet v 1 in the mono-preparation. Therefore, the individual decision regarding the composition of the preparation prior to AIT is generally based on pragmatic considerations:

- 100 % birch pollen extract is frequently used for AIT when symptoms are confined exclusively to April (or the equivalent period of main birch pollen exposure).
- Combined tree pollen preparations (specifically hazel, alder, and birch pollen – one third each) may be appropriate if symptoms also occur during the winter months.

2.4.2 Bet v 1-Associated Cross-Allergies to Plant-Derived Foods

Clinical Presentation and Symptoms

Approximately two thirds of birch pollen-allergic individuals develop a diversity of rapid onset (sometimes immediate but usually after several minutes), predominantly oropharyngeal symptoms of a transient nature (◉ Table 2.2) following the consumption of raw plant-based foods as a result of traces of Bet v 1-homologous proteins (◉ Table 2.1). This complex of symptoms is often referred to as oral allergy syndrome (OAS), implying a singular disease entity. This is not the case, because:

- Oropharyngeal symptoms manifest in many variations and degrees of severity (◉ Table 2.2, symptom complex A).
- More pronounced symptoms sometimes develop in the head area (eyes, ears, nose, and throat) due to the diffusion of inflammatory mediators (e.g., histamine) and/or neuronal reflexes (◉ Table 2.2, symptom complex B).
- Although rare, systemic manifestations, including anaphylaxis, can occur (◉ Table 2.2, symptom complex C).

Moreover, oropharyngeal symptoms are by no means specific to Bet v 1-induced cross-reactivity or to particular foods, having also been described for many other water-soluble food allergens of varying stability:

- In profilin-containing plant-derived foods (▶ Chap. 3)
- In lipid transfer protein (LTP)-containing plant-based foods (▶ Chap. 4)
- In many other (including animal-derived) water-soluble food allergens (▶ Chap. 16)

Therefore, OAS is much less a specific syndrome than it is a variable complex of oropharyngeal symptoms. Finally, oropharyngeal symptoms alone are merely a manifestation of the physicochemical characteristics of the respective food allergen, caused in the case of Bet v 1-homologous PR-10 proteins by:

- Metabolic instability (significant absorption after passing through the gastrointestinal tract is rare)
- Hydrophilicity (rapid onset of symptoms following contact with the mucosa)

Raw apples and hazelnuts are frequently the triggers of local symptoms, an indication of their major allergen's structural relatedness (Bet v 1/Mal d 1 similarity) or their potentially somewhat higher allergen content (Cor a 1 in hazelnuts).

Again, the individual pattern of symptom-triggering foods mirrors an individual's Bet v 1-specific IgE repertoire: the more widely and strongly (avidly) the specific IgE binds possible Bet v 1 epitopes, the more likely the allergic cross-reactivity and the broader the range of relevant foods.

From a clinical perspective, the growing number of foods in the Bet v 1 cluster reported as not tolerated (◉ Fig. 2.2 and ◉ Table 2.1) is likely to be:

- Linked to the severity of Bet v 1 sensitization
- Associated with particularly severe symptoms triggered by foods in the Bet v 1 cluster

The following variables are relevant in relation to rare cases of severe reactions to foods in the Bet v 1 cluster:

1. Marked IgE sensitization to Bet v 1 (high specific IgE in relation to total IgE)
2. Broad Bet v 1-specific IgE repertoire (inferred from the particularly high number of foods not tolerated)

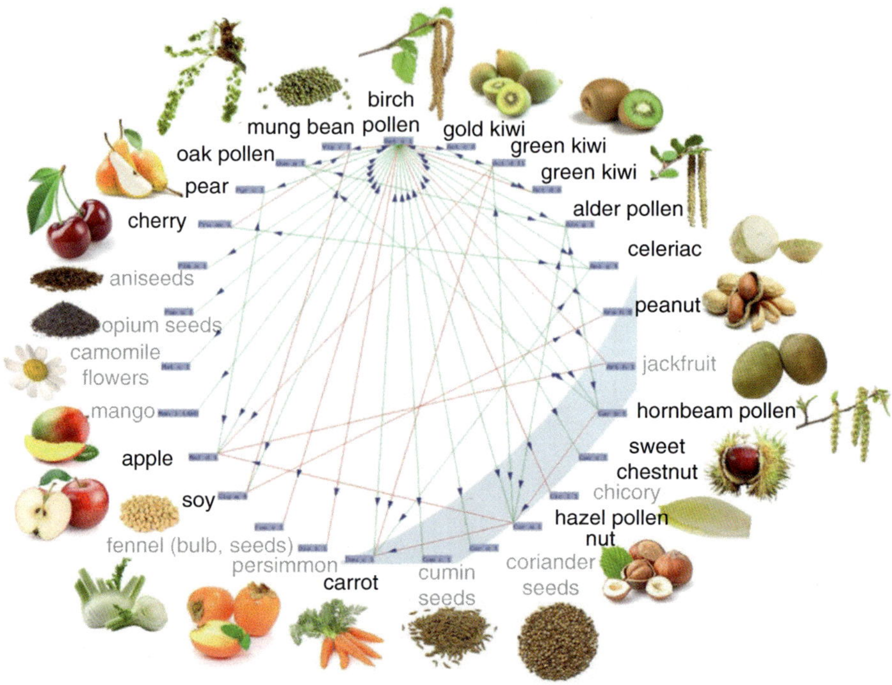

Fig. 2.2 IgE cross-reactivity between the major birch pollen allergen Bet v 1 (shown at 12 o'clock) and its homologous relatives in other pollen plants, pome and stone fruits, nuts, and legumes (not a complete list). Other Bet v 1 homologs are also found in, e.g., peaches, nectarines, apricots, strawberries, raspberries, figs, mangoes, kaki fruit, jackfruit, walnuts, potatoes, tomatoes, and parsley (◉ Table 2.1). Reciprocal cross-reactivity is indicated by double-sided *red arrows* and unilateral cross-reactivity with *green arrows*. Allergens not listed in the IUIS allergen database are *gray* (Represented using the "Allergome O-ring" and dynamically generated on March 10, 2015 using the Allergome database; www.allergome.org)

3. Quantity of the food consumed
4. Possible differences in the metabolic stability of Bet v 1-homologous food allergens (systemic reactions more likely due to hazelnut, soy, carrot, and/or celery than to apple)
5. Lower allergen relatedness to Bet v 1 (e.g., systemic or severe local reactions have been observed more frequently following consumption of celery, carrot, unprocessed soybean products, and occasionally kiwi)
6. Matrix effects of certain foods (e.g., soy), which "protect" Bet v 1-homologous food allergens from rapid degradation

An increase in oropharyngeal symptoms during or shortly after the birch pollen season is a typical clinical observation. A Bet v 1-specific IgE immune response boosted by natural birch pollen exposure (and with a possibly wider IgE repertoire) is likely to be responsible for this phenomenon.

In rare cases, the oropharyngeal symptoms occur following consumption of the relevant food, despite affected individuals not reporting allergic symptoms in the concurrent birch pollen season. This phenomenon, a hitherto silent Bet v 1 sensitization, can result in unexpected reactions following the initial consumption of foods in the Bet v 1 cluster. The complexity of the molecular relationships at play here often delays the diagnosis of birch pollen (Bet v 1)-associated food allergy as well as the urgent counseling required by affected individuals.

Detection of Sensitization

Proven IgE sensitization to Bet v 1 is crucial for confirming the suspicion of birch pollen-associated food allergy. Therefore, diagnostics manufacturers offer major birch pollen allergen(s) in recombinant or purified form for in vitro IgE testing.

Similar confirmation can be obtained in tree pollen-allergic individuals with an unequivocally positive prick test (mean wheal diameter of >3 mm, but ideally ≥5 mm) to birch pollen or pollen from other spring bloomers (hazel, alder, beech, oak), as their extracts contain significant amounts of Bet v 1-homologous allergens.

The same applies to IgE specific to birch pollen extract, however, only when no other birch pollen allergen (e.g. Bet v 2, Bet v 4, Bet v 6) is involved and leads to a positive extract result. Parallel sensitization to birch pollen profilin (Bet v 2) can also cause oropharyngeal symptoms from a number of plant-derived food allergens.

Commercial food extracts (both in prick testing and in specific IgE testing) frequently produce false-negative results due to the low content and lability of Bet v 1-homologous food proteins and are not recommended for diagnostic purposes. Prick-to-prick tests with the suspected fresh, raw food are often useful in equivocal cases (◉ Fig. 2.3). Despite the lack of standardization, this approach often succeeds in achieving a qualitative detection of sensitization. Dose-dependent skin reactions following the application of freshly produced, serial 1:3 to 1:10 dilutions of extracts of foods with water-soluble allergens (e.g., kiwi, peach) can help to differentiate between true sensitizations and unspecific reactions.

Food extracts "spiked" with the associated Bet v 1-homologous allergen represent an exception here, e.g., hazelnut extract with added Cor a 1 (ImmunoCAP Singleplex, PHADIA Thermo Fisher). They permit sensitive IgE detection in the case of suspected Bet v 1-associated, Cor a 1-mediated hazelnut sensitization.

Is it worthwhile to detect other IgE sensitizations/cross-reactions to Bet v 1-homologous food allergens (e.g., specific IgE to the responsible allergens Mal d 1, Cor a 1, Pru p 1, among many others; ◉ Table 2.1)? Probably not, since multiple positive (cross-)reactions can be expected in the presence of Bet v 1-specific IgE (Villalta and Asero 2010) – reactions that permit no conclusions to be drawn on clinical relevance in the absence of symptoms (Matricardi et al. 2016).

IgE sensitization/cross-reaction, and, hence, also a clinically relevant food allergy due to Bet v 1 cross-reactivity, can only reliably be ruled out by an

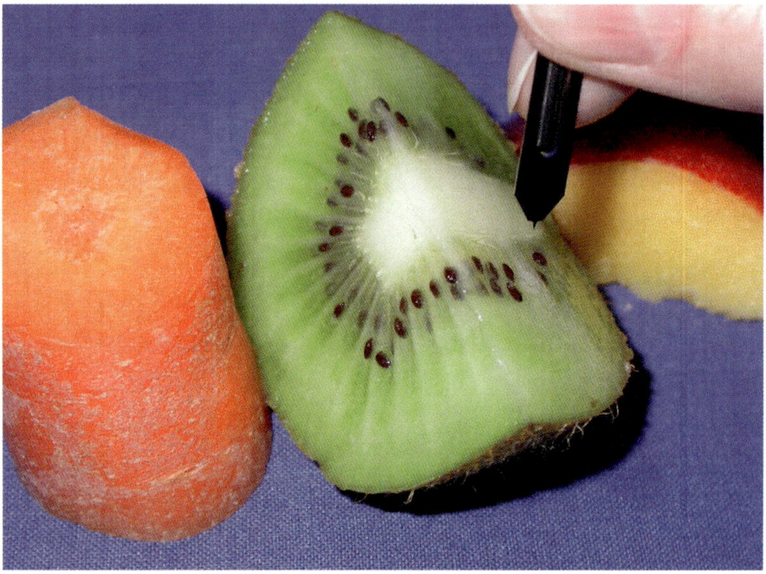

Fig. 2.3 The prick-to-prick test: an important in vivo diagnostic instrument in birch pollen-associated food allergy. Fruit, vegetables, and legumes often contain only traces of Bet v 1 homologs. Due to their instability, commercial food extracts are often not suitable for the diagnosis of birch pollen-associated cross-reactions. Better results are generally obtained using raw, fresh plant-based materials for prick testing

unequivocally negative IgE result to a Bet v 1-homologous single allergen (e.g., Dau c 1, Gly m 4, Pru p 1). This requires a sensitive IgE test method (specific IgE detection limit 0.1 kU_A/l) that is only available with singleplex and not multiplex assays. Unfortunately, this construct is primarily theoretical and rarely occurs in practice.

For certain foods (e.g., unprocessed soybean products, ▶ overview "Fact Sheet on Bet v 1-Associated Soy Allergy"), the associated Bet v 1-homologous protein (in soy: Gly m 4) was developed as a reagent for specific IgE diagnostics and the extract (soybean extract) not spiked. The reason for this is the low Gly m 4 content of the soybean extract, which results in false negatives or excessively low IgE concentrations in Gly m 4 sensitizations (Matricardi et al. 2016). It is important to bear in mind that probably >70 % of individuals with Bet v 1-specific IgE show serological cross-reactions to Gly m 4, whereas only 10–20 % also exhibit clinically relevant allergic reactions. Therefore, nontargeted IgE testing without taking patient history into consideration can be expected to produce numerous Gly m 4 sensitizations/cross-reactions of no clinical relevance.

This problem can be avoided by well-founded and targeted testing (e.g., specific IgE only to Bet v 1). Utilize the diagnostic rule of thumb: sensitization tests are only meaningful in Bet v 1-induced cross-reactions if the results could have clinical relevance and consequences.

Fact Sheet on Bet v 1-Associated Soy Allergy (Kleine-Tebbe et al. 2008)
What every allergist should know:

- The most common form of soy allergy in adolescents and adults in Central Europe is due to a birch pollen-associated cross-reaction.
- The structural similarity between the major birch pollen allergen Bet v 1 and the soy allergen Gly m 4 is the primary cause of birch pollen-soy cross-reactions.
- Reactions predominantly occur following the consumption of large quantities of soy products subjected to no or mild processing: soy milk, soy-containing (diet) powder, and other products with fresh soy protein.
- As with other birch pollen-associated food allergies, local oropharyngeal symptoms are often seen and can become serious due to pronounced swelling in the facial, head, and throat area.
- In individual cases, Gly m 4-induced soy allergy can also cause systemic reactions (skin, gastrointestinal tract, airways, circulatory system).
- According to patient histories, approximately 10 % of birch pollen-allergic individuals react to soy products. The serological cross-reactivity between Bet v 1 and Gly m 4 is >70 %.
- Since primary sensitization to Bet v 1 occurs via inhalation of pollen, consuming a soy-containing product for the first time can cause allergic reactions.
- In individual cases, soy allergy has been observed in individuals with "silent" (clinically irrelevant) birch pollen/Bet v 1 sensitization.
- In the case of an allergic reaction following consumption of a soy product, presumably subjected to mild processing (soy milk, diet powder), an additional history of birch pollen allergy and/or detection of sensitization in skin testing or specific IgE to birch pollen/Bet v 1 renders the diagnosis of a Gly m 4-induced soy allergy highly likely.
- The direct detection of Gly m 4-specific IgE (ImmunoCAP, Phadia Thermo Fisher) is well suited to diagnosing sensitization.
- Due to the low fraction of Gly m 4 in soy extracts, skin testing or measurements of IgE to soy (extract) may be negative or only mildly positive.
- On the basis of likely Gly m 4 content, products that contain unprocessed soy protein should be introduced with caution in birch pollen-associated allergy if the patient has a history of previous severe reactions.
- It is not known whether successful AIT using a birch pollen extract provides protection against a Gly m 4-induced soy allergy.
- Due to the increased use of soy protein in our food and the growing relevance of birch pollen sensitization and associated cross-reactions, Gly m 4-induced soy allergy will be observed more frequently in the future.
- Knowledge on birch pollen-associated soy allergy needs to be more widely disseminated and used to complement counseling for birch pollen-allergic individuals with associated food allergies.

Interpretation

The clinical relevance of proven Bet v 1 sensitization can only be established in conjunction with the patient's symptomatology. For this reason, patient history is of considerable importance in the context of suspected birch pollen-associated food allergy due to Bet v 1-induced cross-reactions (Matricardi et al. 2016).

In practice, the clinical relevance of sensitization tests is determined as follows:

1. The patient is systematically questioned about the possible occurrence of oropharyngeal and/or other allergic symptoms (◉ Table 2.2) following the consumption of relevant foods in raw form (◉ Table 2.1). In order to obtain a complete picture, they should be asked not only about typical foods (apple, hazelnut) but also about all possible potentially Bet v 1 cross-reactive plant-derived foods.
2. In equivocal cases, when data is lacking or history unclear, oral challenge tests serve to verify or exclude clinical cross-reactions. Occasionally, they also help to predict tolerability of a potentially cross-reactive but as yet unconsumed food.

Food challenge tests in Bet v 1-associated food allergy are only rarely performed in routine practice, as they:

- Are extensive, given the multitude of potential cross-reactive foods.
- Are not urgently indicated in the case of oropharyngeal symptoms only.
- Are difficult to evaluate when symptoms are predominantly subjective.
- Have been infrequently validated as dose-dependent tests.
- Only few validated challenge protocols with Bet v 1-associated foods have been described (Ballmer-Weber et al. 2012; Bauermeister et al. 2009).

Only those foods in the Bet v 1 cluster that triggered relevant symptoms are to be avoided in raw form. To avoid all potentially cross-reactive foods would be excessive and unjustified from an allergological perspective. The same applies to foods demonstrating positive IgE sensitizations either indirectly in prick-to-prick testing or directly in serum. Even if all Bet v 1-homologous food proteins (◉ Table 2.1) were available for IgE diagnostics, this would still not permit a differentiation between silent sensitizations and clinically relevant reactions.

Theoretically, different concentrations of specific IgE to Bet v 1-homologous food allergens could provide an indication of dominant and less pronounced IgE sensitizations/cross-reactions. However, the single allergens used for this purpose would need to be optimized, i.e., their isoform(s) would need to be capable of, in effect, binding all Bet v 1 cross-reactive specific IgE. The ratios of specific IgE to the Bet v 1-homologous food protein (e.g., Mal d 1, Cor a 1, or Gly m 4) and the Bet v 1-specific IgE could serve as a measure of serological cross-reactivity. It remains debatable, however, whether ratios of this kind permit reliable clinical conclusions to be drawn.

Thus, the following rule of thumb also applies to the diagnosis to Bet v 1-associated reactions: "the physician establishes the clinical relevance of test findings together with the patient on the basis of symptoms, not the test itself."

Diagnostics in Summary

- Bet v 1 homologs in tree pollen extracts used for diagnostic purposes in skin prick testing testing or IgE determinations cause positive reactions to numerous tree pollens (◉ Table 2.1) that are not necessarily clinically relevant.
- Due to the lability of Bet v 1-homologs, prick-to-prick tests (◉ Fig. 2.3) with fresh foodstuffs are superior to commercial food extracts in the case of birch pollen-associated food allergy.
- By adding recombinant Bet v 1 homologs (e.g., hazelnut extract with Cor a 1) to extracts of birch pollen-associated foods, the extracts are able to bind significantly more IgE, increase test sensitivity (providing a lower limit of quantitation (LoQ)), and yield higher IgE values.
- On the other hand, this "spiking" leads to more positive but potentially clinically irrelevant sensitization tests, which is likely to have a negative impact on extract diagnostics (e.g., high rate of putatively positive peanut sensitization in areas of birch or related tree pollen exposure due to cross-reactive natural Bet v 1 homolog Ara h 8 in the peanut extract).
- Bet v 1-specific IgE is considered a reliable marker for potential serological cross-reactions to numerous plant-derived foods (◉ Table 2.1). The physician establishes the relevance of possible cross-reactions together with the patient on the basis of symptoms (◉ Table 2.2) elicited by foods in the Bet v 1 cluster (◉ Table 2.1).
- Positive IgE to Bet v 1-homologous food allergens (e.g., Pru p 1, ◉ Table 2.1) indicates a sensitization that is only of clinical relevance when accompanied by corresponding symptoms (◉ Table 2.2).
- However, a negative IgE test (e.g., to Gly m 4 from soy, occurring only in around 25 % of cases of Bet v 1 sensitization) would reliably rule out a serological cross-reaction (and hence also a clinically relevant cross-reaction).

2.4.3 Added Benefits of Molecular Diagnostics

The potential benefits of molecular diagnostics in Bet v 1-specific IgE sensitizations/cross-reactions are illustrated by the following generally accepted criteria (see also ▶ Chap. 7):

A. Increased test sensitivity (i.e., lower LoQ).
B. Improved analytical specificity (assuming a single allergen with a known associated clinical risk is used).
C. Indicator allergens for serological cross-reactions exist.
D. Marker allergens for species-specific (primary) sensitizations are available.

2.4.3.1 Advantages of Bet v 1 in Molecular Diagnostics

If one extrapolates these criteria (which primarily increase test utility and are not mutually exclusive to the determination of specific IgE to Bet v 1), one obtains the following paradigm:

Criterion A

Since Bet v 1 is the major allergen component of birch pollen, it is likely that it only marginally improves test sensitivity compared with high-quality (whole) birch pollen extracts.

Criterion B

The analytical specificity of sensitization tests is undoubtedly improved by Bet v 1. Using it precludes the possibility that other potential allergens in the birch pollen extract obscure the identification of sensitization to this important major allergen.

Criterion C

Bet v 1 is the prototype of an indicator for (serological) cross-reactions. Herein lies the great advantage of targeted determinations of IgE to Bet v 1, by means of which a negative test reliably rules out and a positive test unequivocally confirms Bet v 1-specific IgE sensitization.

Criterion D

Bet v 1 is also a reliable marker of primary sensitization. There is no evidence to date that its homologs are able to initiate genuine sensitization to any significant extent. The situation becomes more complicated with the concept of "species-specific" sensitization: indeed, not only pollen from diverse birch and beech families but also from a wide variety of plant-derived foods contain a structurally similar Bet v 1-homologous stress protein.

Overall, the potential advantages of Bet v 1 for the detection of IgE sensitization can be weighted as follows: B > A and C > D.

2.4.3.2 Possibilities of Diagnostics Using Bet v 1-Homologous Allergens

The next question relates to the potential advantages conferred by using Bet v 1-homologous single allergens (i.e. PR-10 proteins from tree pollen or plant-derived foods) for specific IgE diagnostics:

Criterion A

Due to the in vivo lability of Bet v 1-homologous allergen fractions contained in extracts, their use considerably increases test sensitivity but possibly at the expense of specificity. This is often reflected in the significantly higher IgE values for the Bet v 1-homologous single allergens compared with the associated food extracts. Moreover, this puts the exclusion of sensitization (in the case of a negative result to a Bet v 1-homologous allergen) on solid footing. However, it raises the question of whether the greater test sensitivity is actually necessary and/or useful.

Criterion B

The use of Bet v 1-homologous single allergens fundamentally increases analytical specificity compared with extracts of variable composition. However, this alone does not mandate their use, which is only justified when a defined clinical risk is linked to the sensitization. This is not the case for many cross-reactive foods in the Bet v 1 cluster. Thus, the utility of molecular diagnostics is questionable. Severe reactions following the consumption of plant-derived foods, which can be triggered by other food proteins (e.g., storage proteins, LTP, thaumatins), however, may justify single allergen testing.

Criterion C

All Bet v 1-homologous single allergens, whether present in pollen or food, are less predictive of serological cross-reactions than Bet v 1. Therefore, allergen-specific IgE to Bet v 1 is clearly superior in this situation.

Criterion D

There is no evidence to date that Bet v 1-homologous single allergens are suitable as markers for primary sensitization. On the other hand, when positive, they reflect species-specific cross-reactivity, which can, thus, be reliably ruled out by a negative test.

In conclusion, the potential advantages of Bet v 1-homologous single allergens for the detection of IgE sensitization can be weighted as follows: A>B>C and D.

Research conducted over the last three decades into the major birch pollen allergen Bet v 1 and its homologs in other tree pollen and plant-derived foods has substantially enhanced our diagnostic capabilities. This knowledge base is being actively utilized in modern clinical allergology to assess and interpret potential Bet v 1-associated cross-reactivity. However important the use of all Bet v 1-homologs for IgE diagnostics has become, the concept of molecular allergology "in the mind" of the user has brought about the greatest advances in the clinical evaluation of Bet v 1-associated reactions to tree pollen and foods.

2.5 Therapy and Recommendations

Due to the cross-reactivity of the major birch, hazel, and alder pollen allergens (Bet v 1, Cor a 1, Aln g 1), both birch pollen mono-extracts and combinations made up of hazel, alder, and birch pollen are generally suitable for the AIT of tree pollen allergy. The selection is often based on the clinical presentation (individual timing and nature of symptoms).

The extent to which AIT using tree pollen extracts effectively treats pollen-associated food allergy is controversial. The majority of studies have focused on birch pollen-associated apple allergy. Since the major allergen of apple (Mal d 1) exhibits the highest sequence and structural homology to Bet v 1 (Jenkins et al. 2005), the highest level of treatment success would theoretically be expected from AIT. Nevertheless, various studies have yielded mixed results on birch pollen-associated apple allergy (Bolhaar et al. 2004; Hansen et al. 2004; Mauro et al. 2011). AIT with a birch pollen extract for an associated hazelnut allergy achieved no clinical effect at 1 year after treatment (van Hoffen et al. 2011). Thus, based on the available studies, it is not possible to recommend AIT with tree pollen extracts in Bet v 1-associated food allergy in the absence of pollen-induced respiratory symptoms.

2.6 Perspectives

Bet v 1 has been recombinantly produced in recent years (see Cromwell et al. 2011 for an overview) as a folding variant for the subcutaneous and, in unmodified form, for the sublingual AIT of tree pollen allergy; this methodology, however, has not been commercially developed.

2.7 Conclusions for Clinical Practice

Bet v 1 homologs are the most important allergens in the birch and beech family (including birch, alder, hazel, beech, oak, and hornbeam). They are found in a great variety of plant-derived foods (pome and stone fruits, tree nuts, vegetables, and legumes) and frequently cause oropharyngeal symptoms as well as, on occasion, severe allergic reactions in Bet v 1-sensitized individuals. Birch pollen (Bet v 1)-associated reactions to plant foods are considered the most common form of adult food allergy in Central and Northern Europe.

References

Ballmer-Weber BK, Hoffmann-Sommergruber K. Molecular diagnosis of fruit and vegetable allergy. Curr Opin Allergy Clin Immunol. 2011;11:229–35.

Ballmer-Weber BK, Skamstrup Hansen K, Sastre J, et al. Component-resolved in vitro diagnosis of carrot allergy in three different regions of Europe. Allergy. 2012;67:758–66.

Bauermeister K, Ballmer-Weber BK, Bublin M, et al. Assessment of component-resolved in vitro diagnosis of celeriac allergy. J Allergy Clin Immunol. 2009;124:1273–81.

Berkner H, Neudecker P, Mittag D, et al. Cross-reactivity of pollen and food allergens: soybean Gly m 4 is a member of the Bet v 1 superfamily and closely resembles yellow lupine proteins. Biosci Rep. 2009;29:183–92.

Berkner H, Seutter von Loetzen C, Hartl M, et al. Enlarging the toolbox for allergen epitope definition with an allergen-type model protein. PLoS One. 2014;9:e111691.

Bolhaar ST, Tiemessen MM, Zuidmeer L, et al. Efficacy of birch-pollen immunotherapy on cross-reactive food allergy confirmed by skin tests and double-blind food challenges. Clin Exp Allergy. 2004;34:761–9.

Bousquet PJ, Chinn S, Janson C, et al. Geographical variation in the prevalence of positive skin tests to environmental aeroallergens in the European Community Respiratory Health Survey I. Allergy. 2007;62:301–9.

Breiteneder H, Pettenburger K, Bito A, et al. The gene coding for the major birch pollen allergen Betv1, is highly homologous to a pea disease resistance response gene. EMBO J. 1989;8:1935–8.

Bublin M, Eiwegger T, Breiteneder H. Do lipids influence the allergic sensitization process? J Allergy Clin Immunol. 2014;134:521–9.

Chruszcz M, Ciardiello MA, Osinski T, et al. Structural and bioinformatic analysis of the kiwifruit allergen Act d 11, a member of the family of ripening-related proteins. Mol Immunol. 2013;56:794–803.

Cromwell O, Niederberger V, Horak F, et al. Clinical experience with recombinant molecules for allergy vaccination. Curr Top Microbiol Immunol. 2011;352:27–42.

D'Avino R, Bernardi ML, Wallner M, et al. Kiwifruit Act d 11 is the first member of the ripening-related protein family identified as an allergen. Allergy. 2011;66:870–7.

Gajhede M, Osmark P, Poulsen FM, et al. X-ray and NMR structure of Bet v 1, the origin of birch pollen allergy. Nat Struct Biol. 1996;3:1040–5.

Gepp B, Lengger N, Bublin M, et al. Chimeras of Bet v 1 and Api g 1 reveal heterogeneous IgE responses in patients with birch pollen allergy. J Allergy Clin Immunol. 2014;134:188–94.

Guhsl EE, Hofstetter G, Hemmer W, et al. Vig r 6, the cytokinin-specific binding protein from mung bean (Vigna radiata) sprouts, cross-reacts with Bet v 1-related allergens and binds IgE from birch pollen allergic patients' sera. Mol Nutr Food Res. 2014;58:625–34.

Haftenberger M, Laussmann D, Ellert U, et al. Prävalenz von Sensibilisierungen gegen Inhalations- und Nahrungsmittelallergene. Ergebnisse der Studie zur Gesundheit Erwachsener in Deutschland (DEGS1). Bundesgesundheitsblatt Gesundheitsforschung Gesundheitsschutz. 2013;56:687–97.

Hansen KS, Khinchi MS, Skov PS, et al. Food allergy to apple and specific immunotherapy with birch pollen. Mol Nutr Food Res. 2004;48:441–8.

Hurlburt BK, Offermann LR, McBride JK, et al. Structure and function of the peanut panallergen Ara h 8. J Biol Chem. 2013;288:36890–901.

Jenkins JA, Griffiths-Jones S, Shewry PR, et al. Structural relatedness of plant food allergens with specific reference to cross-reactive allergens: an in silico analysis. J Allergy Clin Immunol. 2005;115:163–70.

Kleine-Tebbe J, Herold D, Vieths S. Sojaallergie durch Kreuzreaktionen gegen Birkenpollen-Majorallergen Bet v 1. Allergologie. 2008;31:303–13.

Kleine-Tebbe J, Meißner A-M, Jappe U, et al. Allergenfamilien und molekulare Diagnostik IgE-vermittelter Nahrungsmittelallergien: von der Theorie zur Praxis. Allergo J. 2010;19:251–63.

Kleine-Tebbe J, Vogel L, Crowell DN, et al. Severe oral allergy syndrome and anaphylactic reactions caused by a Bet v 1- related PR-10 protein in soybean, SAM22. J Allergy Clin Immunol. 2002;110:797–804.

Markovic-Housley Z, Basle A, Padavattan S, et al. Structure of the major carrot allergen Dau c 1. Acta Crystallogr D Biol Crystallogr. 2009;65:1206–12.

Matricardi PM, Kleine-Tebbe J, Hoffmann HJ, Valenta R, Hilger C, Hofmaier S, Aalberse RC, Agache I, Asero R, Ballmer-Weber B, Barber D, Beyer K, Biedermann T, Biló MB, Blank S, Bohle B, Bosshard PP, Breiteneder H, Brough HA, Caraballo L, Caubet JC, Crameri R, Davies JM, Douladiris N, Ebisawa M, Eigenmann PA, Fernandez-Rivas M, Ferreira F, Gadermaier G, Glatz M, Hamilton RG, Hawranek T, Hellings P, Hoffmann-Sommergruber K, Jakob T, Jappe U, Jutel M, Kamath SD, Knol EF, Korosec P, Kuehn A, Lack G, Lopata AL, Mäkelä M, Morisset M, Niederberger V, Nowak-Wezgrzyn AH, Papadopoulos NG, Pastorello EA, Pauli G, Platts-Mills T, Posa D, Poulsen LK, Raulf M, Sastre J, Scala E, Schmid JM, Schmid-Grendelmeier P, van Hage M, van Ree R, Vieths S, Weber R, Wickman M, Muraro A, Ollert M. EAACI molecular allergology user's guide. Pediatr Allergy Immunol. 2016;27 Suppl 23:1–250.

Mauro M, Russello M, Incorvaia C, et al. Birch-apple syndrome treated with birch pollen immunotherapy. Int Arch Allergy Immunol. 2011;156:416–22.

Neudecker P, Schweimer K, Nerkamp J, et al. Allergic cross-reactivity made visible: solution structure of the major cherry allergen Pru av 1. J Biol Chem. 2001;276:22756–63.

Osterballe M, Hansen TK, Mortz CG, et al. The clinical relevance of sensitization to pollen-related fruits and vegetables in unselected pollen-sensitized adults. Allergy. 2005;60:218–25.

Pasternak O, Bujacz GD, Fujimoto Y, et al. Crystal structure of Vigna radiata cytokinin-specific binding protein in complex with zeatin. Plant Cell. 2006;18:2622–34.

Radauer C, Lackner P, Breiteneder H. The Bet v 1 fold: an ancient, versatile scaffold for binding of large, hydrophobic ligands. BMC Evol Biol. 2008;8:286.

Schirmer T, Hoffimann-Sommergrube K, Susani M, et al. Crystal structure of the major celery allergen Api g 1: molecular analysis of cross-reactivity. J Mol Biol. 2005;351:1101–9.

Schmitz R, Ellert U, Kalcklosch M, et al. Patterns of sensitization to inhalant and food allergens – findings from the German Health Interview and Examination Survey for Children and Adolescents. Int Arch Allergy Immunol. 2013;162:263–70.

Seutter von Loetzen C, Hoffmann T, Hartl MJ, et al. Secret of the major birch pollen allergen Bet v 1: identification of the physiological ligand. Biochem J. 2014;457:379–90.

van Hoffen E, Peeters KA, van Neerven RJ, et al. Effect of birch pollen-specific immunotherapy on birch pollen-related hazelnut allergy. J Allergy Clin Immunol. 2011;127:100–1.

Villalta D, Asero R. Is the detection of IgE to multiple Bet v 1-homologous food allergens by means of allergen microarray clinically useful? J Allergy Clin Immunol. 2010;125:1158–61.

Wangorsch A, Jamin A, Foetisch K, et al. Identification of Sola l 4 as Bet v 1 homologous pathogenesis related-10 allergen in tomato fruits. Mol Nutr Food Res. 2014;59:582–92.

Worm M, Jappe U, Kleine-Tebbe J, et al. Food allergies resulting from immunological cross-reactivity with inhalant allergens: guidelines from the German Society for Allergology and Clinical Immunology (DGAKI), the German Dermatology Society (DDG), the Association of German Allergologists (AeDA) and the Society for Pediatric Allergology and Environmental Medicine (GPA). Allergo J Int. 2014;23:1–16.

The Concept of Pollen Panallergens: Profilins and Polcalcins

3

M. Wallner, F. Ferreira, H. Hofer, M. Hauser, V. Mahler, and J. Kleine-Tebbe

3.1 Introduction

Because of their ubiquitous distribution and their high level of cross-reactivity, profilins and polcalcins are classified as panallergens. To date, 43 profilin and 15 polcalcin allergens have been identified as allergens (for review see also Matricardi et al. 2016). Profilins are actin-binding proteins, which explain their functionality in many essential cellular processes. They can be identified in various plant-derived foods, pollen, and latex. Polcalcins are expressed exclusively in pollen, and, as indicated by the name, they function in the regulation of intracellular Ca^{++} levels.

This article is based on a publication of the authors published in 2012 in the *Allergo Journal* (Hauser M, Wallner M, Ferreira F, Mahler V, Kleine-Tebbe J (2012): Das Konzept der Pollen-Panallergerne. Allergo J 21: 291–293) which has now been updated, extended, and translated as a book chapter.
The authors gratefully thank Dr. Steve Love, PhD, Laguna Niguel, CA, USA, for reading the manuscript, helpful suggestions, and editorial assistance with the English translation.

M. Wallner, PhD (✉) • F. Ferreira, PhD, Prof. • H. Hofer, PhD • M. Hauser, PhD
Department of Molecular Biology, University of Salzburg, Salzburg, Austria
e-mail: michael.wallner@sbg.ac.at; fatima.ferreira@sbg.ac.at; heidi.hofer@sbg.ac.at; michael.hauser@mynet.at

V. Mahler, MD, Prof.
Department of Dermatology, University Hospital Erlangen, Friedrich-Alexander-University Erlangen-Nuremberg, Erlangen, Germany

Allergology, Paul-Ehrlich Institute, Federal Institute for Vaccines and Biomedicines, D-63225 Langen, Germany
e-mail: vera.mahler@uk-erlangen.de; vera.mahler@fau.de; vera.mahler@pei.de

J. Kleine-Tebbe, MD, Prof.
Allergy and Asthma Center Westend, Outpatient Clinic Hanf, Ackermann and Kleine-Tebbe, Berlin, Germany
e-mail: kleine-tebbe@allergie-experten.de

J. Kleine-Tebbe, T. Jakob (eds.), *Molecular Allergy Diagnostics*,
DOI 10.1007/978-3-319-42499-6_3

In skin prick tests, panallergens frequently cause a pattern of multiple sensitizations. Moreover, IgE specific for a variety of biologically unrelated allergen sources exists. These sensitizations and cross-reactivities are usually irrelevant, and only in rare cases panallergens do represent clinically relevant major allergens.

In some clinical reports of profilin-allergic patients, especially those with grass or weed pollen allergies in areas with high pollen exposure, severe allergic reactions toward certain foods (e.g., melon) have been observed. Pronounced sensitization to polcalcins could possibly be linked to an elevated risk of asthma (i.e., in cedar or cypress pollen-allergic individuals). Moreover, panallergens also affect the analytical specificity of pollen and food allergen extracts in skin prick tests and IgE-based diagnosis. Sensitization to panallergens (i.e., Bet v 2 or Ph p 12), which are accompanied by multiple reactions toward biologically unrelated pollen extracts (i.e., in skin prick tests), requires further allergy diagnosis with source-related, species-specific marker major allergens (i.e., Bet v 1, Ole e 1, Phl p 1/Phl p5, Art v 1, or Amb a 1). These marker allergens contribute significantly to the analytical specificity necessary for identifying the disease-eliciting allergen sources (tree, grass, or weed pollen) used for allergen-specific immunotherapy (AIT).

3.2 Allergen Nomenclature

Because of their ubiquitous distribution and high structural similarity, panallergens are responsible for widespread cross-reactions, even between botanically unrelated plant species. Profilins as well as polcalcins (Ca^{++}-binding proteins found in pollen) are generally classified as panallergens. Numerous molecules belonging to the families of profilins and polcalcins have already been identified and described as allergens. Due to their fundamental roles in cell function, these proteins are highly conserved and widely distributed. While the occurrence of polcalcins is restricted to tree, grass, and weed pollen, profilins have been identified in pollen, plant-derived foods (fruits, vegetables, legumes, nuts), and latex, but also in animal organisms.

3.3 Structure and Function of Profilins

Profilins are ubiquitous, cytosolic proteins present in all eukaryotic cells. Despite a relatively variable amino acid sequence and polypeptide chain length, the structure of profilins is highly conserved. This provides the molecular basis for high serologic cross-reactivity. Structurally, the center of the molecule is a compact beta-sheet which is surrounded by alpha-helices (Fig. 3.1a). Profilins are actin-binding proteins and can also bind other ligands, such as phosphoinositides or poly-L-proline. Phosphoinositides constitute only a small fraction of cellular phospholipids; however they control many essential processes during the life of a cell. These lipids regulate ion channels and vesicular transport and are capable of modulating lipid

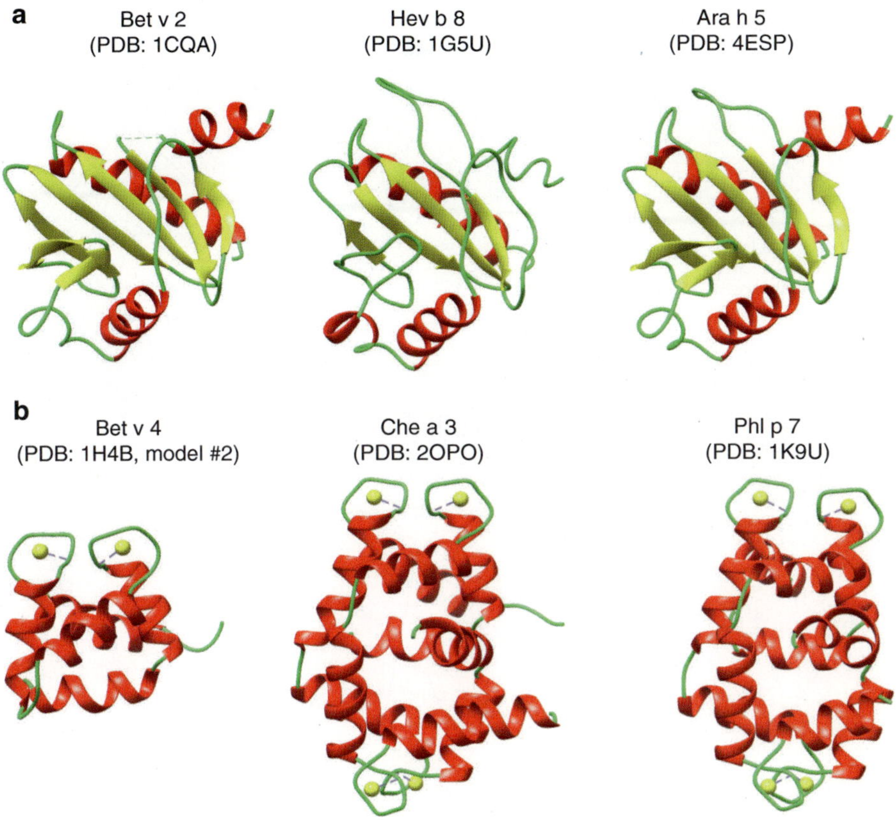

Fig. 3.1 3D ribbon structures of (**a**) allergenic profilins and (**b**) allergenic polcalcins. The accession numbers of the protein database (PDB, www.rcsb.org) are given in parentheses. Alpha-helices are depicted in red, beta-sheets in yellow, and unordered structures in green. Bound Ca^{++} are indicated by yellow spheres

metabolism via a close interplay with lipid transfer proteins (Balla 2013). This suggests a role of profilins in processes such as endo- and exocytosis, as well as intracellular signaling.

Profilins regulate actin polymerization and, thus, cell mobility and are, therefore, also involved in cell separation, cell elongation, outgrowth of pollen tube or root hairs, and rapid cytoplasmic streaming (Hauser et al. 2010). Consequently, profilin-deficient plants display phenotypes of dwarfism or reduced fruit setting (Le et al. 2006).

Additionally, 50 ligands of profilins have been identified, suggesting that profilins are key regulators of molecular processes of complex intracellular networks (Witke 2004). Profilins share the property of binding to poly-L-proline with prolyl hydroxylases. It was this binding property that led to the initial identification of profilins as contaminants during purification of prolyl hydroxylase enzymes (Tanaka

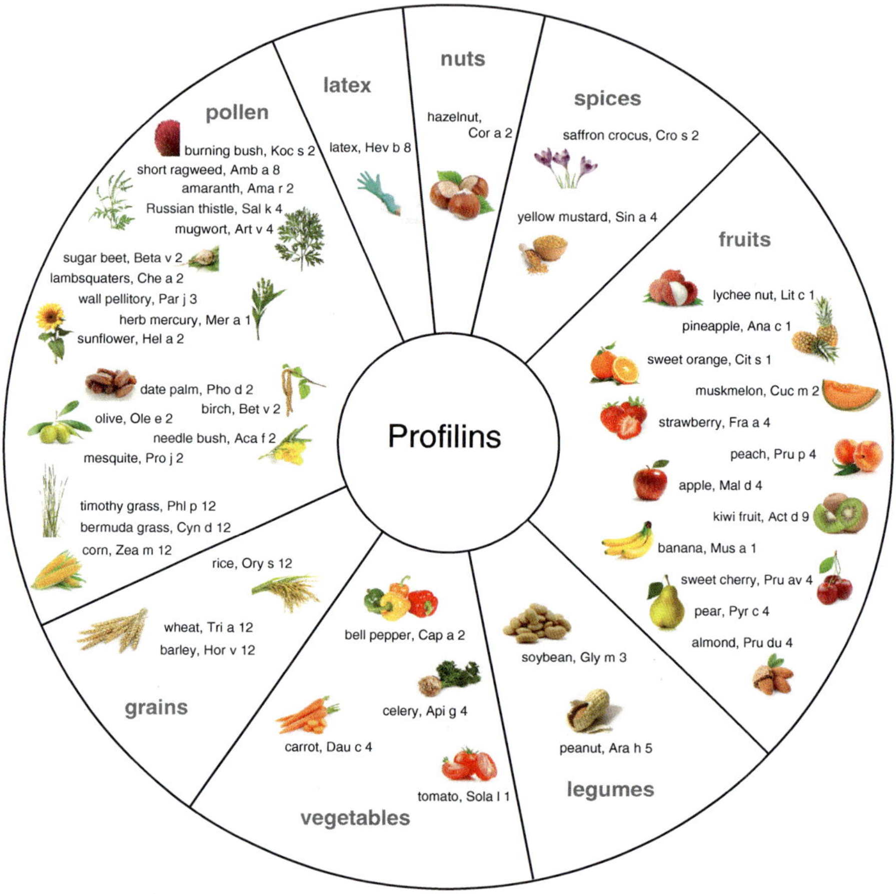

Fig. 3.2 List of cross-reactive allergenic profilins officially acknowledged by the WHO/IUIS allergen nomenclature subcommittee (Photos were obtained from www.fotolia.com)

and Shibata 1995). Now, however, poly-L-proline is successfully used to purify allergenic profilins (Wopfner et al. 2008).

The strongly IgE cross-reactive profilins represent cytosolic proteins with conserved structures, found in all eukaryotic cells. They regulate actin polymerization and are involved in the control of multiple molecular processes within intracellular networks.

3.4 Relevance of Profilins

In 1991, Bet v 2 was identified as the first allergenic profilin in birch pollen (Valenta et al. 1991). Since then, a series of tree, grass, and weed pollen profilins as well as profilins from plant-derived foods and latex have been described as allergens (reviewed also in Matricardi et al. 2016). At present, 43 allergenic profilins have officially been acknowledged by the WHO/IUIS allergen nomenclature subcommittee (Fig. 3.2), including 20 profilin allergens from pollen and latex and 23 profilins from foods (www.allergen.org).

Sensitization rates to pollen profilin allergens are, in general, highly related to geography, with 5–40 % of the allergic population affected. In Germany, sensitization rates of 10–15 % have been reported. IgE to Phl p 12 was observed in 23 % of a large Italian children's cohort. The prevalence, being associated with sensitizations to grass and olive pollen major allergens, declined from northern to southern Italy (Asero et al. 2015). Sensitization rates to mugwort (Art v 4) and ragweed (Amb a 8) profilins among weed pollen-allergic patients in Italy were about 20 %, while Austrian weed pollen allergics showed sensitization rates of 45–50 % (Wopfner et al. 2008). On average, sensitization to pollen profilins is around 30 %, while certain weed pollen, e.g., from *Chenopodium album* (white goosefoot) or *Mercurialis annua* (annual mercury) but also the pollen from date palm (*Phoenix dactylifera*), evoke sensitization rates to profilins of more than 50 % (Asturias et al. 2005; Barderas et al. 2004; Vallverdu et al. 1997).

Profilins have also been identified as potential allergens in plant foods; 70–90 % of melon- and orange-allergic patients are sensitized to profilins. However, most food profilins have been described as minor allergens with sensitization rates below 50 %. Depending on the study, between 12 and 42 % of latex-allergic patients have been found to be sensitized to profilin (Santos and van Ree 2011).

3.5 Sensitization to Profilins

The high IgE cross-reactivity of profilins from different allergen sources (i.e., pollen and fruits) is based on the highly conserved three-dimensional structure of the molecules. Interestingly, sensitization to food profilins is restricted to pollen sensitized atopic individuals. IgE epitopes of profilins are dependent on the proper conformation of the allergens. Thus, antibodies cannot bind to denatured or structurally modified proteins. Profilins are heat labile and unstable in the presence of digestive enzymes (Hauser et al. 2010; Rodriguez-Perez et al. 2003).

Inhibition experiments revealed that pollen profilins could effectively inhibit IgE binding to food profilins. However, the opposite was only partially the case. These results, combined with the fact that profilins are quite susceptible to proteolytic degradation, suggest that pollen profilins are the primary sensitizers of profilin allergies. This hypothesis is further supported by studies, which have demonstrated a relation of IgE antibodies to birch and grass pollen profilins with IgE against profilins from hazelnut or various fruits of the Rosaceae family (e.g., strawberry Fra a 4, apple Mal d 4, cherry Pru av 4, almond Pru du 4, peach Pru p 4, or pear Pyr c 4) (Hauser et al. 2010; van Ree et al. 1995). In addition, association of birch and mugwort pollen allergies with reactions to celery or carrot and also the so-called ragweed-banana-melon syndrome were connected to profilin sensitization (Hauser et al. 2010).

In a study of 106 grass pollen-allergic children, including 50 sensitized to grass pollen panallergens and latex, a positive correlation between sensitization to the profilins Phl p 12 and Hev b 8 was reported; however, the authors did not find evidence for clinical relevance of this cross-reactivity (Casquete-Roman et al. 2012). Despite the fact that profilins are highly cross-reactive in vitro, the clinical relevance of this cross-reactivity is controversial. Thus, only some of the profilin-sensitized patients develop allergic symptoms (Matricardi et al. 2016). These allergic reactions are usually mild among pollen-allergic patients, and only in rare cases of food-allergic individuals may severe allergic reactions be triggered (Hauser et al. 2010; Santos and van Ree 2011).

To date, 43 allergenic profilins have been identified in pollen, plant foods, and latex. In Germany, 10–15 % of pollen-allergic patients display sensitization toward profilins; worldwide, the prevalence of profilin sensitization varies from 5 to 40 %. These sensitization rates can be considerably higher with some allergenic food profilins.

3.6 Structure and Function of Polcalcins

In addition to parvalbumin (Kühn et al. 2012), polcalcins (monomer 8–9 kDa) constitute the majority of allergenic calcium-binding proteins. However, calcium-binding allergens have not only been identified in food and pollen but also in house dust mite, cockroach, and cattle. Consistent with the name, the expression of polcalcins is restricted to pollen. Characteristic to polcalcins is the EF-hand domain, a helix-loop-helix structure which can bind calcium thus forming the dominant structural motif of the mostly alpha-helical proteins. Binding of calcium changes and stabilizes the structure of polcalcins, which concomitantly increases the interactions with IgE antibodies (Kühn et al. 2012). Based on the number of EF-hand motifs, at least three types of polcalcins can be distinguished:

1. Allergens with two calcium-binding domains (i.e., alder Aln g 4, ragweed Amb a 9, mugwort Art v 5, or birch Bet v 4)
2. Allergens with three calcium-binding domains (i.e., ragweed Amb a 10, and birch Bet v 3)
3. Allergens with four calcium-binding domains (i.e., Jun o 4 from prickly juniper or Ole e 8 from olive)

Moreover, polcalcins may occur as monomeric units (Bet v 4) or form dimeric structures (i.e., Phl p 7 from timothy grass or Che a 3 from white goosefoot) (Verdino et al. 2008). Recently, it has been reported that also the per se monomeric Bet v 4 can form reversible dimers or oligomers in a temperature-dependent manner (Magler et al 2010). However, the exact biological role of polcalcins still remains elusive. Due to their localization in pollen and their ability to regulate intracellular calcium levels, it has been suggested that polcalcins play a crucial role in pollen tube outgrowth (Wopfner et al. 2007).

3.7 Relevance of Polcalcins

For calcium-binding proteins, two distinct conformations can be distinguished:

- The closed calcium-free (apo)structure
- The open calcium-bound (holo)form

The latter has been reported to be more stable and shows stronger IgE reactivity. Polcalcins are highly cross-reactive allergens with a sensitization prevalence ranging from 5 to 10 % among pollen-allergic patients (Hauser et al. 2010). Similar to profilins, the clinical relevance of polcalcin sensitization seems highly dependent on geographic factors as well as the allergen source itself. Thus, it has been reported that the sensitization rates to the polcalcins Art v 5 from mugwort and Amb a 9 and 10 from ragweed were, as expected, approximately 10 % in an Austrian cohort, but in an Italian population, reached almost 30 % (Wopfner et al. 2008).

Among all allergenic polcalcins, Phl p 7 from timothy grass pollen is the most cross-reactive molecule. Thus, it can be used as a marker to identify multiple pollen cross-reactivities. The increased IgE binding capacity of Phl p 7 could be a consequence of the dimeric structure of the allergen. This can be explained by the fact that monomeric polcalcins are very small proteins with a molecular weight of 8 kDa. Considering that an antibody epitope covers an area of approximately 1000 $Å^2$ on the surface of a protein (Mirza et al. 2000), an effective IgE cross-linking by the simultaneous binding of multiple IgE antibodies on the surface of such a small protein seems unlikely. However, comparative IgE-binding studies of Phl p 7 dimers with other polcalcins such as monomeric Bet v 4 from birch pollen or the likewise dimeric Che a 3 from white goosefoot are lacking (Tinghino et al. 2002). To date, 15 allergenic polcalcins have officially been acknowledged by the WHO/IUIS allergen nomenclature subcommittee (www.allergen.org) (Fig. 3.3).

Polcalcins are Ca^{++}-binding proteins, but their expression is restricted to pollen. As mentioned in detail above, the number of Ca^{++}-binding motifs is used to distinguish three types of allergenic polcalcins. The allergens are highly cross-reactive, inducing sensitization rates between 5 and 10 % among pollen-allergic patients.

3.8 Diagnosis of Relevant Multi-Sensitizations to Pollen

As panallergens, polcalcins and profilins are responsible for multiple pollen sensitizations; profilins are additionally associated with cross-reactivities of pollen, plant foods and latex (Raulf-Heimsoth and Rihs 2011).

Problems in the specific diagnosis of pollen sensitizations are induced by both profilins and polcalcins because of their high degree of similarity as well as their potential to evoke clinically relevant cross-reactivities. Thus, they reduce the analytical specificity of allergen extracts and interfere with specific allergy diagnosis:

- In skin prick tests, there can be a characteristic pattern of multiple sensitizations to a variety of botanically distinct or even unrelated pollen sources.
- In individual cases, pollen extracts would lead to unexpected results (e.g., hazel and alder positive but birch negative skin prick test) suggesting a different context (as, for instance, Bet v 1-mediated cross-reactivity).
- Concomitant sensitizations to profilins and polcalcins may induce positive test results in any of the tested pollen extracts (in skin prick tests as well as in specific IgE tests using allergen extracts).

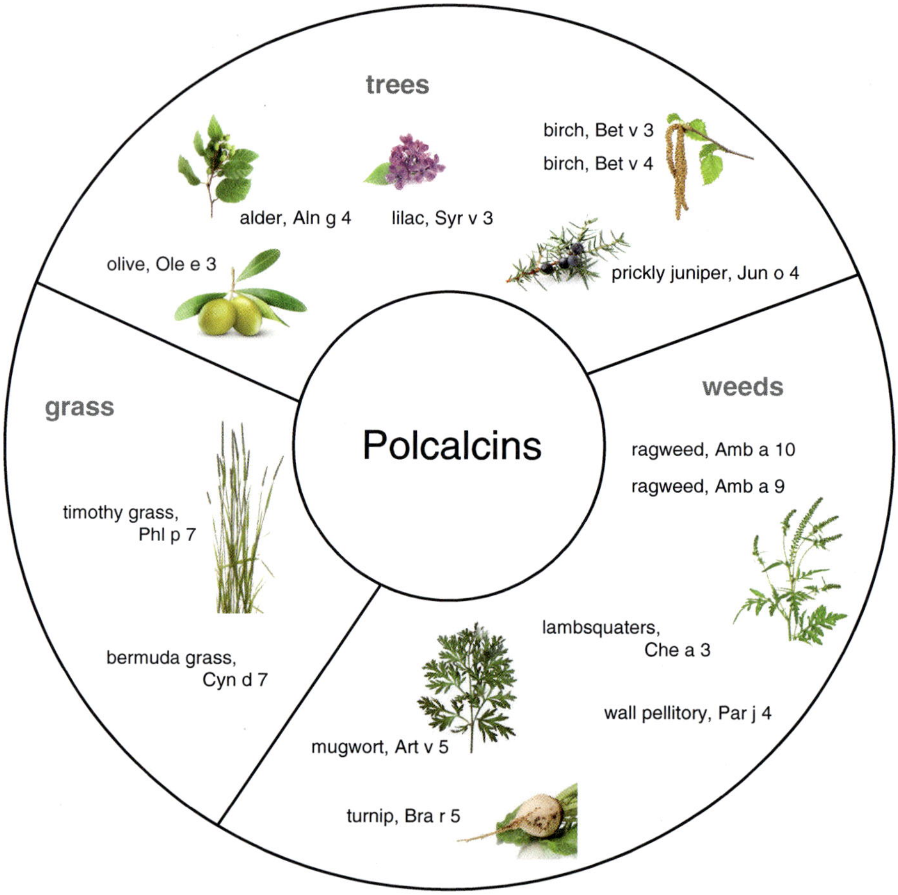

Fig. 3.3 List of allergenic polcalcins acknowledged by the WHO/IUIS allergen nomenclature subcommittee (Photos were obtained from www.fotolia.com)

- Reactions to food plants with a high profilin content (i.e., melon, banana, citrus fruits, tropical fruits, cucumbers, or various vegetables) aside from the typical Bet v 1 homologous foods would serve as an additional indication of a profilin sensitization (Kleine-Tebbe et al. 2010).

In that event, it is recommended to test the sensitization to a (recombinant) member of either of the two panallergens, such as:

- IgE specific to the timothy grass polcalcin Phl p 7 (recommended panallergen) or the birch polcalcin Bet v 4
- IgE specific to the timothy grass profilin Phl p 12 or the birch pollen profilin Bet v 2 (both suitable as panallergens)

An affordable alternative is the simultaneous panallergen detection in specific IgE assays, which are available either as a combination of profilin/polcalcin from birch pollen (t221) or grass pollen (g214, ImmunoCAP, Thermo Fisher). However, this will not allow the discrimination between the two panallergens.

In conclusion, panallergens may cause multiple sensitizations against biologically unrelated allergen sources in skin prick tests as well as in specific IgE tests with allergen extracts. Frequently, these sensitizations remain without symptoms and are therefore considered irrelevant, although clinically relevant cross-reactivities may occur.

3.9 Component-Resolved Diagnosis of Panallergen Sensitizations

With a positive test result for a profilin, polcalcin, or both panallergens, neither skin prick tests nor IgE-based assays with allergen extracts allow a reliable determination of the allergen source. Specific allergy diagnosis with allergen extracts is impossible under those circumstances. Thus, for the exact determination of the sensitizing pollen source, species-specific marker allergens are mandatory (Fig. 3.4) for the correct extract selection for AIT.

3.10 Clinical Relevance of Panallergens

Panallergen-allergic patients are usually only sensitized to the major allergens of the particular allergen source (i.e., Bet v 1 from birch or Phl p 1/Phl p 5 from timothy grass) and not the whole panel of major allergens from all allergen sources. Similarly, for extract-based diagnosis, clinical relevance is only indicated when the patients show appropriate symptoms. However, based on the pollen extracts available for the diagnosis of panallergens (profilin, polcalcin), this is very difficult to determine, since minor allergens are frequently underrepresented in commercial pollen extracts (Focke et al. 2009).

Persistent moderate symptoms during the whole pollen season could indicate a sensitization to panallergens. Conjunctival provocation tests with profilin-containing extracts (i.e., date pollen, ALK-Abelló, Spain) induce positive reactions in some of the affected patients (Tehrani et al. 2011). Moreover, a sensitization to panallergens can be an indication of the severity of the allergy.

Studies with children elucidated the typical sequence of allergic sensitization to various proteins of an allergen source. Allergic sensitization is triggered by a so-called initiator allergen (i.e., Phl p 1 for timothy grass). With progressing sensitization, additional allergens will be recognized by the immune system in a distinct order. First, the major allergens followed by the minor allergens of the source, i.e., grass pollen Phl p 4 and Phl p 5, followed by Phl p 2, Phl p 6, and Phl p 11; thereafter, sensitization to the panallergens Phl p 12 (profilin) and Phl p 7 (polcalcin) can be observed (Hatzler et al. 2012).

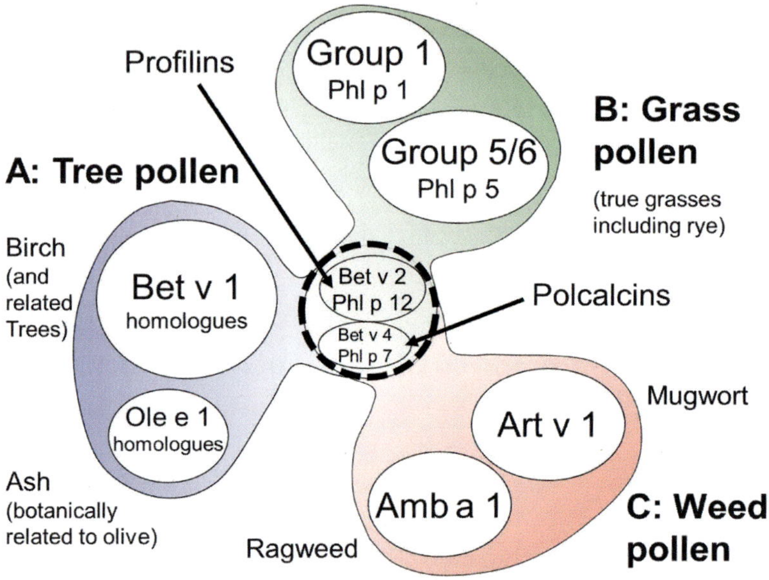

Fig. 3.4 Propeller model of cross-reactivity between pollen allergens. Propeller blades: species-specific, genuine marker allergens; propeller center: highly cross-reactive panallergens. In case of allergic sensitization to the panallergens profilin and/or polcalcin (propeller center), extract-based allergy diagnosis does not allow a precise determination of the allergen source. Tree, grass, and weed pollen sensitization can only be verified via specific sensitization tests (i.e., specific IgE determination) using genuine marker allergens

It has been demonstrated in a study on 891 pollen-allergic patients from Spain that sensitization to grass pollen profilin correlates with the severity of the allergic disease (Barber et al. 2008). With certain pollens, e.g., *Chenopodium album* (white goosefoot), extraordinarily high sensitization rates of 55 % and 46 % to profilin and polcalcin, respectively, have been reported (Barderas et al. 2004). Another study, investigating the sensitization rates to Che a 2, reported that an exceedingly high 81 % of the patients had IgE against the profilin allergen. Thus, it seems necessary to include both panallergens Che a 2 and 3 in the component-resolved determination of goosefoot allergy sensitization patterns (Nouri et al. 2012). Quite high sensitization rates (47 %) have also been reported for the pollen profilins of Russian thistle (*Salsola kali* Sal k 4), 33 % for redroot pigweed (*Amaranthus retroflexus* Ama r 2), and 64 % for date palm (*Phoenix dactylifera* Pho d 2) (Assarehzadegan et al. 2010; Asturias et al. 2005; Tehrani et al. 2011).

Profilins may represent clinically relevant major allergens of certain plant-derived foods. Although profilins may sporadically evoke severe allergic reactions, such as gastrointestinal anaphylaxis, nausea, pruritus, or dyspnea, allergic symptoms are usually restricted to the oropharyngeal region. This is in accordance with the known degradation of profilins by digestive enzymes. The apple profilin Mal d 4, for instance, loses its IgE-binding properties within 10 s of pepsin treatment (Ma et al. 2006). This could also explain the generally mild oropharyngeal allergic symptoms elicited by melon, where profilin has been described as a major allergen (Rodriguez-Perez et al. 2003). Although food processing affects the allergenicity of profilins, it has been reported that cooking diminishes but does not abolish IgE binding to the celery profilin Api g 4 (Ballmer-Weber et al. 2002). It may be that heat treatment initially destroys IgE epitopes of the Api g 4, but that the cooling process might lead to a partial renaturation. In a case report of lychee allergy anaphylaxis induced by profilin, either fresh or canned lychee fruits were of comparable potency. As profilin was the only detectable allergen in lychee, the severe reactions were explained by the significant amount of profilin in the fruits (Santos and van Ree 2011).

In a Spanish study, grass pollen-allergic patients sensitized to profilin were exposed to purified profilin from date palm pollen (Pho d 2) in oral provocation tests using amounts from 0.074 to 740 µg. The study demonstrated that these quantities induced mild to severe allergic reactions, the latter with as little as 7.4 µg of Pho d 2 (Alvarado et al. 2014). The authors concluded that a high grass pollen exposure would eventually lead to a broad sensitization to multiple grass pollen allergens and that these patients would then be at risk for profilin-associated food allergies. In individual cases, sufficient amounts of the allergen could be absorbed via the mucosa to lead not only to oropharyngeal but also more severe systemic reactions.

3.11 Extract Selection for Allergen Immunotherapy (AIT)

The rare patients who are sensitized exclusively to pollen panallergens or minor pollen allergens are probably not suitable for AIT. Thus, before selecting an AIT extract for patients with a history of profilin and/or polcalcin sensitization, one should determine the specific IgE levels to the primary pollen major allergens (Fig. 3.4) to complement allergen-specific diagnosis.

The extent to which pollen AIT is less promising in those patients has only been examined retrospectively (Schmid-Grendelmeier 2010), but has not yet been investigated prospectively. Consider, for example, a pollen-allergic patient who shows only weak skin prick test reactivity to birch pollen extracts: If there is no sensitization to the major birch pollen allergen Bet v 1 but only to the birch pollen profilin Bet v 2, birch pollen AIT would seem to be contraindicated. In Central Europe, such patients are usually sensitized to the grass pollen profilin Phl p 12, leading to cross-reactivity with Bet v 2.

To avoid the undue cost of incorrect extract selection, patients in Central Europe (e.g., Austria and Switzerland, possibly a consequence of the high local prevalence of profilin sensitization) are routinely tested for sensitization to profilins and polcalcins prior to any extract-based AIT. In case of positive results, further tests with the respective major pollen allergens are performed (Pfaar et al. 2014).

Multiple positive results in skin prick tests and/or specific IgE tests with pollen extracts are usually indicative of panallergen sensitization. Thus, it is highly recommended that one investigates the influence of panallergens by molecule-based diagnosis using purified, natural, or recombinant major and minor allergens (Schmid-Grendelmeier 2010).

In component-resolved diagnosis for the selection of pollen extracts for AIT in patients with panallergen sensitization, the major allergens include the following depending on the geographic region:

- Bet v 1 (major birch pollen allergen: sensitization marker for birch, hazel, alder, beech, and oak pollen allergies)
- Cup a 1 (major cypress pollen allergen, marker for sensitization to cypress pollen) *or closely related*
- Jun a 1 (major mountain cedar pollen allergen, marker for sensitization to cedar pollen)
- Ole e 1 (major olive pollen allergen: sensitization marker for olive and ash pollen allergies)
- Phl p 1 and Phl p 5 (major grass pollen allergens: sensitization markers for grass and rye pollen allergies)
- Art v 1 (major mugwort pollen allergen)
- Amb a 1 (major ragweed pollen allergen)

3.12 Conclusions from a Clinical Perspective

Allergy diagnosis based on pollen extracts (skin prick tests, specific IgE tests) is impeded by the fact that, worldwide, 5–40 % of pollen-allergic patients are sensitized to the highly cross-reactive panallergens, profilin and polcalcin. Such sensitization/cross-reactivity patterns do not induce false-positive test results, but are usually clinically irrelevant. Only rarely does sensitization to profilins and polcalcins evoke clinically relevant allergic reactions, e.g., after the ingestion of profilin-rich foods such as melon, tomato, orange, or various tropical fruits.

Molecule-based diagnosis and specific IgE tests against single pollen allergens represent a targeted approach to determining sensitization to important major and minor allergens. The clinical relevance of such sensitization profiles needs to be carefully evaluated by linkage to the associated symptoms. In case of ambiguity, provocation tests are indicated to aid in selecting AIT extracts for pollen-allergic patients.

References

Alvarado MI, Jimeno L, De La Torre F, Boissy P, Rivas B, Lazaro M, Barber D. Profilin as a severe food allergen in allergic patients overexposed to grass pollen. Allergy. 2014;69(12):1610–6. Epub 2014/08/16.

Asero R, Tripodi S, Dondi A, Di Rienzo Businco A, Sfika I, Bianchi A, Candelotti P, Caffarelli C, Povesi Dascola C, Ricci G, Calamelli E, Maiello N, Miraglia Del Giudice M, Frediani T, Frediani S, Macrì F, Moretti M, Dello Iacono I, Patria MF, Varin E, Peroni D, Comberiati P, Chini L, Moschese V, Lucarelli S, Bernardini R, Pingitore G, Pelosi U, Tosca M, Cirisano A, Faggian D, Plebani M, Verga C, Matricardi PM; Italian Pediatric Allergy Network (I-PAN). Prevalence and Clinical Relevance of IgE Sensitization to Profilin in Childhood: A Multicenter Study. Int Arch Allergy Immunol. 2015;168:25–31.

Assarehzadegan MA, Amini A, Sankian M, Tehrani M, Jabbari F, Varasteh A. Sal k 4, a new allergen of Salsola kali, is profilin: a predictive value of conserved conformational regions in cross-reactivity with other plant-derived profilins. Biosci Biotechnol Biochem. 2010;74:1441–6.

Asturias JA, Ibarrola I, Fernandez J, Arilla MC, Gonzalez-Rioja R, Martinez A. Pho d 2, a major allergen from date palm pollen, is a profilin: cloning, sequencing, and immunoglobulin E cross-reactivity with other profilins. Clin Exp Allergy. 2005;35:374–81.

Balla T. Phosphoinositides: tiny lipids with giant impact on cell regulation. Physiol Rev. 2013;93:1019–137.

Ballmer-Weber BK, Hoffmann A, Wuthrich B, Luttkopf D, Pompei C, Wangorsch A, Kastner M, Vieths S. Influence of food processing on the allergenicity of celery: DBPCFC with celery spice and cooked celery in patients with celery allergy. Allergy. 2002;57:228–35.

Barber D, de la Torre F, Feo F, Florido F, Guardia P, Moreno C, Quiralte J, Lombardero M, Villalba M, Salcedo G, Rodriguez R. Understanding patient sensitization profiles in complex pollen areas: a molecular epidemiological study. Allergy. 2008;63:1550–8.

Barderas R, Villalba M, Pascual CY, Batanero E, Rodriguez R. Profilin (Che a 2) and polcalcin (Che a 3) are relevant allergens of Chenopodium album pollen: isolation, amino acid sequences, and immunologic properties. J Allergy Clin Immunol. 2004;113:1192–8.

Casquete-Roman E, Rosado-Gil T, Postigo I, Guisantes JA, Fernandez M, Torres HE, Martinez-Quesada J. Profilin cross-reactive panallergen causes latex sensitization in the pediatric population allergic to pollen. Ann Allergy Asthma Immunol. 2012;109:215–9.

Focke M, Marth K, Valenta R. Molecular composition and biological activity of commercial birch pollen allergen extracts. Eur J Clin Invest. 2009;39:429–36.

Hatzler L, Panetta V, Lau S, Wagner P, Bergmann RL, Illi S, Bergmann KE, Keil T, Hofmaier S, Rohrbach A, Bauer CP, Hoffman U, Forster J, Zepp F, Schuster A, Wahn U, Matricardi PM. Molecular spreading and predictive value of preclinical IgE response to Phleum pratense in children with hay fever. J Allergy Clin Immunol. 2012;130:894–901 e5.

Hauser M, Roulias A, Ferreira F, Egger M. Panallergens and their impact on the allergic patient. Allergy Asthma Clin Immunol. 2010;6:1.

Kleine-Tebbe J, Balmer-Weber B, Breiteneder H, Vieths S. Bet v 1 und Homologe – Verursacher der Baumpollenallergie und birkenpollenassoziierter Kreuzreaktionen. Allergo J. 2010;19:462–4.

Kühn A, Radauer C, Swoboda I, Kleine-Tebbe J. Molekulare Diagnostik der Fischallergie: Parvalbumine und andere Allergene. Allergo J. 2012;21:16–8.

Le LQ, Mahler V, Lorenz Y, Scheurer S, Biemelt S, Vieths S, Sonnewald U. Reduced allergenicity of tomato fruits harvested from Lyc e 1-silenced transgenic tomato plants. J Allergy Clin Immunol. 2006;1180:1176–83.

Ma Y, Zuidmeer L, Bohle B, Bolhaar ST, Gadermaier G, Gonzalez-Mancebo E, Fernandez-Rivas M, Knulst AC, Himly M, Asero R, Ebner C, van Ree R, Ferreira F, Breiteneder H, Hoffmann-Sommergruber K. Characterization of recombinant Mal d 4 and its application for component-resolved diagnosis of apple allergy. Clin Exp Allergy. 2006;36:1087–96.

Magler I, Nuss D, Hauser M, Ferreira F, Brandstetter H. Molecular metamorphosis in polcalcin allergens by EF-hand rearrangements and domain swapping. FEBS J. 2010;277:2598–610.

Matricardi PM, Kleine-Tebbe J, Hoffmann HJ, Valenta R, Hilger C, Hofmaier S, Aalberse RC, Agache I, Asero R, Ballmer-Weber B, Barber D, Beyer K, Biedermann T, Biló MB, Blank S, Bohle B, Bosshard PP, Breiteneder H, Brough HA, Caraballo L, Caubet JC, Crameri R, Davies JM, Douladiris N, Ebisawa M, Eigenmann PA, Fernandez-Rivas M, Ferreira F, Gadermaier G, Glatz M, Hamilton RG, Hawranek T, Hellings P, Hoffmann-Sommergruber K, Jakob T, Jappe U, Jutel M, Kamath SD, Knol EF, Korosec P, Kuehn A, Lack G, Lopata AL, Mäkelä M, Morisset M, Niederberger V, Nowak-Wezgrzyn AH, Papadopoulos NG, Pastorello EA, Pauli G, Platts-Mills T, Posa D, Poulsen LK, Raulf M, Sastre J, Scala E, Schmid JM, Schmid-Grendelmeier P, van Hage M, van Ree R, Vieths S, Weber R, Wickman M, Muraro A, Ollert M. EAACI molecular allergology user's guide. Pediatr Allergy Immunol. 2016;27 Suppl 23:1–250.

Mirza O, Henriksen A, Ipsen H, Larsen JN, Wissenbach M, Spangfort MD, Gajhede M. Dominant epitopes and allergic cross-reactivity: complex formation between a Fab fragment of a monoclonal murine IgG antibody and the major allergen from birch pollen Bet v 1. J Immunol. 2000;165:331–8.

Nouri HR, Sankian M, Vahedi F, Afsharzadeh D, Rouzbeh L, Moghadam M, Varasteh A. Diagnosis of Chenopodium album allergy with a cocktail of recombinant allergens as a tool for component-resolved diagnosis. Mol Biol Rep. 2012;39:3169–78.

Pfaar O, Bachert C, Bufe A, Buhl R, Ebner C, Eng P, Friedrichs F, Fuchs T, Hamelmann E, Hartwig-Bade D, Hering T, Huttegger I, Jung K, Klimek L, Kopp MV, Merk H, Rabe U, Saloga J, Schmid-Grendelmeier P, Schuster A, Schwerk N, Sitter H, Umpfenbach U, Wedi B, Wöhrl S, Worm M, Kleine-Tebbe J. Guideline on allergen-specific immunotherapy in IgE-mediated allergic diseases – S2k Guideline of the German Society for Allergology and Clinical Immunology (DGAKI), the Society for Pediatric Allergy and Environmental Medicine (GPA), the Medical Association of German Allergologists (AeDA), the Austrian Society for Allergy and Immunology (ÖGAI), the Swiss Society for Allergy and Immunology (SGAI), the German Society of Dermatology (DDG), the German Society of Oto-Rhino-Laryngology, Head and Neck Surgery (DGHNO-KHC), the German Society of Pediatrics and Adolescent Medicine (DGKJ), the Society for Pediatric Pneumology (GPP), the German Respiratory Society (DGP), the German Association of ENT Surgeons (BV-HNO), the Professional Federation of Paediatricians and Youth Doctors (BVKJ), the Federal Association of Pulmonologists (BDP) and the German Dermatologists Association (BVDD). Allergo J Int. 2014;23:282–319. doi:10.1007/s40629-014-0032-2.

Raulf-Heimsoth M, Rihs HP. Latexallergene: Sensibilisierungsquellen und Einzelallergenprofile erkennen. Allergo J. 2011;20:241–3.

Rodriguez-Perez R, Crespo JF, Rodriguez J, Salcedo G. Profilin is a relevant melon allergen susceptible to pepsin digestion in patients with oral allergy syndrome. J Allergy Clin Immunol. 2003;111:634–9.

Santos A, Van Ree R. Profilins: mimickers of allergy or relevant allergens? Int Arch Allergy Immunol. 2011;155:191–204.

Schmid-Grendelmeier P. Recombinant allergens. For routine use or still only science? Hautarzt. 2010;61:946–53.

Tanaka M, Shibata H. Poly(L-proline)-binding proteins from chick embryos are a profilin and a profilactin. Eur J Biochem. 1995;151:291–7.

Tehrani M, Sankian M, Assarehzadegan MA, Falak R, Noorbakhsh R, Moghadam M, Jabbari F, Varasteh A. Identification of a new allergen from Amaranthus retroflexus pollen, Ama r 2. Allergol Int. 2011;60:309–16.

Tinghino R, Twardosz A, Barletta B, Puggioni EM, Iacovacci P, Butteroni C, Afferni C, Mari A, Hayek B, Di Felice G, Focke M, Westritschnig K, Valenta R, Pini C. Molecular, structural, and immunologic relationships between different families of recombinant calcium-binding pollen allergens. J Allergy Clin Immunol. 2002;109:314–20.

Valenta R, Duchene M, Pettenburger K, Sillaber C, Valent P, Bettelheim P, Breitenbach M, Rumpold H, Kraft D, Scheiner O. Identification of profilin as a novel pollen allergen; IgE autoreactivity in sensitized individuals. Science. 1991;253:557–60.

Vallverdu A, Garcia-Ortega P, Martinez J, Martinez A, Esteban MI, de Molina M, Fernandez-Tavora L, Fernandez J, Bartolome B, Palacios R. Mercurialis annua: characterization of main allergens and cross-reactivity with other species. Int Arch Allergy Immunol. 1997;112:356–64.

van Ree R, Fernandez-Rivas M, Cuevas M, van Wijngaarden M, Aalberse RC. Pollen-related allergy to peach and apple: an important role for profilin. J Allergy Clin Immunol. 1995;95:726–34.

Verdino P, Barderas R, Villalba M, Westritschnig K, Valenta R, Rodriguez R, Keller W. Three-dimensional structure of the cross-reactive pollen allergen Che a 3: visualizing cross-reactivity on the molecular surfaces of weed, grass, and tree pollen allergens. J Immunol. 2008;180:2313–21.

Witke W. The role of profilin complexes in cell motility and other cellular processes. Trends Cell Biol. 2004;14:461–9.

Wopfner N, Dissertori O, Ferreira F, Lackner P. Calcium-binding proteins and their role in allergic diseases. Immunol Allergy Clin North Am. 2007;27:29–44.

Wopfner N, Gruber P, Wallner M, Briza P, Ebner C, Mari A, Richter K, Vogel L, Ferreira F. Molecular and immunological characterization of novel weed pollen pan-allergens. Allergy. 2008;63(7):872–81.

Stable Plant Food Allergens I: Lipid-Transfer Proteins

4

A. Petersen, J. Kleine-Tebbe, and S. Scheurer

4.1 Introduction

Nonspecific lipid-transfer proteins (nsLTPs, short term LTPs) exist ubiquitously in various tissues of both mono- and dicotyledonous plants and have functions both in the cytoplasmic transport of lipids and the creation of the plant cuticle (a waxy protective film covering the epidermis of leaves). Besides their role in lipophilic binding and transport, LTPs are involved in plant defense (for review see Kader 1996) and have been assigned to the class of plant stress proteins as PR-14 proteins (PR, pathogenesis-related) (van Loon and van Stein 1999).

This article is based on a publication of the authors published in 2011 in the *Allergo Journal* (Petersen A, Kleine-Tebbe J, Scheurer S (2011): Stabile pflanzliche Nahrungsmittelallergene – Lipid-Transfer-Proteine. Allergo J 20: 384–386) which has now been updated, extended, and translated as a book chapter.

The authors gratefully thank Dr. Stefan Schülke, PhD, Paul-Ehrlich-Institute, Research Group Molecular Allergology, Langen, Germany, for his initial English translation and Dr. Steve Love, PhD, Laguna Niguel, CA, USA, for reading the manuscript, his helpful suggestions, and his final editorial assistance.

A. Petersen, PhD (✉)
Research Center Borstel, Borstel, Germany
e-mail: apetersen@fz-borstel.de

J. Kleine-Tebbe, MD, Prof.
Allergy & Asthma Center Westend, Outpatient Clinic Hanf, Ackermann & Kleine-Tebbe, Berlin, Germany
e-mail: kleine-tebbe@allergie-experten.de

S. Scheurer, PhD, Assoc Prof.
Paul-Ehrlich-Institut, Federal Institute for Vaccines and Biomedicines, Langen, Germany
e-mail: stephan.scheurer@pei.de

J. Kleine-Tebbe, T. Jakob (eds.), *Molecular Allergy Diagnostics*,
DOI 10.1007/978-3-319-42499-6_4

LTPs are characterized by a strongly conserved, three-dimensional (3D) protein structure. Along with the structurally closely related 2S albumins and α-amylase/protease inhibitors, LTPs belong to the prolamin protein superfamily (Radauer et al. 2008), which includes alcohol-soluble and glutamine-rich storage proteins.

LTPs were first described as food allergens in 1992 in Spanish patients with a stone fruit-peach allergy. As an IgE-reactive protein (original designation Pru p 1) with a molecular mass of 8–10 kDa, it was found to be predominantly expressed in peach skin (Lleonart et al. 1992). An IgE cross-reactivity of this low molecular weight allergen in patients with food allergies was first demonstrated using extracts from stone fruit (Pastorello et al. 1994).

In 1999 peach and apple LTPs were first described on a molecular level as allergenic LTPs (Pastorello et al. 1999) and designated as Pru p 3 and Mal d 3, respectively (Sánchez-Monge et al. 1999). To date (November 2016) 41 plant LTPs have been accepted as allergens by the IUIS (International Union of Immunological Sciences) Allergen Nomenclature Subcommittee. Furthermore, other LTPs with allergenic properties have been described (www.allergome.org). As LTPs are common proteins in the plant kingdom, they are referred to as panallergens (Asero et al. 2000; for review see also van Winkle and Chang 2014).

Structurally homologous allergens have not been described in allergen sources from non-plants. Food-derived LTPs were described as major allergens in Southern Europe (Matricardi et al. 2016), especially in the Mediterranean area and in Asia, while sensitization to LTPs is much more rare in Central and Northern Europe. The reason for this geographic difference in the sensitization profile is unknown. Food-derived LTPs are highly stable proteins and can elicit severe systemic reactions. Allergen-specific immunotherapy has not been established to date for LTPs.

4.2 Structure of Allergens

LTPs are globular, non-glycosylated proteins composed of four α-helical domains connected by flexible loops. LTPs have a molecular mass of approximately 6–10 kDa (91 to 93 amino acids) and a basic isoelectric point of approximately 9. They are divided into two subfamilies: LTP1 (9–10 kDa) and LTP2 (6–7 kDa) (Lin et al. 2004). To date, almost all known LTPs belong to the LTP1 subfamily. The existence of both subfamilies in one organism was shown for celery plants. Api g 2 (LTP1) is expressed in the celery stalks (American celery, *Apium graveolens* var. *dulce*), while Api g 6 (LTP2) is expressed in celeriac tuber (European celery, *Apium graveolens* var. *rapaceum*) (Vejvar et al. 2013). LTPs form a multigene family (Richard et al. 2007). LTP isoforms (>67 % sequence identity) as well as variants (>97 % sequence identity) within one species are known, for example, Ara h 9 (peanut), Art v 3 (mugwort), Aspa a 1 (asparagus), Fra a 3 (strawberry), Mal d 3 (apple), Par j 1 and Par j 2 (pellitory, abundant in the Mediterranean, formerly used as medical plant (diuretic)), Pha v 3 (green bean), Pun g 1 (pomegranate), Tri a 14 (wheat), Zea m 14 (corn), and Pru p 3 (peach).

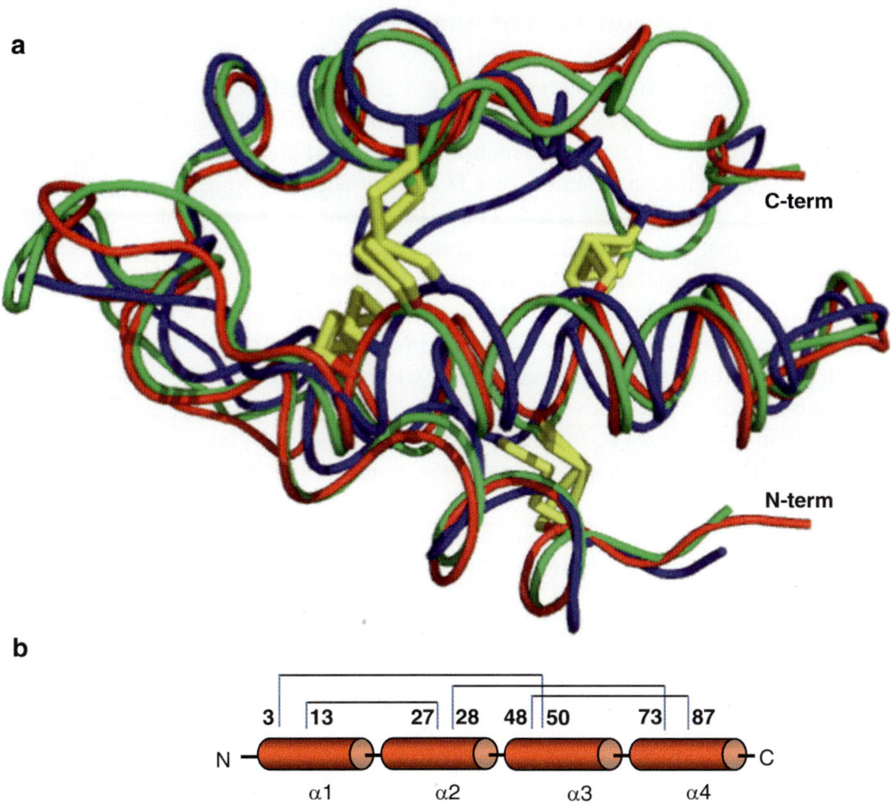

Fig. 4.1 (**a**) 3D protein structure of peach LTP Pru p 3 (PDB 2ALG, *red*) in comparison with wheat LTP Tri a 14 (PDB 1GH1, *blue*) and a model of Par j 1 from pellitory (*green*). Amino acid sequence identity to Pru p 3: Tri a 14 = 47.3 %, Par j 1 = 18.6 %. Intramolecular disulfide bonds are depicted in *yellow*. (**b**) Schematic representation of the four highly conserved disulfide bonds connecting the four α-helices (Fig. 4.1a generated with PyMol v 0.99 and kindly provided by Dr. Kay Fötisch, Paul-Ehrlich-Institut, Langen)

The LTP protein structure is compact and stabilized in four positions by strongly conserved intramolecular disulfide bonds, contributing to a high thermal and proteolytic stability (Asero et al. 2000; Gaier et al. 2008).

Although LTPs belong to different taxonomic plant families and display only partial (<30 %) amino acid sequence identity, the 3D protein structure is highly conserved (Fig. 4.1). LTP-mediated IgE reactivity is determined by the 3D protein structure (conformational epitopes). Here, the highly stable nature of the molecule allows it to come in contact with effector cells in a non-fragmented, IgE-reactive form and cause allergic reactions. This occurs despite high-temperature food processing and contact with gastrointestinal enzymes such as pepsin.

4.3 Biological Function of Allergens

Analysis of the protein structure of Pru p 3 contributed to the elucidation of the biological function of LTPs (Pasquato et al. 2006). The LTP protein scaffold forms a central hydrophobic tunnel in which fatty acids and phospholipids can be bound nonspecifically. Thus, a function of LTPs in intracellular lipid transport between organelles has been hypothesized. The existence of an N-terminal signal peptide also suggests that these proteins are secreted to the extracellular compartment.

LTPs contribute to the extracellular assembly and stabilization of both cell membrane and cuticle (Kader 1996). The outer surface of fruits (pericarp) contains especially high concentrations of LTPs. Peach skin contains a 7 times higher concentration of Pru p 3 than the pulp (Carnés et al. 2002). Furthermore, LTPs also accumulate in the seeds of fruits such as kiwi – Act d 10 and Act c 10 (Bernardi et al. 2011).

As members of the PR-14 family, LTPs participate in plant pathogen defense (biotic stress) (García-Olmedo et al. 1995). Furthermore, the proteins are upregulated under conditions of abiotic stress such as temperature extremes or drought (Guo et al. 2013). Systematic quantification of the LTP content of organic in comparison to conventionally cultivated foods is not available.

4.4 Frequency of Sensitization and Geographic Distribution

A total of 35 allergenic LTPs from food sources are described in the IUIS allergen database (reviewed in Matricardi et al. 2016). Source plant materials are fruits (stone, e.g., peach, and accessory, e.g., apple and strawberry, fruits), vegetables (e.g., lentil, green bean), spices (e.g., white mustard), and seeds (e.g., cereals, peanuts, and tree nuts). Additionally, allergenic LTPs are described for pollen (Amb a 6 *Ambrosia*, ragweed; Art v 3 *Artemisia*, mugwort; Ole e 7 *Olea*, olive; Par j 1, Par j 2, and Par o 1 from *Parietaria*, pellitory; Pla a 3 and Pla or 3 from *Platanus*, plane tree), chloroplasts (Can s 3 *Cannabis*, marihuana), and latex (Hev b 12 *Hevea*, latex).

LTPs are clinically relevant food allergens that may induce primary gastrointestinal sensitization. Therefore, in contrast to birch pollen-associated food allergens, they are considered to be in class I, referring to primary sensitizers. Patients sensitized to LTPs, however, often tolerate foods such as carrot, potato, banana, and melon (Asero et al. 2007).

Most LTPs are only known as major allergens in Southern Europe (Egger et al. 2010). In Mediterranean areas, more than 90 % of patients with reactions to foods, especially within the Rosaceae family, are sensitized to the respective LTPs. Almost all peach-allergic patients with severe systemic reactions are sensitized to peach LTP Pru p 3 (Pastorello et al. 1999), the clinically most important and best characterized food LTP. Outside of the Mediterranean areas, Pru p 3 was described as major allergen in peach-allergic individuals with associated mugwort allergy (Gao et al. 2013). In contrast, sensitization to LTPs is infrequent in Northern and Central Europe. Here, predominantly Bet v 1-homologous allergens frequently induce mild oropharyngeal reactions. In these areas, only individual cases of food allergy and sensitization to the respective LTPs have been described, for example, to Cor a 8, Ara h 9, Mal d 3, Tri a 14, Act d 10, Api g 6, Len c 3, Pru av 3, Vit v 1, and Vac m 3 (Table 4.1). It is known

Table 4.1 Frequency of sensitization against LTPs outside of Southern Europe

LTP	Prevalence of sensitization	Patient category		Reference
Pru p 3 (peach)	96 % (23/24)	Peach allergics with mugwort allergy	(Northern) China	Gao et al. (2013)
Cor a 8 (hazelnut)	5 % (1/20)	Adult hazelnut allergics (DBPCFC+)	Denmark	Skamstrup Hansen et al. (2009)
	15 % (3/20)		Switzerland	
	8 % (3/40) vs. 5 % (2/39)	Pediatric (DBPCFC+) vs. adult hazelnut allergics with objective symptoms	The Netherlands	Masthoff et al. (2013)
	14 % (4/29)	Hazelnut allergics with or without apple allergy, positive sIgE or SPT+	The Netherlands	Le et al. (2013a)
	100 % (8/8)[a] vs. 6 % (1/18)	Hazelnut-sensitized pediatric patients with ($n=8$) and without ($n=18$) objective symptoms in a DBPCFC controlled study	The Netherlands	Flinterman et al. (2008)
Ara h 9 (peanut)	67 % (4/6)	Positive case history and positive sIgE to peanut	USA	Lauer et al. (2009)
	17 % (2/12)		Germany	
	20 % (38/192)	Pediatric patients with positive case history to peanut	Great Britain	Arkwright et al. (2013)
	14.3 % (5/35)	Positive case history to peanut	Sweden	Vereda et al. (2011)
	7.7 % (2/30)		USA	
Mal d 3 (apple)	95 % (20/21) with reactivity against putative LTP in extract	Pediatric patients with birch pollen allergy and positive sIgE to birch and apple	Poland	Cudowska et al. (2008)
	1 % (1/99)	Positive case history and SPT+	The Netherlands	Fernández-Rivas et al. (2006)
	2 % (2/94)		Austria	
Tri a 14 (wheat)	2.5 % (1/40)	Patients with baker's asthma, positive sIgE to wheat	Germany	Sander et al. (2011)

(continued)

Table 4.1 (continued)

LTP	Prevalence of sensitization	Patient category		Reference
Act d 10 (kiwi fruit)	3 %	Positive case history to kiwifruit	Iceland	Le et al. (2013b)
	9 %		Eastern Europe	
	11 %		Western/Middle Europe	
Api g 6 (celery)	38 % (12/32)	Celeriac allergics and positive sIgE and/or SPT	Austria	Vejvar et al. (2013)
Len c 3 (lentil)	3-Feb	Adult patients with positive case history to lentils or other legumes, positive sIgE to lentils	The Netherlands	Akkerdaas et al. (2012)
Pru av 3 (cherry)	3 % (3/101)	Positive case history and positive sIgE	Germany	Scheurer et al. (2001)
	4 % (1/24)	Adult cherry allergics (DBPCFC+), 23/24 SPT+	Switzerland	Ballmer-Weber et al. (2002)
	5 % (1/21)	Adult cherry allergics (DBPCFC+)	(middle) Europe (Germany and Switzerland)	Reuter et al. (2006)
	14 % (12/87)	Adult cherry allergics (pos. case history)		
Vit v 1 (grape)	Case report (*n* = 1)	Positive case history, positive sIgE and SPT+	Germany	Schäd et al. (2005)
Vac m 3 (blueberry)	Case report (*n* = 1)	Positive case history, positive sIgE and SPT+	Germany	Gebhardt et al. (2009)

[a]False positive?; *DBPCFC* double-blind placebo-controlled food challenge

that in Southern Europe approximately 60 % of patients with "baker's asthma" are sensitized to the wheat LTP Tri a 14 (Palacin et al. 2007). In Central Europe this is only the case for approximately 2.5 % of such patients (Sander et al. 2011). Thus, sensitization to LTPs clearly causes work-related diseases in some areas.

The reasons for the observed differences in geographic distribution patterns of sensitization to LTPs are unclear. Differences in nutrition habits, greater exposure to pollen LTPs in Southern Europe, and genetic predisposition are probably relevant to allergic sensitization rates (Schocker et al. 2004). The influence of respiratory exposure to pollen LTPs (especially Art v 3 from mugwort and Pla a 3 from plane tree) on the development of food allergies is controversial. Some authors describe LTP-mediated respiratory allergies as a consequence of primary sensitization to peach

Pru p 3 and subsequent cross-reactivity with Art v 3 from mugwort pollen (Pastorello et al. 2002; Sánchez-López et al. 2014). In contrast, others postulate pollen LTPs as having primary sensitizing properties (Lombardero et al. 2004). Gao et al. (2013) speculate that high exposure to mugwort pollen (in Northern China) can lead to primary sensitization against Art v 3, which promotes the subsequent development of peach allergy by cross-reactivity with Pru p 3 in some patients.

4.5 Clinical Relevance

Because of their high thermal and proteolytic stability, intact LTPs can act directly on the immune system of the gastrointestinal mucosa.

Allergic reactions are not only caused by the consumption of foods but also in individual cases by skin contact (Asero 2011b; Gandolfo-Cano et al. 2014) or airway exposure, e.g., by Tri a 14 (wheat) and Ory s 14 (rice) (Borghesan et al. 2008; García et al. 2004).

Besides the primary sensitization to food LTPs and subsequent cross-reactivity with homologous LTPs from pollen, the converse is also possible: Pollen LTPs can induce sensitization leading to a subsequent cross-reactivity with food LTPs (Zuidmeer and van Ree 2007).

Food-allergic patients with IgE reactivity to LTPs often suffer from oropharyngeal allergic symptoms (oral allergy syndrome, OAS), urticaria, or anaphylactic reactions. Food LTPs can elicit symptoms in LTP-sensitized patients within 5 min of exposure (Arkwright et al. 2013). Pru p 3 from peach is described as clinically relevant to this syndrome.

Pru p 3 can elicit severe allergies even during infancy, while allergies caused by pollen LTPs usually have a later-onset cause and milder symptoms (Pastorello et al. 2013).

Pru p 3-specific IgE titers are inversely correlated with patient's age and are especially high in pediatric patients (Pastorello et al. 2013). However, no significant correlation could be established between specific IgE titers and the type or severity of reaction (Novembre et al. 2012). The occurrence of contact urticaria after contact with plant foods with a high surface LTP content (e.g., melon rind) is significantly more frequent in patients sensitized to Pru p 3 than in patients with pollen-associated food allergies (Asero 2011a). This finding was not correlated with specific IgE values (Asero 2011a). Pru p 3 exhibits both a stronger IgE-binding capacity than pollen or food LTPs (Pastorello et al. 2013) and strong T-cell stimulating properties (Schulten et al. 2011). Human Cor a 8-specific T-cell lines were stimulated more effectively with Pru p 3 than Cor a 8, possibly due to a dominant Pru p 3-specific T-cell peptide. Schulten et al. (2011) and Tordesillas et al. (2013) tried to explain the high allergenicity of Pru p 3 in two ways: first, by its high T-cell immunogenicity and, second, by its efficient transepithelial transport and subsequent presentation to the gastrointestinal immune system, which leads to the secretion of cytokines by epithelial cells promoting allergic Th2 immune responses. Another explanation for the high prevalence of Pru p 3 sensitization compared to other food LTPs is, besides

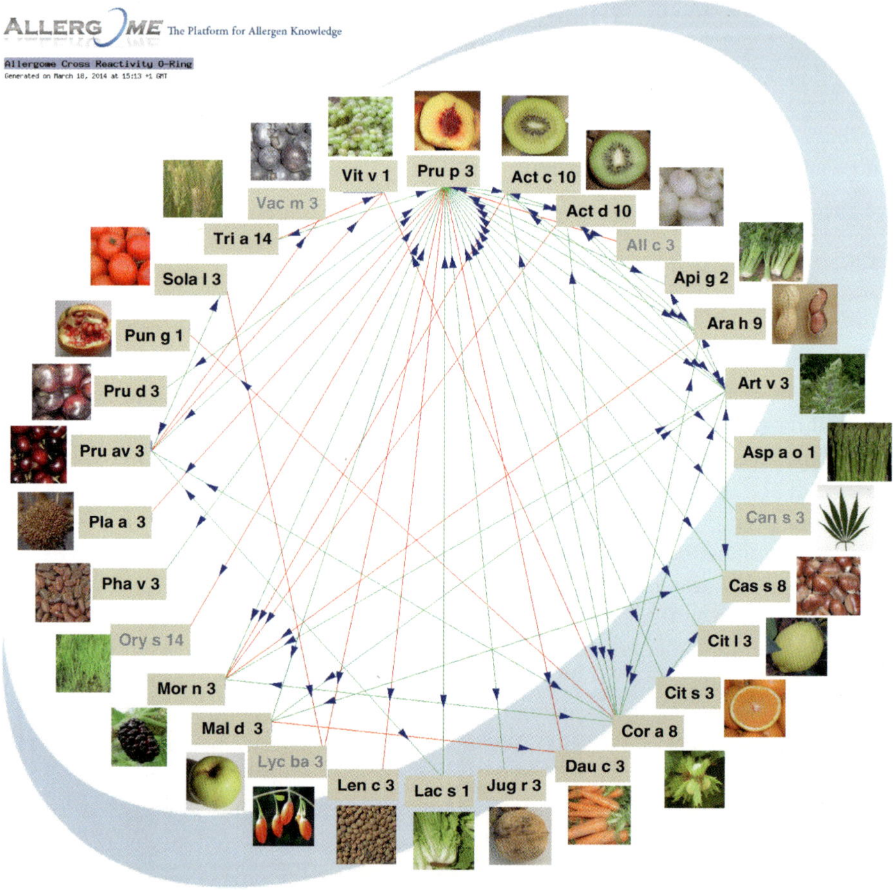

Fig. 4.2 IgE cross-reactivity between allergenic LTPs, displayed using the "Allergome O-ring." Bidirectional cross-reactivity is highlighted with double-sided *red arrows*, unidirectional, with *green arrows*. Allergens not included in the IUIS allergen database are depicted in *gray*

the suggested high frequency of peach consumption, the high accumulation of the allergen in peach skin, which is much higher than in the skin of pears (Ramazzina et al. 2012).

4.6 IgE Cross-Reactivity Between LTPs

LTPs are plant allergens which are ubiquitously expressed in foods (fruits, vegetables, and seeds), in pollen (tree, grass, and weed pollen), and in latex. Among LTPs, there is a high degree of IgE cross-reactivity. The peach LTP Pru p 3 shows the most pronounced cross-reactivity. Figure 4.2 shows, in an O-ring, confirmed cross-reactivities between LTPs from various food sources. Strongly cross-reactive are members of the Prunoideae (stone fruits) family, a subfamily of the Rosaceae that shows high sequence identity to Pru p 3:

- plum LTP Pru d 3
- cherry LTP Pru av 3
- apricot LTP Pru ar 3 (Pastorello et al. 1994)

Additional cross-reactivity exists among fruits of the Pomoideae subfamily: apple and pear (Borges et al. 2006), but also with botanically non-related families (Asero et al. 2002). Here, individual cross-reactivities can refer to single or multiple LTPs (Asero 2010). In contrast to the severity of clinical manifestations, the degree of cross-reactivity in Pru p 3 mono-sensitized patients correlates positively with peach-specific IgE titers (Fig. 4.3). The reason for this correlation probably is an extensive Pru p 3-specific IgE repertoire and cross-reactive epitopes in other LTPs.

Pru p 3 is known to be the clinically most important and most allergenic food LTP. The clinical relevance is correlated with a strong cellular and humoral immune response directed against Pru p 3. For example, the IgE reactivity to food LTPs (e.g., the hazelnut LTP Cor a 8) is usually associated with sensitization to the peach LTP Pru p 3, while the converse is not the case. Supporting this concept, IgE binding to walnut (Jug r 3) and peanut (Ara h 9) LTP was completely abolished by Pru p 3 in inhibition studies (Asero et al. 2002). Conversely, IgE binding to Pru p 3 was only partly inhibited by other food LTPs, suggesting a high avidity of Pru p 3-specific antibodies and/or a high IgE epitope density for Pru p 3. Systematic investigation of the T-cell immunogenicity of various food LTPs have not yet been performed. Therefore, Pru p 3 is the most important marker of sensitization to other food LTPs. This well-described IgE cross-reactivity is attributed to conserved, conformational (discontinuous) epitopes, whereas sequential (linear) epitopes are of lesser importance. In addition to the cross-reactive epitopes, species-specific epitopes exist. This explains why some patients are sensitized to certain pollen LTPs, but not Pru p 3. In regard to structural similarities of food and pollen LTPs, a classification into two groups was suggested by Salcedo et al. (2007):

- *Group 1:* Pollen LTPs of ambrosia (Amb a 6), olive (Ole e 7), and pellitory (Par j 1 and 2) with a sequence identity to Pru p 3 of <35 % and, therefore, no cross-reactivity
- *Group 2:* LTPs of plane tree (sycamore in the USA) and mugwort pollen (Pla a 3 and Art v 3) with a sequence identity to Pru p 3 of >45 % conducive of cross-reactivity

Up to now, exposure to plane tree (sycamore) pollen has not been shown to be responsible for a primary respiratory sensitization and subsequent clinical reaction to Pru p 3 (Lauer et al. 2007). Although nasal challenge with mugwort LTP Art v 3 was shown to elicit respiratory symptoms in Pru p 3-sensitized patients, the pollen LTP was not considered as primary sensitizer (Sánchez-López et al. 2014). More likely, a primary sensitization to Pru p 3 triggers respiratory

Patient	**Peach**	**Apple**	**Walnut**	**Hazelnut**	**Peanut**	**Lentil**	**Maize**	*Soy*	**Tomato**	**Kiwi**	*Sesame*	*Mustard*	**Melon**	*Celery*
1	58.1	59.2	43.3	7.66	20.9	23	21.9	12.9	7.37	1.92	7.21	2.54	1.07	2
2	16.6	12	11.1	1.17	0.65	0.82	0	0.39	0	1.18	0	0	0	0
3	12.1	9.1	4.93	1.12	1.9	0.83	0.79	0.58	0.47	0.68	0	0.49	0	0
4	11.6	9.25	4.52	3.05	3.75	2.94	2.23	1.37	1.1	1.1	0	0.42	0	0
5	11.4	11.9	6.61	6.29	2.05	1.77	3.85	0.75	0.67	2.01	0.71	0	0	0.36
6	7.04	5.34	4.39	1.86	2.14	0.61	3.92	1.14	2.8	0.76	0.67	0	0	1.08
7	4.58	2.57	2.05	0	0	0.37	1.53	0	0	0.41	0	0	0	0
8	3.81	2.33	1.32	0.49	1.86	1.18	1.73	0.79	1.02	0	0.55	0	0	0
9	3.12	1.44	0.38	0	0	0	0	0	0	0	0	0	0	0
10	2.75	1.92	1.59	1.18	0.86	0.75	0.43	0.47	0	0.74	0.56	0	0	0
11	1.75	0.74	0	0	0	0	0	0	0	0	0	0	0	0
12	1.44	0.77	0	0	0	0.42	0	0	0	0	0	0	0	0
13	1.11	0.84	0	0	0	0	0	0	0	0.83	0	0	0	0
14	1.08	0.39	0	0	0	0	0	0	0	0	0	0	0	0
15	0.41	0	0	0	0	0	0	0	0	0	0	0	0	0

Fig. 4.3 Allergen-specific IgE (kU_A/l) and clinical symptoms (*red* systemic reactions, *yellow* local reactions) of 15 peach-allergic patients (*left column*) with LTP mono-sensitization after consumption of the respective food (headline: *bold text* clinical data on the reaction pattern documented for at least one patient, *italic text* no clinical information available for these plant foods) (Modified from Asero 2014)

symptoms by Art v 3 due to IgE cross-reactivity. Nevertheless, the clinical relevance of cross-reactivity between food and homologous pollen LTPs (e.g., plane tree (sycamore), mugwort, and olive) for the manifestation of LTP-mediated allergies is still unclear.

4.7 Diagnosis by Sensitization Tests with LTPs and LTP-Containing Extracts

Due to their stability, sensitization to LTPs can be determined both by prick-to-prick tests using fresh plant material and commercial prick test solutions (Asero et al. 2001; Reuter et al. 2006). However, the LTP concentration in prick test solutions can be highly variable depending on the extraction method used (Akkerdaas et al. 2003). In vitro test systems using purified LTPs support discrimination between birch pollen-associated food allergies and the LTP-mediated allergies. Both recombinant and natural LTPs are available for diagnosis (Thermo Fisher Scientific: rPru p 3, rAra h 9, rCor a 8, rTri a 14, rJug r 3, rMal d 3 in ImmunoCAP and nArt v 3, nOle e 7, and rPla a 3 in the ISAC-Chip). It has been shown that recombinant Pru p 3 is comparable to the natural allergen in regard to both structure and IgE reactivity (García-Casado et al. 2003). Although Pru p 3 is described as a marker allergen for LTP sensitization, some patients react to isolated, species-specific LTPs due to a micro-heterogenicity of the relevant epitopes (Bernardi et al. 2011). Therefore, the authors suggest testing a broad spectrum of LTPs to cover sources other than peach as possible causes for the primary sensitization. Moreover, it was shown for pomegranate that LTP isoforms within one plant species could have different IgE-binding properties in individual patients (Bolla et al. 2014). These should be considered when selecting recombinant molecules for component-resolved diagnosis.

Molecular diagnosis has shown that patients who react to LTPs frequently do not react to other allergens derived from the same food source and, thus, are considered mono-sensitized. Twenty (20) of 22 (91 %) Spanish, cherry-allergic patients were sensitized to Pru av 3, but less than 10 % of patients were sensitized to the other known cherry allergens. Fifty percent of these patients reported systemic reactions after consumption of cherries (Reuter et al. 2006). Mono-sensitization, rather than poly-sensitization, possibly results in stronger clinical reactions because the IgE receptors on the effector cells are bound primarily by LTP-specific IgE (Asero 2011a). In this case, one must consider the ratio of LTP-specific IgE (e.g., against Pru p 3) to total IgE that is also present on the surface of mast cells and basophils.

If sensitization to peach occurs at an early age, it is very likely to be primarily directed against Pru p 3. In most cases these patients have higher IgE titers than patients sensitized later in life that have already developed cross-reactivity to Bet v 1-homologs (Pastorello et al. 2013). By contrast, Bernardi et al. (2011) found that LTP-specific IgE titers do not correlate with the probability of cross-reactivity to other LTPs.

4.8 Clinical Relevance of LTP Sensitization

Because of its high IgE reactivity and cross-reactive properties, peach LTP Pru p 3 is used as a reliable biomarker for sensitization to LTPs. Although peach extracts are suitable for determining LTP sensitization/cross-reactivity (Fig. 4.3), the sensitivity of the assay is enhanced when using Pru p 3 (or other individual LTPs) for IgE diagnostics.

For the detection of specific IgE to Pru p 3 compared to peach extract, the pure allergen considerably enhances analytical specificity. The same holds true for other LTPs and their respective allergen sources. If available for in vitro diagnosis, suspected LTPs are in general preferred over the respective extracts for detecting allergen-specific IgE. But even the detection of specific IgE sensitization is not always clinically relevant, as approximately 50 % of LTP-sensitized individuals are asymptomatic (Asero 2011a).

The usage of LTPs for diagnostic purposes delivers high diagnostic sensitivity but low specificity (Ballmer-Weber et al. 2005). Clinical reactions with normally asymptomatic LTP sensitization can occur in the presence of cofactors (Asero and Pravettoni 2013), e.g.:

- Physical activity (Romano et al. 2012)
- Food processing, e.g., potential glycation of proteins by heat treatment (Sancho et al. 2005)
- Drinking of alcoholic beverages
- Usage of nonsteroidal anti-inflammatory drugs (NSAIDs) (Cardona et al. 2012)

Oral provocation testing for suspected LTP allergy carries the risk of severe reactions and is, thus, rarely used for the confirmation of LTP sensitization. Despite this general precaution, in individual cases oral provocation may be necessary:

- To provide a basis for advising the patient on food avoidance
- To provide individual allergen elimination strategies
- To provide guidance for the makeup of individual diets (Crespo et al. 2002)
- If applicable, to establish strategies for the handling of cofactors mentioned above
- To determine LTP-related thresholds for the development of symptoms

The diagnostic interpretation of a positive LTP sensitization is a real challenge for the physician. The difficulties of judging the clinical relevance are well known to allergists in the Mediterranean area due to the high prevalence of LTP-allergic patients there (Matricardi et al. 2016). They are the following:

- *Is the determined LTP sensitization clinically relevant?*
- Tip: Clarification only possible by detailed history, including symptoms of an OAS and/or systemic allergic reactions.

- *Are cofactors such as physical activity, drinking of alcoholic beverages, or NSAID intake involved in the reaction?*
- Tip: In the case of an uncertain history, provocation in the presence of the respective cofactors may be necessary, but only if an unambiguous diagnosis is mandated.
- *Which LTP-containing foods are also potential triggers of OAS and/or systemic reactions?*
- Tip: Question in detail previous tolerance of LTP-containing foods (Fig. 4.2); when a clear history cannot be obtained, provocation may be justified, again only if an absolute diagnosis is necessary.
- *Is it worthwhile to determine IgE levels against other available LTPs?*
- Answer: Probably not, since additional IgE determinations with positive results for other LTPs cannot determine clinical relevance; only in the case of unambiguously negative IgE levels against certain LTPs, a sensitization and/or cross-reactivity and, consequently, a clinical reaction also are unlikely.
- *Is it worthwhile to determine IgE levels against other LTP-containing foods or extracts that are suspected to induce the allergic reactions?*
- Evaluation: Probably not, as additional positive IgE findings (for examples, see Fig. 4.3) cannot clarify whether the results obtained are clinically relevant; even in the case of unambiguous negative IgE levels against these foods, a sensitization and/or cross-reactivity cannot be excluded with absolute certainty. The (possibly low) LTP content in the respective foods and their extracts is usually unknown.

Conclusions for Diagnostics in Clinical Routine

As allergic reactions to plant foods such as grapes, blueberries, citrus fruits, or vegetables not belonging to the Bet v 1 cluster are rare in Central Europe, LTPs should be considered as triggering allergens.

Determining IgE levels against the peach LTP Pru p 3 (designated as a marker allergen) is an elegant way to identify LTP sensitizations and questionable cross-reactivities.

LTP sensitization should usually be suspected in case of a positive reaction to peach extract, as in contrast to the unstable Bet v 1 homolog Pru p 1, Pru p 3 is present in sufficient amounts in diagnostic extracts.

In the event of negative IgE levels against Pru p 3, a possible LTP sensitization or cross-reactivity can be virtually excluded.

The actual challenge when detecting IgE against Pru p 3 (or another food LTP) is to determine the clinical relevance of the sensitization and possible cross-reactivities. Here, only a careful history or oral provocations, but not extended IgE diagnostics, can help to determine how well the LTP sensitization is correlated with either clinical symptoms or additional LTP-mediated cross-reactivities.

4.9 Therapeutic Recommendations

In order to reduce allergen exposure, peeling of peaches and apples is recommended. Peach skin has a sevenfold higher LTP content than the pulp (Borges et al. 2006). Thermal processing of foods is not an adequate preventive measure due to the heat stability of the allergens. IgE-reactive LTPs have been detected in thermally processed foods such as jam or pasteurized fruit juice (Scheurer et al. 2004). For food allergies, specific immunotherapy has not yet been established in clinical practice. However, promising results were obtained by sublingual immunotherapy in LTP-allergic patients using hazelnut (Enrique et al. 2005) and peach extracts (Fernández-Rivas et al. 2009).

4.10 Other Perspectives

Using RNAi (RNA interference)-mediated gene suppression, it has been possible to generate transgenic foods that express significantly lower amounts of LTPs. A proof-of-concept study was performed with tomatoes. Here, RNAi-mediated suppression of the tomato LTP Lyc e 3 (renamed as Sola l 3) resulted in tomatoes that elicited considerably lower or no skin reactions in LTP-sensitized allergic patients (Lorenz et al. 2006). In principle, this method can be applied to other foods, but has not been further implemented, probably because of the antagonism of the general public toward genetically engineered foods.

Other approaches aim at the causative treatment of LTP-allergic patients. Currently, a hypoallergenic Pru p 3 variant for allergen-specific immunotherapy is in preclinical testing. It has been shown that irreversible unfolding Pru p 3 by cleavage and alkylation of disulfide bonds abrogated IgE reactivity, while preserving T-cell recognition in mice (Toda et al. 2011). Furthermore, the development of recombinant hypoallergenic Pru p 3 for sublingual immunotherapy is one aim of the EU project "Food Allergy Specific ImmunoTherapy" known as the FAST project (Zuidmeer-Jongejan et al. 2012).

4.11 Implications for Routine Clinical Practice

Food LTPs are thermally and proteolytically stable allergens, which cause frequent and sometimes severe reactions, mainly in Southern Europe. Sensitization to LTPs has been described outside of the Mediterranean area, but with lower prevalence. When the history is unclear, LTP-mediated allergic reactions should also be considered for patients in Central and Northern Europe. This is especially the case if a birch pollen-associated food allergy can be excluded or the triggering plant food does not belong to the Bet v 1 cluster (including grapes, blueberries, citrus fruits, and cabbage). Pru p 3 can be used as a suitable biomarker in serologic diagnostics, albeit with high sensitivity but low specificity. As for other IgE sensitizations, positive in vitro results should be checked for clinical relevance. When one is utilizing the results to give recommendations for food elimination from the diet, the key question is which LTP-containing foods actually caused the allergic symptoms. One therapeutic option currently undergoing clinical development is the use of recombinant, hypoallergenic Pru p 3.

References

Akkerdaas JH, Wensing M, Knulst AC, Krebitz M, Breiteneder H, de Vries S, Penninks AH, Aalberse RC, Hefle SL, van Ree R. How accurate and safe is the diagnosis of hazelnut allergy by means of commercial skin prick test reagents? Int Arch Allergy Immunol. 2003;132: 132–40.

Akkerdaas J, Finkina EI, Balandin SV, Santos Magadán S, Knulst A, Fernandez-Rivas M, Asero R, van Ree R, Ovchinnikova TV. Lentil (Lens culinaris) lipid transfer protein Len c 3: a novel legume allergen. Int Arch Allergy Immunol. 2012;157:51–7.

Arkwright PD, Summers CW, Riley BJ, Alsediq N, Pumphrey RS. IgE sensitization to the nonspecific lipid-transfer protein Ara h 9 and peanut-associated bronchospasm. Biomed Res Int. 2013;2013:746507.

Asero R. Co-recognition of lipid transfer protein in pollen and foods in northern Italy: clinician's view. Eur Ann Allergy Clin Immunol. 2010;42:205–8.

Asero R. Lipid transfer protein cross-reactivity assessed in vivo and in vitro in the office: pros and cons. J Investig Allergol Clin Immunol. 2011a;21:129–36.

Asero R. Peach-induced contact urticaria is associated with lipid transfer protein sensitization. Int Arch Allergy Immunol. 2011b;154:345–8.

Asero R. In patients with LTP syndrome food-specific IgE show a predictable hierarchical order. Eur Ann Allergy Clin Immunol. 2014;46:142–6.

Asero R, Pravettoni V. Anaphylaxis to plant-foods and pollen allergens in patients with lipid transfer protein syndrome. Curr Opin Allergy Clin Immunol. 2013;13:379–85.

Asero R, Mistrello G, Roncarolo D, de Vries SC, Gautier MF, Ciurana CL, Verbeek E, Mohammadi T, Knul-Brettlova V, Akkerdaas JH, Bulder I, Aalberse RC, van Ree R. Lipid transfer protein: a pan-allergen in plant-derived foods that is highly resistant to pepsin digestion. Int Arch Allergy Immunol. 2000;122:20–32.

Asero R, Mistrello G, Roncarolo D, Casarini M, Falagiani P. Allergy to nonspecific lipid transfer proteins in Rosaceae: a comparative study of different in vivo diagnostic methods. Ann Allergy Asthma Immunol. 2001;87:68–71.

Asero R, Mistrello G, Roncarolo D, Amato S, Caldironi G, Barocci F, van Ree R. Immunological cross-reactivity between lipid transfer proteins from botanically unrelated plant-derived foods: a clinical study. Allergy. 2002;57:900–6.

Asero R, Mistrello G, Roncarolo D, Amato S. Detection of some safe plant-derived foods for LTP-allergic patients. Int Arch Allergy Immunol. 2007;144:57–63.

Ballmer-Weber BK, Scheurer S, Fritsche P, Enrique E, Cistero-Bahima A, Haase T, Wüthrich B. Component-resolved diagnosis with recombinant allergens in patients with cherry allergy. J Allergy Clin Immunol. 2002;110:167–73.

Ballmer-Weber BK, Wangorsch A, Bohle B, Kaul S, Kündig T, Fötisch K, van Ree R, Vieths S. Component-resolved in vitro diagnosis in carrot allergy: does the use of recombinant carrot allergens improve the reliability of the diagnostic procedure? Clin Exp Allergy. 2005;35:970–8.

Bernardi ML, Giangrieco I, Camardella L, Ferrara R, Palazzo P, Panico MR, Crescenzo R, Carratore V, Zennaro D, Liso M, Santoro M, Zuzzi S, Tamburrini M, Ciardiello MA, Mari A. Allergenic lipid transfer proteins from plant-derived foods do not immunologically and clinically behave homogeneously: the kiwifruit LTP as a model. PLoS One. 2011;6:e27856.

Bolla M, Zenoni S, Scheurer S, Vieths S, San Miguel Moncin MM, Olivieri M, Antico A, Ferrer M, Berroa F, Enrique E, Avesani L, Marsano F, Zoccatelli G. Pomegranate (Punica granatum L.)

expresses several nsLTP isoforms characterized by different IgE-binding properties. Int Arch Allergy Immunol. 2014;164:112–21.

Borges JP, Jauneau A, Brulé C, Culerrier R, Barre A, Didier A, Rougé P. The lipid transfer proteins (LTP) essentially concentrate in the skin of Rosaceae fruits as cell surface exposed allergens. Plant Physiol Biochem. 2006;44:535–42.

Borghesan F, Mistrello G, Roncarolo D, Amato S, Plebani M, Asero R. Respiratory allergy to lipid transfer protein. Int Arch Allergy Immunol. 2008;147:161–5.

Cardona V, Luengo O, Garriga T, Labrador-Horrillo M, Sala-Cunill A, Izquierdo A, Soto L, Guilarte M. Co-factor-enhanced food allergy. Allergy. 2012;67:1316–8.

Carnés J, Fernández-Caldas E, Gallego MT, Ferrer A, Cuesta-Herranz J. Pru p 3 (LTP) content in peach extracts. Allergy. 2002;57:1071–5.

Crespo JF, Rodríguez J, James JM, Daroca P, Reaño M, Vives R. Reactivity to potential cross-reactive foods in fruit-allergic patients: implications for prescribing food avoidance. Allergy. 2002;57:946–9.

Cudowska B, Kaczmarski M, Restani P. Lipid transfer protein in diagnosis of birch-apple syndrome in children. Immunobiology. 2008;213:89–96.

Egger M, Hauser M, Mari A, Ferreira F, Gadermaier G. The role of lipid transfer proteins in allergic diseases. Curr Allergy Asthma Rep. 2010;10:326–35.

Enrique E, Pineda F, Malek T, Bartra J, Basagaña M, Tella R, Castelló JV, Alonso R, de Mateo JA, Cerdá-Trias T, San Miguel-MoncínMdel M, Monzón S, García M, Palacios R, Cisteró-Bahíma A. Sublingual immunotherapy for hazelnut food allergy: a randomized, double-blind, placebo-controlled study with a standardized hazelnut extract. Allergy Clin Immunol. 2005;116:1073–9.

Fernández-Rivas M, Bolhaar S, González-Mancebo E, Asero R, van Leeuwen A, Bohle B, Ma Y, Ebner C, Rigby N, Sancho AI, Miles S, Zuidmeer L, Knulst A, Breiteneder H, Mills C, Hoffmann-Sommergruber K, van Ree R. Apple allergy across Europe: how allergen sensitization profiles determine the clinical expression of allergies to plant foods. J Allergy Clin Immunol. 2006;118:481–8.

Fernández-Rivas M, Garrido Fernández S, Nadal JA, Díaz de Durana MD, García BE, González-Mancebo E, Martín S, Barber D, Rico P, Tabar AI. Randomized double-blind, placebo-controlled trial of sublingual immunotherapy with a Pru p 3 quantified peach extract. Allergy. 2009;64:76–83.

Flinterman AE, Akkerdaas JH, den Hartog Jager CF, Rigby NM, Fernandez-Rivas M, Hoekstra MO, Bruijnzeel-Koomen CA, Knulst AC, van Ree R, Pasmans SG. Lipid transfer protein-linked hazelnut allergy in children from a non-Mediterranean birch-endemic area. J Allergy Clin Immunol. 2008;121:423–8.

Gaier S, Marsh J, Oberhuber C, Rigby NM, Lovegrove A, Alessandri S, Briza P, Radauer C, Zuidmeer L, van Ree R, Hemmer W, Sancho AI, Mills C, Hoffmann-Sommergruber K, Shewry PR. Purification and structural stability of the peach allergens Pru p 1 and Pru p 3. Mol Nutr Food Res. 2008;52 Suppl 2:S220–9.

Gao ZS, Yang ZW, Wu SD, Wang HY, Liu ML, Mao WL, Wang J, Gadermaier G, Ferreira F, Zheng M, van Ree R. Peach allergy in China: a dominant role for mugwort pollen lipid transfer protein as a primary sensitizer. J Allergy Clin Immunol. 2013;131:224–6.

Gandolfo-Cano M, Bartra J, González-Mancebo E, Feo-Brito F, Gómez E, Bartolomé B, Muñoz-García E, Sanz Maroto A, Vivanco F, Cuesta-Herranz J, Pastor-Vargas C. Molecular characterization of contact urticaria in patients with melon allergy. Br J Dermatol. 2014;170:651–6.

García BE, Lombardero M, Echechipía S, Olaguibel JM, Díaz-Perales A, Sánchez-Monge R, Barber D, Salcedo G, Tabar AI. Respiratory allergy to peach leaves and lipid-transfer proteins. Clin Exp Allergy. 2004;34:291–5.

García-Casado G, Pacios LF, Díaz-Perales A, Sánchez-Monge R, Lombardero M, García-Selles FJ, Polo F, Barber D, Salcedo G. Identification of IgE-binding epitopes of the major peach allergen Pru p 3. J Allergy Clin Immunol. 2003;112:599–605.

García-Olmedo F, Molina A, Segura A, Moreno M. The defensive role of nonspecific lipid-transfer proteins in plants. Trends Microbiol. 1995;3:72–4.

Gebhardt C, Vieths S, Gubesch M, Averbeck M, Simon JC, Treudler R. 10 kDa lipid transfer protein: the main allergenic structure in a German patient with anaphylaxis to blueberry. Allergy. 2009;64:498–9.

Guo L, Yang H, Zhang X, Yang S. Lipid transfer protein 3 as a target of MYB96 mediates freezing and drought stress in Arabidopsis. J Exp Bot. 2013;64:1755–67.

Kader JC. Lipid transfer proteins in plants. Annu Rev Plant Physiol Plant Mol Biol. 1996;47:627–54.

Lauer I, Miguel-Moncin MS, Abel T, Foetisch K, Hartz C, Fortunato D, Cistero-Bahima A, Vieths S, Scheurer S. Identification of a plane pollen lipid transfer protein (Pla a 3) and its immunological relation to the peach lipid-transfer protein, Pru p 3. Clin Exp Allergy. 2007;37:261–9.

Lauer I, Dueringer N, Pokoj S, Rehm S, Zoccatelli G, Reese G, Miguel-Moncin MS, Cistero-Bahima A, Enrique E, Lidholm J, Vieths S, Scheurer S. The non-specific lipid transfer protein, Ara h 9, is an important allergen in peanut. Clin Exp Allergy. 2009;39:1427–37.

Le TM, van Hoffen E, Lebens AF, Bruijnzeel-Koomen CA, Knulst AC. Anaphylactic versus mild reactions to hazelnut and apple in a birch-endemic area: different sensitization profiles? Int Arch Allergy Immunol. 2013a;160:56–62.

Le TM, Bublin M, Breiteneder H, Fernández-Rivas M, Asero R, Ballmer-Weber B, Barreales L, Bures P, Belohlavkova S, de Blay F, Clausen M, Dubakiene R, Gislason D, van Hoffen E, Jedrzejczak-Czechowicz M, Kowalski ML, Kralimarkova T, Lidholm J, DeWitt AM, Mills CE, Papadopoulos NG, Popov T, Purohit A, van Ree R, Seneviratne S, Sinaniotis A, Summers C, Vázquez-Cortés S, Vieths S, Vogel L, Hoffmann-Sommergruber K, Knulst AC. Kiwifruit allergy across Europe: clinical manifestation and IgE recognition patterns to kiwifruit allergens. J Allergy Clin Immunol. 2013b;131:164–71.

Lin CH, Li L, Lyu PC, Chang JY. Distinct unfolding and refolding pathways of lipid transfer proteins LTP1 and LTP2. Protein J. 2004;23:553–66.

Lleonart R, Cisteró A, Carreira J, Batista A, Moscoso del Prado J. Food allergy: identification of the major IgE-binding component of peach (Prunus persica). Ann Allergy. 1992;69:128–30.

Lombardero M, García-Sellés FJ, Polo F, Jimeno L, Chamorro MJ, García-Casado G, Sánchez-Monge R, Díaz-Perales A, Salcedo G, Barber D. Prevalence of sensitization to Artemisia allergens Art v 1, Art v 3 and Art v 60 kDa. Cross-reactivity among Art v 3 and other relevant lipid-transfer protein allergens. Clin Exp Allergy. 2004;34:1415–21.

Lorenz Y, Enrique E, Lequynh L, Fötisch K, Retzek M, Biemelt S, Sonnewald U, Vieths S, Scheurer S. Skin prick tests reveal stable and heritable reduction of allergenic potency of gene-silenced tomato fruits. J Allergy Clin Immunol. 2006;118:711–8.

Masthoff LJ, Mattsson L, Zuidmeer-Jongejan L, Lidholm J, Andersson K, Akkerdaas JH, Versteeg SA, Garino C, Meijer Y, Kentie P, Versluis A, den Hartog Jager CF, Bruijnzeel-Koomen CA, Knulst AC, van Ree R, van Hoffen E, Pasmans SG. Sensitization to Cor a 9 and Cor a 14 is highly specific for a hazelnut allergy with objective symptoms in Dutch children and adults. J Allergy Clin Immunol. 2013;132:393–9.

Matricardi PM, Kleine-Tebbe J, Hoffmann HJ, Valenta R, Hilger C, Hofmaier S, Aalberse RC, Agache I, Asero R, Ballmer-Weber B, Barber D, Beyer K, Biedermann T, Biló MB, Blank S, Bohle B, Bosshard PP, Breiteneder H, Brough HA, Caraballo L, Caubet JC, Crameri R, Davies JM, Douladiris N, Ebisawa M, Eigenmann PA, Fernandez-Rivas M, Ferreira F, Gadermaier G, Glatz M, Hamilton RG, Hawranek T, Hellings P, Hoffmann-Sommergruber K, Jakob T, Jappe U, Jutel M, Kamath SD, Knol EF, Korosec P, Kuehn A, Lack G, Lopata AL, Mäkelä M, Morisset M, Niederberger V, Nowak-Wezgrzyn AH, Papadopoulos NG, Pastorello EA, Pauli G, Platts-Mills T, Posa D, Poulsen LK, Raulf M, Sastre J, Scala E, Schmid JM, Schmid-Grendelmeier P, van Hage M, van Ree R, Vieths S, Weber R, Wickman M, Muraro A, Ollert M. EAACI Molecular Allergology User's Guide. Pediatr Allergy Immunol. 2016; 27(Suppl23):1–250.

Novembre E, Mori F, Contestabile S, Rossi ME, Pucci N. Correlation of anti-Pru p 3 IgE levels with severity of peach allergy reactions in children. Ann Allergy Asthma Immunol. 2012; 108:271–4.

Palacin A, Quirce S, Armentia A, Fernández-Nieto M, Pacios LF, Asensio T, Sastre J, Diaz-Perales A, Salcedo GJ. Wheat lipid transfer protein is a major allergen associated with baker's asthma. J Allergy Clin Immunol. 2007;120:1132–8.

Pasquato N, Berni R, Folli C, Folloni S, Cianci M, Pantano S, Helliwell JR, Zanotti G. Crystal structure of peach Pru p 3, the prototypic member of the family of plant non-specific lipid transfer protein pan-allergens. J Mol Biol. 2006;356:684–94.

Pastorello EA, Ortolani C, Farioli L, Pravettoni V, Ispano M, Borga A, Bengtsson A, Incorvaia C, Berti C, Zanussi C. Allergenic cross-reactivity among peach, apricot, plum, and cherry in patients with oral allergy syndrome: an in vivo and in vitro study. J Allergy Clin Immunol. 1994;94:699–707.

Pastorello EA, Farioli L, Pravettoni V, Ortolani C, Ispano M, Monza M, Baroglio C, Scibola E, Ansaloni R, Incorvaia C, Conti AJ. The major allergen of peach (Prunus persica) is a lipid transfer protein. J Allergy Clin Immunol. 1999;103:520–6.

Pastorello EA, Pravettoni V, Farioli L, Rivolta F, Conti A, Ispano M, Fortunato D, Bengtsson A, Bianchi M. Hypersensitivity to mugwort (Artemisia vulgaris) in patients with peach allergy is due to a common lipid transfer protein allergen and is often without clinical expression. J Allergy Clin Immunol. 2002;110:310–7.

Pastorello EA, Farioli L, Stafylaraki C, Mascheri A, Scibilia J, Pravettoni V, Primavesi L, Piantanida M, Nichelatti M, Asero R. Anti-rPru p 3 IgE levels are inversely related to the age at onset of peach-induced severe symptoms reported by peach-allergic adults. Int Arch Allergy Immunol. 2013;162:45–9.

Radauer C, Bublin M, Wagner S, Mari A, Breiteneder H. Allergens are distributed into few protein families and possess a restricted number of biochemical functions. J Allergy Clin Immunol. 2008;121:847–52.

Ramazzina I, Amato S, Passera E, Sforza S, Mistrello G, Berni R, Folli C. Isoform identification, recombinant production and characterization of the allergen lipid transfer protein 1 from pear (Pyr c 3). Gene. 2012;491:173–81.

Reuter A, Lidholm J, Andersson K, Ostling J, Lundberg M, Scheurer S, Enrique E, Cistero-Bahima A, San Miguel-Moncin M, Ballmer-Weber BK, Vieths S. A critical assessment of allergen component-based in vitro diagnosis in cherry allergy across Europe. Clin Exp Allergy. 2006; 36:815–23.

Richard C, Leduc V, Battais F. Plant lipid transfer proteins (LTP): biochemical aspect in panallergen – structural and functional features, and allergenicity. Eur Ann Allergy Clin Immunol. 2007;39:76–84.

Romano A, Scala E, Rumi G, Gaeta F, Caruso C, Alonzi C, Maggioletti M, Ferrara R, Palazzo P, Palmieri V, Zeppilli P, Mari A. Lipid transfer proteins: the most frequent sensitizer in Italian subjects with food-dependent exercise-induced anaphylaxis. Clin Exp Allergy. 2012;42: 1643–53.

Salcedo G, Sánchez-Monge R, Barber D, Díaz-Perales A. Plant non-specific lipid transfer proteins: an interface between plant defence and human allergy. Biochim Biophys Acta. 2007; 1771:781–91.

Sánchez-López J, Tordesillas L, Pascal M, Muñoz-Cano R, Garrido M, Rueda M, Vilella R, Valero A, Díaz-Perales A, Picado C, Bartra J. Role of Art v 3 in pollinosis of patients allergic to Pru p 3. J Allergy Clin Immunol. 2014;133:1018–25.

Sánchez-Monge R, Lombardero M, García-Sellés FJ, Barber D, Salcedo G. Lipid-transfer proteins are relevant allergens in fruit allergy. J Allergy Clin Immunol. 1999;103:514–9.

Sancho AI, Rigby NM, Zuidmeer L, Asero R, Mistrello G, Amato S, González-Mancebo E, Fernández-Rivas M, van Ree R, Mills EN. The effect of thermal processing on the IgE reactivity of the non-specific lipid transfer protein from apple, Mal d 3. Allergy. 2005;60:1262–8.

Sander I, Rozynek P, Rihs HP, van Kampen V, Chew FT, Lee WS, Kotschy-Lang N, Merget R, Brüning T, Raulf-Heimsoth M. Multiple wheat flour allergens and cross-reactive carbohydrate determinants bind IgE in baker's asthma. Allergy. 2011;66:1208–15.

Schäd SG, Trcka J, Vieths S, Scheurer S, Conti A, Brocker EB, Trautmann A. Wine anaphylaxis in a German patient: IgE-mediated allergy against a lipid transfer protein of grapes. Int Arch Allergy Immunol. 2005;136:159–64.

Scheurer S, Pastorello EA, Wangorsch A, Kästner M, Haustein D, Vieths S. Recombinant allergens Pru av 1 and Pru av 4 and a newly identified lipid transfer protein in the in vitro diagnosis of cherry allergy. J Allergy Clin Immunol. 2001;107:724–31.

Scheurer S, Lauer I, Foetisch K, San Miguel Moncin M, Retzek M, Hartz C, Enrique E, Lidholm J, Cistero-Bahima A, Vieths S. Strong allergenicity of Pru av 3, the lipid transfer protein from cherry, is related to high stability against thermal processing and digestion. J Allergy Clin Immunol. 2004;114:900–7.

Schocker F, Lüttkopf D, Scheurer S, Petersen A, Cisteró-Bahima A, Enrique E, San Miguel-Moncín M, Akkerdaas J, van Ree R, Vieths S, Becker WM. Recombinant lipid transfer protein Cor a 8 from hazelnut: a new tool for in vitro diagnosis of potentially severe hazelnut allergy. J Allergy Clin Immunol. 2004;113:141–7.

Schulten V, Nagl B, Scala E, Bernardi ML, Mari A, Ciardiello MA, Lauer I, Scheurer S, Briza P, Jürets A, Ferreira F, Jahn-Schmid B, Fischer GF, Bohle B. Pru p 3, the nonspecific lipid transfer protein from peach, dominates the immune response to its homolog in hazelnut. Allergy. 2011; 66:1005–13.

Skamstrup Hansen K, Ballmer-Weber BK, Sastre J, Lidholm J, Andersson K, Oberhofer H, Lluch-Bernal M, Ostling J, Mattsson L, Schocker F, Vieths S, Poulsen LK. Component-resolved in vitro diagnosis of hazelnut allergy in Europe. J Allergy Clin Immunol. 2009; 123:1134–41.

Toda M, Reese G, Gadermaier G, Schulten V, Lauer I, Egger M, Briza P, Randow S, Wolfheimer S, Kigongo V, Del Mar San Miguel Moncin M, Fötisch K, Bohle B, Vieths S, Scheurer S. Protein unfolding strongly modulates the allergenicity and immunogenicity of Pru p 3, the major peach allergen. J Allergy Clin Immunol. 2011;128:1022–30.

Tordesillas L, Gómez-Casado C, Garrido-Arandia M, Murua-García A, Palacín A, Varela J, Konieczna P, Cuesta-Herranz J, Akdis CA, O'Mahony L, Díaz-Perales A. Transport of Pru p 3 across gastrointestinal epithelium – an essential step towards the induction of food allergy? Clin Exp Allergy. 2013;43:1374–83.

van Loon LC, van Stein EA. The families of pathogenesis-related proteins, their activities, and comparative analysis of PR-1 type proteins. Phys Mol Plant Pathol. 1999;55:85–97.

van Winkle RC, Chang C. The biochemical basis and clinical evidence of food allergy due to lipid transfer proteins: a comprehensive review. Clin Rev Allergy Immunol. 2014;46:211–24.

Vejvar E, Himly M, Briza P, Eichhorn S, Ebner C, Hemmer W, Ferreira F, Gadermaier G. Allergenic relevance of nonspecific lipid transfer proteins 2: Identification and characterization of Api g 6 from celery tuber as representative of a novel IgE-binding protein family. Mol Nutr Food Res. 2013;57:2061–70.

Vereda A, van Hage M, Ahlstedt S, Ibañez MD, Cuesta-Herranz J, van Odijk J, Wickman M, Sampson HA. Peanut allergy: clinical and immunologic differences among patients from 3 different geographic regions. J Allergy Clin Immunol. 2011;127:603–7.

Zuidmeer L, van Ree R. Lipid transfer protein allergy: primary food allergy or pollen/food syndrome in some cases. Curr Opin Allergy Clin Immunol. 2007;7:269–73.

Zuidmeer-Jongejan L, Fernandez-Rivas M, Poulsen LK, Neubauer A, Asturias J, Blom L, Boye J, Bindslev-Jensen C, Clausen M, Ferrara R, Garosi P, Huber H, Jensen BM, Koppelman S, Kowalski ML, Lewandowska-Polak A, Linhart B, Maillere B, Mari A, Martinez A, Mills CE, Nicoletti C, Opstelten DJ, Papadopoulos NG, Portoles A, Rigby N, Scala E, Schnoor HJ, Sigurdardottir ST, Stavroulakis G, Stolz F, Swoboda I, Valenta R, van den Hout R, Versteeg SA, Witten M, van Ree R. FAST: towards safe and effective subcutaneous immunotherapy of persistent life-threatening food allergies. Clin Transl Allergy. 2012;2:5.

Stable Plant Food Allergens II: Storage Proteins

5

C. Radauer, J. Kleine-Tebbe, and K. Beyer

5.1 Introduction

Seeds are among the most important foods of plant origin. Based on botanical relatedness, type, and use of seeds, a distinction can be made between cereal grains (e.g., wheat, rye, rice, corn, oats), legumes (e.g., peanuts, beans, lentils, chickpeas), tree nuts (e.g., walnut, hazelnut, almond), and others not classifiable into any of these groups (e.g., buckwheat, sesame, mustard). Seeds are rich in proteins – chiefly storage proteins – which, after germination, serve as a nutrient supply for the seedling. These storage proteins are of similar composition for all seeds except the grains, with the majority belonging to three protein families: 2S albumins, 7S globulins, and 11S globulins. These groups are also the major allergens in seeds and are responsible for most cases of primary allergies to nuts, legumes, and other seeds

This contribution is based on a publication that appeared in the *Allergo Journal* in 2012 (Radauer C, Kleine-Tebbe J, Beyer K: Stabile pflanzliche Nahrungsmittelallergene: Speicherproteine. Allergo J 2012; 21: 155–158) and which has now been updated, expanded, and translated into English as a chapter for this book.
The authors gratefully thank Dr. Steve Love, PhD, Laguna Niguel, CA, USA, for reading the manuscript, helpful suggestions, and editorial assistance with the English translation.

C. Radauer, MD, Prof. (✉)
Department of Pathophysiology and Allergy Research, Center for Pathophysiology, Infectiology and Immunology, Medical University of Vienna, Vienna, Austria
e-mail: christian.radauer@meduniwien.ac.at

J. Kleine-Tebbe, MD, Prof.
Allergy & Asthma Center Westend, Outpatient Clinic Hanf, Ackermann & Kleine-Tebbe, Berlin, Germany
e-mail: kleine-tebbe@allergie-experten.de

K. Beyer, MD, Prof.
Department of Pediatric Pneumology and Immunology, Charité-Universitätsmedizin, Berlin, Germany
e-mail: kirsten.beyer@charite.de

J. Kleine-Tebbe, T. Jakob (eds.), *Molecular Allergy Diagnostics*,
DOI 10.1007/978-3-319-42499-6_5

except grains. This chapter addresses the biochemical and immunological properties of these proteins as well as their relevance in molecular allergy diagnostics. The chief storage proteins of the grain seeds (gliadins and glutenins) will not be addressed here.

5.2 Allergen Nomenclature

The 2S albumins belong to the prolamin superfamily, as do the bifunctional amylase and protease inhibitors in grains and the nonspecific lipid transfer proteins (nsLTPs). Important members of this family are Ara h 2 and Ara h 6 from peanut, Jug r 1 from walnut, and Ses i 1 and Ses i 2 from sesame (◉ Table 5.1). The 7S globulins (vicilins) and the 11S globulins (legumins) are distantly related and belong to the cupin superfamily. Important allergenic vicilins are Ara h 1 from peanut, Gly m 5 from soybean, and Jug r 2 from walnut. Legumins with allergenic properties are Ara h 3 from peanut, Gly m 6 from soybean, and Cor a 9 from hazelnut (◉ Table 5.1).

The biochemical characterization of storage proteins began as early as the nineteenth century, when they were fractionated by solubility, which also lead to their designations. Albumins are soluble in water, whereas globulins dissolve only when salt is added. Additionally, common names have been designated for many storage proteins. Examples are conglutin, conarachin, and arachin for the 2S albumin, 7S and 11S globulins from peanut, β-conglycinin and glycinin for the 7S and 11S globulins from soybean, and napin for the 2S albumin from rapeseed. In one instance, the names are particularly confusing: storage proteins from lupins – 11S globulins, 7S globulins, and 2S albumins – are designated α-, β-, and δ-conglutins, respectively.

5.3 Protein Structures

The 2S albumins, like all members of the prolamin superfamily, fold to form a compact bundle of 4–5 α-helices, stabilized by 4–5 conserved disulfide bonds (◉ Fig. 5.1a). The helices are connected by long, variable loops. Most 2S albumins consist of two polypeptide chains of about 9 and 5 kDa, covalently cross-linked by disulfide bonds.

The 7S and 11S globulins belong to the cupin superfamily. These proteins fold to create stable pairs of barrel-like structures formed from β-sheets (◉ Fig. 5.1b). The 7S globulins consist of one polypeptide chain per subunit and are often glycosylated. The subunits of 11S globulins are posttranslationally cleaved into two chains covalently linked by a disulfide bond. Globulins attain additional stability through formation of oligomers: 7S globulins form trimers (◉ Fig. 5.1c) and 11S globulins are mainly found as hexamers (◉ Fig. 5.1d).

Storage proteins present in seeds are a diverse mixture of molecules (Chassaigne et al. 2009). This complexity has various roots:

Table 5.1 Seed storage proteins identified as allergens

Source	2S albumins	7S globulins	11S globulins
Legumes (Fabaceae)			
Peanut (*Arachis hypogaea*)	**Ara h 2** [r, 1, 2] **Ara h 6** [n, 2] Ara h 7	**Ara h 1** [r, 1, 2]	**Ara h 3** [r, 1, 2]
Soybean (*Glycine max*)	Gly m 8	**Gly m 5** [n, 1, 2]	**Gly m 6** [n, 1, 2]
Mung bean (*Vigna radiata*)		Vig r 2	
Green bean (*Phaseolus vulgaris*)		(Pha v phaseolin)	
Pea (*Pisum sativum*)		Pis s 1 Pis s 2	
Lentil (*Lens culinaris*)		Len c 1	
Chickpea (*Cicer arietinum*)	(Cic a 2S albumin)	(Cic a 1)	(Cic a 6)
White lupin (*Lupinus albus*)	(Lup a δ-conglutin)	(Lup a 1)	(Lup a α-conglutin)
Narrow-leaved blue lupin (*Lupinus angustifolius*)	(Lup an δ-conglutin)	Lup an 1	(Lup an α-conglutin)
Fenugreek (*Trigonella foenum-graecum*)	(Tri fg 2)	(Tri fg 1)	(Tri fg 3)
Birch family (Betulaceae)			
Hazelnut (*Corylus avellana*)	**Cor a 14** [r, 1]	Cor a 11	**Cor a 9** [n, 1, 2]
Walnut family (Juglandaceae)			
English walnut (*Juglans regia*)	**Jug r 1** [r, 1, 2]	**Jug r 2** [n, 2]	Jug r 4
Black walnut (*Juglans nigra*)	Jug n 1	Jug n 2	
Pecan (*Carya illinoinensis*)	Car i 1		Car i 4
Sumac family (Anacardiaceae)			
Cashew (*Anacardium occidentale*)	**Ana o 3** [r, 1]	Ana o 1	**Ana o 2** [r, 2]
Pistachio (*Pistacia vera*)	Pis v 1	Pis v 3	Pis v 2 Pis v 5
Lecythidaceae			
Brazil nut (*Bertholletia excelsa*)	**Ber e 1** [r, 1, 2]		Ber e 2
Rose family (Rosaceae)			
Almond (*Prunus dulcis*)	(Pru du 2S albumin)		Pru du 6
Palm family (Arecaceae)			
Coconut (*Cocos nucifera*)		Coc n 1	(Coc n 4)
Pine family (Pinaceae)			
Stone pine (*Pinus pinea*)	Pin p 1	(Pin p vicilin)	
Knotweed family (Polygonaceae)			
Common buckwheat (*Fagopyrum esculentum*)	**Fag e 2** [n, 2]	Fag e 3	(Fag e 1)
Tartarian buckwheat (*Fagopyrum tataricum*)	Fag t 2		(Fag t 1)

(continued)

Table 5.1 (continued)

Source	2S albumins	7S globulins	11S globulins
Pedalium/sesame family (Pedaliaceae)			
Sesame (*Sesamum indicum*)	**Ses i 1** [n, 2] Ses i 2	Ses i 3	Ses i 6 Ses i 7
Crucifer family (Brassicaceae)			
Yellow mustard (*Sinapis alba*)	Sin a 1		Sin a 2
Oriental mustard (*Brassica juncea*)	Bra j 1		
Rapeseed (*Brassica napus*)	Bra n 1		
Turnip (*Brassica rapa*)	Bra r 1		
Composite plants (Asteraceae)			
Sunflower (*Helianthus annuus*)	(Hel a 2S albumin)		
Spurge family (Euphorbiaceae)			
Castor bean (*Ricinus communis*)	Ric c 1 (Ric c 3)		(Ric c 2)
Mallow family (Malvaceae)			
Upland cotton (*Gossypium hirsutum*)		(Gos h vicilin)	
Chinese gooseberry family (Actinidiaceae)			
Kiwi fruit (*Actinidia deliciosa*)	Act d 13		Act d 12

Allergens with official IUIS allergen nomenclature (www.allergen.org); additional allergens without official IUIS allergen designation (www.allergome.org), provisional names in parentheses

Bold and[1, 2]: available for in vitro diagnostics (Thermo Fisher Scientific, formerly Phadia: [1] ImmunoCAP and [2] ISAC; www.phadia.com)

[n]Purified, natural allergen

[r]Recombinant allergen

- *Isoforms*: many storage proteins are encoded by several genes with similar sequences. For example, the UniProt database contains 14 sequences of Ara h 3, the 11S globulin of the peanut.
- *Posttranslational modifications*: storage proteins are extensively modified in plant cells following synthesis. Several amino acids are cleaved from the N- and C-termini. In the case of 2S albumins and 11S globulins, the process of cleaving the immature protein into two polypeptide chains is accompanied by the removal of several amino acids. Moreover, the 7S globulins are often glycosylated.
- *Modifications caused by processing of seeds*: roasting and other methods of processing are associated with chemical degradation that further increase complexity. Modifications of amino acids are found, as are cleavages of peptide bonds and macromolecular aggregates (Hebling et al. 2013).

A detailed molecular characterization of Sin a 1 and Cor a 14, the 2S albumins from mustard and hazelnut, by mass spectrometry confirmed a considerable extent of heterogeneity due to multiple isoforms and posttranslational modifications

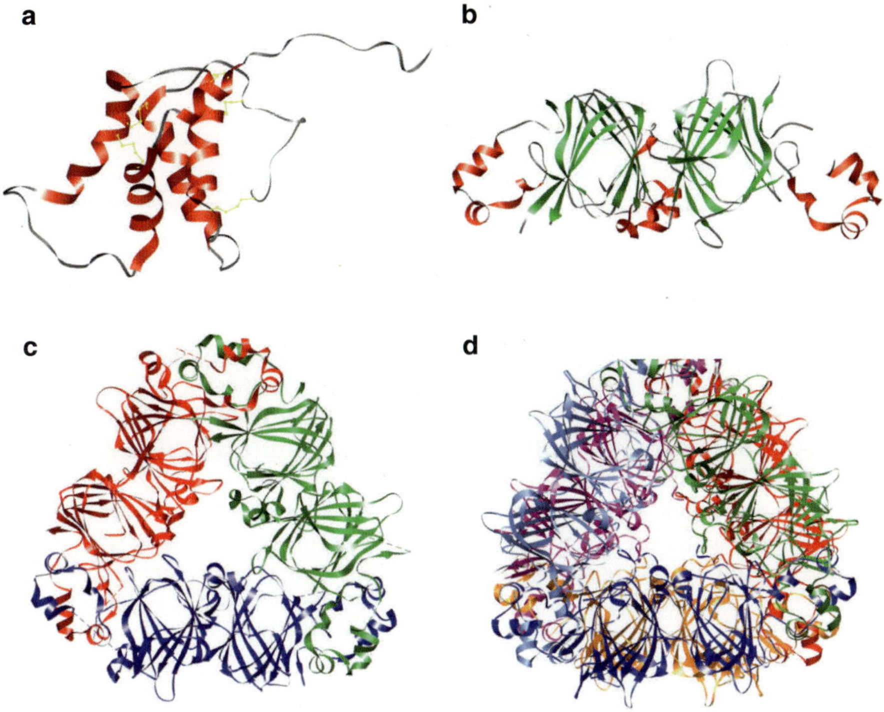

Fig. 5.1 (**a–d**) Structures of typical storage protein allergens: (**a**) Ara h 6 from peanut, a 2S albumin. Five α-helices (*red*) are stabilized by five disulfide bonds (*yellow*). (**b**) Monomer of Gly m 5 from soybean, a 7S globulin. The β-strands, which form two cupin barrels (*green*), are connected by variable, α-helical loops (*red* and *gray*). (**c**) Trimer of Gly m 5. (**d**) Hexamer of Gly m 6 from soybean, an 11S globulin. Each subunit is shown in a different color

(Hummel et al. 2015; Pfeifer et al. 2015). This complexity of natural storage proteins must always be considered when recombinant allergens are to be used for diagnostic purposes. The recombinant allergen must contain the entire repertoire of potential IgE epitopes.

5.4 Functions

Storage proteins are produced in plant seeds as energy and nutrient reserves, supplying the seedling until roots and leaves are formed. This biochemical function accounts for many properties of this group of proteins.

Quantity

Seeds have a protein content between 10 % (cereal grains) and 40 % (some legumes and oilseeds) of dry weight (Shewry et al. 1995), with storage proteins accounting for a large proportion of total protein. This is why sensitized patients may experience allergic symptoms even when they ingest only extremely small amounts of the food concerned. In studies, some individuals reacted to as little as 0.1 mg of peanut flour or 0.5 mg of lupin flour after placebo-controlled double-blind oral provocation (Peeters et al. 2009). Small amounts of these substances are also often found as impurities in processed foods. These "hidden" allergens pose a real risk to allergic individuals, who may react with dangerously severe symptoms.

Stability
Plant seeds often remain viable for many years, surviving even unfavorable environmental conditions. One reason for this is the high stability of storage proteins. Heating and other food-processing methods have little impact on the allergenic activity of storage proteins (Vissers et al. 2011). One extreme example is the peanut, whose allergenicity is actually increased by dry roasting due to the formation of stable aggregates (Beyer et al. 2001). Because of their stability, storage proteins are digested only partially in the stomach, so that immunologically active allergens can reach the small intestine and enter the bloodstream. Patients allergic to storage proteins from legumes, nuts, or seeds may thus react with systemic symptoms and even life-threatening anaphylaxis.

5.5 Relevance

Storage proteins are the major allergens in legumes (e.g., peanut, lupin, soybean), nuts (e.g., walnut, hazelnut), and other seeds of dicotyledonous plants (e.g., buckwheat, sesame, mustard) (◉ Table 5.1, ◉ Fig. 5.2). Along with nsLTPs (see Chap. 4), storage proteins are chiefly responsible for primary allergies to legumes, nuts, and seeds, frequently causing severe reactions.

Storage proteins may also play a role in allergic reactions to fruits. The seeds of some fruits such as kiwi and tomato are generally eaten, and the storage proteins they contain are released in the stomach. For kiwifruit, it has been demonstrated that many kiwi-allergic patients with a negative skin test to commercial kiwi extract are sensitized to Act d 12 and Act d 13 – an 11S globulin and a 2S albumin, respectively (Sirvent et al. 2014a).

5.6 Complex Cross-Reactivity Among Storage Proteins

There are few studies in which cross-reactivity between legumes, nuts, and other seeds has been investigated at the level of single allergens (Bublin and Breiteneder 2014). IgE cross-reactivity has been detected between 2S albumins and 7S as well as 11S globulins from distantly related plants.

2S Albumins
Most of the immunodominant IgE epitopes of 2S albumins are located in the surface-exposed loops that connect the α-helical scaffold of these proteins. As the sequences of these loops are highly variable, only a low level of cross-reactivity

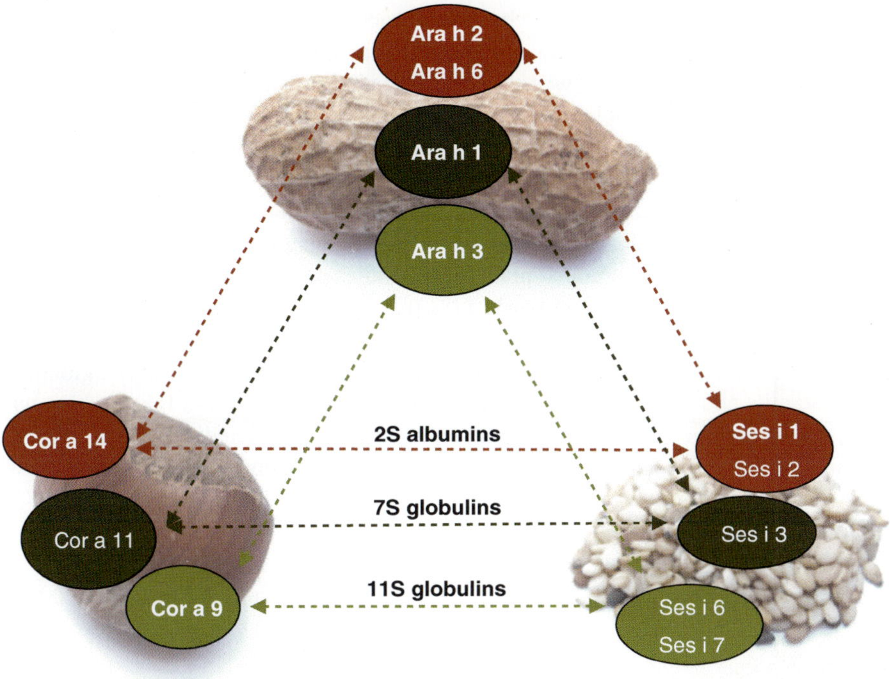

Fig. 5.2 Storage proteins as stable food allergens. Allergens in legumes (e.g., peanut, Ara h), tree nuts (e.g., hazelnut, Cor a), and other seeds (e.g., sesame, Ses i) can be assigned to three protein families and may induce severe IgE-mediated reactions. **Bold**: available for IgE diagnostics. *Arrows*: structural relatedness, but limited serological/clinical cross-reaction

among 2S albumins from different plant families can be expected. There are, however, a few examples of such cross-reactivity. In one investigation, marked cross-reactivity was shown between Ara h 2 from peanut and 2S albumins in extracts of almond and Brazil nut. Cross-reactivity between Ara h 2 and hazelnuts or cashews was, in contrast, only minimal (de Leon et al. 2007). A similarly selective cross-reactivity pattern has been demonstrated for Act d 13 from kiwifruit seeds, which cross-reacted with peanut, almond, and walnut, but not with hazelnut (Sirvent et al. 2014b). The clinically important cross-reactivity between peanut and lupins was partially caused by cross-reactivity between the 2S albumins (Ara h 2 and δ-conglutin; Dooper et al. 2009).

7S Globulins

There are few studies of the cross-reactivity between 7S globulins using purified proteins. The 7S globulins (Ara h 1 and β-conglutin) are also involved in cross-reactivity between peanut and lupin (Dooper et al. 2009). Pistachio and cashew nuts (both from the sumac family) contain the cross-reactive 7S globulins Pis v 3 and Ana o 1 (Willison et al. 2008). Where natural 7S globulins are used diagnostically, the glycosylation of these allergens must be taken into account. In one investigation, it was shown that many patients whose IgE reacted in an ISAC test to natural purified Jug r 2 as the only walnut allergen did not have a walnut allergy. In those patients, reactions to Jug r 2 were generally caused by clinically nonrelevant binding to cross-reactive carbohydrates (Villalta et al. 2013).

11S Globulins

Of the protein families discussed here, the 11S globulins exhibit the most pronounced cross-reactivity among unrelated plants. The studies mentioned represent only a few examples of recently published work. Sera from mustard-allergic individuals sensitized to Sin a 2 (Sirvent et al. 2012) and kiwifruit-allergic patients with IgE reactivity to Act d 12 (Sirvent et al. 2014b) showed marked cross-reactivity with 11S globulins from peanuts and tree nuts. In a child with buckwheat allergy, the IgE – which was directed against the 11S globulin from buckwheat – also reacted to 11S globulins of sesame, poppy, and hazelnut (Varga et al. 2011). The structural basis of these cross-reactions has been investigated. In this study, the previously identified linear IgE epitopes of Ara h 3 (peanut), Cor a 9 (hazelnut), Jug r 4 (walnut), and Ana o 2 (cashew nut) were mapped onto the protein structures. These epitopes were observed to be exposed to the surface and to exhibit similar conformations (Barre et al. 2007).

Cross-Reactivity Across Families

It has recently been demonstrated that the peanut allergens Ara h 1 (vicilin), Ara h 2 (2S albumin), and Ara h 3 (legumin) are mutually cross-reactive, although 2S albumin is not related to 7S and 11S globulins, and no similarities in structure or the overall amino acid sequence are evident (Bublin et al. 2013). It was shown that the cross-reactive IgE antibodies bind to unstructured loops that are exposed at the allergen's surface and whose sequences exhibit similarities between these unrelated proteins. This observation also explains why the majority of peanut-allergic individuals showed sensitization to all three major allergens. Similar cross-reactivity across protein families has also been demonstrated between Ara h 2 and Jug r 2, a 7S globulin from walnut (Maleki et al. 2011), and the α-conglutin (an 11S globulin) from lupin (Dooper et al. 2009).

Clinical Relevance

In diagnostics involving total extracts, it is common to find serological cross-reactivity among various legumes and between legumes, nuts, and seeds (◉ Fig. 5.2). This significantly decreases the analytical specificity (selectivity) of these extracts. However, the clinical relevance of this cross-reactive IgE is low (Sicherer 2001). The greatest discrepancy between serological and clinical cross-reactivity is observed between peanut and soybean. Although more than half of peanut-allergic individuals with systemic reactions show positive IgE tests to soybean, fewer than 10 % react in placebo-controlled provocation (Sicherer 2001). By contrast, up to one-third of patients with peanut allergy also exhibit allergic reactions to lupin, probably triggered by storage proteins (Peeters et al. 2009). In most studies, however, IgE cross-reactivity was tested only using total extracts, with no differentiation between single allergens, including storage proteins.

5.7 Diagnostic Challenges

Component-resolved diagnostics with storage proteins for distinguishing between primary and pollen-associated sensitivity to legumes, nuts, and seeds:

- In the temperate zones of Europe and North America, pollen-associated IgE cross-reactions to legumes, nuts, and seeds are frequently caused by labile allergens from the families of Bet v 1-related proteins (▶ Chap. 2) and profilins (▶ Chap. 3). They are clinically manifested in a completely different manner than primary allergies to stable allergens: these allergic reactions do not usually occur in children under 5 years of age as they are the consequence of a primary sensitization to pollen. Primarily induced by raw, non-heat-treated foods, they are often limited to mild, predominantly oropharyngeal symptoms.

Assessment of the risk of potentially dangerous sensitization to storage proteins (e.g., peanut 2S albumin, Ara h 2, and hazelnut 11S globulin, Cor a 9):

- For most allergen sources – with the exception of peanut – few storage proteins are currently available for IgE diagnostics (◉ Table 5.1). Diagnosis of peanut and tree nut allergy is covered in greater detail in ▶ Chaps. 11 and 12.
- The as-yet-unclarified role of component-resolved diagnostics in defining the clinical relevance of serological cross-reactivity among storage proteins from different legumes and also among legumes, nuts, and other seeds. This is due to a paucity of:
  - Components for diagnostics
  - Controlled studies with clinically well-characterized patients

Cautious interpretation is necessary where diagnosis is based solely on components and where evidence of sensitization to storage proteins is lacking:

- For component-resolved diagnosis, both purified natural and recombinant single allergens (◉ Table 5.1) are used. Due to the presence of isoforms and considerable posttranslational modifications (proteolytic cleavage of short peptides and glycosylation), the use of a recombinant storage protein may result in a restricted spectrum of potential IgE epitopes, with a consequent diminution of diagnostic sensitivity of the test (◉ Fig. 5.3).
- Varying test outcomes due to distinctive methodological features of IgE testing: instead of specific IgE testing to individual components (i.e., singleplex), lower costs and a lower requirement for serum make multiplex approaches attractive. However, the microarray techniques developed thus far deliver only semiquantitative results and are analytically less sensitive than singleplex testing procedures, in which the allergen is present in excess.

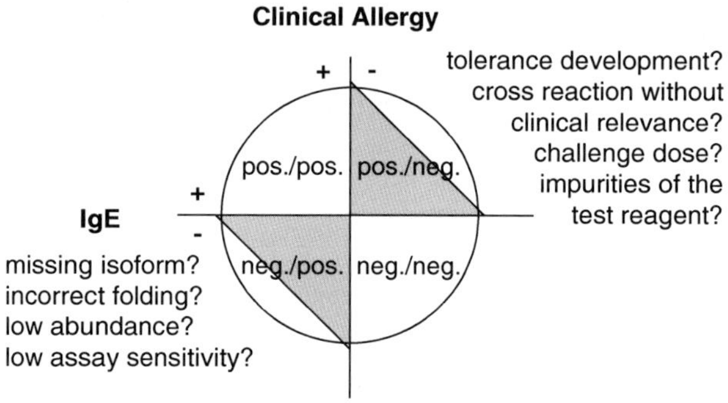

Fig. 5.3 Diagnostic dilemmas relating to storage proteins. Thus far, only a few storage proteins are available for component-resolved diagnostics, and in many cases clinical data on their use are scarce. There are several explanations for the mismatch (indicated in *gray*) between detection of sensitization (e.g., IgE) and clinical allergy (e.g., after oral provocation); this also applies to many other protein allergens

5.8 Additional Possible Benefits from Molecular Diagnostics

Potential advantages in the use of storage proteins for IgE diagnostics can be assessed with reference to the following general criteria (▶ Chap. 7):

A. Increased test sensitivity (lower limit of quantification, LoQ)
B. Increased test specificity (selectivity)
C. Indicators for cross-reactivity
D. Markers for primary, genuine (possibly species-specific) IgE sensitization

The following sections argue for the suitability of storage proteins for diagnostic goals:

Ad A
Because storage proteins generally are highly concentrated and stable in allergen extracts from legumes, nuts, and other seeds, IgE sensitivity to these proteins can usually be assessed fairly reliably. Only in specific cases, therefore, can pure storage proteins improve in vitro diagnostics by enhancing sensitivity to IgE testing:

- Rarely, sera with very low specific IgE to storage proteins, resulting in negative IgE to the corresponding allergen source (extracts from legumes, nuts, or other seeds).
- Sera with relatively low specific IgE to storage proteins (relative to total IgE) and/or a very low total IgE (<20 kU/l, <10 kU/l, 5 kU/l). The latter situation is also highly unusual, as the food-allergic individuals affected – frequently atopic infants, toddlers, and children, possibly with severe eczema – usually show markedly *elevated* (as opposed to *lower*) total IgE concentrations in serum.

Ad B

The use of storage proteins in IgE diagnostics should, in principle, improve analytical specificity, as positive test signals relate to clearly defined molecules rather than to complex protein mixtures.

- This criterion would, by itself, not suffice as an argument. It is only when the special properties of storage proteins are considered (high levels in the allergen source and very high stability), along with the associated risks of systemic reactions, that they are so useful for selectively detecting or ruling out sensitizations.
- This relationship between IgE sensitization and an increased risk of systemic allergic symptoms has been impressively demonstrated for storage proteins from various allergen sources, particularly 2S albumins from peanut and hazelnut (Beyer et al. 2015; Eller and Bindslev-Jensen 2013; Klemans et al. 2013; Masthoff et al. 2013).
- Therefore, other potentially IgE-binding proteins, such as Bet v 1 homologs or profilins (as the variable composition of extracts of legumes or nuts adversely affects their analytical specificity), are not relevant here and can be considered separately. The analytical specificity of storage proteins with regard to selective detection/ruling out of IgE is likely to fulfill the objective of "allergen-specific" diagnostics and is a compelling argument for their routine use.

Ad C

Storage proteins are suitable only to some extent as cross-reaction markers. Although allergens from different species can be grouped into distinct families (2S albumins, 7S and 11S globulins), storage proteins from different legumes, nuts, and other seeds may differ considerably in their extent of cross-reactivity as follows:

- Numerous isoforms of each storage protein with, possibly, variable IgE binding
- Restricted cross-reactivity due to limited and variable sequence identity
- Hard-to-predict cross-reactivity between storage proteins from different families due to surface-exposed loops with similar amino acid sequence (shown for Ara h 1, 2, and 3)

This results in heterogeneous IgE repertoires with individual patterns of sensitivity, which generally limits the reliability of storage proteins as markers for cross-reactions. In summary, the storage proteins are unsuitable as a marker of cross-reactivity within their entire protein family.

Ad D

Storage proteins, owing to their partial cross-reactivity, are only somewhat suitable as markers of species-specific IgE sensitization. This results in variable test outcomes that can be interpreted only on a case-by-case basis:

- If specific IgE to storage protein A and storage protein B (from the same protein family) is elevated by about the same amount, it remains unclear whether this is the consequence of a double sensitization or a cross-reaction with an unknown primary source of sensitization.

- If specific IgE to storage protein A is considerably higher than that to storage protein B (from the same protein family), then A is probably the primary source of sensitization. The relevance of the cross-reaction with B can, however, be determined only clinically by patient history or provocation test.
- If specific IgE to storage protein A is positive and that to storage protein B (from the same protein family) is negative, cross-reaction and the clinical relevance of B may be virtually ruled out.

These examples illustrate that the individual IgE repertoire can be assessed only indirectly, by comparing the levels of specific IgE to other storage proteins from the same family. Ideally, therefore, all structurally related storage proteins would be needed for IgE diagnostics in order to identify or rule out a primary source of sensitization and/or potential cross-reactions.

5.9 Outlook

The future will see a progressive increase in the number of seed storage proteins available for the molecular diagnostics of allergies. Ultimately, their diagnostic value will need to be verified by large-scale trials of subjects with well-defined symptomatology. Component-resolved diagnostics has now been extended to include epitope-based diagnosis, and serum samples have been tested for IgE binding to short peptides known to be IgE-binding sites. IgE of peanut-allergic children with relatively severe symptoms was directed against an increased number of peptides of Ara h 1, Ara h 2, and Ara h 3 (Flinterman et al. 2008). Epitope-based diagnostics is, however, not yet a routine clinical tool.

5.10 Conclusion: Potential for Routine Clinical Practice

In Central and Northern Europe as well as in North America, most primary allergies to legumes, nuts, and seeds involving systemic, sometimes severe, reactions are caused by storage proteins. Currently, the greatest potential for molecular allergy diagnostics lies in distinguishing these primary allergies from pollen-associated food allergies, especially where the history is inconclusive. As yet, the clinical relevance of serologic cross-reactivity among various legumes, nuts, and seeds cannot be deduced with certainty, even on the basis of component-resolved diagnostics. In most cases, therefore, oral food provocation testing remains essential for defining clinical reactivity (Nicolaou and Custovic 2011).

References

Barre A, Jacquet G, et al. Homology modelling and conformational analysis of IgE-binding epitopes of Ara h 3 and other legumin allergens with a cupin fold from tree nuts. Mol Immunol. 2007;44:3243–55.

Beyer K, Morrow E, et al. Effects of cooking methods on peanut allergenicity. J Allergy Clin Immunol. 2001;107:1077–81.
Beyer K, Grabenhenrich L, et al. Predictive values of component-specific IgE for the outcome of peanut and hazelnut food challenges in children. Allergy. 2015;70:90–8.
Bublin M, Kostadinova M, et al. IgE cross-reactivity between the major peanut allergen Ara h 2 and the nonhomologous allergens Ara h 1 and Ara h 3. J Allergy Clin Immunol. 2013; 132:118–24.
Bublin M, Breiteneder H. Cross-reactivity of peanut allergens. Curr Allergy Asthma Rep. 2014; 14:426.
Chassaigne H, Tregoat V, et al. Resolution and identification of major peanut allergens using a combination of fluorescence two-dimensional differential gel electrophoresis, Western blotting and Q-TOF mass spectrometry. J Proteomics. 2009;72:511–26.
de Leon MP, Drew AC, et al. IgE cross-reactivity between the major peanut allergen Ara h 2 and tree nut allergens. Mol Immunol. 2007;44:463–71.
Dooper MM, Plassen C, et al. Immunoglobulin E cross-reactivity between lupine conglutins and peanut allergens in serum of lupine-allergic individuals. J Invest Allergol Clin Immunol. 2009;19:283–91.
Eller E, Bindslev-Jensen C. Clinical value of component-resolved diagnostics in peanut-allergic patients. Allergy. 2013;68:190–4.
Flinterman AE, Knol EF, et al. Peanut epitopes for IgE and IgG4 in peanut-sensitized children in relation to severity of peanut allergy. J Allergy Clin Immunol. 2008;121:737–43.
Hebling CM, McFarland MA, et al. Global proteomic screening of protein allergens and advanced glycation endproducts in thermally processed peanuts. J Agric Food Chem. 2013;61:5638–48.
Hummel M, Wigger T, et al. Characterization of mustard 2S albumin allergens by bottom-up, middle-down, and top-down proteomics: a consensus set of isoforms of Sin a 1. J Proteome Res. 2015;14:1547–56.
Klemans RJ, Otte D, et al. The diagnostic value of specific IgE to Ara h 2 to predict peanut allergy in children is comparable to a validated and updated diagnostic prediction model. J Allergy Clin Immunol. 2013;131:157–63.
Maleki SJ, Teuber SS, et al. Computationally predicted IgE epitopes of walnut allergens contribute to cross-reactivity with peanuts. Allergy. 2011;66:1522–9.
Masthoff LJ, Mattsson L, et al. Sensitization to Cor a 9 and Cor a 14 is highly specific for a hazelnut allergy with objective symptoms in Dutch children and adults. J Allergy Clin Immunol. 2013;132:393–9.
Nicolaou N, Custovic A. Molecular diagnosis of peanut and legume allergy. Curr Opin Allergy Clin Immunol. 2011;11:222–8.
Peeters KA, Koppelman SJ, et al. Clinical relevance of sensitization to lupine in peanut-sensitized adults. Allergy. 2009;64:549–55.
Pfeifer S, Bublin M, et al. Cor a 14, the allergenic 2S albumin from hazelnut, is highly thermostable and resistant to gastrointestinal digestion. Mol Nutr Food Res. 2015;59:2077–86.
Shewry PR, Napier JA, et al. Seed storage proteins – structures and biosynthesis. Plant Cell. 1995;7:945–56.
Sicherer SH. Clinical implications of cross-reactive food allergens. J Allergy Clin Immunol. 2001;108:881–90.
Sirvent S, Akotenou M, et al. The 11S globulin Sin a 2 from yellow mustard seeds shows IgE cross-reactivity with homologous counterparts from tree nuts and peanut. Clin Transl Allergy. 2012;2:23.
Sirvent S, Canto B, et al. Act d 12 and Act d 13: two novel, masked, relevant allergens in kiwifruit seeds. J Allergy Clin Immunol. 2014a;133:1765–7.
Sirvent S, Cantó B, et al. Detailed characterization of Act d 12 and Act d 13 from kiwi seeds: implication in IgE cross-reactivity with peanut and tree nuts. Allergy. 2014b;69:1481–8.
Varga EM, Kollmann D, et al. Anaphylaxis to buckwheat in an atopic child: a risk factor for severe allergy to nuts and seeds? Int Arch Allergy Immunol. 2011;156:112–6.

Villalta D, Conte M, et al. Isolated IgE reactivity to native walnut vicilin-like protein (nJug r 2) on ISAC microarray is due to cross-reactive carbohydrate epitopes. Clin Chem Lab Med. 2013; 51:1991–5.

Vissers YM, Blanc F, et al. Effect of heating and glycation on the allergenicity of 2S albumins (Ara h 2/6) from peanut. PLoS One. 2011;6:e23998.

Willison LN, Tawde P, et al. Pistachio vicilin, Pis v 3, is immunoglobulin E-reactive and cross-reacts with the homologous cashew allergen, Ana o 1. Clin Exp Allergy. 2008;38:1229–38.

Cross-Reactive Carbohydrate Determinants: Diagnostic and Clinical Relevance

6

U. Jappe and M. Raulf

List of Abbreviations

α-gal	Galactose-α-1,3-galactose
CAP	Capsulated hydrophilic carrier polymer
CCD	Cross-reactive carbohydrate determinant
Fab	Fragment antigen binding
FEIA	Fluorescent enzyme immunoassay
HSA	Human serum albumin
HRP	Horseradish peroxidase
MBP	Maltose-binding protein

This contribution is based on a publication by the authors that appeared in the *Allergo Journal* in 2013 (Jappe U, Petersen A, Raulf-Heimsoth M: Allergische Soforttypreaktionen und kreuzreaktive Kohlenhydratepitope (CCD). Allergo J 2013; 22: 25–32) and which has now been updated, expanded, and translated into English as a chapter for this book.
We are grateful to Dr. Ozan Angün of Lübeck University's Department of Dermatology, Dr. Arne Homann, Div. of Clinical and Molecular Allergology, Research Center Borstel, for the graphics used in Fig. 6.1, and Professor Arnd Petersen of Research Center Borstel for preparing Fig. 6.2 and reviewing the manuscript.
The authors gratefully thank Dr. Steve Love, PhD, Laguna Niguel, CA, USA, for reading the manuscript, helpful suggestions, and editorial assistance with the English translation.

U. Jappe, MD, Prof. (✉)
Division of Clinical and Molecular Allergology, Research Center Borstel, Airway Research Center North (ARCN), Member of the German Center for Lung Research (DZL), Borstel, Germany

Interdisciplinary Allergy Unit, Department of Pneumology, University Medical Center, University of Lübeck, Lübeck, Germany
e-mail: ujappe@fz-borstel.de

M. Raulf, PhD, Prof.
Center Allergology/Immunology, Institute for Prevention and Occupational Medicine of the German Social Accident Insurance, Institute of the Ruhr-Universität Bochum, Bochum, Germany
e-mail: raulf@ipa-dguv.de

J. Kleine-Tebbe, T. Jakob (eds.), *Molecular Allergy Diagnostics*,
DOI 10.1007/978-3-319-42499-6_6

MMX	Man α-1,6 (Man α-1,3) (Xyl β-1,2) Man β-1,4 GlcNAc β-1,4 GlcNAc α-D-mannosyl-(1->6)-[α-D-mannosyl-(1->3)]-[β-D-xylosyl-(1->2)]-β-D-mannosyl-(1->4)-N-acetyl-β-D-glucosaminyl-(1->4)-N-acetyl-D-glucosamine
MMXF3	Man α-1,6 (Man α-1,3)-(Xyl β-1,2) Man β-1,4 GlcNAc β-1,4 (Fuc α-1,3) GlcNAc α-D-mannosyl-(1->6)-[α-D-mannosyl-(1->3)]-[β-D-xylosyl-(1->2)]-β-D-mannosyl-(1->4)-N-acetyl-β-D-glucosaminyl-(1->4)]-N-acetyl-D-glucosamine
MUXF	Man α-1,6 (Xyl β-1,2) Man β-1,4 GlcNAc β-1,4 (Fuc α-1,3) GlcNAc α-D-mannosyl-(1->6)-[β-D-xylosyl-(1->2)]-β-D-mannosyl-(1->4)-N-acetyl-β-D-glucosaminyl-(1->4)]-[α-L-fucosyl-(1->3)]-N-acetyl-D-glucosamine
MMF3F6	Man α-1,6 (Man α-1,3) Man β-1,4 GlcNAc β-1,4 (Fuc α-1,3) (Fuc α-1,6) GlcNAc α-D-mannosyl-(1->6)-[α-D-mannosyl-(1->3)]-β-D-mannosyl-(1->4)-N-acetyl-β-D-glucosaminyl-(1->4)]-[α-L-fucosyl-(1->3)]-[α-L-fucosyl-(1->6)]-N-acetyl-D-glucosamine

6.1 Introduction

The most allergologically relevant protein families are the Bet v 1 superfamily, the cupins, the lipid transfer proteins (LTPs), the profilins, and the cross-reactive carbohydrate determinants (CCDs), thus named as they are responsible for a variety of cross-reactions. The term cross-reaction refers to the binding of antibodies to – or the activation of – T lymphocytes specifically sensitized to various molecules (proteins, carbohydrates, glycoproteins) that have identical or similar antigenic determinants. This property may be due to a high degree of sequence similarity (linear epitopes), but also to the similarity of the 3D structure (conformation, conformational epitopes).

As plant allergens are usually glycoproteins, which often occur in high concentrations in pollen, especially grass pollen, as well as in foods of plant origin and latex, IgE antibodies directed against CCDs are found primarily in sera of patients with multiple sensitizations to plant allergens. Carbohydrate moieties are present in the form of side chains, which are usually exposed to their milieu and may present a binding site for substances such as IgE antibodies. This frequently complicates the identification of the substances that cause severe allergic reactions. The detection of IgE antibodies to CCDs is specific and yields true positives, but it often does not correlate with clinical findings.

Recombinant allergens, which are being much more frequently used in allergy laboratory diagnostics, have no CCDs when they are expressed in *E. coli*. The reason is that *E. coli,* the bacterium used for mass-producing recombinant proteins, including allergens, is not able to produce proteins with posttranslational modifications such as glycosylation. This must be considered in diagnostics, especially in attempting to elucidate cross-reactions.

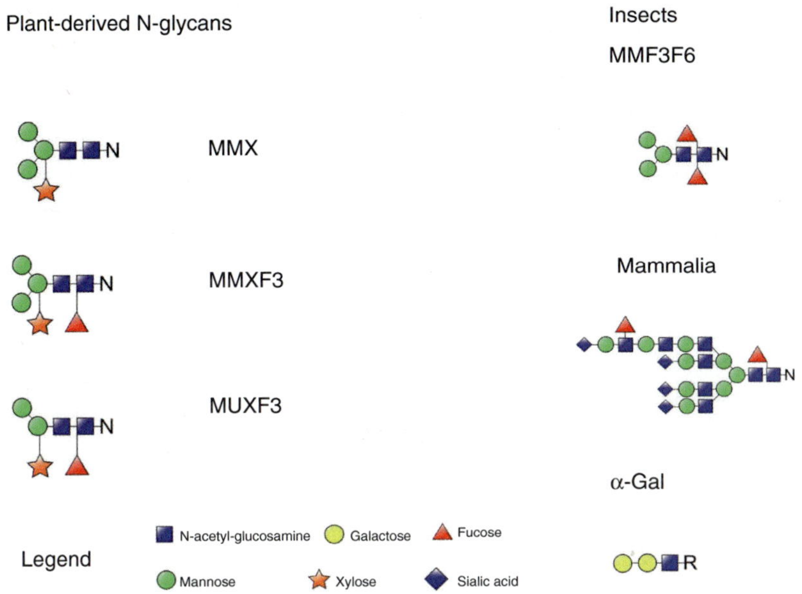

Fig. 6.1 Graphical overview of the various glycan structures Plant for abbreviations see list of abbreviations on previous page (Adapted from Malandain 2005, mod. after www.ncbi.nlm.nih.gov/books/NBK1917/)

6.1.1 Cross-Reactive Carbohydrate Determinants

Glycosylation of proteins is the commonest form of modification in most organisms. During the biosynthesis of glycoproteins, carbohydrate chains are progressively synthesized and covalently bound to various amino acid residues of a glycoprotein. However, the carbohydrate moieties vary greatly in complexity, from mono-, di-, and oligosaccharides to polysaccharides. These carbohydrate chains serve various purposes. They may afford protection from proteases; they can also influence functionality, folding, solubility, and/or intercellular transport of the glycoprotein. Depending on whether the carbohydrate side chain is linked to the amino acid by reaction with a hydroxyl group (in the case of serine or threonine) or an amino group (asparagine), the resulting bond is described as O-glycosidic or N-glycosidic. The best-studied carbohydrate determinants are based on the monosaccharides fucose (a hexose) and xylose (a pentose); the carbohydrates are epitopes of the MMXF and MUXF type (◉ Fig. 6.1).

Glycoproteins from plants and invertebrates contain similar fucosylated and/or xylosylated N-glycans. As this type of modification does not occur in mammals, it exhibits pronounced immunogenicity in man. The widespread presence of fucose and xylose on plant-derived N-glycans, as well as those from invertebrates, explains the marked cross-reactivity of these molecules and has led to the name, "cross-reactive carbohydrate determinants" – CCDs (Aalberse et al. 1981). The first allergenic CCD investigated in detail was the phospholipase A_2 from bee venom which carries an α-1,3 fucosylated N-glycan but no xylose (Weber et al. 1987). It is now widely accepted that xylose and fucose residues constitute important elements both for IgE binding to invertebrate- and plant-derived glycoproteins and for cross-reactivity (Jappe and Raulf-Heimsoth 2007, 2008; van Ree et al. 2000).

A recently identified allergen in domestic mammalian meat – an allergen associated with severe reactions (in some cases with delayed-type anaphylaxis; Chung et al. 2008) – is also a carbohydrate epitope rather than a non-glycosylated protein. This phenomenon, discovered comparatively recently, has brought about a paradigm shift regarding the clinical significance of carbohydrate epitopes (which had been regarded as relatively minor).

The most important characteristics of the allergologically relevant carbohydrate determinants are described below.

6.2 Allergen Sources

6.2.1 "Classical" CCDs

"Classical" CCDs are commonly present in pollen, food plants, arthropods, mollusks, and some pathogenic helminths (◉ Fig. 6.2).

6.2.2 Galactose-α-1,3-Galactose

Galactose-α-1,3-galactose (α-gal) is an ubiquitous carbohydrate, a disaccharide, in cells and tissues of most non-primate mammals and New World monkeys, however, not in Old World monkeys, apes, and human beings (Jappe 2012). The primary source of this CCD allergen is, therefore, mammalian meat, not fish or poultry. A second source can be therapeutic antibodies partly derived from mammals. The Fab part of the heavy chain of cetuximab, a treatment for cancer of the head and neck, is glycosylated with a sequence of carbohydrates on aspartate residue N88, including α-gal and the sialic acid, N-glycolylneuraminic acid (Qian et al. 2007). It has also been reported that some patients with allergy to cat dander have IgE specific to α-gal, a carbohydrate epitope on cat IgA (Adedoyin et al. 2007).

6.3 Structural Considerations

6.3.1 "Classical" CCDs

CCDs in plants, arthropods, and mollusks can essentially be divided into two types: MMXF and MUXF. These are N-glycans, containing α-1,3-linked fucose, which are widespread, particularly in insects and throughout the plant kingdom, but not in mammals. Additionally, in plants, xylose can be β-1,2 linked to the first mannose of the N-glycan core and constitute an antigenic determinant (◉ Fig. 6.1).

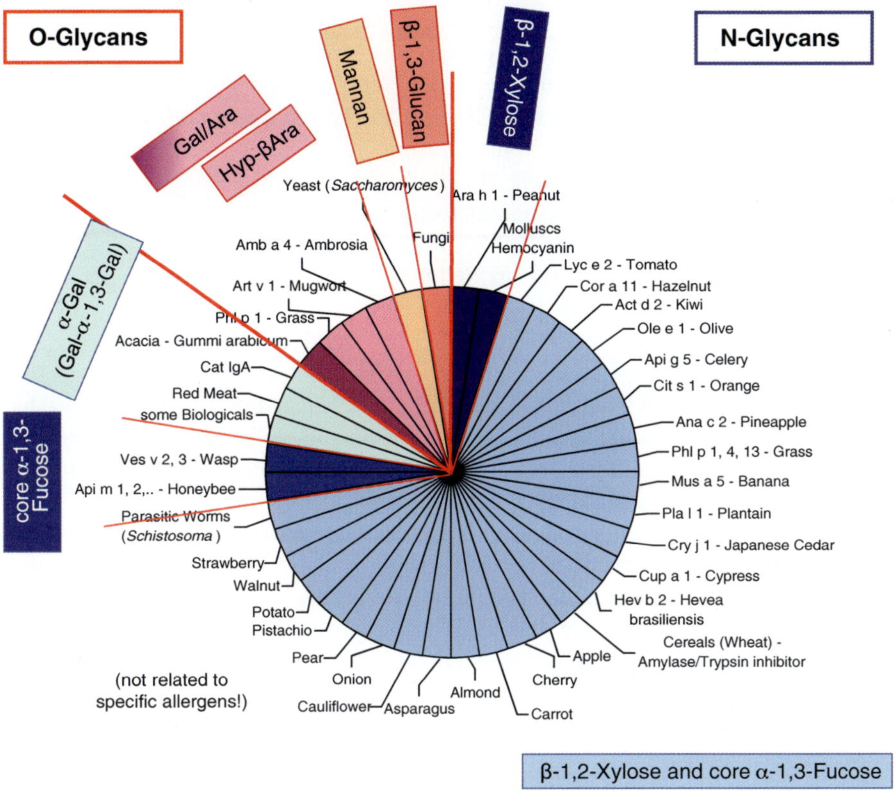

Fig. 6.2 Allergen sources and single allergens with IgE-binding carbohydrate moieties. The allergen sources have been grouped into N- and O-glycans and related subgroups where the IgE-binding epitopes have been identified

6.3.2 Galactose-α-1,3-Galactose

The α-gal epitope is a disaccharide that itself is a constituent of some oligosaccharides. α-Gal linkages are also present in blood group antigen B of humans.

6.4 Frequency of Sensitization and Allergenicity

6.4.1 "Classical" CCDs

Carbohydrate side chains may account for up to 30 % of an allergenic glycoprotein molecule. The CCDs of MMXF and MUXF type are panallergens, and therefore, anti-CCD IgE antibodies are found in sera of patients sensitized to various allergens. Current data from Holzweber et al. (2013) show the incidence of anti-CCD IgE to be 22 % among 6,000 sera from allergic individuals. There are, to date, no published findings on whether CCDs are a cause of primary sensitization. To date, the inhalation of grass and ragweed pollen, which contain allergens especially rich in glycoproteins (Jappe and Raulf-Heimsoth 2008), is known to lead to the production of IgE antibodies specific to CCDs, as do Hymenoptera venoms (Jappe and Raulf-Heimsoth 2008). Insect venoms appear to have greater potential for sensitization, as natural exposure, i.e., via "field stings," evidently leads to a temporary increase in anti-CCD IgE, while natural exposure to pollen allergens does not cause a corresponding increase (Jappe and Raulf-Heimsoth 2007).

Data on the prevalence of IgE to CCDs in insect venom-allergic persons vary across studies. The present authors' own investigations show that up to 72 % of insect venom-allergic patients are anti-CCD IgE positive (Jappe et al. 2006).

Few data exist on the prevalence of anti-CCD IgE in sera of patients with food allergies. Of those sensitized to zucchini, celery, carrot, and/or tomato, 10–50 % had anti-CCD IgE in the serum (Jappe and Raulf-Heimsoth 2008).

Data are also scarce on the prevalence and clinical relevance of anti-CCD IgE in patients with occupational allergy. Whereas only a very low percentage of latex-allergic persons working in the healthcare sector (due to natural rubber gloves) exhibited specific IgE reactions to CCDs (Raulf-Heimsoth et al. 2007), polysensitized individuals that have latex-specific IgE antibodies without known exposure to natural rubber latex often are anti-CCD IgE positive. Specific IgE antibodies to CCDs have also been detected among workers in the wood-processing industry with IgE antibodies to beech and pine wood dust, especially in all those individuals IgE positive to both woods (Kespohl et al. 2010). Further characterization showed that, in employees without allergic symptoms, IgE binding depended primarily on glycan structures. In symptomatic individuals, IgE binding to wood dust allergens occurred in three different variants: exclusively to proteins, mixed to proteins and glycan containing moieties, and solely to glycan structures (Kespohl et al. 2012). Palacin et al. (2008) ascribed the possible association between respiratory allergy to grain flours (baker's asthma) and kiwifruit allergy to cross-reactive carbohydrate determinants and thiol proteases. In addition, Sander et al. (2011) studied the frequency of sensitization to 17 recombinant wheat flour allergens and 2 CCDs (HRP and MUXF) in 40 German bakers with work-related asthma/rhinitis and 10 controls with pollinosis. The group found that IgE binding to HRP and MUXF was as frequent (25 %) as to the most relevant recombinant allergen Tri a 28.0101 in the bakers' group and nearly as frequent (40–60 %) as to the panallergen profilin in the control group, confirming previous observations that xylose- and fucose-containing complex glycans are relevant for cross-reactive IgE binding (Garcia-Casado et al. 1996).

6.4.2 Galactose-α-1,3-Galactose

Galactose-α-1,3-galactose (α-gal) is a carbohydrate ubiquitous in cells and tissues of all mammals other than primates, as well as in New World monkeys and prosimians. In higher primates and humans, the gene coding for α-1,3-galactosyltransferase is not functional. By contrast, α-gal-negative organisms can produce IgG antibodies specific to this oligosaccharide (Jappe 2012). The naturally occurring IgG to α-gal is responsible for the hyperacute rejection response following xenografting from pigs to primates (Jappe 2012). Its allergenicity became evident when, in the USA, anaphylactic reactions occurred after the first dose of the therapeutic antibody cetuximab and were assigned to IgE antibodies to α-gal (Chung et al. 2008). Cetuximab – a chimeric mouse-human IgG1 monoclonal antibody directed against the epidermal growth factor receptor produced in mouse myeloma cells – carries α-gal on its murine part. Anti-α-gal IgE was found in patients even before therapy, and a geographical cluster of reactivity to cetuximab was observed in Tennessee, Arkansas, North Carolina, Missouri, and Virginia, prompting investigations into the sensitization pathway. The fact that α-gal is present on both Fab fragments of the cetuximab antibody suggests the efficient, pairwise cross-linking of IgE antibodies on mast cells.

Recent studies point to tick bites and helminth infestation in addition to the consumption of mammalian red meat as causal agents in the sensitization to α-gal (Jappe 2012, 2015). α-Gal, for example, was shown to be present in the gastrointestinal tract of ticks (*Ixodes ricinus*) in Sweden, which was reactive with IgE from patients allergic to red meat implying host exposure to α-gal during tick bite (Hamsten et al. 2013).

Classification as Major or Minor Allergens

Categorization into major or minor allergens has not yet been undertaken for CCDs of the MMXF and MUXF type but has been done for the corresponding glycosylated allergens (glycoproteins) such as Ara h 1, a storage protein from peanut (◉ Fig. 6.2). Act d 2 from kiwifruit, recently identified as a major allergen in adults in Spain (Palacin et al. 2008), is a glycoprotein with complex asparagine-linked glycans, as is the thaumatin-like allergen from apple, Mal d 2. Allergens in rubber plant latex (Hev b 2: Palacin et al. 2011) and in olive pollen (Ole e 9: Palacin et al. 2011), however, are N-glycosylated glucanases. They appear to be involved in cross-reactivity between natural rubber latex, pollen, and food allergens of plant origin and are generally minor allergens. However, sensitization to Ole e 9 in geographical areas with very high exposure to olive pollen is increasing significantly (Palacin et al. 2011).

A subdivision of this kind has not yet been undertaken for α-gal. With an increasing abundance of data, the tendency is toward classifying it as a major allergen in delayed meat allergy.

6.5 Clinical Assessment of Allergenicity

6.5.1 "Classical" CCDs

CCDs are, according to Altmann (2007), those epitopes to which humans are most frequently exposed but which do not occur in vertebrates. It is this foreign nature that renders them highly immunogenic.

Allergenicity (i.e., sensitization with the potential to become clinically relevant) is partly determined by the multivalent occurrence of carbohydrate determinants in a protein. This allows for cross-linking by IgE antibodies with specificity for this structure and hence release of mediators.

An additional factor in sensitization appears to be alcohol consumption. Sera of alcoholics display a high prevalence of IgE antibodies to pollen, insect venoms (Gonzalez-Quintela et al. 2008), and natural rubber latex (Coutinho et al. 2008); the sera also frequently exhibit positive reactions in multiallergen IgE testing (González-Quintela et al. 2009). Several studies have established an increased IgE titer to CCDs in alcoholics (Coutinho et al. 2008; Gonzalez-Quintela et al. 2008; Vidal et al. 2009), although the mechanism and clinical relevance of this observation remain unclear. Ethyl alcohol (ethanol) is a strong immunomodulator, capable of switching the balance of immune reactions toward Th2 responses (Heinz and Waltenbaugh 2007; Linneberg et al. 2008). Chronic consumption of ethanol is associated with an increasing concentration of total IgE in serum, both in humans and (in the context of research) in animals. In theory, the glycoprotein content of some alcoholic drinks may play a part. Grapes and wines contain glycoproteins that can, in rare cases, induce clinically relevant sensitizations (Pastorello et al. 2003; Vassilopoulou et al. 2007). Additionally, Hymenoptera venom allergens may have entered the wine during the initial processing stages (Armentia et al. 2007).

A study by Gonzalez-Quintela et al. (2011) suggests that a considerable proportion of hospitalized alcoholics exhibit IgE reactivity to N-glycans of wine glycoproteins. Moreover, N-glycans and wine glycoprotein extracts were able to trigger basophil activation in alcoholics highly sensitized to N-glycans. Methodologically, however, it is important to note that it was not the N-glycans that were used but glycan conjugates (N-glycans attached to a carrier protein). Specific mechanisms that increase CCD exposure in alcoholics – and, thus, sensitization to foods – may be related to increased intestinal GI permeability and/or reduced gastric digestion of proteins, both a consequence of chronic alcohol exposure (Untersmayr and Jensen-Jarolim 2008). Endothelial dysfunction may also be involved in CCD sensitization of alcoholics (Di Gennaro et al. 2007). Experimental alcohol-induced gastritis increases sensitization to food allergens in mice (Andrade et al. 2006). Overall, however, data from Gonzalez-Quintela et al. (2011) substantiate the observation that CCDs tend to exhibit low-level biological activity in vivo. None of the CCD-sensitized patients in this study had allergic symptoms following consumption of foods containing CCDs or of alcoholic drinks (Gonzalez-Quintela et al. 2011). Furthermore, prick tests with allergens carrying CCDs were negative in individuals with IgE specific to these allergens. The discrepancy between pronounced in vitro activity in basophil activation tests and an absence of in vivo activity part of anti-CCD IgE was ascribed by Gonzalez-Quintela to unknown tolerance mechanisms.

Although there is conflicting evidence, there is some support for the idea that chronic alcohol consumption accompanied by asymptomatic sensitization to foods may be associated with symptomatic food allergy (Serghini-Idrissi et al. 2001).

6.5.2 Galactose-α-1,3-Galactose

Commins et al. (2009) tested patients with allergic reactions to beef for IgE antibodies to α-gal. They identified 24 individuals who had repeated occurrences of anaphylaxis, angioedema, and urticaria several hours after consumption of bovine meat and had developed IgE to α-gal. Only 3 of the 24 sera were IgE positive to the "classical" CCD of the pineapple protease, bromelain. However, sera that were strongly IgE positive to bromelain did not exhibit IgE to α-gal. Laminin-γ1 (240 kDa) and the α1(VI) collagen chain (140 kDa) in extract of beef (*Bos taurus*) are the dominant IgE-reactive proteins in Japanese patients with meat allergy. Inhibition experiments have shown that the α-gal present in these proteins is responsible for IgE reactivity (Takahashi et al. 2014).

6.6 Unresolved Issues

In view of the fact that chronic alcohol consumption appears to be a contributing factor, it remains to be seen whether the "classical" CCDs of glycoproteins in food allergen sources will become major allergens.

With regard to anti-α-gal IgE antibodies, it remains unclear in which situation and at which concentration they cause allergy symptoms. Additionally, the association between α-gal and adjacent peptide structures appears relevant for IgE binding (Jappe, unpublished data). The cause of anti-α-gal IgE-associated, delayed-type anaphylaxis upon consumption of muscle and/or visceral meat also remains elusive. An impact of alcohol consumption, as described for "classical" CCDs, has yet to be shown. A possible lipid association has been posited as a cause of the delayed anaphylaxis (Jappe 2015). The fattier a meat-based meal, the more reliably positive were the provocation tests with meat and the more severe the reactions (Commins and Platts-Mills 2013).

A clear relationship exists between the route of administration and the rate of reaction to α-gal: intravenous administration of cetuximab or drugs containing gelatin induces immediate-type anaphylaxis, whereas delayed anaphylaxis develops upon consumption of mammalian meat or meat-containing products (Chung et al. 2008; Commins et al. 2009; Mullins et al. 2012). Elucidation of the sensitization pathways has not yet been completed.

The question of whether these patients should completely avoid mammalian meat is not yet resolved. There are indications that meat allergy is dose dependent and maybe the fat content is a relevant aggravating factor. What remains unclear, however, is the effect of portion size and the influence of processing and preparation methods, on the occurrence and severity of the clinical reaction.

6.7 Relevance for Allergy Diagnostic Tests and Availability of Reagents for *In Vitro* or *In Vivo* Testing

6.7.1 "Classical" CCDs

CCDs are not, per se, available for in vivo testing. For in vitro diagnostics, the natural glycoproteins, bromelain, horseradish peroxidase (HRP), and ascorbate oxidase have proven of value as screening tools, with HRP having the greatest sensitivity (Jappe et al. 2006). MUXF, the glycan component of bromelain, which (without the

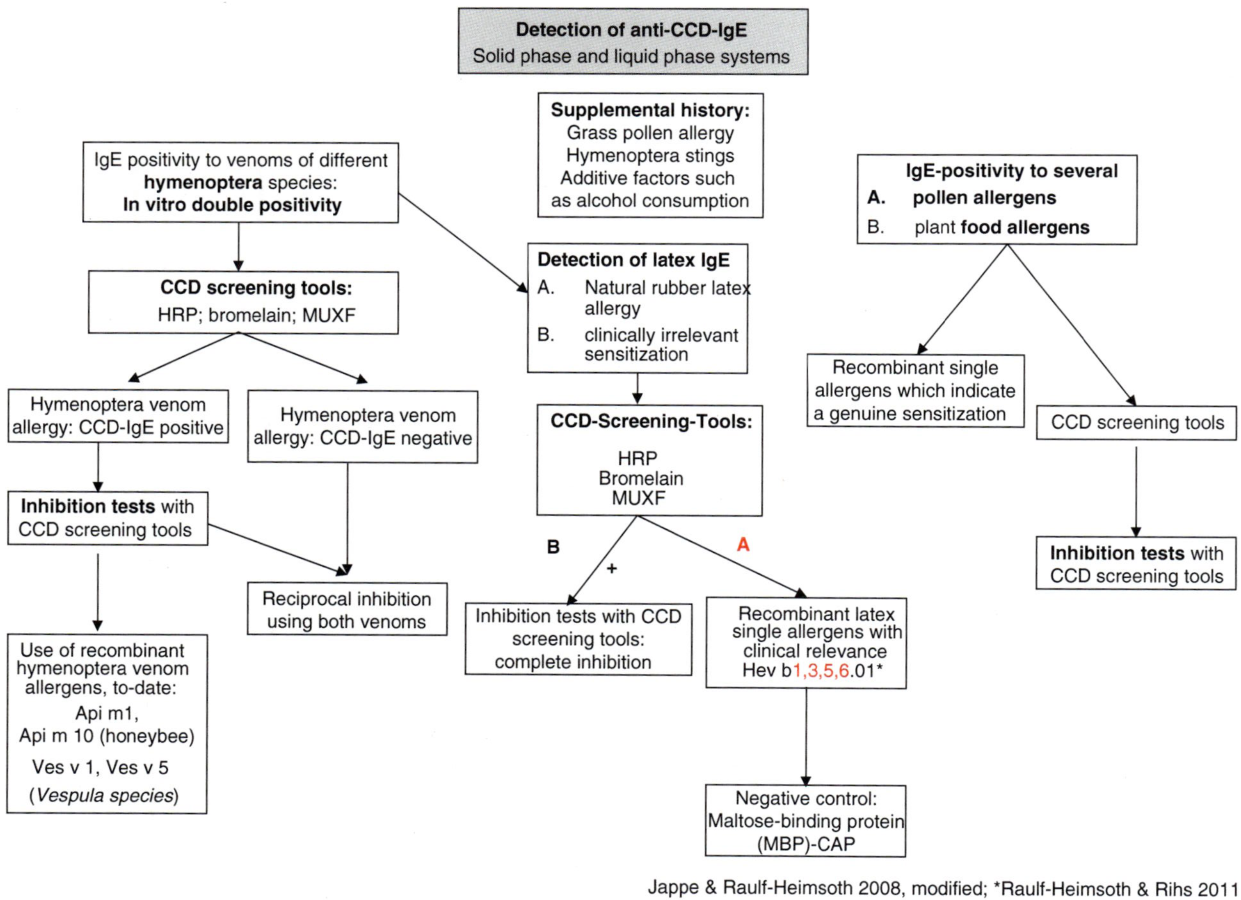

Fig. 6.3 Flow chart of the diagnostic approach to detecting anti-CCD IgE in serum. The single allergens of natural rubber latex, highlighted in *red*, support the clinical diagnosis of latex allergy (from Raulf-Heimsoth and Rihs 2011)

peptide portion) is already available for in vitro diagnostics, is inferior to HRP in respect to sensitivity and specificity (Jappe, unpublished data). The abovementioned CCD tools make specific detection of anti-CCD IgE possible. However, it cannot be established from their application alone whether IgE binding is based solely on a specific allergen source, whether additional peptide epitopes are recognized, or whether protein-specific IgE antibodies are involved. Although inhibition tests enhance the specificity of testing, they are cost- and effort-intensive and have not become established in routine clinical practice (◉ Fig. 6.3).

The research team headed by Friedrich Altmann in Vienna has produced semi-synthetic conjugates, the first of which is a CCD (without a peptide component), linked to bovine serum albumin, and the second, MUXF, linked to human serum albumin. The latter was purified so that no extraneous peptides are present. The "CCD blocker" is a synthetic, well-defined neoglycoprotein composed of human serum albumin (HSA, Sigma-Aldrich) and a highly purified plant glycopeptide, extracted and purified from bromelain, with all existing protein epitopes having proteolytically been destroyed.

Holzweber et al. (2013) reported that 8–10 MUXF molecules can be linked to a single HSA molecule. They were unable to detect other antigen determinants in their CCD blocker, so that there is negligible risk that it will induce clinically relevant IgE-allergen binding. The polyvalence of this CCD blocker allows a low working concentration of 20 mg per liter (or 10 μg in 0.5 ml of serum) for the use of this serum in standard, routine IgE detection. According to the authors, a preincubation period prior to the use of the serum is not necessary, a clear practical advantage (Aberer et al. 2014).

In the first comprehensive analysis of more than 6,000 serum samples, it was found that – for the 43 patient sera that were fully evaluable – total inhibition of the anti-CCD IgE was not achieved in all cases by administration of the CCD blocker. Thus, additional prospective studies are required, with larger numbers of subjects and better-defined sera.

In particular, when multiallergen (strip) tests are utilized and with all assays in which both recombinant allergens and naturally purified (especially food) allergens are used, the CCD issue remains of great significance. It follows that the differentiation between anti-CCD IgE and protein-specific or peptide-specific IgE is also crucial.

Thus, the use of total extracts remains relevant, especially for food allergen sources. The same applies, therefore, to the glycosylated moieties they contain. For these allergen sources all is not yet in place for component-resolved diagnostics. In other words, not all allergens are identified, isolated, and/or available for diagnostic purposes. For example, when the allergens are available in recombinant form from *E. coli*, they generally lack a CCD component.

Using sera pretreated with CCD blockers, Aberer et al. (2014) and Holzweber et al. (2013) observed when applying the ISAC test (Thermo Fisher Scientific, Freiburg) that the binding of serum-IgE antibodies to recombinant, CCD-free allergens occurred. Both investigators considered this to be evidence for the specificity of the CCD blocker. The CCD inhibitor has proven effective in both singleplex and multiplex arrays, as well as in multiallergen strips and component arrays. Other advantages are that it does not dilute the samples or trigger unwanted inhibition of interactions not involving CCDs, but peptides (Holzweber et al. 2013). The authors of this chapter wish to note from personal experience, however, that 100 % inhibition may not occur in all cases, as only one type of CCD, namely, MUXF, is used, and not MMXF.

Holzweber et al. (2013) also noted that the CCD blocker worked better in the ISAC system than with ImmunoCAP testing, an observation which may be related to the higher concentration of antigens in the ImmunoCAP matrix.

Another interesting finding of research by Holzweber et al. during their examination of over 6,000 sera was an age association for the presence of anti-CCD IgE. In childhood its concentration is relatively low, in adolescence it increases markedly, but, after the age of 40, it begins to revert to a lower level. Their hypothesis is that anti-CCD IgE is the result of a normal sensitization process. Additionally, the onset of CCD sensitization in childhood is an argument against a general link between CCD positivity and alcoholism (Holzweber et al. 2013).

6.7.2 Galactose-α-1,3-Galactose

Recently anti-α-gal IgE antibodies have been detected in the serum of German patients with suspected meat allergy. Detection was by immunoblot using the therapeutic antibody cetuximab as the target antigen (Jappe et al. 2011); CAP-FEIA is another diagnostic option for these antibodies which is commercially available on the basis of bovine thyroglobulin.

6.8 Evaluating the Clinical Relevance of CCDs

6.8.1 "Classical" CCDs

The clinical significance of IgE antibodies that are specifically directed against CCDs of the MMXF and MUXF type lies principally in their reduction of the specificity of in vitro allergologic diagnostics.

In individual cases, "classical" CCDs appear to be associated with severe anaphylactic reactions, as for example, to Hymenoptera stings (Jappe et al. 2006), and also to some foods.

Alcoholics have been shown to have heightened IgE reactivity to peanut. However, none of the alcoholic patients in this study exhibited symptoms of peanut allergy following consumption of this legume (Vidal et al. 2009). This suggests that IgE reactivity to peanuts in alcoholics is attributable to CCDs. Vidal et al. believe the particular significance of this diagnostic phenomenon lies in the fact that peanut consumption is widespread and peanut is a high-risk allergen source: when dealing with high-risk allergens, clinicians chiefly rely on in vitro diagnosis, since allergen challenge is clearly too high risk. In some alcoholics, however, IgE antibodies reach concentrations with a >95 % positive predictive value for clinical reactions upon provocation with peanut in patients who have a consistent history of peanut allergy (Sampson 2001; Sampson and Ho 1997). Consideration of high concentrations of anti-peanut-IgE in patients with chronic alcohol consumption as hazardous may lead to a recommendation of avoidance and prescription of an emergency kit, although the IgE value is totally explained by binding to CCDs and is clinically of very little relevance. In this situation, the adverse effect that CCDs have on the specificity of laboratory diagnostics becomes very evident. Apart from the use of CCD screening tools to assess clinical relevance, a potential solution is the application of inhibition tests and/or the use of the CCD inhibitor.

The banana allergen β-1,3-glucanase (Mus a 5) is, along with the thaumatin-like protein, one of the components with highest IgE-binding capacity in banana extract; its in vivo potency, however, is minimal (Palacin et al. 2011). Mus a 5 is glycosylated. The fact that CCDs play a major role in the IgE-binding capacity of Mus a 5 accounts, in part, for the great difference between its in vitro and in vivo reactivity. Banana allergy is clinically important as this fruit is introduced very early in the diet of infants, and consumption by adults is also widespread. The banana is also of importance in the latex-fruit syndrome. A situation comparable to bananas was observed for other glycosylated allergens in foods of plant origin, such as the germin-like glycoprotein from orange (Cit s 1) (cited in Palacin et al. 2011).

Palacin et al. (2011) found patients with monosensitization to Mus a 5 and IgE-reactive peptide epitopes on Mus a 5; this is a further indication of its allergenic potency. Additionally, cross-reactivity via other allergenic plant β-1,3-glucanases, which are also N-glycosylated – such as Hev b 2 in natural rubber latex and Ole e 9 in olive pollen – could be relevant and so far unknown factors in cosensitization between plant-derived foods and pollen. However, both CCD and protein epitopes should be taken into account always. In general, most of the children with banana allergy have IgE antibodies to allergens from many different protein families, and a particularly large number is sensitized to CCDs.

Among the occupational immediate-type allergies, no clinical relevance has been shown for anti-CCD IgE in connection with allergy to wood dust inhalation (Kespohl et al. 2010) or to natural rubber latex (Raulf-Heimsoth et al. 2007). Moreover, CCDs do not generally appear to be relevant in "latex-fruit syndrome". However, there have been individual cases of clinically relevant cross-reaction between latex, kiwifruit, and banana (see below). In that they bind to CCDs, IgE antibodies specific for natural rubber latex are involved in reducing the specificity of IgE-detection assays with serum from patients with Hymenoptera venom allergy. Thus, individuals who had natural rubber latex-specific IgE owing to CCD specificity do in general not report allergic reactions to latex (Jappe, personal communication).

A Polish study included 81 workers (bakers, farmers, woodworkers, and health-care workers) with suspected occupationally related, allergic respiratory disease. In the study, identification of anti-CCD IgE in serum did not prove that the workers had developed true occupational allergic asthma. Rather, an independent sensitization to common inhalant allergens (such as tree and grass pollen) was the reason for the presence of IgE antibodies, and not the phenomenon of cross-reactivity itself (Wiszniewska et al. 2010). In a Spanish investigation of baker's asthma, patients with a high prevalence (35 %) of concomitant thiol proteases, and CCDs were, for the first time, identified as possible inducers of a wheat-kiwifruit cross-reaction (Palacin et al. 2008). The role CCDs play in wheat allergens – in the sensitization and severity of clinical symptoms among persons with occupational allergy to wheat flour – is yet to be clarified (Palacin et al. 2008; Sander et al. 2011).

Indications of possible biological activity of glycan moieties in certain allergens were provided by tests of cellular function. In the basophil activation test, trials with natural Lyc e 2 – a glycosylated allergen of tomato – were positive; the opposite was the case with recombinant Lyc e 2 which does not contain CCDs (Jappe and Raulf-Heimsoth 2007). There are other such examples where clinical relevance of CCD is predicted on the basis of the outcome of cellular functional diagnostics (Jappe and Raulf-Heimsoth 2007).

The limitation regarding clinical relevance is due not to the low binding affinity of anti-CCD IgE, but to the high affinity shown by IgG antibodies that act as blocking antibodies and inhibit the clinical activity of anti-CCD IgE. This IgG affinity is more important than the relative concentrations of these CCD-specific antibodies (Jin et al. 2008). There is also a hypothesis concerning tolerance toward CCDs, put forward in response to investigations of serum samples from beekeepers, of whom only 7.7 % had anti-CCD IgE. It was proposed that the high venom exposure caused by repeated bee stings induced tolerance to CCDs, as indicated by the presence of anti-CCD IgG antibodies in the majority of the serum samples (Carballada et al. 2011). Altmann (2007) proposed a model of natural glycoimmunotherapy, which states that all individuals develop a general tolerance to CCDs, mediated by IgG antibodies, through oral intake and inhalation, possibly on a daily basis, of various plant glycoproteins.

A special case would appear to be that of IgE-mediated reaction to mannitol, a hexitol added for various reasons to many drug preparations. Roncati et al. (2013) reported a fatality due to anaphylaxis occurring concurrently with the intravenous administration of 250 mg of thymoglobulin with mannitol as additive. The patient immediately developed anaphylaxis with cardiovascular failure and, despite maximal intervention, died. Postmortem examination revealed IgE antibodies to CCDs of the MUXF type, but not to natural rubber latex, and highly elevated serum tryptase levels indicating an allergic reaction. IgE-mediated reactions to mannitol were known, but none fatal until this case. Roncati et al. concluded that this individual's anti-CCD IgE antibodies were also directed against mannitol, and not against the active ingredient, anti-thymocyte globulin.

(*Note from the authors of this chapter*: Given the anti-CCD IgE to MUXF, it is unusual that the patient was anti-latex IgE negative. Mannitol itself is immunologically inert and hence unable alone to trigger an immune response (Hegde and Venkatesh 2007). Hedge et al. demonstrated the main properties of mannitol, reporting that only linking to a carrier protein induces mannitol-specific antibodies – although these are, unlike "classical" anti-CCD IgE antibodies, not very cross-reactive. The authors hypothesize that mannitol, being a hapten, can bind to autologous proteins in humans (*note from the authors of this chapter*) or possibly also to pharmacologically active proteins and thus can induce IgE antibodies with subsequent anaphylaxis.

6.8.2 Galactose-α-1,3-Galactose

The anti-α-gal-IgE-associated allergy to mammalian muscle and visceral meat is not limited to certain regions of the USA and Australia; it has also been observed in

France, Spain, and Germany (Jappe 2012, 2015). As well as the unusual occurrence of delayed anaphylaxis, it appears that those patients who have anti-α-gal IgE and milk allergy constitute a separate subgroup: α-gal-associated reactions to milk occur in children over the age of 5, many of whom do not have a history of food allergy, or, indeed, any allergy at all (Commins et al. 2009). A factor may be involved that differs from normal protein-based milk allergy.

α-Gal has also been detected in beef gelatin-based colloids. A study by Mullins et al. (2012) showed that most meat-allergic individuals had sensitization to gelatin; a subpopulation had clinical allergy to both. The authors posit anti-α-gal IgE as the cause of gelatin reactivity (Mullins et al. 2012).

In cases of α-gal-mediated meat allergy, it is important, when taking a history, to attempt to obtain correct information with regard to all foods (this may be difficult) and medications containing gelatin (colloids, vaccines, oral preparations with gelatin as a filler or a capsule component (Caponetto et al. 2013)). Patients should be warned to avoid consumption of gelatin-containing substances, but this will be very difficult to achieve in practice.

6.9 Conclusion: Implications for Everyday Clinical Practice

While the number of reports of the association between anti-α-gal IgE and severe and/or delayed reactions is growing, to the authors' knowledge no case has yet been reported in which clinical relevance could be clearly attributed to anti-CCD IgE. Respected allergists, however, believe that this may occur (Altmann 2010; Jappe et al. 2006).

Anti-CCD IgE antibodies can cause false-positive IgE results in various utilized complex allergen extracts as target antigens for IgE detection. The principal downside appears to be that of limiting diagnostic specificity. Thus, modifications need to be made in in vitro diagnostics to enhance specificity (◉ Fig. 6.3).

In individual cases, anti-CCD IgE antibodies seem to be associated with anaphylactic reactions, such as those to Hymenoptera stings and also to some foods.

References

Aalberse RC, Koshte V, Clemens JG. Immunoglobulin E antibodies that crossreact with vegetable foods, pollen, and hymenoptera venom. J Allergy Clin Immunol. 1981;68:356–64.

Aberer W, Holzweber F, Hemmer W, Koch L, Bokanovic S, Fellner W, Altmann F. Inhibition kreuzreaktiver Kohlenhydratdeterminanten (CCDs) erhöht die Treffsicherheit der In-vitro-Allergiediagnostik. Allergologie. 2014;37:45–53.

Adedoyin J, Grönlund H, Öman H, Johansson SGO, van Hage M. Cat IgA, representative of new carbohydrate cross-reactive allergens. J Allergy Clin Immunol. 2007;119:640–5.

Altmann F. The role of protein glycosylation in allergy. Int Arch Allergy Immunol. 2007; 142:99–115.

Altmann F. Basophil activation test is better but not good enough for the diagnosis of hymenoptera venom allergy: the problem of cross-reactive carbohydrate determinants. Clin Exp Allergy. 2010;40:1290–2.

Andrade MC, Menezes JS, Cassali GD, Martins-Filho OA, Cara DC, Faria AM. Alcohol-induced gastritis prevents oral tolerance induction in mice. Clin Exp Immunol. 2006;146:312–22.

Armentia A, Pineda F, Fernández S. Wine-induced anaphylaxis and sensitization to hymenoptera venom. N Engl J Med. 2007;357:719–20.

Caponetto P, Fischer J, Biedermann T. Gelatin-containing sweets can elicit anaphylaxis in a patient with sensitization to galactose-α-1,3-galactose. J Allergy Clin Immunol Pract. 2013;1:302–3.

Carballada FJ, Gonzalez-Quintela A, Nuñez R, Vidal C, Boquete M. Low prevalence of IgE to cross-reactive carbohydrate determinants in bee-keepers. J Allergy Clin Immunol. 2011; 128:1350–2.

Chung CH, Mirakhur B, Chan E, Le QT, Berlin J, Morse M, Murphy BA, Satinover SM, Hosen J, Mauro D, Slebos RJ, Zhou Q, Gold D, Hatley T, Hicklin DJ, Platts-Mills TA. Cetuximab-induced anaphylaxis and IgE specific for galactose-alpha-1,3-galactose. N Engl J Med. 2008;358:1109–17.

Commins SP, Satinover SM, Hosen J, Mozena J, Borish L, Lewis BD, Woodfolk JA, Platts-Mills TA. Delayed anaphylaxis, angioedema, or urticaria after consumption of red meat in patients with IgE antibodies specific for galactose-alpha-1,3-galactose. J Allergy Clin Immunol. 2009; 123:426–33.

Commins SP, Platts-Mills TA. Delayed anaphylaxis to red meat in patients with IgE specific for galactose alpha-1,3-galactose (α-GAL). Curr Allergy Asthma Rep. 2013;13:72–7.

Coutinho V, Vidal C, Garrido M, Gude F, Lojo S, Linneberg A, Gonzalez-Quintela A. Interference of cross-reactive carbohydrates in the determination of specific IgE in alcohol drinkers and strategies to minimize it: the example of latex. Ann Allergy Asthma Immunol. 2008;101:394–401.

Di Gennaro C, Biggi A, Barilli AL, Fasoli E, Carra N, Novarini A, Delsignore R, Montanari A. Endothelial dysfunction and cardiovascular risk profile in long-term withdrawing alcoholics. J Hypertens. 2007;25:367–73.

Garcia-Casado G, Sanchez-Monge R, Chrispeels MJ, Armentia A, Salcedo G, Gomez L. Role of complex asparagine-linked glycans in the allergenicity of plant glycoproteins. Glycobiology. 1996;6:471–7.

Gonzalez-Quintela A, Garrido M, Gude F, Campos J, Linneberg A, Lojo S, Vidal C. Sensitization to cross-reactive carbohydrate determinants in relation to alcohol consumption. Clin Exp Allergy. 2008;38:152–60.

González-Quintela A, Garrido M, Gude F, Campos J, Lojo S, Linneberg A, Vidal C. Discordant positive results of multiallergen immunoglobulin E tests in relation to crossreactive carbohydrate determinants and alcohol consumption. J Investig Allergol Clin Immunol. 2009;19:70–1.

Gonzalez-Quintela A, Valcarcel C, Campos J, Alonso M, Sanz ML, Vidal C. Biologic activity of cross-reactive carbohydrate determinants in heavy drinkers. Clin Exp Allergy. 2011;41:759–61.

Hamsten C, Starkhammar M, Tran TAT, Johansson M, Bengtsson U, Ahlen G, Sällberg M, Grönlund H, van Hage M. Identification of galactose-a-1,3-galactose in the gastrointestinal tract of the tick Ixodes ricinus; possible relationship with red meat allergy. Allergy. 2013;68:549–52.

Hegde VL, Venkatesh YP. Generation of antibodies specific to D-mannitol, a unique haptenic allergen, using reductively aminated d-mannose-bovine serum albumin conjugate as the immunogen. Immunobiology. 2007;212:119–28.

Heinz R, Waltenbaugh C. Ethanol consumption modifies dendritic cell antigen presentation in mice. Alcohol Clin Res. 2007;31:1759–71.

Holzweber F, Svehla W, Fellner W, Dalik T, Stubler S, Hemmer W, Altmann F. Inhibition of IgE binding to cross-reactive carbohydrate determinants enhances diagnostic selectivity. Allergy. 2013;68:1269–77.

Jappe U. Allergy to red meat. α-Gal: new epitope, new entity? Hautarzt. 2012;63:299–306.

Jappe U. Delayed anaphylaxis due to hidden food allergens. Allergologie. 2015;37:265–74.

Jappe U, Raulf-Heimsoth M, Hoffmann M, Burow G, Hübsch-Müller C, Enk A. In vitro hymenoptera venom allergy diagnosis: improved by screening for cross-reactive carbohydrate determinants and reciprocal inhibition. Allergy. 2006;61:1220–9.

Jappe U, Raulf-Heimsoth M. Allergologische In-vitro-Diagnostik und die kreuzreaktiven Kohlenhydratepitope. Allergo J. 2007;16:264–74.

Jappe U, Raulf-Heimsoth M. Kreuzreagierende Kohlenhydratdeterminanten (cross-reactive carbohydrate determinants, CCD) und ihre Bedeutung für die Allergiediagnostik. Allergologie. 2008;31:82–90.

Jappe U, Kreft B, Ludwig A, Przybilla B, Walker A, Biedermann T, Raulf-Heimsoth M, Sültz J, Becker WM, Petersen A. Aufbau und Anwendung eines sensitiven Verfahrens zum Nachweis von IgE-Antikörpern gegen das Kohlenhydratepitop Galactose-α-1,3-Galactose. Abstract Allergo J. 2011;20:33.

Jin C, Hantusch B, Hemmer W, Stadlmann J, Altmann F. Affinity of IgE and IgG against cross-reactive carbohydrate determinants on plant and insect glycoproteins. J Allergy Clin Immunol. 2008;121:185–90.

Kespohl S, Schlünssen V, Jacobsen G, Schaumburg I, Maryska S, Meurer U, Brüning T, Sigsgaard T, Raulf-Heimsoth M. Impact of cross-reactive carbohydrate determinants on wood dust sensitization. Clin Exp Allergy. 2010;40:1099–106.

Kespohl S, Kotschy-Lang N, Tomm JM, von Bergen M, Maryska S, Brüning T, Raulf-Heimsoth M. Occupational IgE-mediated softwood allergy: characterization of the causative allergen. Int Arch Allergy Immunol. 2012;157:202–8.

Linneberg A, Berg ND, Gonzalez-Quintela A, Vidal C, Elberling J. Prevalence of self-reported hypersensitivity symptoms following intake of alcoholic drinks. Clin Exp Allergy. 2008;38:145–51.

Malandain H. IgE-reactive carbohydrate epitopes – classification, cross-reactivity, and clinical impact. Eur Ann Allergy Clin Immunol. 2005;37:122–8.

Mullins RJ, James H, Platts-Mills TA, Commins S. Relationship between red meat allergy and sensitization to gelatin and galactose-α-1,3-galactose. J Allergy Clin Immunol. 2012;129:1334–42.

Palacin A, Quirce S, Sánchez-Monge R, Fernández-Nieto M, Varela J, Sastre J, Salcedo G. Allergy to kiwi in patients with baker's asthma: identification of potential cross-reactive allergens. Ann Allergy Asthma Immunol. 2008;101:200–5.

Palacin A, Quirce S, Sanchez-Monge R, Bobolea I, Diaz-Perales A, Martin-Muñoz F, Pascual C, Salcedo G. Sensitization profiles to purified plant food allergens among pediatric patients with allergy to banana. Pediatr Allergy Immunol. 2011;22:186–95.

Pastorello EA, Farioli L, Pravettoni V, Ortolani C, Fortunato D, Giuffrida MG, Perono Garoffo L, Calamari AM, Brenna O, Conti A. Identification of grape and wine allergens as an endochitinase 4, a lipid-transfer protein, and a thaumatin. J Allergy Clin Immunol. 2003;111:350–9.

Qian J, Liu T, Yang L, Daus A, Crowley R, Zhou Q. Structural characterization of N-linked oligosaccharides on monoclonal antibody cetuximab by the combination of orthogonal matrix-assisted laser desorption/ionization hybrid quadrupole-quadrupole time-of-flight tandem mass spectrometry and sequential enzymatic digestion. Anal Biochem. 2007;364:8–18.

Raulf-Heimsoth M, Rihs HP, Rozynek P, et al. Quantitative analysis of immunoglobulin E reactivity profiles in patients allergic or sensitized to natural rubber latex (*Hevea brasiliensis*). Clin Exp Allergy. 2007;37:1657–67.

Raulf-Heimsoth M, Rihs HP. Latexallergene: Sensibilisierungsquellen und Einzelallergenprofile erkennen. Allergo J. 2011;20:241–3.

van Ree R, Cabanes-Macheteau M, Akkerdaas J, Milazzo JP, Loutelier-Bourhis C, Rayon C, Villalba M, Koppelman S, Aalberse R, Rodriguez R, Faye L, Lerouge P. Beta(1,2)-xylose and alpha(1,3)-fucose residues have a strong contribution in IgE binding to plant glycoallergens. J Biol Chem. 2000;275:11451–8.

Roncati L, Barbolini G, Scacchetti AT, Busani S, Maiorana A. Unexpected death: anaphylactic intraoperative death due to thymoglobulin carbohydrate excipient. Forensic Sci Int. 2013; 228:e28–32.

Sampson HA, Ho D. Relationship between food-specific IgE-concentration and the risk of positive food challenges in children and adolescents. J Allergy Clin Immunol. 1997;100:444–51.

Sampson HA. Utility of food-specific IgE-concentrations in predicting symptomatic food allergy. J Allergy Clin Immunol. 2001;107:891–6.

Sander I, Rozynek P, Rihs HP, van Kampen V, Chew FT, Lee WS, Kotschy-Lang N, Merget R, Brüning T, Raulf-Heimsoth M. Multiple wheat flour allergens and cross-reactive carbohydrate determinants bind IgE in baker's asthma. Allergy. 2011;66:1208–15.

Serghini-Idrissi N, Ravier I, Aucouturier H, Ait Tahar H, Sonneville A. Food allergy in the chronic alcoholic and alcohol in food allergy: apropos of 38 cases. Allergy Immunol (Paris). 2001;33:378–82.

Takahashi H, Chinuki Y, Tanaka A, Morita E. Laminin γ-1 and collagen α-1 (VI) chain are galactose-α-1,3-galactose-bound allergens in beef. Allergy. 2014;69:199–207.

Untersmayr E, Jensen-Jarolim E. The role of protein digestibility and antacids on food allergy outcomes. J Allergy Clin Immunol. 2008;121:1301–8.

Vassilopoulou E, Zuidmeer L, Akkerdaas J, Tassios I, Rigby NR, Mills EN, van Ree R, Saxoni-Papageorgiou P, Papadopoulos NG. Severe immediate allergic reactions to grapes: part of a lipid transfer protein-associated clinical syndrome. Int Arch Allergy Immunol. 2007;143:92–102.

Vidal C, Vizcaino L, Díaz-Peromingo JA, Garrido M, Gomez-Rial J, Linneberg A, Gonzalez-Quintela A. Immunoglobulin-E reactivity to a glycosylated food allergen (peanuts) due to interference with cross-reactive carbohydrate determinants in heavy drinkers. Alcohol Clin Exp Res. 2009;33:1322–8.

Weber A, Schröder H, Thalberg K, März L. Specific interaction of IgE antibodies with a carbohydrate epitope of honey bee venom phospholipase A2. Allergy. 1987;42:464–70.

Wiszniewska M, Zgorzelska-Kowalik J, NowakowskaSwirta E, Palczynski C, Walusiak-Skorupa J. Cross – reactive carbohydrate determinants in diagnostics of occupational allergy – preliminary results. Allergy. 2010;65:664–6.

Part II

Test Systems, Singleplex Analysis and Multiplex Analysis

Molecular Allergy Diagnostics Using IgE Singleplex Assays: Methodological and Practical Considerations

7

J. Kleine-Tebbe, T. Jakob, and R.G. Hamilton

7.1 Introduction

7.1.1 Atopy and Allergen-Specific IgE

The number of atopic diseases, such as allergic rhinoconjunctivitis, allergic bronchial asthma, atopic eczema, and food allergies, has increased worldwide in recent years. Atopy is a genetic predisposition to develop IgE antibodies (IgE), against otherwise harmless, widely distributed environmental allergens. Once sensitized (IgE antibody positive), atopic individuals can develop the aforementioned atopic diseases following subsequent exposure to corresponding allergens.

The present chapter is based on, and modified from, an article by the authors that appeared in 2015 in *Allergo Journal International* (Kleine-Tebbe J, Jakob T: Molecular allergy diagnostics using IgE singleplex determinations: methodological and practical consideration for the use in clinical practice. Allergo J Int 2015;24:185–197. doi: 10.1007/s40629-015-0057-1).

J. Kleine-Tebbe, MD, Prof. (✉)
Allergy & Asthma Center Westend, Outpatient Clinic Hanf, Ackermann & Kleine-Tebbe, Berlin, Germany
e-mail: kleine-tebbe@allergie-experten.de

T. Jakob, MD, Prof.
Department of Dermatology and Allergology, University Medical Center Giessen (UKGM), Justus-Liebig-University, Giessen, Germany
e-mail: thilo.jakob@derma.med.uni-giessen.de

R.G. Hamilton, PhD, Prof.
Department of Medicine, Johns Hopkins University School of Medicine, Baltimore, MD, USA

Johns Hopkins Dermatology, Allergy and Clinical Immunology Reference Laboratory, Baltimore, MD, USA

Johns Hopkins Asthma and Allergy Center, Baltimore, MD, USA
e-mail: rhamilto@jhmi.edu

J. Kleine-Tebbe, T. Jakob (eds.), *Molecular Allergy Diagnostics*,
DOI 10.1007/978-3-319-42499-6_7

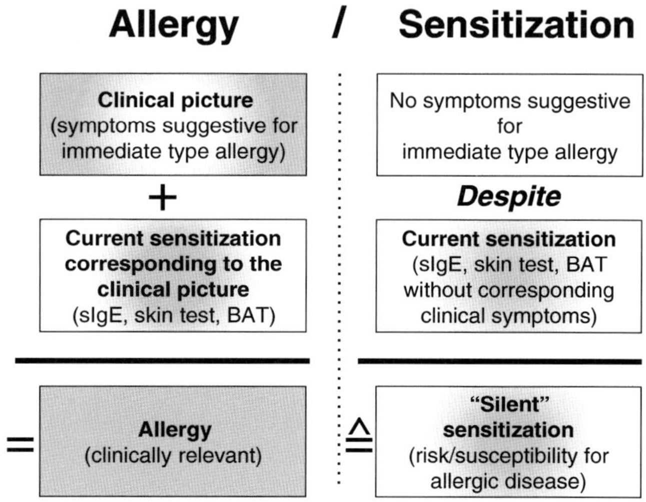

Fig. 7.1 Basic concept in allergy: Relationship between sensitization and clinically relevant allergy. One speaks of a clinically relevant allergy only when specific IgE triggers symptoms in a reproducible manner following allergen exposure. The detection of sIgE in the absence of clinical symptoms is consistent with a silent sensitization, which reveals a risk factor or susceptibility for allergic disease, but one that is not as yet manifested clinically. Abbreviations: BAT: basophil activation test; sIgE: allergen-specific IgE

Recent epidemiological studies have shown that 46.5 % of the adolescent population between the ages of 14 and 17 years (42 % of girls and 51 % of boys; Schmitz et al. 2013) and 48.6 % of the adult population (45 % of women and 52 % of men; Haftenberger et al. 2013) in Germany are sensitized with specific IgE to at least one allergen source (pollen, mites, animal dander, molds, and food).

Diagnostic tests that either directly or indirectly detect IgE antibodies in the context of an increased susceptibility to allergies (*sensitization*) are referred to as sensitization tests. In the presence of allergic symptoms that are consistent with IgE sensitization, one speaks of a *clinically relevant allergy* (⦿ Fig. 7.1). (Kleine-Tebbe and Jakob 2015)

7.1.2 IgE, IgE Receptors, and the Effector Phase of Allergic Reactions: Background Information and Relevance in IgE Antibody Diagnostics

As the least abundant human antibody, IgE was not discovered until 1966 [see Johansson (2011) for a historical summary]. Approximately half of IgE is found as free IgE in the vascular circulation, while the other half is bound by IgE receptors on a variety of cells. The high-affinity IgE receptor (FcεRI) on tissue-bound mast cells and circulating basophils is the most important binding partner (approximately 100,000–250,000 FcεRI/basophilic leukocyte; ⦿ Fig. 7.2) in immediate-type allergic reactions. Although free serum IgE has a half-life of only a few days,

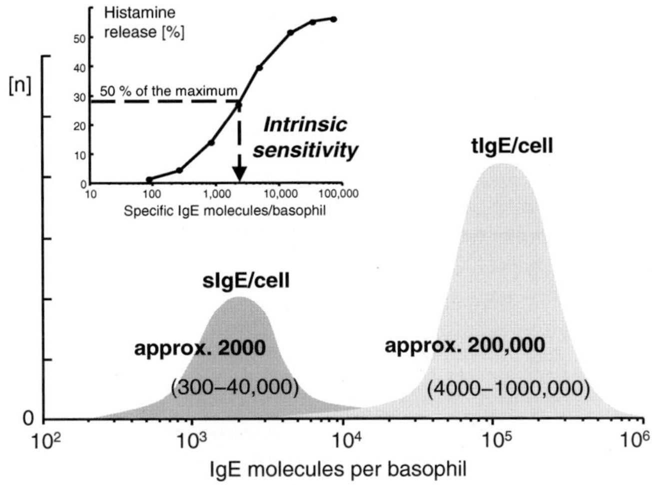

Fig. 7.2 Population-based FcεRI-bound IgE on effector cells. *Light gray area*, total bound IgE/cell (number of FcεRI occupied by IgE with population-based distribution) on basophilic leukocytes. *Dark gray area*, specific IgE/cell required for half-maximal cell activation (intrinsic sensitivity of basophils with population-based distribution). The distribution of both variables is approximately normal and can differ significantly; a fraction (approx. 1 %) of bound total IgE is sufficient for half-maximal allergen-specific activation. For this reason, the specific IgE to total IgE ratio is interesting in the interpretation. *n*: Frequency. *Inset top left*, individual mediator release as a function of cell-bound specific IgE; basis for the population-based normal distributions illustrated in the lower part of the figure

FcεRI-bound IgE persists for approximately 2 weeks due its slow off-rate. It takes approximately 2 months to remove the majority of cell-bound IgE by therapeutic biological drugs such as anti-IgE (omalizumab). Thus, it is not free but rather cell-bound IgE that is essential for the effector phase of the allergic reaction. Upon renewed allergen exposure, specific IgE antibodies are cross-linked, either in pairs or as a large aggregates. It takes an average of 2000 cross-linked IgE molecules to induce a half-maximal cell response (e.g., histamine release; ⦿ Fig. 7.2) only a fraction of total cell-bound IgE (200,000 molecules/basophil). For this reason, basophil tests have an extremely high analytical sensitivity. Phosphorylation of tyrosine kinases (e.g., Syk) activates intracellular signal cascades involving:

- Release of preformed mediators
- De novo synthesis of lipid mediators from the plasma membrane
- Production and release of cytokines

The activation status of effector cells is quantified by the expression of specific surface markers using flow cytometry; basophilic leukocytes from fresh blood are generally used, since they are easier to isolate (basophil activation test, BAT). (for review: Hoffmann et al. 2015).

It was possible to elucidate the effect of the individual IgE repertoire on the effector phase (basophil activation) using polyclonal synthetic Der p 2-specific IgE antibodies of varying epitope specificity and affinity (Christensen et al. 2008). The following variables have a significant effect on the dose-dependent activation of basophilic leukocytes:

- The total amount of cell-bound IgE.
- The ratio of specific IgE to total IgE (as little as 1 % is sufficient for half-maximal activation of effector cells, see above).
- The number of epitope-specific antibodies capable of binding to a defined allergen (clonality).
- The binding strength between individual IgE antibodies and the allergen (affinity).
- The total number of multivalent specific IgE binding sites that bind strongly to the allergen (avidity).
- The ratio of low- to high-affinity IgE antibodies directed to a defined allergen.

IgE stabilizes the continuously newly synthesized FcεRI receptors at the cell surface (MacGlashan et al. 2001). In this way, the level of total IgE passively regulates the number of its receptors and thus also the amount of cell-bound IgE (MacGlashan 2005). These relationships, which have been studied using basophils since the end of the 1990s, similarly apply to tissue-bound mast cells. The latter, with their cutaneous population (skin mast cells), form the basis for sensitization testing on skin (skin prick test, intradermal skin test). The complex variables involved (Kleine-Tebbe et al. 2006), besides the allergen-specific IgE level, explain why various sensitization tests (specific IgE, titrated skin test, dose-dependent BAT) correspond well qualitatively (concordance between positive or negative results) but not quantitatively (Purohit et al. 2005).

7.1.3 The IgE Repertoire: A Phenomenon with Complex Variables

The IgE synthesized by plasma cells is directed against (glyco)protein surface structures. The more alike and abundant the common binding sites (epitopes) are, the likelier it is that specific IgE will cross to allergens of similar structure—this is the basis of *cross-reactivity* or *cross-sensitization*.

Polyclonally produced IgE antibodies differ in terms of their binding strength (avidity/affinity) and recognition of specific epitopes (Lund et al. 2012). The resulting IgE repertoire, e.g., against *one* allergen molecule, is therefore made up of a multitude of antibodies with differing epitope specificity and binding strength. In the course of the immune response to an allergen, the repertoire can expand and the binding strength will increase through the recognition of further epitopes. To date, it has only been possible to investigate the variables described (epitope specificity, avidity, polyclonality) under experimental conditions, not in routine tests (Christensen et al. 2008). Thus, even modern quantitative singleplex tests for specific IgE determination using individual allergen molecules can recognize only the *total quantity of the polyclonal IgE response* ("the scale of the iceberg") in the best case, while additional parameters of the allergen-specific repertoire ("the number and height of the various tips of the iceberg") continue to remain hidden to routine diagnostics (Kleine-Tebbe 2012).

7.1.4 Techniques to Detect Sensitization in Routine Diagnostics

In routine diagnostics, sensitization tests serve to detect IgE either (⊙ Fig. 7.3):

- Directly
- Indirectly

The following methods are available to detect sensitization in IgE-mediated reactions and diseases (Matricardi et al. 2016):

1. Skin tests (skin prick testing, in selected cases intradermal testing; Bousquet et al. 2012; Worm et al. 2015)
2. Serum IgE determination (allergen-specific IgE, total IgE; Matricardi et al. 2016; Hamilton et al. 2016)

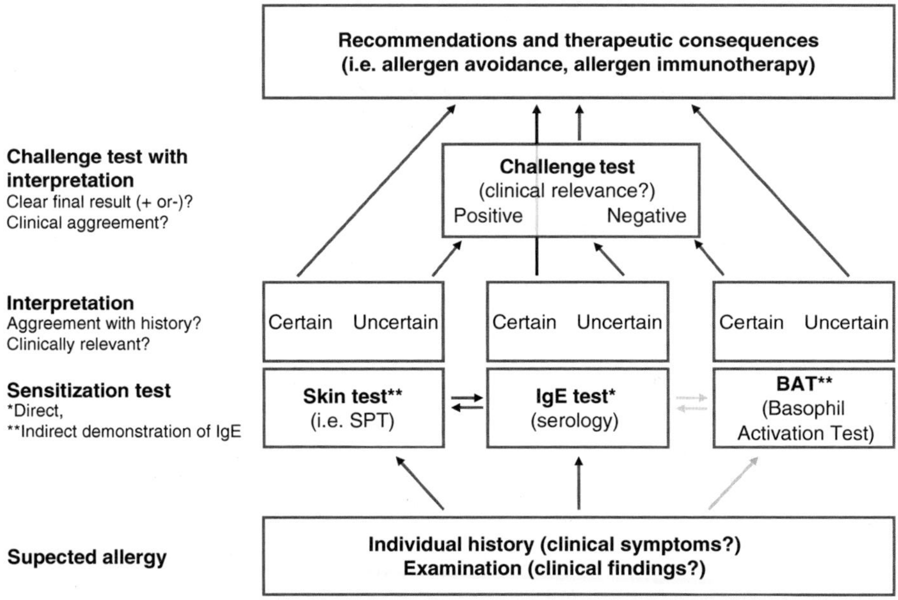

Fig. 7.3 Diagnostic algorithm in IgE-mediated allergies. Following collection of an allergy history and performance of an examination of the patient, their susceptibility risk for allergy (IgE sensitization) to potential allergen sources (e.g., pollen, mites, animal components, mold spores, food, insect venom) is evaluated. To this end, skin prick testing, followed by targeted allergen-specific IgE testing, is usually performed. In rare cases (*gray arrows*, e.g., negative skin prick test and specific IgE results in the case of low total IgE despite strong suspicion of an IgE-mediated reaction), cellular tests with basophil leukocytes, due to their extremely high analytical sensitivity (Kleine-Tebbe et al. 2006), represent an additional option to detect indirectly IgE sensitization. In the ideal case, sensitization tests agree well qualitatively (susceptibility to allergy: yes or no), but poorly on the quantitative level (how strongly positive?) due to additional cellular variables in skin and basophil tests for the indirect detection of IgE. Results are interpreted with reference to the previous clinical history and, in the case of good agreement with the patient history (reliable interpretation), form the basis for further treatment measures. In cases of doubt, challenge testing can help to determine the clinical relevance of IgE sensitizations

3. Basophil function tests (BAT and cellular antigen stimulation test, CAST) only in selected indications (Uyttebroek et al. 2014)

While serum IgE determination directly measures free IgE, the skin prick test and BAT yield indirect information on mast cell- and basophil-bound IgE. As such, they are comparable in terms of the diagnostic (qualitative) information they yield, even though there can be significant quantitative variation between results, particularly in the case of different allergen sources and due to the variables mentioned above (Purohit et al. 2005).

For historical reasons, skin prick testing with allergen extracts has become established as a common and robust screening method in routine practice (Bousquet et al. 2012; Worm et al. 2015). However, allergen molecules are easier to apply to laboratory assays than to in vivo testing (e.g., skin tests), since they are classified as a drug when used directly on humans and need to meet the stringent requirements associated with gaining market authorization for in vivo diagnostic agents of this kind. For this reason, allergen molecules are currently—and will probably remain—predominantly used in serological in vitro diagnostics.

7.2 Technological Basis of IgE Determination

Solid-phase immunoassays for the routine diagnosis of specific IgE have been available since the early 1970s. Initially, radioimmunological methods (radioallergosorbent test, RAST) consisted of coupling allergen extracts to activated paper disks in order to bind specific IgE from the sera of allergy sufferers. Today, measurements are no longer red by means of a radioactive tag, but rather by means of enzyme labeling or fluorimetry; moreover, allergenic molecules are also increasingly used in this context (⊙ Table 7.1 provides a selection of single allergens available for singleplex IgE analysis).

7.2.1 Test Design and Test Components

Modern immunoassays to determine allergen-specific IgE antibodies (overview in ⊙ Table 7.2) comprise the following components (Hamilton et al. 2016; Matricardi et al. 2016):

(a) Reaction vessel: plastic (polyethylene) or glass test tubes, plastic microtiter plate with wells, plastic rods or pellets, polyethylene cap with spongelike matrix
(b) Allergen-containing reagent: allergen adsorbed to a solid phase or labeled allergen in the liquid phase
(c) Anti-IgE-Fc antibody (detection antibody specific to the constant Fc fragment of IgE)
(d) Calibration system: e.g., reference serum with defined IgE volume in order to generate a total IgE calibration curve

Table 7.1 Single allergens available for allergen-specific IgE determination using a singleplex assay

Allergen source	Allergen[a]	Protein family/function	Relevance in clinical diagnostics
Tree pollen (see ▶ Chap. 10 for more details)			
Birch	**rBet v 1**	PR-10	Major allergen, marker for sensitization to birch pollen and the Fagales group (alder, hazel, beech, oak), varying cross-reactivity with other members of the PR-10 proteins, e.g., in birch pollen-related food allergy
Birch	**rBet v 2**	Profilin	Minor allergen, Cross-reactive allergen, indicator of cross-reactivity with other profilins in tree, grass, or weed pollen or plant-based foods
Birch	**rBet v 4**	Polcalcin	Minor allergen, Cross-reactive allergen, indicator of cross-reactivity with other polcalcins in tree, grass, or weed pollen
Plane (maple-leaved)	**rPla a 1**	Invertase inhibitor	Major allergen, marker for sensitization to plane pollen
Olive tree	**rOle e 1**	Oleaceae group 1	Major allergen, marker for sensitization to olive and ash pollen and other members of the Lamiales (lilac, privet)
Cypress (Arizona)	**nCup a 1**	Pectate lyase	Major allergen, marker for sensitization to cypress, cedar, and juniper; IgE reactivity can be partially based on reactivity to the CCD component
Grass pollen (see ▶ Chap. 10 for more details)			
Meadow foxtail	**nCyn d 1**	Grass group 1	Major allergen, marker for sensitization to meadow foxtail pollen and other grass pollens of the Chlorideae subfamily; IgE reactivity can be partially based on reactivity to the CCD component
Timothy grass	**rPhl p 1**	Grass group 1	Major allergen, marker for sensitization to timothy grass pollen and all other grass pollens (Poaceae)
Timothy grass	**rPhl p 2**	Grass group 2	Minor allergen, marker for sensitization to timothy grass pollen and other grass pollens of the Pooideae subfamily (e.g., rye, smooth meadow grass, rye grass)
Timothy grass	**rPhl p 4**	Berberine bridge enzyme	Minor allergen, marker for sensitization to timothy pollen and other grass pollens; IgE reactivity can be partially based on reactivity to the CCD component
Timothy grass	**rPhl p 5**	Unknown	Major allergen, marker for sensitization to timothy pollen and other grass pollens of the Pooideae subfamily (e.g., rye, smooth meadow grass, rye grass)

(continued)

Table 7.1 (continued)

Allergen source	Allergen[a]	Protein family/function	Relevance in clinical diagnostics
Timothy grass	**rPhl p 6**	Unknown	Minor allergen, marker for sensitization to timothy grass and other grass pollens of the Pooideae subfamily (e.g., rye, smooth meadow grass, rye grass)
Timothy grass	**rPhl p 7**	Polcalcin	Minor allergen, Cross-reactive allergen, indicator of cross-reactivity with other polcalcins in tree, grass, or weed pollen
Timothy grass	**rPhl p 12**	Profilin	Minor allergen, Cross-reactive allergen, indicator of cross-reactivity with other profilins in tree, grass, or weed pollen or plant-based foods
Weed pollen (see ▶ Chap. 11 for more details)			
Mugwort	**nArt v 1**	Defensin-like protein	Major allergen, marker for sensitization to mugwort pollen
Mugwort	**nArt v 3**	nsLTP	Major allergen, marker for sensitization to mugwort pollen, Cross-reactive allergen, indicator of potential cross-reactivity with other members of the LTP family, e.g., in mugwort pollen-associated food allergy
Wall pellitory	**rPar j 2**	nsLTP	Major allergen, marker for sensitization to wall pellitory pollen, Cross-reactive allergen, indicator of potential cross-reactivity with other members of the LTP family
Tumbleweed	**nSal k 1**	Pectin methyl esterase	Major allergen, marker allergen for sensitization to tumbleweed pollen
Ribwort	**rPla l 1**	Trypsin inhibitor	Major allergen, marker allergen for sensitization to ribwort pollen
Ragweed (*Ambrosia artemisiifolia*)	**nAmb a 1**	Pectate lyase	Major allergen, marker allergen for sensitization to ragweed pollen (*Ambrosia*)
Legume allergens (see ▶ Chap. 12 for more details)			
Peanut	**rAra h 1**	7S globulin (vicilin)	Marker allergen, indicator of high-risk sensitization
Peanut	**rAra h 2**	2S albumin (conglutin)	Marker allergen, indicator of high-risk sensitization
Peanut	**rAra h 3**	11S globulin (glycinin)	Marker allergen, indicator of high-risk sensitization
Peanut	rAra h 6	2S albumin (conglutin)	Marker allergen, indicator of high-risk sensitization
Peanut	**rAra h 8**	PR-10 protein (Bet v 1 homolog)	Cross-reactive allergen, cross-reactivity generally caused by Bet v 1 sensitization, no high-risk sensitization
Peanut	**rAra h 9**	nsLTP	Cross-reactive allergen, indicator of cross-reactivity with other nsLTPs
Soybean	**rGly m 4**	PR-10 protein (Bet v 1 homolog)	Cross-reactive allergen, cross-reactivity generally caused by Bet v 1 sensitization, local oropharyngeal reactions common, severe local or systemic reactions in isolated cases

Soybean	**Gly m 5**	7S globulin	Marker allergen, indicator of high-risk sensitization
Soybean	**Gly m 6**	11S globulin	Marker allergen, indicator of high-risk sensitization
Soybean	**rGly m 8** (from 2016)	2S albumin	Marker allergen, indicator of high-risk sensitization
Nut allergens (see ▶ Chap. 13 for more details)			
Hazelnut	**rCor a 1.0401**	PR-10 protein (Bet v 1 homolog)	Cross-reactive allergen, cross-reactivity generally caused by Bet v 1 sensitization, no high-risk sensitization, severe clinical reactions uncommon
Hazelnut	**rCor a 8**	nsLTP	Cross-reactive allergen, moderate indicator of cross-reactivity with other nsLTPs
Hazelnut	**Cor a 9**	11S globulin	Marker allergen, indicator of high-risk sensitization
Hazelnut	**rCor a 14**	2S albumin	Marker allergen, indicator of high-risk sensitization
Cashew nut	rAna o 2	11S globulin	Marker allergen, indicator of high-risk sensitization
Brazil nut	**rBer e 1**	2S albumin	Marker allergen, indicator of high-risk sensitization
Walnut	**Jug r 1**	2S albumin	Marker allergen, indicator of high-risk sensitization
Walnut	Jug r 2	7S globulin	Marker allergen, indicator of high-risk sensitization
Walnut	**Jug r 3**	nsLTP	Cross-reactive allergen, indicator of cross-reactivity with other nsLTPs
Fruit and vegetable allergens (see ▶ Chap. 14 for more details)			
Apple	**rMal d 1**	PR-10 protein	Cross-reactive allergen, varying cross-reactivity with other members of the PR-10 proteins, e.g., in birch pollen-associated food allergy
Apple	**rMal d 3**	nsLTP	Marker allergen, cross-reactivity with other nsLTPs, indicator of high-risk sensitization
Carrot	Dau c 1	PR-10 protein	Cross-reactive allergen, varying cross-reactivity with other members of the PR-10 proteins, e.g., in birch pollen-associated food allergy, also potential high-risk sensitization
Carrot	Dau c 4	Profilin	Cross-reactive allergen, high cross-reactivity with other profilins
Carrot	Dau c 5	Isoflavone reductase	
Celery	**Api g 1**	PR-10 protein	Cross-reactive allergen, varying cross-reactivity with other members of the PR-10 proteins, e.g., in birch pollen-associated food allergy, also potential high-risk sensitization
Celery	Api g 10	nsLTP	Marker allergen, cross-reactivity with other nsLTPs, indicator of high-risk sensitization

(continued)

Table 7.1 (continued)

Allergen source	Allergen[a]	Protein family/function	Relevance in clinical diagnostics
Kiwi	Act d 1	Actinidin (cysteine protease)	Marker allergen for primary kiwi sensitization, indicator of high-risk sensitization
Kiwi	Act d 2	Thaumatin-like protein	Minor allergen, potential systemic reactions due to stability to digestion
Kiwi	Act d 5	Kiwellin	Major allergen, marker allergen for primary kiwi sensitization, indicator of high-risk sensitization
Kiwi	**Act d 8**	PR-10 protein	Cross-reactive allergen, varying cross-reactivity with other members of the PR-10 proteins, e.g., in birch pollen-associated food allergy
Peach	**Pru p 1**	PR-10 protein	Cross-reactive allergen, varying cross-reactivity with other members of the PR-10 proteins, e.g., in birch pollen-associated food allergy
Peach	**Pru p 3**	nsLTP	Marker allergen, cross-reactivity with other nsLTPs, indicator of high-risk sensitization, particularly in the Mediterranean region
Peach	**Pru p 4**	Profilin	Cross-reactive allergen, high cross-reactivity with other profilins
Wheat allergens and other food allergens in FDEIA (see ▶ Chap. 15 for more details)			
Wheat	**rTri a 14**	LTP	Minor allergen, Cross-reactive allergen with other LPTs
Wheat	**rTri a 19**	ω-5-Gliadin	Major allergen, marker allergen for WDEIA
Wheat	nTri a 21	α/β-Gliadin	Major allergen, marker allergen for WDEIA
Wheat	nTri a 26	HMW glutenin	Major allergen, marker allergen for WDEIA
Wheat	rTri a 36	LMW glutenin GluB3-23	Major allergen, marker allergen for WDEIA
Wheat	nTri a γ-Gliadin	γ-Gliadin	Major allergen, marker allergen for WDEIA
Wheat	**nGliadin**	α/βγ/ω-Gliadin	Major allergens, marker allergens for WDEIA
Shrimp	**rPen a 1**	Tropomyosin	Major allergen, marker allergen for sensitization to crustaceans, N.B. high cross-reactivity with tropomyosin from other sources
Soy	**rGly m 5**	β-Conglycinin	Marker allergen for genuine soy sensitization
Peach	**rPru p 3**	nsLTP	Marker allergen for peach sensitization, cross-reactivity with various other nsLTPs
Meat (red), innards	**α-Gal**	Galactose-α-1,3-galactose	Marker allergen for delayed meat allergy

Insect venom (see ▶ Chap. 16 for more details)			
Honey bee	**rApi m 1**	Phospholipase A_2	Major allergen, marker for bee venom sensitization
Honey bee	**rApi m 2**	Hyaluronidase	Minor allergen, marker for bee venom sensitization, cross-reactivity with hyaluronidase of wasp venom (Ves v 2) possible
Honey bee	**rApi m 3** (from 2016)	Acid phosphatase	Major allergen, marker for bee venom sensitization
Honey bee	nApi m 4	Melittin	Minor allergen, marker for bee venom sensitization
Honey bee	**rApi m 5** (from 2016)	Vitellogenin	Major allergen, Cross-reactive allergen, cross-reactivity with vitellogenin of wasp venom Ves v 3
Honey bee	**rApi m 10** (from 2015)	Icarapin	Major allergen, marker for bee venom sensitization
Wasp	**rVes v 1**	Phospholipase A_1	Major allergen, marker for wasp venom sensitization
Wasp	rVes v 2	Hyaluronidase	Minor allergen, Cross-reactive allergen, most cross-reactivity with bee venom hyaluronidase (Api m 2)
Wasp	rVes v 3	Vitellogenin	Minor allergen, Cross-reactive allergen, cross-reactivity with bee venom vitellogenin (Api m 5)
Wasp	**rVes v 5**	Antigen 5	Major allergen, marker for wasp venom sensitization
Paper wasp	**rPol d 5**	Antigen 5	Major allergen, marker for paper wasp sensitization, high cross-reactivity with other antigen-5 allergens such as Ves v 5
Animal dander (see ▶ Chap. 17 for more details)			
Cat	**rFel d 1**	Uteroglobin	Major allergen, marker for sensitization to cat dander
Cat	**nFel d 2**	Serum albumin	Minor allergen, Cross-reactive allergen, indicator of cross-reactivity with other animal danders
Cat	**rFel d 4**	Lipocalin	Minor allergen, Cross-reactive allergen, cross-reactivity with other lipocalins (e.g., Can f 6 or Equ c 1)
Dog	**rCan f 1**	Lipocalin	Marker for sensitization to dog dander
Dog	**rCan f 2**	Lipocalin	Marker for sensitization to dog dander
Dog	**nCan f 3**	Serum albumin	Cross-reactive allergen, indicator of cross-reactivity with other animal danders and components

(continued)

Table 7.1 (continued)

Allergen source	Allergen[a]	Protein family/function	Relevance in clinical diagnostics
Dog	**rCan f 5**	Arginine esterase	Marker for sensitization to dog dander
Horse	**rEqu c 1**	Lipocalin	Major allergen, marker for sensitization to horse dander, cross-reactivity with other lipocalins (e.g., Can f 6 or Fel d 4)
Horse	rEqu c 3	Serum albumin	Minor allergen, Cross-reactive allergen, cross-reactivity with other lipocalins (e.g., Can f 6 or Equ c 1)
Animal food allergens			
Hen's egg	**Gal d 1**	Ovomucoid	Major allergen and marker allergen for chicken egg sensitization, associated with persistent chicken egg allergy
Hen's egg	**Gal d 2**	Ovalbumin	Marker allergen for hen's egg sensitization
Hen's egg	**Gal d 3**	Conalbumin/ovotransferrin	Marker allergen for hen's egg sensitization
Hen's egg	Gal d 5	Livetin/serum albumin	Allergen in egg yolk and chicken meat, indicator of bird egg syndrome
Cow's milk	**Bos d 4**	α-Lactalbumin	Major allergen (whey protein) in cow's milk
Cow's milk	**Bos d 5**	β-Lactoglobulin	Major allergen (whey protein) in cow's milk
Cow's milk	Bos d 6	Serum albumin	Minor allergen, Cross-reactive allergen, indicator of cross-reactivity with other albumins in animal dander or (uncooked) meat
Cow's milk	**Bos d 8**	Casein	Major allergen in cow milk and cheese, cross-reactions with sheep and goat milk products
Fish allergens (see ▶ Chap. 18 for more details)			
Cod	**rGad c 1**	Parvalbumin	Major allergen, Cross-reactive allergen, high cross-reactivity with parvalbumins from various fish species
Carp	**rCyp c 1**	Parvalbumin	Major allergen, Cross-reactive allergen, high cross-reactivity with parvalbumins from various fish species
House dust mites (see ▶ Chap. 19 for more details)			
House dust mite	**rDer p 1**	Cysteine protease	Major allergen, marker for sensitization to house dust mites
House dust mite	**rDer p 2**	NPC2 family	Major allergen, marker for sensitization to house dust mites
House dust mite	**rDer p 10**	Tropomyosin	Minor allergen, Cross-reactive allergen, indicator of cross-reactivity with tropomyosin from crustaceans, cockroaches
House dust mite	rDer p 23	Chitin-binding protein	Major allergen, marker for sensitization to house dust mites

Mold (see ▶ Chap. 21 for more details)			
Alternaria alternata	**rAlt a 1**	Unknown function	Marker for sensitization to outside air mold *Alternaria*
Aspergillus fumigatus	**rAsp f 1**	Enolase	Marker for sensitization to *Aspergillus fumigatus*
Aspergillus fumigatus	**rAsp f 2**	Mitogillin	Marker for sensitization to *Aspergillus fumigatus*, evidence of allergic bronchopulmonary aspergillosis (ABPA) in conjunction with positive values for Asp f 2, 4, 6
Aspergillus fumigatus	**rAsp f 3**	Fibrinogen-binding protein	Marker for sensitization to *Aspergillus fumigatus*
Aspergillus fumigatus	**rAsp f 4**	Peroxisomal protein	Marker for sensitization to *Aspergillus fumigatus*, evidence of allergic bronchopulmonary aspergillosis (ABPA) in conjunction with positive values for Asp f 2, 4, 6
Aspergillus fumigatus	**rAsp f 6**	Mn-superoxide dismutase	Marker for sensitization to *Aspergillus fumigatus*, evidence of allergic bronchopulmonary aspergillosis (ABPA) in conjunction with positive values for Asp f 2, 4, 6
Latex (see ▶ Chap. 22 for more details)			
Latex	**rHev b 1**	Rubber elongation factor	Marker for latex sensitization, major allergen for patients with spina bifida
Latex	**rHev b 3**	Small rubber particle protein	Marker for latex sensitization, major allergen for patients with spina bifida
Latex	**rHev b 5**	Unknown	Marker for latex sensitization, major allergen for patients with spina bifida and healthcare personnel
Latex	**rHev b 6.01**	Hevein precursor	Marker for latex sensitization, major allergen for healthcare personnel
Latex	**rHev b 8**	Profilin	Cross-reactive allergen, indicator of cross-reactivity with other profilins in tree, grass, and weed pollen or plant-based foods

[a]**Boldface**: available as singleplex assays for IgE determinations

Table 7.2 Various test principles for determining specific IgE antibodies in a singleplex assay

IgE assay format	Short description	Advantages	Disadvantages
Solid-phase assay	Solid-phase assays for IgE determination have been established for many years. The allergens coupled to a solid phase directly bind all allergen-specific antibodies (e.g., IgE, IgG); washing removes unbound antibodies. The bound specific IgE antibodies are then determined using radiolabeled anti-IgE antibodies. The latter are marked with suitable reagents (fluorescence, chemiluminescence) and substrates that enable quantification of bound specific IgE antibodies	In the case of a large surface area of the solid phase used and surplus allergens/allergen sources, complete binding of all specific IgE antibodies is possible (prerequisite of true quantitation) However, low-affinity IgE antibodies are also bound	In the case of low surface area of the solid phase (e.g., paper disk) and no surplus allergens/allergen sources, true quantitation of specific IgE is not possible and competitive inhibition of the IgE signal by allergen-specific IgG antibodies occurs (particularly in high titers, e.g., after allergen-specific immunotherapy)
Liquid-phase assay	This test format involves the use of liquid and labeled allergens to bind allergen-specific IgE. Following the appropriate washing procedure, the allergen–IgE marker complexes are bound by immobilized reagents (e.g., the biotin–streptavidin system). The use of appropriate substrates likewise enables quantitation of primarily bound specific IgE on the allergens used	Rapid binding kinetics due to the liquid phase	True quantitation of specific IgE not possible in the absence of surplus allergens/allergen sources
Reverse IgE assay	With this test system, all IgE antibodies (e.g., contained in serum) are bound by immobilized anti-IgE antibodies in a first step. Following the removal of unbound antibodies (e.g., IgG), allergen-specific IgE can be identified by adding appropriately labeled liquid allergens. By labeling the allergens, it is possible to quantify specific bound antibodies	No inhibition caused by the high proportion of allergen-specific IgG antibodies	Limited binding capacity particularly in the case of extremely high total IgE (>2000 kU/l)

(e) Reaction buffer: mineral- and protein-containing solutions for constant pH values and constant protein matrix to ensure minimal nonspecific binding
(f) Human serum with specific IgE antibodies and negative serum controls
(g) Data processing system (software or algorithm)

The *allergen-containing reagent* (b) is considered the most complex component of the test materials, irrespective of whether extracts of biological origin or single defined allergen molecules are involved.

The second and equally important component is the *anti-IgE reagent* (c), generated either polyclonally in various animal hosts (rabbit, goat, horse) or as monoclonal mouse antibodies with defined binding to epitopes on the Fc region of human IgE antibodies. Monoclonal and polyclonal antibodies to IgE are often used in combination in order to achieve parallelism and linearity in the test system over a broad concentration range.

The *calibration system* (d) is the third key component of IgE determination. Since there are no internationally accepted standards for allergen-specific IgE tests, a total IgE calibration curve enables the units measured to be expressed as quantitative allergen-specific IgE antibody levels (⦿ Fig. 7.4): kU_A/l (where "A" stands for "allergen specific," thereby distinguishing units from the internationally standardized kU/l = IU/ml for total IgE determination). The randomly assigned "classes" that have evolved over time serve to semiquantitatively and broadly categorize IgE concentrations and, in the authors' view, play only a minor role today. The test systems currently available, as well as their test principles, are shown in ⦿ Table 7.2.

7.2.2 Detection Thresholds in sIgE Determination

The lower detection threshold limit for specific IgE was formerly 0.35 kU_A/l. The analytical sensitivity of IgE assays is now enhanced thanks to more sensitive calibration and improved resolution of low IgE values. Thus, modern specific IgE antibody immunoassays now produce values below 0.35 down to 0.1 kU_A/l (⦿ Fig. 7.4). This range is particularly informative and relevant when total IgE is extremely low (<20 kU/l). The upper detection limit is 100 kU_A/l for most specific

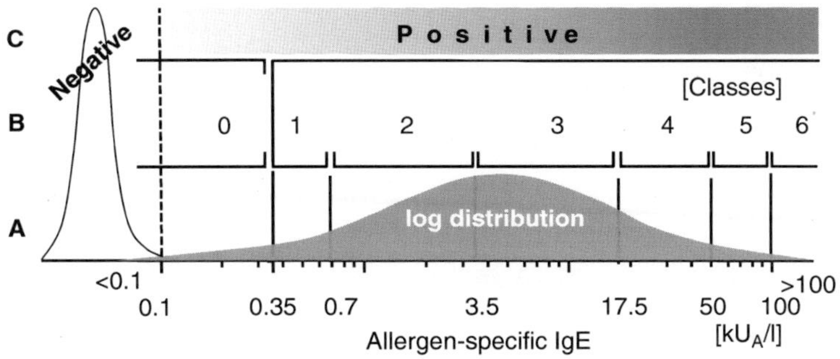

Fig. 7.4 Options for the evaluation of logarithmically distributed allergen-specific IgE levels. *A* quantitative, *B* semiquantitative (in the German Medical Association guidelines, this term is no longer used; specific IgE levels given in classes are considered as qualitative evaluations), *C* qualitative. Allergen-specific IgE levels expressed as units of specific IgE, kU_A/l (*A* stands for allergen specific), using WHO standards for total IgE determination (heterologous calibration). *white area under the curve*, population of serum samples with no allergen-specific IgE (levels fall below the detection limit of 0.1 kU_A/l). *Dark gray area*, population of positive serum samples with logarithmic (hypothetically normal) distribution of allergen-specific IgE levels above the detection limit of 0.1 kU_A/l

IgE detection methods. Therefore, sera with higher specific IgE levels should be measured in a diluted form (1:10) in order to determine the actual value after multiplying ×10.

7.2.3 Specific IgE–Total IgE Ratio

A number of modern assays have shown that the unit for total IgE (kU/l) corresponds to the heterologously calibrated units for allergen-specific IgE (kU_A/l) (Kober and Perborn 2006). Working on this assumption, both variables, specific and total IgE, can be directly compared and used to improve interpretation (Hamilton et al. 2010) The ratio of specific IgE to total IgE (also referred to as *antibody-specific activity*; Hamilton et al. 2010) is given particular significance in the case of:

- Extremely low total IgE levels (e.g., <20 kU/l), for instance, in:
  - Some atopic patients with unusually low total serum IgE levels
  - Non-atopic patients with IgE sensitization to particular allergens, e.g., insect venom or occupational allergens
- Extremely high total IgE levels, for instance, in:
  - Atopic patients with currently or previously manifest atopic dermatitis
  - Patients with other causes of extremely high total IgE such as allergic bronchopulmonary aspergillosis (Renz et al. 2010)

It is important to bear in mind that normal distribution of IgE is not linear, but rather logarithmic, and thus it needs to be represented using a logarithmic scale (⊙ Fig. 7.4).

The ratio of specific IgE to total IgE in serum is found in the same way on effector cells (mast cells, basophils). If specific IgE is given relative (e.g., in percent) to total IgE (see ⊙ Fig. 7.5 for a more detailed explanation) (Hamilton et al. 2010), the values relating to individual total IgE levels are normalized: By taking this step, one can expect better concordance between the relative specific IgE proportion (in percent) and the quantitative analysis of other sensitization tests (skin prick test, BAT).

7.2.4 Isoforms: Natural Variants of Allergen Molecules

Points of criticism on the use of allergen molecules relate to their origin or production:

When derived from natural sources, even defined allergens are variable mixtures with multiple molecule variants (isoforms), which bind IgE with varying strength depending on the individual IgE repertoire. Mixing isoforms potentially has the advantage of covering all IgE specificities; however, complex mixtures of this kind are challenging to purify and standardize.

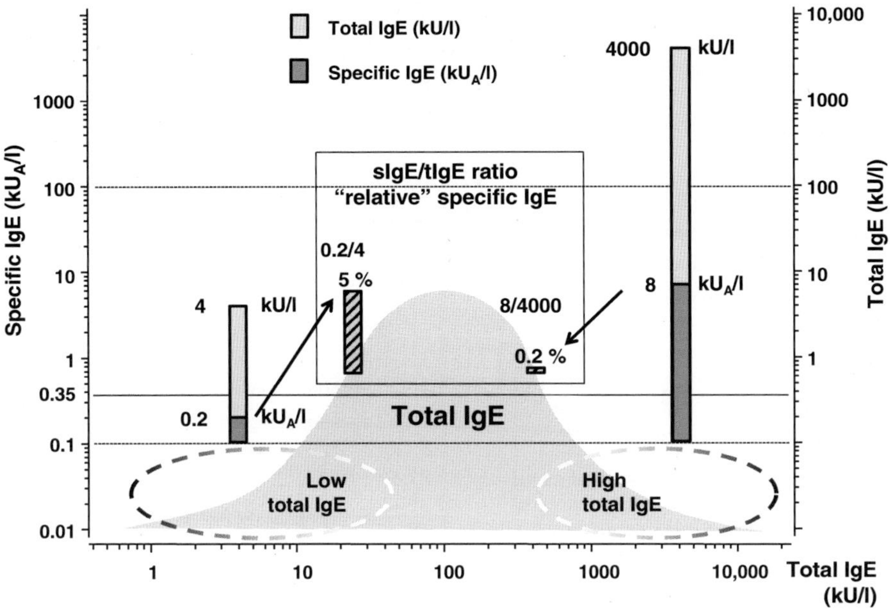

Fig. 7.5 Significance of the total and specific immunoglobulin E ratio. Due to the variability of total IgE levels, logarithmically distributed specific IgE (*dark gray bars*) can also be expressed as a relative quantity of total IgE (*light gray bars*) (Hamilton et al. 2010). This process "normalizes" specific IgE to total IgE on a percentage basis (*hatched bars*). Primarily the borderline cases (see numerical examples) with particularly low (normal distribution curve, far left) or extremely high total IgE (normal distribution curve, far right) make it clear that specific IgE can only be correctly interpreted once total IgE is known. This ratio of specific to total IgE is also found on the surface of effector cells (mast cells, basophil granulocytes), thereby providing the basis for diagnostic ex vivo (basophil activation test, BAT) and in vivo tests (skin prick test, provocation test)

Therefore, allergen molecules are predominantly used in recombinant form for molecular IgE diagnostics (Matricardi et al. 2016). This presupposes the selection of a representative isoform that determines as many (ideally all) specific IgE antibodies to the allergen in question. A further condition is correct protein folding that corresponds to the natural allergen. If both these prerequisites are fulfilled, the quality of this type of reagent can be considerably better controlled by means of process-integrated standardization.

7.3 Possible Applications for Allergen Molecules in IgE Diagnostics

Serological in vitro diagnosis can be modified in different ways using single allergens (⦿ Fig. 7.6):

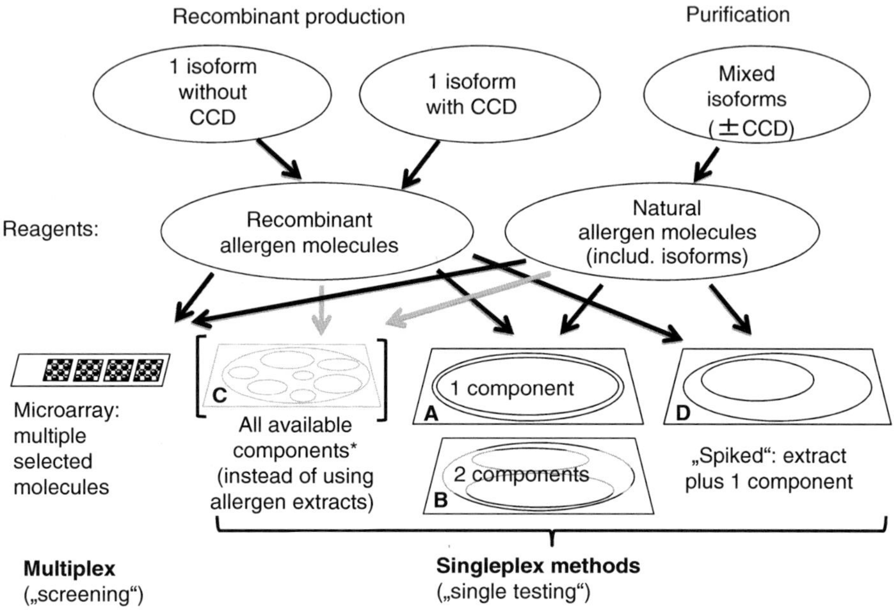

Fig. 7.6 Selection and application of allergen molecules for diagnostic purposes. *A*, *B*, *C*, and *D*: Variants of the test system for IgE singleplex assays (singleplex) using purified or recombinantly produced single allergens.

(a) Allergen molecules are used individually as reagents for specific IgE determination (currently the most frequent application).
(b) Selected allergens are combined as reagents for specific IgE determination (combination of important marker allergens, such as Phl p 1 and Phl p 5, or cross-reactive allergens such as Phl p 7 and Phl p 12).
(c) All available individual components of an allergen source can be used as a mix instead of a complex allergen extract (theoretically possible, but not yet implemented due to complexity, costs, and questionable use).
(d) Individual components can be added to allergen extracts ("spiking") to increase assay sensitivity (e.g., in the case of underrepresented components) (▸ Chap. 8).

Variant (a) enables the targeted and precise differentiation of sensitizations by means of single allergens. This procedure has also known as component-specific or component-resolved diagnostics (CRD) (Valenta et al. 1999) and currently plays the largest role in molecular allergy diagnostics (typical case studies in Kleine-Tebbe and Jappe 2014).

7.3.1 Distinction Between Purified and Recombinantly Produced Components

An important crossroads for the manufacturers of diagnostic products is the decision whether to use purified natural single allergens with all their variants (isoforms) or whether to select a single, recombinantly produced protein.

The latter should be representative and have the major IgE binding sites in order to be able to cover, as far as possible, all allergy sufferers sensitized to this allergen molecule.

This problem does not apply when natural components are used, since these generally contain all molecule variants occurring in natural allergen sources. It is only important to ensure here that the preparations do not contain any impurities with other allergens. This is particularly challenging if the allergen to be purified is available in very small quantities in the allergen source, while other allergens are present in high concentrations. A typical example would be allergens in bee venom (Api m 3, Api m 5, and Api m 10), which are present at less than 1 % of the venom dry weight, while Api m 4 (melittin), with more than 40 % of the venom dry weight, render clean purification of the abovementioned allergens virtually impossible.

Another problem with purified natural allergens is encountered when glycoproteins with N-glycan sugar side chains are involved, which are recognized as cross-reactive carbohydrate determinants (CCD) by CCD-specific IgE, thereby falsifying results (▶ Chap. 6).

In contrast to the purification of allergens from natural sources, the recombinant production of allergens by selecting the appropriate expression system enables one to circumvent the problem of cross-reactive carbohydrate side chains (CCD). Thus, expressing allergens in *Escherichia coli* bacteria permits their production without CCD, while production in yeast cells or certain insect cells makes allergens with normal or modified carbohydrate side chains possible.

Due to patent protection, some manufacturers are not permitted to use recombinant allergen molecules, meaning that they are only able to offer purified allergens for molecular allergy diagnostics (⊙ Table 7.3 lists a selection of single allergens, commonly available test platforms, and manufacturers of diagnostic agents).

Table 7.3 A (by no means exhaustive) selection of single allergens for specific IgE diagnostics

Allergen source	Species	Allergen component	Suppliers in Germany				
			Euroimmun	Dr. Fooke Laboratorien	Omega Diagnostics	Siemens Healthcare	Thermo Fisher Phadia
			Test systems				
			Euroline	Allergo-o-liq	Allergozyme IgE	Immulite 2000	(a) ImmunoCAP[5] (b) ImmunoCAP ISAC112[6]
			Test principle and Internet information				
			Enzyme allergo sorbent strip test[1]	Reversed enzyme allergo sorbent test[2]	Enzyme allergo sorbent test[3]	Chemiluminescence enzyme immunoassay with allergens in fluid phase[4]	(a) Fluorescence enzyme allergo sorbent test[5] (b) Multiple fluorescence enzyme allergo sorbent test[6]
Tree pollen	Birch	Bet v 1 (major allergen)	r (DPA-Dx[a])	r (RT301)	n (x901)	n (A89)	r (t215)
		Bet v 2 (profilin)	r (DPA-Dx)	r (RT302)	n (x907)	r (A127)	r (t216)
	Ash/olive	Ole e 1 (major allergen)	–	r (RT901)	–	n (A482)	r (t224)
Grass pollen	Timothy grass	Phl p 1 (major allergen)	r (DPA-Dx)	r (RG601)	n (x903)	–	r (g205)
		Phl p 5 (major allergen)	r (DPA-Dx)	r (RG605)	n (x902)	–	r (g215)
		Phl p 7 (polcalcin)	r (DPA-Dx)	r (RG607)	–	–	r (g210)
		Phl p 12 (profilin)	r (DPA-Dx)	r (RG612)	–	–	r (g212) among others

Weed pollen	Mugwort	Art v 1 (major allergen)	–	r (RW601)	–	n (A753)	n (w231)
	Ragweed (*Ambrosia*)	Amb a 1 (major allergen)	–	n (NW101)	–	–	n (w230)
Rosaceae fruits	Apple	Mal d 1 (Bet v 1H)	–	r (RF491)	–	r (A464L2)	r (f434)
		Mal d 4 (profilin)	–	–	–	r (A796L2)	–
	Peach	Pru p 3 (LTP)	–	r (RF533)	–	n (A603L2)	r (f420)
	Cherry	Pru av 1 (Bet v 1H)	–	–	–	r (A597L2)	–
		Pru av 3 (LTP)	–	–	–	r (A599L2)	–
		Pru av 4 (profilin)	–	–	–	r (A600L2)	–
Tree nuts	Hazelnut	Cor a 1 (Bet v 1H)	–	r (RF171)	–	–	r (f428)
		Cor a 9 (11S legumin)	–	–	–	–	r (f440)
		Cor a 14 (2S albumin)	–	–	–	–	r (f439)
Pulses	Peanut	Ara h 1 (7S globulin)	r (f422) DPA-Dx[b]	n (NF131)	–		r (f422)
		Ara h 2 (2S albumin)	r (f423) DPA-Dx[b]	n (NF132)	–	–	r (f432)
		Ara h 3 (11S globulin)	r (f424) DPA-Dx[b]	–	–	–	r (f424)
		Ara h 9 (LTP)	r (f427) DPA-Dx[b]	r (RF139)	–	–	r (f427)

(continued)

Table 7.3 (continued)

Insect venom	Bee venom	Api m 1	r (i208) DPA-Dx[c]	r (RI101)	–	r (A45)	r(i208)
		Api m 2	r (i213) DPA-Dx[c]	r (RI102)	–	r (A46)	–
		Api m 10	r (i216) DPA-Dx[c]		–	–	r(i217)
	Wasp venom	Ves v 1	r (i211) DPA-Dx[c]	–	–	r (A668)	r(i211)
		Ves v 5	r (i209) DPA-Dx[c]	r (RI305)	–	r (A670)	r(i209)

r recombinant component, *n* natural component, purified from extracts, *in parentheses* company-specific laboratory codes
Bet v 1H Bet v 1 homologous PR-10 protein, *2S albumin* storage protein, *11S legumin* storage protein
[a]DPA-Dx: Defined partial allergen diagnostics, panel strip test (DP 3210-1601-1 E) with Bet v 4 and Bet v 6, as well as birch pollen and timothy grass extract
[b]Panel strip test for peanut sensitizations (DPA-Dx Peanut 1) with rAra h 1, 2, 3, 5, 6, 7, 9, rBet v 1 and carbohydrate side chain reagent (CCD marker)
[c]Panel strip test for insect venom sensitizations (DP 3850-1601-2 E) with Api m 1, 2, and 10 and Ves v 1 and 5, bee venom and wasp venom extracts, and CCD marker
Internet information on test principles
[1]http://www.euroimmun.com/produkte/indikationen/allergologie/molekulare-allergologie.html
[2]http://www.fooke-labs.com/grobritannien-uk/downloadbereich/index.php
[3]http://www.omegadiagnostics.de/products/by-area/allergozyme-specific-ige/ (only in Germany)
[4]http://healthcare.siemens.com/clinical-specialities/allergy/laboratorian-information
[5]http://www.phadia.com/en-US/Products/Products/ImmunoCAP-Assays/ImmunoCAP-Specific-IgE/Test-Principle-ImmunoCAP-Specific-IgE/
[6]http://www.phadia.com/en-US/Products/Products/ImmunoCAP-ISAC/Test-Principle-ImmunoCAP-ISAC/

7.3.2 Laboratory-Scale Evaluation: Assay Sensitivity and Analytical Specificity (Selectivity)

Test method efficacy is investigated on an international basis using the variables "sensitivity and specificity". As part of this process, a distinction is made between two pairs of definitions: analytical and diagnostic sensitivity and specificity.

Definition of Terms Used to Measure Test Method Efficacy

Analytical sensitivity is defined as the slope of an (immuno)assay's calibration curve. The *actual sensitivity* (*lower detection limit*) of a test, on the other hand, is determined and expressed today using the following variables (Armbruster and Pry 2008):

- Limit of blank (LoB)
- Limit of detection (LoD)
- Limit of quantitation (LoQ)

LoB: LoB is defined as the highest test signal obtained from repeated blank measurements (serum sample without IgE): $LoB = Mean_{Blank} + 1.645\ (SD_{blank})$.

LoD: LoD refers to the weakest signal or lowest concentration of specific IgE antibodies reliably determined from the test: $LoD = LoB + 1.645\ (SD_{lowest\ concentration\ sample})$.

LoQ: LoQ is the lowest concentration of specific IgE antibodies that can be reliably detected within a predefined range. LoQ may be equivalent to or higher than LoD.

These definitions have been introduced in international laboratory guidelines (Hamilton et al. 2016) for IgE determination methods and are particularly important when single allergens are used (Matricardi et al. 2016).

Assay sensitivity is often enhanced (i.e., LoQ is lower) when using allergen molecules, particularly if these allergens are underrepresented in the natural extract or are entirely absent due to their instability. Greater assay sensitivity (lower LoQ) is thus an important argument in support of the use of allergen molecules for the diagnosis of specific IgE (⊙ Fig. 7.7 and ⊙ Table 7.4).

Example

Sensitization to wheat extract is found in only 20–30 % of patients with wheat-dependent exercise-induced anaphylaxis (WDEIA), while sIgE to Tri a 19 (ω-5 gliadin) is detected in 80–90 % of cases. Since the gliadins responsible for WDEIA are not water soluble, they are not present in sufficient quantities in

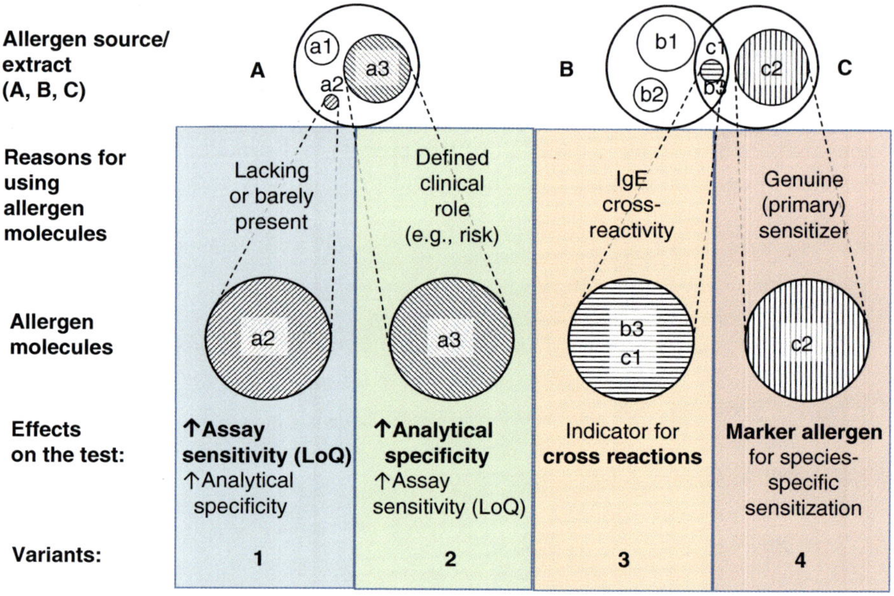

Fig. 7.7 Methodological rationales for molecular allergy diagnostics. The variants *1–4* shown in the figure (see also ⊙ Table 7.4) reflect universal arguments for the methodological use of allergen molecules. They move (virtually) exclusively on the test (sensitization) level, irrespective of the patient's clinical status. Thus, they improve only the sensitization test per se, without affecting clinical test findings/interpretation, which must always be performed by the treating physician (or person requesting the test) based on clinical information provided by the patient (history/provocation) on a case-by-case basis (Adapted from Hamilton et al. 2016)

Table 7.4 Improved test characteristics due to using defined allergen molecules for specific immunoglobulin E (IgE) determination in a singleplex assay (see also ⊙ Fig. 7.7 for variants)

Variants	1	2	3	4
Examples (allergen source, allergen carrier)	Greater assay sensitivity due to lower limit of quantitation (LoQ)	Improved analytical specificity (selectivity)	Cross-reactive allergens	Species/ family-specific marker allergens
Cat		Fel d 2	Fel d 2	Fel d 1
Hazelnut	Cor a 1 (Bet v 1 homolog)	Cor a 14 (2S albumin) Cor a 9 (11S globulin) Cor a 8 (LTP, Mediterranean region)		
Kiwi	Act d 8 (Bet v 1 homolog)		Act d 8 (Bet v 1 homolog)	
Peach	Pru p 1 (Bet v 1 homolog)	Pru p 3 (LTP, marker, Mediterranean region)	Pru p 1 (Bet v 1 homolog) Pru p 4 (profilin)	

Table 7.4 (continued)

Variants	1	2	3	4
Examples (allergen source, allergen carrier)	Greater assay sensitivity due to lower limit of quantitation (LoQ)	Improved analytical specificity (selectivity)	Cross-reactive allergens	Species/ family-specific marker allergens
Peanut	Ara h 10 Ara h 11 (oleosins)	Ara h 1 (7S globulin) Ara h 2 (2S albumin) Ara h 3 (11S globulin) Ara h 6/7 (2S albumin) Ara h 9 (LTP, Mediterranean region)	Ara h 8 (Bet v 1 homolog) Ara h 5[a]	
Soy	Gly m 4 (Bet v 1 homolog)	Gly m 5 Gly m 6		
Wheat	Tri a 19 (ω-5 gliadin)			
Meat	α-GAL	α-GAL		
Bee venom	Api m 3 Api m 4 Api m 10	Api m 1 Api m 3 Api m 4 Api m 10		Api m 1 Api m 3 Api m 4 Api m 10
Wasp venom	Ves v 5	Ves v 1 Ves v 5		Ves v 1 Ves v 5
Birch (hazel, alder, birch pollen) and beech family (beech, oak pollen)		Bet v 1	Bet v 2[a] Bet v 4[b]	Bet v 1
Oleaceae (ash, olive pollen)		Ole e 1	Ole e 2[a] Ole e 3[b]	Ole e 1
Poaceae (sweet grass pollen)		Phl p 1 Phl p 5	Phl p 12[a] Phl p 7[b]	Phl p 1 Phl p 5
Mugwort pollen		Art v 1	Art v 4[a] Art v 5[b]	Art v 1
Ragweed pollen		Amb a 1	Amb a 8[a] Amb a 10[b]	Amb a 1

Adapted from Hamilton et al. (2016)

The benefit of allergen molecules as diagnostic reagents from different allergen sources/extracts (left column), the rationales, and potentially improved test characteristics (top line) vary and depend on the individual diagnostic question and the specific allergen used

[a]Profilin family members: widespread, highly conserved, and extremely cross-reactive panallergens in pollen and plant-based foods

[b]Polcalcin family members (Ca^{++} – binding proteins): widespread, highly conserved, and extremely cross-reactive panallergens in pollen

aqueous wheat extracts. This problem can be avoided by using recombinantly produced Tri a 19 in the test system.

The *analytical specificity* of an IgE test method can relate to the specificity of the antibody class on the one hand, whereby the test effectively determines IgE and no antibodies of other classes, such as IgA, IgD, IgG, or IgM (Hamilton et al. 2016).

On the other hand, analytical specificity can relate to a more targeted, more "selective" IgE determination of particular allergen molecules: Whereas an allergen extract, as a complex protein mixture, determines the total IgE repertoire to an allergen source, only a proportion of specific antibodies are determined when using allergen molecules, thereby increasing analytical specificity (selectivity) (Matricardi et al. 2016).

This permits more targeted (more analytically specific) detection or exclusion of sensitization particularly in the case of allergen molecules with special characteristics—such as high stability and a relatively high proportion of total protein (e.g., Ara h 2 or Cor a 14) and thus an increased risk for severe reactions to food (peanut or hazelnut).

Example

More than 10 % of German children and adolescents show specific IgE to peanut extract—caused primarily by pollen-associated cross-reactions. Diagnosis using the stable and risk-related peanut storage protein, Ara h 2, yields elevated values in only a fraction of patients (approx. maximum 0.4 %, Kirsten Beyer, personal communication), thereby affording greater analytical specificity (selectivity) compared with peanut extract.

7.3.3 Universal Arguments for the Use of Molecular Allergens in IgE Diagnostics

Four arguments generally provide plausible support for the use of single allergens (⦿ Table 7.5). In this context, particularly the improved assay sensitivity (LoQ) and the increased analytical specificity mentioned above help to justify the use of allergen molecules (⦿ Fig. 7.7 and examples in ⦿ Table 7.4) (Hamilton et al. 2016; Matricardi et al. 2016):

1. Provided that allergen molecules (e.g., when present in insufficient proportions or absent in the extract) increase the assay sensitivity (LoQ) of IgE determination, their use is both useful and important.
2. Provided that allergen molecules permit improved analytical specificity (selectivity) by binding a partial amount of the specific IgE repertoire, as well as additional clinical findings (e.g., increased burden of risk, degree of clinical severity, other associated clinical characteristics), their use is, once again, useful and recommended from a diagnostic perspective.
3. Certain allergen molecules, by binding cross-reactive IgE antibodies, serve as an indicator for cross-sensitizations. In the case of positive results, they indirectly

Table 7.5 General criteria for optimizing tests and universal arguments to support the use of allergen molecules in specific immunoglobulin E (IgE) determination

	Analytical criteria (for possible test optimization)		Clinical criteria (potential clinical advantages)
1	**Assay sensitivity ↑** **Limit of quantitation (LoQ) ↓**	I	*Diagnostic sensitivity ↑*
2	**Analytical specificity ↑**	II	*Diagnostic specificity ↑*
3	**Indicator for serological cross-reactivity**	III	*Indicator for clinical cross-reactivity*
4	**Marker for primary/genuine sensitizations**	IV	*Prediction of clinically relevant reactions (PPV, NPV)*

Diagnostic methods in allergology can be evaluated analytically, i.e., on the test level (left column) and clinically (right column). The use of allergen molecules for IgE determination primarily improves the analytical criteria (1–4). Using single allergens frequently alters several criteria/variables

To what extent single allergens can optimize diagnostic/clinical criteria (right column, I–IV) depends on the cohort investigated, the single allergens in question, and the study endpoints selected. In general, clinical criteria are based on the individual interpretation of test results on the basis of clinical history and, where appropriate, reproducible symptoms in the affected allergy sufferer. Thus, they go beyond the actual results of allergen-specific IgE tests (sensitization, yes or no). Diagnostic/clinical criteria (right column) are therefore:

Less suited to the evaluation of sensitization tests (hence the italic font)

Often not at all necessary to demonstrate the benefits of single allergens

Fraught with unsatisfactory results due to their limited ability to predict clinical results

illustrate the lack of analytical specificity of IgE tests against allergen extracts (in affected individuals with potential cross-reactions).

4. Depending on findings, particular allergen molecules are suitable as protein family or species-specific IgE-binding marker allergens to detect or exclude genuine ("primary") sensitization.

It should be noted here that all the abovementioned arguments relate primarily to sensitization and do not take the clinical status of the patient into consideration. Examples of and indications for the detection of specific sensitization using single allergens are listed in ⊙ Table 7.6.

7.4 Clinical Evaluation: Diagnostic Sensitivity and Specificity

Diagnostic sensitivity and specificity relate to the symptoms of the affected allergy sufferer. A precondition to assessing and calculating these is unequivocal clinical information from the patient or, in case of doubt, additional provocation tests to confirm the clinical diagnosis (⊙ Table 7.5, right column).

However, allergen-specific IgE diagnostics only cover sensitization (susceptibility to allergy) and cannot per se predict the clinical reaction (Hamilton et al. 2016; Matricardi et al. 2016; Renz et al. 2010). Therefore, concordant results (positive history and positive specific IgE), for instance, are often referred to as *clinically relevant* (instead of correctly positive). The same applies to concordant negative results that

Table 7.6 Examples for the use of single allergens to detect sensitization: typical clinical questions in the case of suspected inhalant, food, and insect venom allergy. Potential advantages of using allergen molecules for IgE singleplex determinations and the significance of results

			Diagnostic advantages compared with extracts					Significance of results		
Indication	Diagnostic question	Allergen	Assay sensitivity	Analytical specificity	Indicator for cross-reactivity	Marker for primary sensitization	Allergen source	Positive	Negative	Comments
Suspected inhalant allergy (aeroallergens)										
Tree pollen sensitization?	Suspicion/exclusion of sensitization to birch, hazel, alder, birch, and oak	Bet v 1	?	↑	(+)	+	Birch pollen extract	Suspicion confirmed; clinically relevant only in the presence of corresponding symptoms	Suspicion excluded, other tree pollen responsible, e.g., ash?	Cross-reactivity to all Fagales pollen and potentially to Bet v 1 cross-reactive foods (e.g., pome and stone fruits, nuts, carrots, celery, and soy) present
Ash or Olive pollen sensitization?	Suspicion/exclusion of sensitization to ash and olive tree pollen	Ole e 1	?	↑	(+)	(+)	Olive pollen extract	Suspicion of olive/ash pollen sensitization confirmed; clinically relevant only in the presence of corresponding symptoms	Suspicion excluded, other tree pollens responsible, e.g., birch, oak, beech?	Cross-reactivity to pollen in the Oleaceae family (olive pollen, ash pollen) present

Grass pollen sensitization?	Suspicion/ exclusion of sensitization to grass pollen	Phl p 1 and Phl p 5	↑	↑	(+)	+	Timothy grass pollen extract	Suspicion confirmed; clinically relevant only in the presence of corresponding symptoms	Suspicion excluded, other seasonal allergens responsible, e.g., *Alternaria* mold or simultaneously flowering weed pollen?	Cross-reactivity to all sweet grasses present
Mugwort pollen sensitization?	Suspicion/ exclusion of sensitization to mugwort pollen	Art v 1	?	↑	(+)	+	Mugwort pollen extract	Suspicion confirmed; clinically relevant only in the presence of corresponding symptoms	Suspicion excluded, other seasonal allergen sources responsible, e.g., *Alternaria*?	Cross-reactivity possible to foods with Art v 1 homologous allergens
Ragweed pollen sensitization?	Suspicion/ exclusion of sensitization to ragweed pollen	Amb a 1	?	↑	–	+	Ragweed pollen extract	Suspicion confirmed; clinically relevant only in the presence of corresponding symptoms	Suspicion excluded, other weed pollens responsible, e.g., mugwort?	

(continued)

Table 7.6 (continued)

Indication	Diagnostic question	Allergen	Diagnostic advantages compared with extracts				Allergen source	Significance of results		Comments
			Assay sensitivity	Analytical specificity	Indicator for cross-reactivity	Marker for primary sensitization		Positive	Negative	
Sensitization to pollen panallergen profilin	Suspicion/exclusion of sensitization to universal pollen and food allergen profilin (e.g., in the case of numerous reactions to pollen extracts in skin tests)?	Phl p 12 or Bet v 2	↑	↑	++	–	Grass pollen or birch pollen	Suspicion confirmed; profilin sensitization evidently possible cause of multiple reactions to pollen extracts: essential to ask about oropharyngeal symptoms elicited by profilin-containing foods	Suspicion excluded	Cross-reactivity to all pollens (tree, grass, weed) and numerous plant-based food allergens present
Sensitization to pollen panallergen polcalcin	Suspicion/exclusion of sensitization to universal pollen allergen polcalcin (e.g., in the case of numerous reactions to pollen extracts in skin tests)?	Phl p 7 or Bet v 4	↑	↑	++	–	Grass pollen or birch pollen	Suspicion confirmed; polcalcin sensitization evidently possible cause of multiple reactions to pollen extracts	Suspicion excluded	Cross-reactivity to all pollens (tree, grass, weed) present

Alternaria sensitization?	Suspicion/ exclusion of sensitization to seasonal mold *Alternaria*	Alt a 1	?	↑	–	+	*Alternaria* extract	Suspicion confirmed; clinically relevant only in the presence of corresponding symptoms	Suspicion excluded, other seasonal allergen responsible, e.g., grass pollen or simultaneously flowering weed pollen (mugwort, ribwort, goosefoot)?	Cross-reactivity to all sweet grasses present
House dust mite sensitization?	Suspicion/ exclusion of sensitization to house dust mites *Dermatophagoides pter./far.*	Der p 1 and Der p 2 or Der f 1 and Der f 2	?	↑	(+)	+	House dust mite extract from *Dermatophagoides pter.* or *Dermatophagoides far.*	Suspicion confirmed; clinically relevant only in the presence of corresponding symptoms	Suspicion of house dust mite sensitization largely excluded; in rare cases, other major allergens, e.g., Der p 23, are responsible for sensitization	No confirmed advantages over extract diagnostics; distinction between *D. pter* and *D. far.* not possible
Cat sensitization?	Suspicion/ exclusion of sensitization to cats	Fel d 1	?	↑	–	+	Cat fur extract	Suspicion confirmed; clinically relevant only in the presence of corresponding symptoms	Suspicion excluded, are other perennial allergens relevant?	

(continued)

Table 7.6 (continued)

Indication	Diagnostic question	Allergen	Diagnostic advantages compared with extracts				Allergen source	Significance of results		Comments
			Assay sensitivity	Analytical specificity	Indicator for cross-reactivity	Marker for primary sensitization		Positive	Negative	
Dog sensitization	Suspicion/exclusion of sensitization to dog	Can f 1	?	↑	–	+	Dog hair extract	Suspicion confirmed; clinically relevant only in the presence of corresponding symptoms	Suspicion excluded, are other perennial allergens relevant?	
Suspected food allergy (marker/Cross-reactive allergen)										
Birch pollen-associated food cross-reactivity?	Suspicion/exclusion of sensitization to cross-reactive plant-based foods (pome and stone fruits, hazelnuts, carrots, celery, soy)	Bet v 1	↑	↑	+	(+)	Birch pollen extract	Suspicion confirmed; clinically relevant only in the presence of corresponding symptoms to the relevant, potentially cross-reactive plant-based food (▶ Chap. 2)	Suspicion excluded, are other cross-reactive allergens in plant-based foods relevant, e.g., profilin or LTP?	Well-suited marker for Bet v 1-associated cross-reactivity; better than commercial fruit, nut, and vegetable extracts

Profilin-associated food cross-reactivity?	Suspicion/ exclusion of sensitization to cross-reactive plant-based foods (fruit including rosaceae fruits, melon, citrus fruits, berries, nuts, vegetables, pulses)	Bet v 2 or Phl p 12	↑	↑	+	(+)	Birch pollen extract or grass pollen extract	Suspicion confirmed; clinically relevant only in the presence of corresponding symptoms to the relevant, potentially cross-reactive plant-based food (▶ Chap. 3)	Suspicion excluded, are other cross-reactive allergens in plant-based foods relevant, e.g., due to Bet v 1 or LTP sensitization?	Potential marker for profilin-associated cross-reactivity; more suitable than commercial fruit, nut, vegetable, pulse extracts
LTP-related food sensitization/ cross-reactivity?	Suspicion/ exclusion of sensitization to cross-reactive plant-based foods (fruit including rosaceae fruits, grapes, citrus fruits, berries, nuts, vegetables, pulses)	Pru p 3	↑	↑	+	(+)	Peach extract	Suspicion confirmed; clinically relevant only in the presence of corresponding symptoms to the relevant, potentially cross-reactive plant-based food (▶ Chap. 4)	Suspicion excluded, are other cross-reactive allergens in plant-based foods relevant, e.g., Bet v 1 or profilin?	Marker for LTP-related cross-reactivity; more suitable than fruit, nut, vegetable, and pulse extracts

(continued)

Table 7.6 (continued)

			Diagnostic advantages compared with extracts					Significance of results		
Indication	Diagnostic question	Allergen	Assay sensitivity	Analytical specificity	Indicator for cross-reactivity	Marker for primary sensitization	Allergen source	Positive	Negative	Comments
Wheat-dependent exercise-induced anaphylaxis?	Suspicion/exclusion of sensitization to wheat protein due to anaphylactic reactions to physical exertion?	Tri a 19	↑↑	↑	–	+	Wheat extract	Suspicion confirmed; clinically relevant only in the presence of corresponding symptoms to wheat-containing foods in conjunction with physical exertion	Suspicion excluded, other potential wheat allergens (Tria a 14?) or food allergens (LTP?) relevant?	Marker for ω-5-gliadin-specific wheat sensitization
Risk-related peanut sensitization?	Suspicion/exclusion of sensitization to peanut proteins based on anaphylactic reactions in the previous history?	Ara h 2, (Ara h 6), Ara h 1, Ara h 3	↑	↑	–	+	Peanut	Suspicion confirmed; clinically relevant only in the presence of corresponding symptoms	Suspicion excluded, are other potential peanut allergens (Ara h 6, oleosins?) or panallergens (LTP?) relevant?	Marker for primary, genuine peanut allergy (assuming IgE levels to other storage proteins are significantly lower); marker for hazardous systemic reactions

Risk-related soy sensitization?	Suspicion/ exclusion of sensitization to soy protein based on anaphylactic reactions in the previous history?	Gly m 5, Gly m 6, Gly m 8 (2017)	↑	↑	–	+	Soybean	Suspicion confirmed; clinically relevant only in the presence of corresponding symptoms	Suspicion excluded, are other potential soy allergens (Gly m 4? oleosins?) or panallergens (LTP?) relevant?	Marker for primary, genuine soy allergy (assuming IgE levels to other storage proteins are significantly lower); marker for hazardous systemic reactions
Risk-related hazelnut sensitization?	Suspicion/ exclusion of sensitization to hazelnut proteins based on systemic/ anaphylactic reactions in the previous history?	Cor a 14, Cor a 9	↑	↑	–	+	Hazelnut	Suspicion confirmed; clinically relevant only in the presence of corresponding symptoms	Suspicion excluded, are other potential hazelnut allergens (Cor a 11?) or panallergens (LTP) relevant?	Marker for primary, genuine hazelnut allergy (assuming IgE levels to other storage proteins are significantly lower); marker for hazardous systemic reactions

(continued)

Table 7.6 (continued)

Indication	Diagnostic question	Allergen	Diagnostic advantages compared with extracts				Allergen source	Significance of results		Comments
			Assay sensitivity	Analytical specificity	Indicator for cross-reactivity	Marker for primary sensitization		Positive	Negative	
Risk-related nut sensitization?	Suspicion/exclusion of sensitization to: (a) Walnut proteins (b) Brazil nut proteins (c) Cashew kernel proteins based on systemic/anaphylactic reactions in the previous history?	(a) Jug r 1, Jug r 2 (b) Ber e 1 (c) Ana o 2	↑	↑	–	+	(a) Walnut (b) Brazil nut (c) Cashew kernel	Suspicion confirmed; clinically relevant only in the presence of corresponding symptoms	Suspicion excluded, are other potential storage proteins or panallergens (LTP) relevant?	Marker for primary, genuine nut allergy (assuming IgE levels to other storage proteins are significantly lower); marker for hazardous systemic reactions
Suspected insect venom allergy (insect venom allergens)										
Bee venom sensitization?	Suspicion/exclusion of sensitization to bee venom proteins based on systemic/anaphylactic reactions in the previous history?	Api m 1, Api m 3, Api m 4, Api m 10,	↑	↑	–	+	Bee venom	Suspicion confirmed; clinically relevant only in the presence of corresponding symptoms	Are other been venom proteins (Api m 2, Api m 3, Api m 4, Api m 5, and Api m 10) relevant?	Marker for genuine, primary been venom sensitization

Wasp venom sensitization?	Suspicion/ exclusion of sensitization to wasp venom proteins based on systemic/ anaphylactic reactions in the previous history?	Ves v 1, Ves v 5	↑	↑	–	+	Wasp venom	Suspicion confirmed; clinically relevant only in the presence of corresponding symptoms	Suspicion largely excluded	Marker for genuine, primary wasp venom sensitization

? Effect on the test statistic (e.g., assay sensitivity) not unequivocally elucidated
↑ Increases the relevant performance (e.g., assay sensitivity, analytical specificity)
\+ Positive differentiation (e.g., as an indicator for cross-reactivity or marker of primary sensitization)
(+) Limited advantages in terms of differentiation (cross-reactivity or primary sensitization)
– No advantages in terms of differentiation (cross-reactivity or primary sensitization)

exclude allergy, and thereby also an underlying sensitization. A positive IgE finding combined with a negative history is often classified as *clinically irrelevant* (instead of false positive). Declaring clinically irrelevant results as false positive does not go to the core of the matter, since ultimately the test result, i.e., the allergen-specific IgE that is present, can very well be valid and cannot be questioned.

A number of clinical studies have investigated the diagnostic sensitivity and specificity of individual allergens from one allergen source (selection in ⊙ Table 7.7). By increasing assay sensitivity (low LoQ), absent or underrepresented allergens were also able to significantly increase diagnostic sensitivity. However, increased sensitizations were reported parallel to this, even in individuals with no clinically relevant reactions.

Table 7.7 Examples of the successful clinical validation of molecular allergy diagnostics (plant allergen sources) (Kleine-Tebbe and Jappe 2013)

Allergen source	Allergens	Comments	References
Hazelnut	rCor a 1.04 rCor a 2 rCor a 8 nCor a 9 rCor a 11	Clinical evaluation of component-specific diagnostics in hazelnut-allergic individuals from various regions (Denmark, Switzerland, and Spain); diagnosis partially confirmed by controlled oral challenge, additional cohorts with pollen allergy, and non-atopics; overall heterogeneous sensitization profiles depending on the region investigated	Hansen et al. (2009)
Carrot	rDau c 1.0104 rDau c 1.0201 rDau c 4 rDau c IFR 1 rDau c IFR 2 rDau c Cyc	(a) Clinical evaluation of three carrot allergens in carrot-allergic individuals (confirmed as such by oral challenge) compared with birch pollen-allergic individuals with no carrot allergy or non-atopic controls (b) Clinical evaluation of component-specific diagnostics in carrot-allergic individuals from various regions (Denmark, Switzerland, and Spain); diagnosis partially confirmed by controlled oral challenge, additional cohorts with pollen allergy, and non-atopics; overall heterogeneous sensitization profiles depending on the region investigated	Ballmer-Weber et al. (2005, 2012)
Cherry	rPru av 1 rPru av 3 rPru av 4	Clinical evaluation of component-specific diagnostics in cherry-allergic individuals from Central and Southern Europe (Spain); diagnosis partially confirmed by controlled oral challenge, additional cohorts with pollen allergy, and non-atopics; heterogeneous sensitization profiles depending on the region investigated and clear superiority of single allergens compared with extract-based diagnostics (skin prick test; specific IgE with cherry extracts)	Reuter et al. (2006)

Table 7.7 (continued)

Allergen source	Allergens	Comments	References
Celery	rApi g 1.01 rApi g 4 nApi g 5	Clinical evaluation of component-specific diagnostics in celery-allergic individuals; diagnosis confirmed by controlled oral challenge, additional cohorts with pollen allergy, and non-atopics; clear superiority of single allergens compared with extract-based diagnostics; nApi g 5-specific IgE is targeted predominantly against CCD	Ballmer-Weber et al. (2000), Bauermeister et al. (2009)

The interdependence between diagnostic sensitivity and specificity is a fundamental problem in testing and is often represented in "receiver operating characteristic" (ROC) curves (⦿ Fig. 7.8). Better diagnostic sensitivity and specificity for the risk assessment of severe clinical reactions has been described for some single allergens, such as Ara h 2 or other high-risk allergens from the 2S-albumin group of storage proteins (overview in Lange et al. 2014). Moreover, predictive specific IgE decision points for positive or negative oral challenge in children with suspected peanut or hazelnut allergy have been defined with the help of risk-related 2S albumins [Beyer et al. (2015); see also ▶ Chaps. 11 and 12].

A clinical reaction (or absence thereof) can never be predicted in a foolproof manner (to 100 %) using sensitization tests such as IgE determination (Beyer et al. 2015). Therefore, methodological arguments first need to be considered for future assessments of the diagnostic suitability of allergen molecules (⦿ Table 7.5, left column). Even without a complete clinical evaluation (including diagnostic sensitivity and specificity, as well as predictive value, ⦿ Table 7.5, right column, study examples in ⦿ Table 7.7), the analytical test's characteristics of IgE diagnostics using allergen molecules are, in many cases, significantly better compared with allergen extracts (▶ Sect. 7.3.3) (Matricardi et al. 2016). This viewpoint is reflected in the updated international laboratory guidelines on IgE test methods (Hamilton et al. 2016) and should serve to ease and accelerate the evaluation and introduction of allergen molecules for diagnostic purposes in the future.

7.5 Interpretation to Establish Clinical Relevance

Ultimately, the central question relates to the clinical relevance of the specific IgE concentrations obtained:

- The following basic rule still applies: a *positive specific IgE result* is consistent with a sensitization that is only clinically relevant in the presence of corresponding symptoms.
- A *negative specific IgE result* (e.g., to an allergen molecule or a mixture of natural isoforms of a single allergen) largely excludes allergic sensitization to the tested allergen, however, only if:
  - Total IgE is sufficiently high.
  - The allergen is available intact and in adequate quantities.

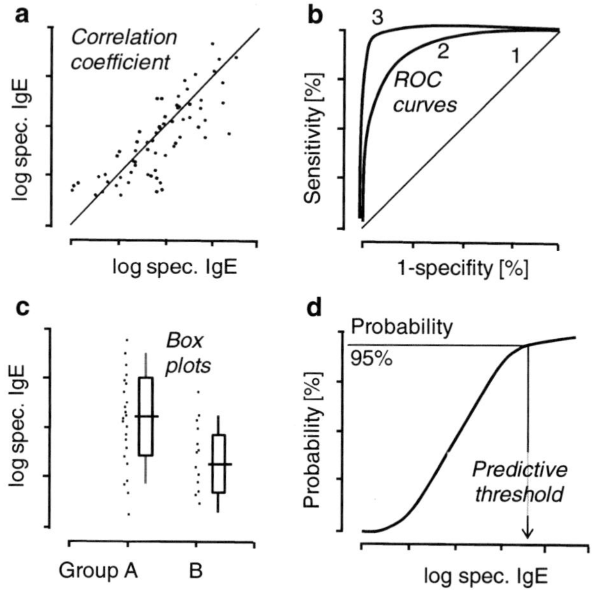

Fig. 7.8 Typical data analysis of IgE laboratory results (e.g., with allergen molecules). (**a**) Concordance between logarithmically distributed specific IgE levels (e.g., to a natural or recombinant allergen molecules). (**b**) Diagnostic efficacy (*ROC* receiver operating curves) when using allergens (allergen molecules). The *line* (*1*) represents a test situation in which diagnostic sensitivity (*y*-axis) and specificity (*x*-axis: 1 specificity) are equally inadequate (corresponding to a pure chance level = "toss of a coin"); the *line* (*2*) and more so the *line* (*3*) represent tests with better diagnostic sensitivity and specificity. A right-angled ROC curve (=100 % diagnostic efficacy) that closely follows the top left corner would be ideal. (**c**) Individual values and median values with 25 and 75 percentiles in the comparison of groups. (**d**) Cut-off values (threshold levels) for the prediction of clinical reactions (e.g., 95 % probability of a positive challenge test)

- The analytical assay sensitivity of the IgE determination method has been optimized and is correspondingly high.

Finally, irrespective of whether allergen extracts or molecules are used for diagnostic purposes, only a physician can determine the clinical relevance of an allergic sensitization, not the test (Kleine-Tebbe and Jakob 2015).

Therefore, all diagnostic findings from sensitization tests—and that applies equally to allergen molecules—need to be evaluated in the clinical context and in conjunction with the individual patient's previous history.

7.6 Potential and Quantitative Concepts of Molecular Allergology

Diagnostic methods using single allergens (Matricardi et al. 2016) open up new opportunities to differentiate the IgE response to certain allergen sources. Some marker allergens are characteristic of certain allergen sources and enable their unequivocal classification. These triggers of genuine, primary sensitization are also referred to as species-specific allergens and can be used as "markers" for certain allergen sources (⦿ Tables 7.4 and 7.6). Thus, in most parts of Europe, for example, it is possible to reliably detect sensitizations to pollen using marker allergens and to exclude potential cross-reactions.

This is particularly useful in the case of additional sensitizations to panallergens from the polcalcin and profilin families (▶ Chap. 3), in order to reestablish the analytical specificity of exclusively extract-based diagnosis that is otherwise inadequate in this setting. Polcalcins and profilins are present in a wide variety of allergen sources and, due to their high structural similarity, are responsible for marked cross-reactions. Although rarely of clinical relevance, they complicate specific diagnosis when extracts alone are used, since the latter contain both markers and cross-reactive allergens.

As part of the test interpretation, primary sensitization in the case of a series of positive IgE results can be deduced from the level of IgE concentrations:

The primary sensitizing allergen has the most epitopes recognized by specific IgE antibodies. In contrast, the number of cross-reactive epitopes of structurally related, similar protein allergens is often lower or of lower affinity.

The following rule of thumb applies: The highest IgE antibody level to a protein compared with other members of the same protein family likely reveals the primary sensitizer.

7.6.1 The Use of Singleplex IgE Assays in Bet v 1-Related Cross-Reactivity

A classic example of this is the PR-10 protein family, in the case of which primary birch pollen sensitization is evidenced by high Bet v 1-specific IgE levels, while Bet v 1-related secondary pollen or food sensitizations are reflected in low IgE values to the relevant Bet v 1 homologous PR-10 proteins (⦿ Fig. 7.9b). Moreover, the structural relationship between allergens in a family can be indirectly ascertained from the level of specific IgE (⦿ Fig. 7.9).

7.6.2 The Use of Singleplex IgE Assays in Profilin Sensitization

In the case of strong structural similarity and marked cross-reactivity within an allergen family, one can expect comparable specific IgE levels to the individual proteins, as observed with profilins, for example (⦿ Fig. 7.9c). Determining IgE to profilins from different allergen sources is unlikely to bring any benefit here. A single IgE measurement, e.g., to grass pollen profilin Phl p 12 or birch pollen profilin Bet v 2, is sufficient. Other profilin sources could also come into question, e.g., latex or annual mercury (Mer a 1, only in multiplex ImmunoCAP ISAC). It is possible to establish the clinical relevance of IgE sensitization by means of detailed patient interviews, e.g., potential symptoms induced by botanically unrelated pollen plants or reactions to plant-based foods that, in particular, do not belong to the Bet v 1 cluster, e.g., melon and banana, as well as exotic and citrus fruits (Santos and van Ree 2011).

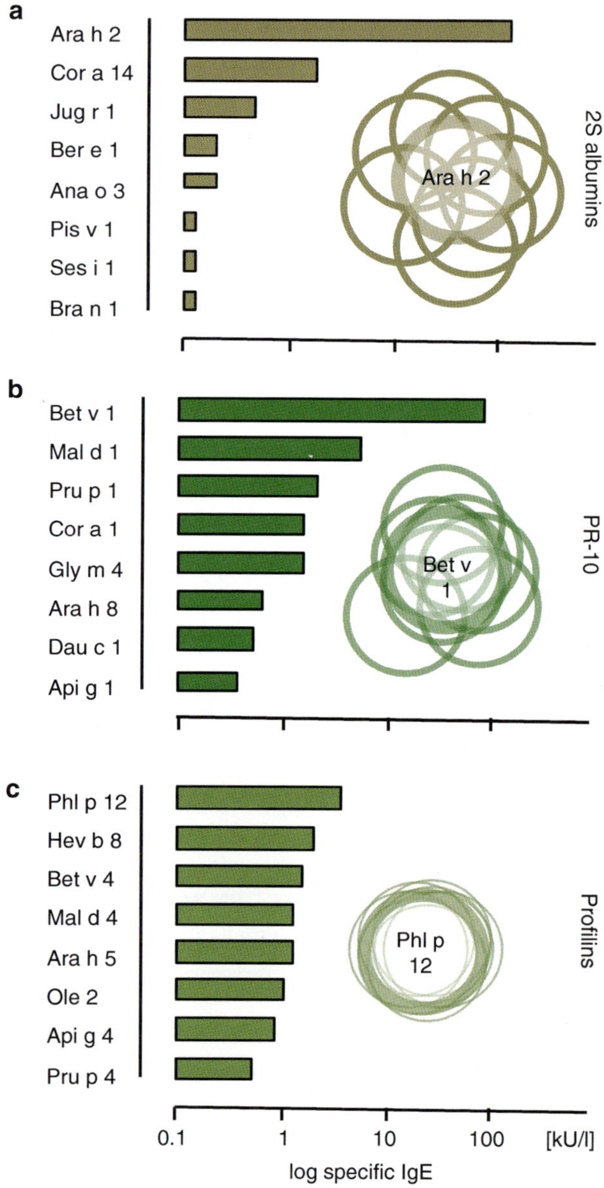

Fig. 7.9 Immunoglobulin E (IgE) levels to allergen molecules depending on structural similarity within an allergen family. (**a**) Variable, limited cross-reactivity between 2S albumins (stable storage proteins in nuts, pulses, and seeds). (**b**) Variable cross-reactivity between Bet v 1 homologous food allergens. (**c**) High cross-reactivity due to the strongly preserved and similar structure of profilins (in pollen, latex, and foods)

7.6.3 The Use of Singleplex IgE Assays Against Storage Proteins

IgE levels against members of the same protein family can vary significantly in the case of low structural similarity and correspondingly low cross-reactivity, as can be seen with the example of storage proteins (⦿ Fig. 7.9a).

Although the typical basic structure of storage proteins, i.e.,:

- 2S albumins
- 7S globulins
- 11S globulins

from different allergen sources—such as legumes (peanut, soybean), tree nuts (hazel and walnut), and seeds—is similar, only partially cross-reactive, potential IgE-binding epitopes are present. As a result, a complex pattern of possible cross-reactivities emerges, depending on the individual IgE repertoire. The IgE response to one storage protein (e.g., Ara h 3 from peanut) does not permit an assessment of IgE reactivity to other members of the 11S globulin family (e.g., Gly m 6 from soybean or Cor a 9 from hazelnut). Thus, strictly speaking, the sensitization pattern to storage proteins can only be determined by using all available proteins from this storage protein family. Unfortunately, not all members of these stable allergens from tree nuts, capsule and stone fruits, as well as seeds are as yet available, meaning that gaps remain in our diagnostic potential for the time being.

As a result, the highest IgE level to a particular storage protein (e.g., Ara h 2 from the 2S albumin group) likely reveals the primary source of sensitization (e.g., peanut). Lower levels, e.g., to corresponding soy (2S albumin Gly m 8) or hazel nut allergens (2S albumin Cor a 14) signal potential IgE cross-reactivity. However, their clinical relevance and the associated risk of reactions following consumption of the respective allergen source cannot be established from the level of specific IgE, but needs instead to be conclusively established by the patient's history or provocation tests.

Higher than expected IgE levels (to a food protein investigated as a secondary allergen source) raise doubts about the suspected primary allergen source and should be carefully investigated for plausibility.

Only when the corresponding proteins from the same protein family yield wholly negative IgE values can one assume that serological cross-reactivity is absent and that no clinical (cross-)reactions are to be expected.

Thus, a negative result is particularly important for the exclusion of an allergic (cross-)reaction.

It is here that the current limitations of molecular allergy diagnostics become apparent, since a structural relationship between allergens, depending on individual IgE repertoires, can determine highly variable cross-reactivities: from completely absent to strong IgE binding of similar epitopes. The various serological and clinical reaction patterns are ultimately based on numerous variables that go beyond the purely structural characteristics of the allergens (Kleine-Tebbe and Jakob 2015):

- Personal IgE repertoires with individual patterns of serological and potential clinical cross-reactions
- Proportion of the allergen relative to the total protein or total weight
- Stability of the relevant allergens, which depends on the processing of the foodstuff
- Volume of the foodstuff consumed
- Cofactors for a systemic or anaphylactic reaction

Against the background of these factors, efforts to make successful clinical predictions on the basis of molecule-specific IgE sensitizations are limited in their scope. It is essential, therefore, to correct overblown expectations of molecular diagnostics. IgE sensitization tests can be optimized using defined allergens and plausible criteria (depending predominantly on the clinical phenotype). The advantages for serological diagnosis, however, lie in testing each allergen separately.

Conclusions

Singleplex determinations of allergen-specific IgE against allergen molecules enable sensitization (i.e., allergic disposition) to be detected or excluded in a targeted manner. The novel opportunities offered by molecular allergology—increased detection sensitivity and heightened analytical specificity, a marker function for primary sensitizations, and an indicator function for serological cross-reactions—improve test characteristics, thereby broadening the opportunities offered hitherto exclusively extract-based diagnostics. Thus, carefully defined allergen molecules serve as a useful complement to the reagents available to date and optimize IgE determinations and the detection of specific sensitization in the context of allergy diagnosis.

Our additional knowledge of molecular relationships enables a more comprehensive and specific interpretation of IgE profiles and sensitization patterns on the basis of singleplex determinations and make counseling easier. A prerequisite of this, however, is that the clinical relevance of these findings continues to be ultimately based on individual symptoms and reactions in the affected patient on a case-by-case basis.

References

Armbruster DA, Pry T. Limit of blank, limit of detection and limit of quantitation. Clin Biochem Rev. 2008;29 Suppl 1:S49–52.

Ballmer-Weber BK, Vieths S, Luttkopf D, et al. Celery allergy confirmed by double-blind, placebo-controlled food challenge: a clinical study in 32 subjects with a history of adverse reactions to celery root. J Allergy Clin Immunol. 2000;106:373–8.

Ballmer-Weber BK, Wangorsch A, Bohle B, et al. Component-resolved in vitro diagnosis in carrot allergy: does the use of recombinant carrot allergens improve the reliability of the diagnostic procedure? Clin Exp Allergy. 2005;35:970–8.

Ballmer-Weber BK, Skamstrup Hansen K, Sastre J, et al. Component-resolved in vitro diagnosis of carrot allergy in three different regions of Europe. Allergy. 2012;67:758–66.

Bauermeister K, Ballmer-Weber BK, Bublin M, et al. Assessment of component-resolved in vitro diagnosis of celeriac allergy. J Allergy Clin Immunol. 2009;124:1273–81.

Beyer K, Grabenhenrich L, Hartl M, et al. Predictive values of component-specific IgE for the outcome of peanut and hazelnut food challenges in children. Allergy. 2015;70:90–8.

Bousquet J, Heinzerling L, Bachert C, et al. Global Allergy and Asthma European Network; Allergic Rhinitis and its Impact on Asthma. Practical guide to skin prick tests in allergy to aero-allergens. Allergy. 2012;67:18–24.

Christensen LH, Holm J, Lund G, et al. Several distinct properties of the IgE repertoire determine effector cell degranulation in response to allergen challenge. J Allergy Clin Immunol. 2008;122:298–304.

Haftenberger M, Laussmann D, Ellert U, et al. Prevalence of sensitisation to aeraoallergens and food allergens: results of the German Health Interview and Examination Survey for Adults (DEGS1). Bundesgesundheitsblatt Gesundheitsforschung Gesundheitsschutz. 2013; 56:687–97.

Hamilton RG, MacGlashan Jr DW, Saini SS. IgE antibody-specific activity in human allergic disease. Immunol Res. 2010;47:273–84.

Hamilton RG, Matsson PNJ, Adkinson F, et al. Analytical performance characteristics, quality assurance, and clinical utility of immunological assays for human immunoglobulin E antibodies of defined allergen specificities. 3rd ed. CLSI report I/LA20-3rd ed. ISBN: 1-56238-948-3 [print]; 1-56238-949 [electronic]; Wayne, PA: Clinical Laboratory Standards Institute; 2016.

Hansen KS, Ballmer-Weber BK, Sastre J, et al. Component-resolved in vitro diagnosis of hazelnut allergy in Europe. J Allergy Clin Immunol. 2009;123:1134–41.

Hoffmann HJ, Santos AF, Mayorga C, et al. The clinical utility of basophil activation testing in diagnosis and monitoring of allergic disease. Allergy. 2015;70:1393–405.

Johansson SG. The history of IgE: from discovery to 2010. Curr Allergy Asthma Rep. 2011;11:173–7.

Kleine-Tebbe J. Old questions and novel clues: complexity of IgE repertoires. Clin Exp Allergy. 2012;42:1142–5.

Kleine-Tebbe J, Jappe U. Molekulare Allergiediagnostik: Entwicklung und Bedeutung für die klinische Praxis. Allergologie. 2013;36:327–49.

Kleine-Tebbe J, Jappe U. Molekulare Allergologie – Einführung mit kommentierten Kasuistiken. München-Deisenhofen: Dustri; 2014.

Kleine-Tebbe J, Jakob T. Molecular allergy diagnostics using IgE singleplex determinations: methodological and practical consideration for the use in clinical practice. Allergo J Int. 2015;24(6):185–97.

Kleine-Tebbe J, Erdmann S, Knol EF, et al. Diagnostic tests based on human basophils: potentials, pitfalls and perspectives. Int Arch Allergy Immunol. 2006;141:79–90.

Kleine-Tebbe J, Meißner A-M, Jappe U, et al. Allergenfamilien und molekulare Diagnostik IgE-vermittelter Nahrungsmittelallergien: von der Theorie zur Praxis. Allergo J. 2010;19:251–63.

Kober A, Perborn H. Quantitation of mouse-human chimeric allergen-specific IgE antibodies with ImmunoCAP technology. J Allergy Clin Immunol. 2006;117:S219 (Abstract 845).

Lange L, Beyer K, Kleine-Tebbe J. Molekulare Diagnostik bei Erdnussallergie. Allergo J Int. 2014;23:158–63.

Lund G, Willumsen N, Holm J, et al. Antibody repertoire complexity and effector cell biology determined by assays for IgE-mediated basophil and T-cell activation. J Immunol Methods. 2012;383:4–20.

MacGlashan Jr D. IgE and FcepsilonRI regulation. Clin Rev Allergy Immunol. 2005;29:49–60.

MacGlashan Jr D, Xia HZ, Schwartz LB, et al. IgE-regulated loss, not IgE-regulated synthesis, controls expression of FcepsilonRI in human basophils. J Leukoc Biol. 2001;70:207–18.

Matricardi PM, Kleine-Tebbe J, Hoffmann HJ, Valenta R, Hilger C, Hofmaier S, Aalberse RC, Agache I, Asero R, Ballmer-Weber B, Barber D, Beyer K, Biedermann T, Biló MB, Blank S, Bohle B, Bosshard PP, Breiteneder H, Brough HA, Caraballo L, Caubet JC, Crameri R, Davies JM, Douladiris N, Ebisawa M, Eigenmann PA, Fernandez-Rivas M, Ferreira F, Gadermaier G, Glatz M, Hamilton RG, Hawranek T, Hellings P, Hoffmann-Sommergruber K, Jakob T, Jappe U, Jutel M, Kamath SD, Knol EF, Korosec P, Kuehn A, Lack G, Lopata AL, Mäkelä M, Morisset M, Niederberger V, Nowak-Wezgrzyn AH, Papadopoulos NG, Pastorello EA, Pauli G, Platts-Mills T, Posa D, Poulsen LK, Raulf M, Sastre J, Scala E, Schmid JM, Schmid-Grendelmeier P, van Hage M, van Ree R, Vieths S, Weber R, Wickman M, Muraro A, Ollert M. EAACI molecular allergology user's guide. Pediatr Allergy Immunol. 2016;27:(suppl 23):1–250.

Purohit A, Laffer S, Metz-Favre C, et al. Poor association between allergen-specific serum immunoglobulin E levels, skin sensitivity and basophil degranulation: a study with recombinant birch pollen allergen Bet v 1 and an immunoglobulin E detection system measuring immunoglobulin E capable of binding to Fc epsilon RI. Clin Exp Allergy. 2005;35:186–92.

Renz H, Biedermann T, Bufe A, et al. In-vitro-Allergiediagnostik. Allergo J. 2010;19:110–28.
Reuter A, Lidholm J, Andersson K, et al. A critical assessment of allergen component-based in vitro diagnosis in cherry allergy across Europe. Clin Exp Allergy. 2006;36:815–23.
Santos A, van Ree R. Profilins: mimickers of allergy or relevant allergens? Int Arch Allergy Immunol. 2011;155:191–204.
Schmitz R, Ellert U, Kalcklosch M, et al. Patterns of sensitization to inhalant and food allergens—findings from the German Health Interview and Examination Survey for Children and Adolescents. Int Arch Allergy Immunol. 2013;162:263–70.
Uyttebroek AP, Sabato V, Faber MA, et al. Basophil activation tests: time for a reconsideration. Expert Rev Clin Immunol. 2014;10:1325–35.
Valenta R, Lidholm J, Niederberger V, et al. The recombinant allergen-based concept of component-resolved diagnostics and immunotherapy (CRD and CRIT). Clin Exp Allergy. 1999;29:896–904.
Worm M, Reese I, Ballmer-Weber B, et al. Guidelines on the management of IgE-mediated food allergies: S2k-Guidelines of the German Society for Allergology and Clinical Immunology (DGAKI) in collaboration with other German Medical Societies including the Association of the Scientific Medical Societies in Germany (AWMF). Allergo J Int. 2015;24:256–293.

8 Spiking with Recombinant Individual Allergens for Improvement of Allergen Extracts

J. Huss-Marp, M. Raulf, and T. Jakob

8.1 Introduction

Molecular allergy diagnostics are based on the philosophy that isolated allergens and not the entire allergen source are relevant for sensitization and clinical manifestation of an allergic reaction. The use of allergen components in diagnostics offers three possibilities for modifying an in vitro IgE singleplex test: (a) allergen components can be used individually for IgE antibody determination, (b) the

This contribution is based on the publication of the authors published 2015 in *Allergo Journal International* (Huss-Marp J, Raulf M, Jakob T: Spiking with recombinant allergens to improve allergen extracts: benefits and limitations for the use in routine diagnostics. Allergo J Int 2015;24:236–243 DOI 10.1007/s40629-015-0058-0) which has now been modified as book chapter.
The authors gratefully thank Prof. Robert G. Hamilton, PhD, Johns Hopkins Dermatology, Allergy and Clinical Immunology (DACI) Reference Laboratory at the Johns Hopkins Asthma & Allergy Center, Baltimore, MD, USA, for reviewing the manuscript, expert editorial assistance, and helpful suggestions regarding this chapter.

J. Huss-Marp, MD, Assoc Prof. (✉)
Therapeutic Area Dermatology, AbbVie Deutschland GmbH & Co KG, Wiesbaden, Germany
e-mail: johannes.huss-marp@abbvie.com

M. Raulf, PhD, Prof.
Center Allergology/Immunology, Institute for Prevention and Occupational Medicine of the German Social Accident Insurance, Institute of the Ruhr-Universität Bochum, Bochum, Germany
e-mail: raulf@ipa-dguv.de

T. Jakob, MD, Prof.
Department of Dermatology and Allergology, University Medical Center Giessen (UKGM), Justus-Liebig-University, Giessen, Germany
e-mail: thilo.jakob@derma.med.uni-giessen.de

J. Kleine-Tebbe, T. Jakob (eds.), *Molecular Allergy Diagnostics*,
DOI 10.1007/978-3-319-42499-6_8

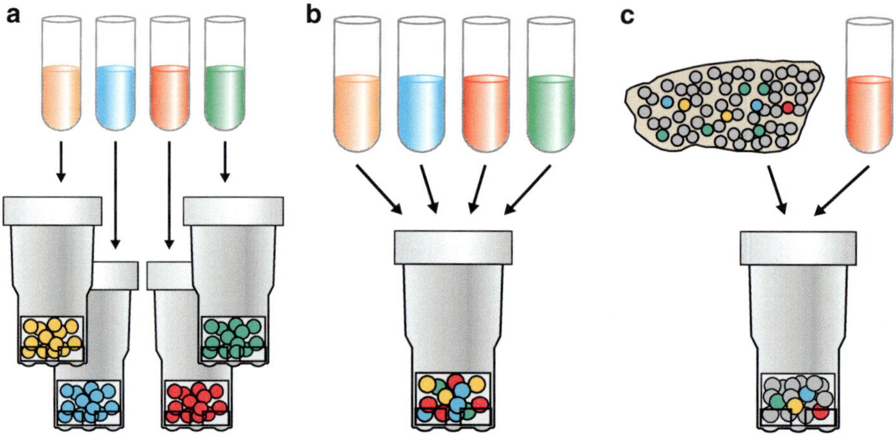

Fig. 8.1 Use of allergen components in allergy diagnostics: (**a**) allergen components used individually, (**b**) allergen components combined as a mixture and used in one test, and (**c**) "spiking" of an allergenic extract with individual allergen components

available allergen components can be combined as a mixture and used in one test to replace a natural extract, and (c) individual allergen components can be specifically added to the extract (◉ Fig. 8.1). While option (a) currently represents the most extensively used application of molecular allergy diagnostics and is described in the remaining chapters of this book in detail, option (b) is rarely used in practice; since selecting the optimal ratios of allergens is challenging, the process is expensive and the benefits are questionable. The last application (c), so-called spiking of an extract with allergen components with the goal of increasing an assay's sensitivity is, however, used in some extract-based in vitro tests. This procedure is particularly useful if allergen components are underrepresented in the conventional extract-based test.

There are a number of reasons why one or several allergen components are underrepresented in an extract-based test. They range from the complex composition and variation of the natural source material with regard to the occurrence of the individual allergen components, the differential solubility and thus extractability of different allergen components from the raw material, and variable stability of the allergenic component molecules after extraction (Matricardi et al. 2016). Test-specific aspects such as the bonding behaviors of allergen components contribute to composition variability.

Since important allergen components have been known to be underrepresented in the conventional reagents used to detect IgE antibodies to latex, hazelnut, and yellow jacket venom, these have been good candidates for component spiking. We will present examples of this process using *Hevea brasiliensis* natural rubber latex, hazelnut, and yellow jacket venom as illustrations and discuss the clinical implications of supplementation.

A modification of ImmunoCAP tests by spiking was performed for latex (09/2001), hazelnut, (05/2006) and yellow jacket venom (06/2012) with the goal of increasing the analytical sensitivity of the assay. The modified ImmunoCAP tests have subsequently replaced the prior non-spiked allergen reagents. A clear communication of this product change is critical for effective interpretation and thus optimal clinical use.

8.2 Improvement of Diagnostics Through Allergen Addition in Latex Allergy

Type I latex allergy represents a classical, IgE-mediated, immediate-type reaction. Proteins in the natural latex milk of the Pará rubber tree *Hevea brasiliensis* are the triggers of latex allergy. Currently 18 latex allergens (including isoforms) have been identified and described as Hev b 1 to Hev b 15 according to the IUIS allergen nomenclature (Hev b is derived from *Hevea brasiliensis*; http://www.allergen.org/List.htm) (Raulf-Heimsoth and Rihs 2011).

Since the skin test extracts to detect sensitization to latex allergens are increasingly limited in their availability, the serological test for latex-specific IgE not only represents an additional, but in some countries the only method to detect sensitization to *Hevea brasiliensis* latex allergens.

As investigations by Chen et al. (2000) or Lundberg et al. (2001) have shown, 16 of 111 latex allergic patients from the healthcare system with a positive latex skin test reaction and the clinical symptoms of a latex allergy tested negative in the specific IgE test with the commonly used *Hevea* latex allergen extract. Through the use of individual recombinant latex allergens, it was possible to show that eight of these patients were monosensitized to Hev b 5. Hev b 5 is an acidic protein that is similar to a protein in kiwi fruit, and it is considered a major latex allergen along with Hev b 1 and Hev b 6.01/6.02. It is recognized by patients in the healthcare system and those with spina bifida who are allergic to latex (Akasawa et al. 1996; Slater et al. 1996). The addition of rHev b 5 to the extracted latex allergen material routinely used for detecting latex-specific IgE produced a new ImmunoCAP ("k82 supplemented with rHev b 5"; Lundberg et al. 2001) which demonstrated improved diagnostic sensitivity – particularly in individual cases (◉ Fig. 8.2). These results demonstrated a new overall strategy for the manufacturing of standardized allergy diagnostics: if relevant allergens are too unstable to withstand the production steps of standardized allergen extracts or if they are missing, stable recombinant proteins can be supplemented into the extract during production.

"k82 enriched with rHev b 5" has been commercially available since spring 2002 in order to enhance the performance of latex-specific IgE measurements. This enriched ImmunoCAP replaced the original ImmunoCAP k82 and continues to be

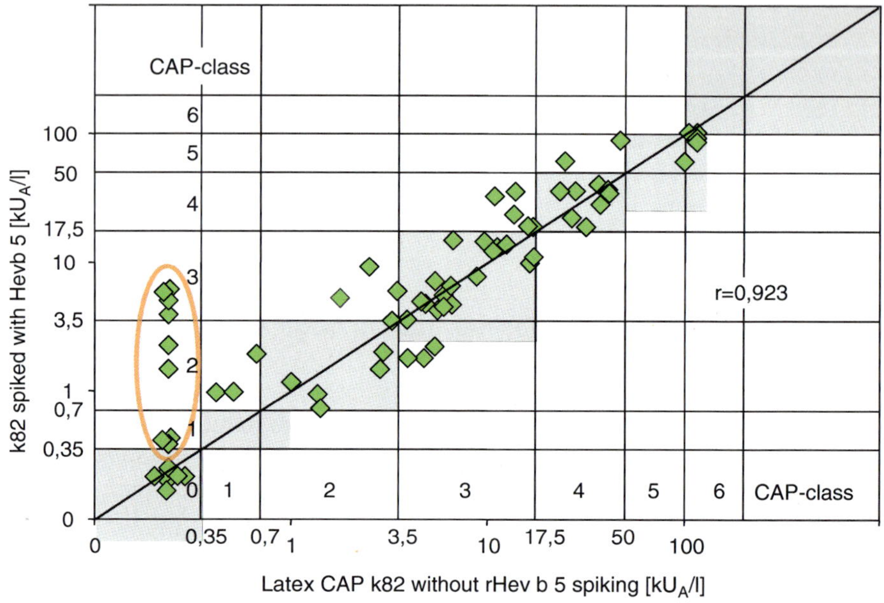

Fig. 8.2 Comparison of latex ImmunoCAP results using an allergosorbent (k82) without rHev b 5 versus enriched with rHev b 5. Study collective: healthcare workers ($n = 68$) with latex allergy were tested with both tests (Modified according to Raulf-Heimsoth et al. (2007))

Table 8.1 Determination of latex-specific IgE with different ImmunoCAP tests

Method	Sensitivity (%)	Specificity (%)	PPV (%)	NPV (%)	Efficacy (%)
k82 "old"	76.0	98.3	98.1	78.7	86.7
k82+rHev b 5	90.0	98.3	98.4	89.4	93.8
rHev b-Mix[a]	83.6	98.3	98.2	84.3	90.6

According to Raulf-Heimsoth et al. (2007)
PPV positive predictive value, *NPV* negative predictive value
[a]rHev-v-Mix consists of rHev b 1, rHev b 5, rHev b 6.01, and rHev b 8

identified as k82. As Table 8.1 shows, the diagnostic sensitivity of the latex-specific IgE determination was increased from 76 % (latex extract without rHev b 5) to 90 % with a test efficiency of 93.75 % using the ImmunoCAP reagent that was supplemented with rHev b 5. The use of an ImmunoCAP manufactured for research purpose, consisting of the latex allergens rHev b 1, rHev b 5, rHev 6.01, and rHev b 8, improved test efficiency compared to the ImmunoCAP without rHev b 5 from 86.7 to 90.6 % (◉ Table 8.1), but ultimately it did not achieve the efficiency of the rHev b 5-supplemented "enriched" ImmunoCAP (Raulf-Heimsoth et al. 2007).

8.3 Benefits and Disadvantages of Allergen Addition in Hazelnut Allergy

Hazelnuts are among the most common triggers of food allergies worldwide. Associated symptoms range from the oral allergy syndrome to severe systemic and even fatal reactions. To date, a number of allergen components of the hazelnut have been identified, which can be categorized into the protein families of:

- PR-10 proteins (Cor a 1)
- Profilins (Cor a 2)
- Nonspecific lipid transfer proteins (nsLTP; Cor a 8)
- Storage proteins (Cor a 9, Cor a 11, Cor a 14) and
- Oleosins (Cor a 12, Cor a 13) (http://www.allergen.org/List.htm)

In this case, as well as in a number of other food allergies, the molecular sensitization profile allows a risk assessment regarding the patient's risk potential upon allergen exposure. Among other things, this depends on the amount of allergen in the allergenic source as well as on its stability following exposure to heat and enzymatic digestion. Storage proteins and nsLTPs are often associated with an increased risk potential for allergic reactions, whereas PR-10 protein sensitizations are frequently associated with birch pollen and suggest cross-reactivity. Sensitization to the heat-stable and digestion-resistant nsLTP or storage proteins of hazelnut is frequently accompanied by severe systemic symptoms. In contrast, the heat-labile hazelnut component Cor a 1 (PR-10 protein) is usually a trigger of mild allergic reactions, such as the oral allergy syndrome (Masthoff et al. 2013). Thus, Cor a 8, Cor a 9, and Cor a 14 are particularly important for estimation of the risk potential in patients with hazelnut allergy (Masthoff et al. 2013). Added value in the diagnosis of hazelnut allergy could be shown recently with Cor a 14-specific IgE analysis: a 90 % probability for a positive oral hazelnut challenge was estimated for Cor a 14-specific IgE at 47.8 kU/l (Beyer et al. 2015). This finding could reduce oral food challenges if implemented in the diagnostic routine workup of hazelnut allergy.

These allergen components were already sufficiently represented in the past in the extract-based IgE test that allowed for recognition of these patients. However, the PR-10 protein Cor a 1 that particularly stands for cross-reactivity to birch pollen was not well represented in the extract. This fact led to clinical studies with the hazelnut ImmunoCAP f17 (Thermo Fisher Scientific, Freiburg, Germany) sometimes only having a low sensitivity for the test, depending on the patient population and the geographical region. For example, a study from the Netherlands detected sensitization in only 18 of 31 patients (58 %) with a confirmed hazelnut allergy using f17 (f17 sIgE $\geq$ 0.35 KU/l) (Wensing et al. 2002). These and comparable results in further studies led the manufacturer to modify the ImmunoCAP f17 by spiking it with Cor a 1 in the hope of increasing its diagnostic sensitivity. The investigations performed in this context were published (Andersson et al. 2007) and ultimately led to a significant increase in test sensitivity: the “old” ImmunoCAP f17 did not detect eight patients with confirmed hazelnut allergy in a group of 50 patients from Central Europe, while the new f17 test supplemented with recombinant Cor a 1 detected IgE antibody to hazelnut in all the sensitized patients. This corresponded to an increase in sensitivity from 84 to 100 % (Andersson et al. 2007). The Cor a 1-supplemented f17 test was introduced to the market in May 2006, and it subsequently replaced the test that was previously used.

The response from allergists to this change was not positive as shown by a publication from Sicherer et al. (2008): many pediatricians in the USA had previously used the f17 test primarily in the diagnosis of hazelnut allergies in infancy and childhood which can generally be attributed to storage proteins. The hazelnut extract supplemented with Cor a 1 now no longer only detected sensitizations to nsLTP and storage proteins but also PR-10 proteins with high sensitivity. These sensitizations are partly clinically irrelevant and can usually be attributed to cross-reactions due to tree pollen allergy. Criticism was particularly focused on the fact that the new Cor a 1-supplemented f17 ImmunoCAP could no longer differentiate between different sensitization patterns, and this change was not communicated by the manufacturer to the laboratories or practicing physicians.

Today, Cor a 1, Cor a 8, Cor a, 9 and Cor a 14 are available as molecular singleplex tests in addition to the Cor a 1-supplemented hazelnut ImmunoCAP f17; they allow for detailed recognition of the patient’s sensitization profile and for the implementation of molecular-based allergy diagnostics in patients with hazelnut allergy.

8.4 Improvement of Test Sensitivity by Allergen Addition in Yellow Jacket Venom Allergy

Another example of improved diagnostics by addition of a recombinant individual allergen to the allergen extract relates to the diagnosis of yellow jacket venom allergy. The serological IgE diagnostics of hymenoptera venom allergy is complicated by a high degree of cross-reactivity between honeybee and yellow jacket venom extracts. For example, up to 45 % of our patients exhibit dual sensitization to both insect venoms (Hofmann et al. 2011). This cross-reactivity is either caused by cross-reactive carbohydrate determinants (CCD) or recognition of proteins with homology between individual honeybee and yellow jacket venom allergens. The introduction of CCD-free species-specific marker allergens (Api m 1 for honeybee venom or Ves v 5 and Ves v 1 for yellow jacket venom) has allowed for more definitive differentiation between sensitization to honeybee and yellow jacket venom allergens. This has significantly improved the serological diagnosis of Hymenoptera venom allergy (Hofmann et al. 2011).

The first report on the benefits of rApi m 1 and rVes v 5 use in the IgE diagnostics of Hymenoptera venom allergy described positive sIgE levels to the marker allergen rVes v 5 (i209) but negative IgE serological results to yellow jacket venom (ImmunoCAP i3) as measured in 5 of 7 patients with a clear history of anaphylaxis after a yellow jacket sting (Hofmann et al. 2011). A larger follow-up examination of

308 patients with yellow jacket venom allergy confirmed these initial findings (Vos et al. 2013). In this study, only 83.4 % of the patients showed sensitization to the wasp yellow jacket (i3), while IgE sensitization (≥0.35 kU_A/L) was detectable in 96 % of the cases using the individual allergens Ves v 1 and Ves v 5. Among patients with yellow jacket venom allergy who tested negative to IgE against yellow jacket venom extract (i3), IgE could be detected against rVes v 5 in 84.4 % (42/51, ≥0,35 kU_A/l). Comparative evaluation of IgE reactivity to yellow jacket venom extract (i3) and rVes v 1 (i211) detected higher values for the total venom than for the individual allergen in almost all patients which suggests that only part of the IgE reactivity is directed against the selected allergen (◉ Fig. 8.3a). In contrast, comparative studies of IgE reactivity to yellow jacket venom extract (i3) and rVes v 5 (i209) detected IgE reactivity to the individual allergen that was on average 2.4 times higher than that to whole venom (◉ Fig. 8.3b). This observation suggested that the IgE immunoreactivity to Ves v 5 is underrepresented when tests were performed using the allergosorbent coupled with yellow jacket venom extract (i3).

Various explanations can be proposed to explain the observed results: (a) a lack of the allergen Ves v 5 in yellow jacket venom extract, (b) poor or insufficient coupling of Ves v 5 in natural yellow jacket venom to the solid phase of the test system, and (c) steric blockade of the IgE epitopes to Ves v 5 by endogenous inhibitors, among others.

The apparently absent IgE immunoreactivity in the conventional ImmunoCAP i3 was compensated by spiking the yellow jacket venom extract with recombinant Ves v 5 (Vos et al. 2013). A direct comparison with the non-enriched yellow jacket venom ImmunoCAP in Ves v 5-positive patients detected significantly higher IgE reactivity for the rVes v 5-supplemented ImmunoCAP (◉ Fig. 8.3c). Both CAP variants delivered comparable results in Ves v 5-negative patients. In comparison to the previous yellow jacket venom ImmunoCAP, the Ves v 5-supplemented ImmunoCAP captured 96.8 % of the patients who were allergic to yellow jacket venom. The test's diagnostic sensitivity increased from 83.4 to 96.8 % through addition of rVes v 5 (◉ Fig. 8.4). Similar results were also reported from other groups (Ebo et al. 2013). The observed increase in the sensitivity was not associated with reduced specificity of the test system. Based on this data, rVes v 5-supplemented yellow jacket venom was introduced for routine diagnostics in June 2012. After a transitional period, the previous (not Ves v 5-supplemented) yellow jacket venom ImmunoCAP (i3) was taken off the market.

Unfortunately the manufacturer failed to adequately communicate this change in the test system and provide the different variants with individual names. This is particularly relevant for follow-up observations in the context of specific immunotherapy. On the whole, it can be presumed that before 2012, sIgE to yellow jacket venom (i3) was measured with the non-supplemented ImmunoCAPs, while all values collected from 2013 onward were analyzed with the new rVes v 5-supplemented ImmunoCAP.

The significant improvement in sensitivity resulting from the addition of rVes v 5 suggests that further individual allergens such as Ves v 1, Ves v 2, or Ves v 3 could possibly be used for improvement of test performance. However, this is not the case,

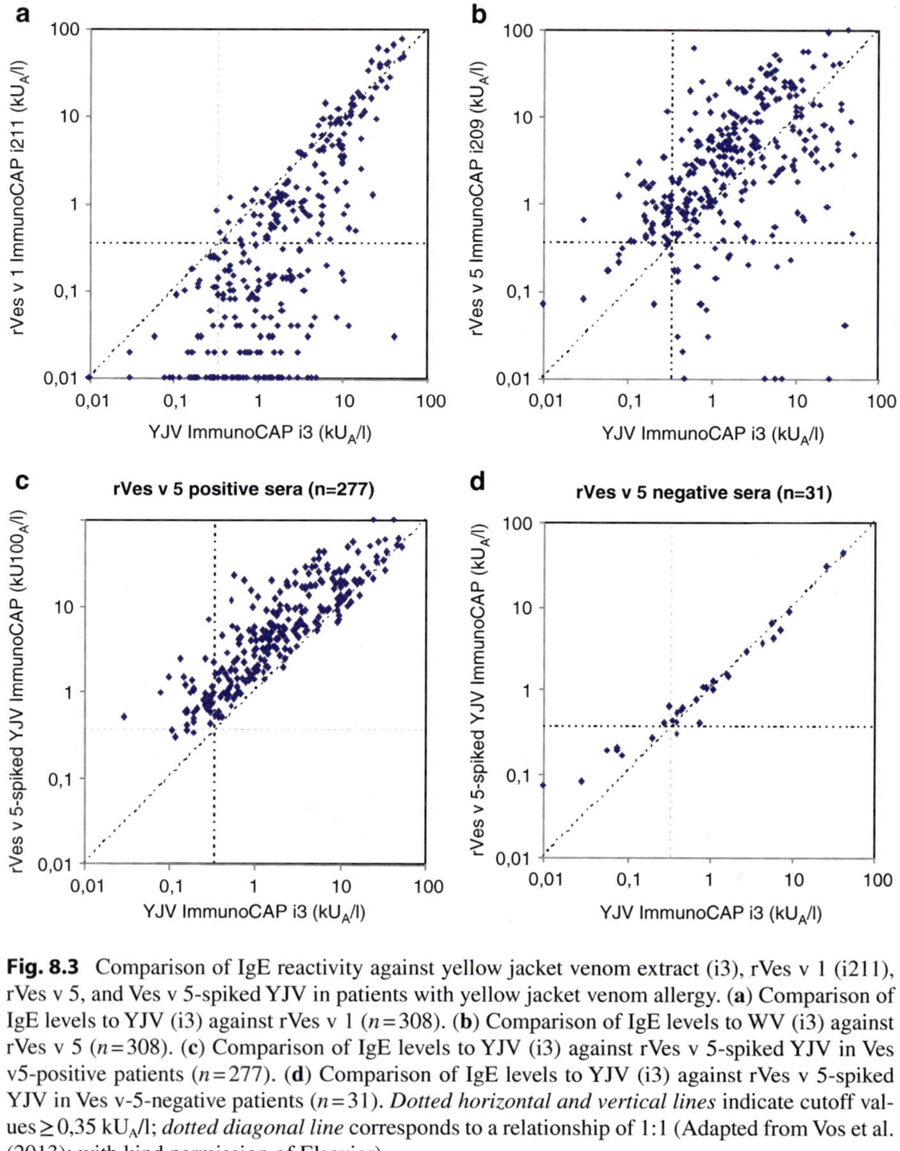

Fig. 8.3 Comparison of IgE reactivity against yellow jacket venom extract (i3), rVes v 1 (i211), rVes v 5, and Ves v 5-spiked YJV in patients with yellow jacket venom allergy. (**a**) Comparison of IgE levels to YJV (i3) against rVes v 1 (n=308). (**b**) Comparison of IgE levels to WV (i3) against rVes v 5 (n=308). (**c**) Comparison of IgE levels to YJV (i3) against rVes v 5-spiked YJV in Ves v5-positive patients (n=277). (**d**) Comparison of IgE levels to YJV (i3) against rVes v 5-spiked YJV in Ves v-5-negative patients (n=31). *Dotted horizontal and vertical lines* indicate cutoff values ≥ 0,35 kU$_A$/l; *dotted diagonal line* corresponds to a relationship of 1:1 (Adapted from Vos et al. (2013); with kind permission of Elsevier)

as investigations on the sera of patients with a clear history of yellow jacket venom allergy but without sIgE to Ves v 5-supplemented yellow jacket venom showed (Rafei-Shamsabadi et al. 2014). The same goes for the individual diagnostic bee venom allergens Api m 1, Api m 2, Api m 3, Api m 4, Api m 5, and Api m 10 that have been characterized to date (Köhler et al. 2014). In patients with a clear history of bee venom allergy but without positive sIgE values to whole honeybee venom extract, the

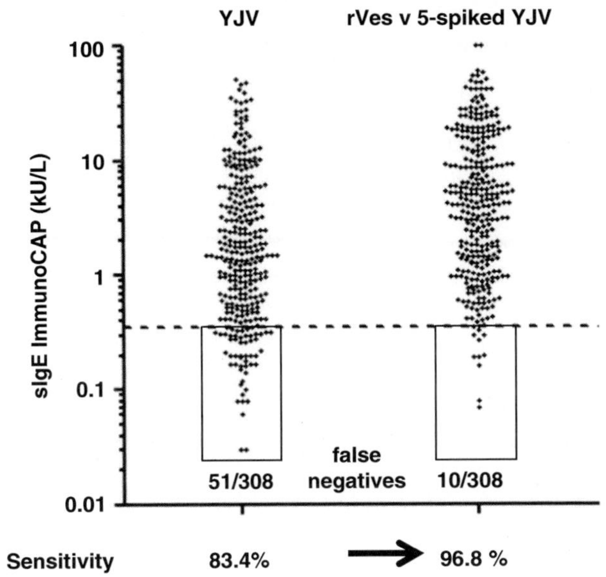

Fig. 8.4 Enhancement of diagnostic sensitivity in yellow jacket venom allergy by spiking with rVes v 5. sIgE reactivity against YJV (i3) without (*left*) and with addition of rVes v 5 (*right*) in 308 patients with YJV allergy (adapted from Vos et al., 2013)

application of Api m 1, Api m 2, Api m 3, Api m 4, Api m 5, and Api m 10 did not lead to an improvement in diagnostic sensitivity (Rafei-Shamsabadi et al. 2014).

8.5 Additional Value of Molecular Diagnostics and Conclusion for Routine Clinical Practice

The examples of addition of recombinant individual allergens to extract-based tests listed in this chapter show the potential of this approach for improved diagnostics but also the associated problems. While the diagnostic sensitivity of the tests was significantly increased for latex, hazelnut, and yellow jacket venom, the example of the hazelnut ImmunoCAP f17 shows that the diagnostic discriminatory power can certainly also be reduced as a result. Today this problem can be overcome by combining further allergen component-based singleplex tests. Based on the broad spectrum of available molecular tests, a detailed sensitization profile can be obtained which, taken together with history and clinical findings, allows more accurate diagnosis and risk assessment. The decision to alter an extract-based in vitro allergy test by adding individual recombinant allergens should always be carefully considered, since the performance and application of the test can be permanently affected all over the world. Not all extract-based IgE tests where allergen components are underrepresented were supplemented in the past by addition of the relevant allergens. For example, the allergen component Tri a 19 (omega-5-gliadin) is underrepresented in the wheat ImmunoCAP and Gly m 4 in the soy ImmunoCAP, but no decision has been made to add these allergens to the extracts in recombinant form. Since these allergen components are available as molecular singleplex tests, there is no diagnostic gap.

Finally, it should be noted that molecular-based allergy diagnostics opens new diagnostic possibilities in allergy through the option of spiking in combination with molecular singleplex tests. Clear communication on the part of the manufacturer, to which test(s) recombinant allergens were added and from what time point on – and also where this was not done despite underrepresented allergen components – is essential in order to allow clinicians to optimally interpret the results and utilize these measurements for improved patient management.

8.6 Conclusion for Clinical Routine

In conclusion, molecular allergy diagnostics is opening up new diagnostic possibilities through the spiking of extracts with molecular allergens that are then used in singleplex tests. A clear communication by the manufacturer about any product changes by spiking is critical for accurate interpretation of the resultant IgE antibody data. It is also important to indicate where this was not performed and why, even though important allergen components may be underrepresented in the native extract-based test. If these prerequisites are met, the clinician has the possibility to make optimal use of molecular allergy testing for the benefit of improved patient care.

Bibliography

Akasawa A, Hsieh LS, Martin BM, Liu T, Lin Y. A novel acidic allergen, Hev b 5, in latex. Purification, cloning and characterization. J Biol Chem. 1996;271:25389–93.

Andersson K, Ballmer-Weber BK, Cistero-Bahima A, Östling J, Lauer I, Vieths S, Lidholm J. Enhancement of hazelnut extract for IgE testing by recombinant allergen spiking. Allergy. 2007;62:897–904.

Beyer K, Grabenhenrich L, Härtl M, Beder A, Kalb B, Ziegert M, Finger A, Harandi N, Schlags R, Gappa M, Puzzo L, Röblitz H, Millner-Uhlemann M, Büsing S, Ott H, Lange L, Niggemann B. Predictive values of component-specific IgE for the outcome of peanut and hazelnut food challenges in children. Allergy. 2015;70:90–8.

Chen Z, Rihs HP, Slater JE, Paupore EJ, Schneider EM, Baur X. The absence of Hev b 5 in capture antigen may cause false-negative results in serologic assays for latex-specific IgE antibodies. J Allergy Clin Immunol. 2000;105:S8.

Ebo DG, Faber M, Sabato V, Leysen J, Bridts CH, De Clerck LS. Component-resolved diagnosis of wasp (yellow jacket) venom allergy. Clin Exp Allergy. 2013;43:255–61.

Hofmann SC, Pfender N, Weckesser S, Huss-Marp J, Jakob T. Added value of IgE detection to rApi m 1 and rVes v 5 in patients with Hymenoptera venom allergy. J Allergy Clin Immunol. 2011;127:265–7.

Köhler J, Blank S, Müller S, Frick M, Bantleon F, Huss-Marp J, Lidholm J, Spillner E, Jakob T. Component resolution reveals additional major allergens in bee venom allergic patients. J Allergy Clin Immunol. 2014;133:1383–9.

Lundberg M, Chen Z, Rihs HP, Wrangsjö K. Recombinant spiked allergen extract. Allergy. 2001;56:794–5.

Masthoff LJ, Mattsson L, Zuidmeer-Jongejan L, Lidholm J, Andersson K, Akkerdaas JH, Versteeg SA, Garino C, Meijer Y, Kentie P, Versluis A, den Hartog Jager CF, Bruijnzeel-Koomen CAFM, Knulst AC, van Ree R, van Hoffen E, Pasmans SGMA. Sensitization to Cor a 9 and Cor a 14 is highly specific for a hazelnut allergy with objective symptoms in Dutch children and adults. J Allergy Clin Immunol. 2013;132:393–9.

Matricardi PM, Kleine-Tebbe J, Hoffmann HJ, Valenta R, Hilger C, Hofmaier S, Aalberse RC, Agache I, Asero R, Ballmer-Weber B, Barber D, Beyer K, Biedermann T, Biló MB, Blank S, Bohle B, Bosshard PP, Breiteneder H, Brough HA, Caraballo L, Caubet JC, Crameri R, Davies JM, Douladiris N, Ebisawa M, Eigenmann PA, Fernandez-Rivas M, Ferreira F, Gadermaier G, Glatz M, Hamilton RG, Hawranek T, Hellings P, Hoffmann-Sommergruber K, Jakob T, Jappe U, Jutel M, Kamath SD, Knol EF, Korosec P, Kuehn A, Lack G, Lopata AL, Mäkelä M, Morisset M, Niederberger V, Nowak-Wezgrzyn AH, Papadopoulos NG, Pastorello EA, Pauli G, Platts-Mills T, Posa D, Poulsen LK, Raulf M, Sastre J, Scala E, Schmid JM, Schmid-Grendelmeier P, van Hage M, van Ree R, Vieths S, Weber R, Wickman M, Muraro A, Ollert M. EAACI molecular allergology user's guide. Pediatr Allergy Immunol. 2016;27(suppl 23):1–250.

Müller U, Schmid-Grendelmeier P, Hausmann O, Helbling A. IgE to recombinant allergens Api m 1, Ves v 1, and Ves v 5 distinguish double sensitization from crossreaction in venom allergy. Allergy. 2012;67:1069–73.

Rafei-Shamsabadi D, Müller S, Pfützner W, Spillner E, Rueff F, Jakob T. Recombinant allergens rarely allow identification of Hymenoptera venom allergic patients with negative specific IgE to whole venom preparations. J Allergy Clin Immunol. 2014;134:493–4.

Raulf-Heimsoth M, Rihs H-P. Latexallergene: Sensibilisierungsquellen und Einzelallergenprofile erkennen. Allergo J. 2011;20:241–3.

Raulf-Heimsoth M, Rihs HP, Rozynek P, Cremer R, Gaspar Â, Pires G, Yeang HY, Arif SAM, Hamilton RG, Sander I, Lundberg M, Brüning T. Quantitative analysis of IgE reactivity profiles in patients allergic or sensitized to natural rubber latex (Hevea brasiliensis). Clin Exp Allergy. 2007;37:1657–67.

Sicherer SH, Dhillon G, Laughery KA, Hamilton RG, Wood RA. Caution: the Phadia hazelnut ImmunoCAP (f17) has been supplemented with recombinant Cor a 1 and now detects Bet v 1–specific IgE, which leads to elevated values for persons with birch pollen allergy. J Allergy Clin Immunol. 2008;122:413–4.

Slater JE, Vedvick T, Arthur-Smith A, Trybul DE, Kekwick RGO. Identification, cloning, and sequence of a major allergen (Hev b 5) from natural rubber latex (Hevea brasiliensis). J Biol Chem. 1996;271:25394–9.

Vos B, Köhler J, Müller S, Stretz E, Ruëff F, Jakob T. Spiking venom with rVes v 5 improves sensitivity of IgE detection in patients with allergy to Vespula venom. J Allergy Clin Immunol. 2013;131:1225–7.

Wensing M, Penninks AH, Hefle SL, Akkerdaas JH, van Ree R, Koppelman SJ, Bruijnzeel-Koomen CA, Knulst AC. The range of minimum provoking doses in hazelnut-allergic patients as determined by double-blind, placebocontrolled food challenges. Clin Exp Allergy. 2002;32:1757–62.

Molecular Allergy Diagnostics Using Multiplex Assays

9

T. Jakob, P. Forstenlechner, P.M. Matricardi, and J. Kleine-Tebbe

The present chapter is based on, and modified from, an article by the authors published in 2015 in *Allergo Journal International* (Jakob T, Forstenlechner P, Matricardi P, Kleine-Tebbe J: Molecular allergy diagnostics using multiplex assays: methodological and practical considerations for use in research and clinical routine. Allergo J Int 2015;24: 320–332 DOI 10.1007/s40629-015-0056-2). The authors gratefully thank Prof. Robert G. Hamilton, PhD, Johns Hopkins Dermatology, Allergy and Clinical Immunology (DACI) Reference Laboratory at the Johns Hopkins Asthma & Allergy Center, Baltimore, MD, USA, for reviewing the manuscript, expert editorial assistance, and many helpful suggestions regarding this chapter.

T. Jakob, MD, Prof. (✉)
Department of Dermatology and Allergology, University Medical Center Giessen (UKGM), Justus-Liebig-University, Giessen, Germany
e-mail: thilo.jakob@derma.med.uni-giessen.de

P. Forstenlechner, PhD
Phadia – Thermo Fisher Scientific, Wien, Austria
e-mail: peter.forstenlechner@thermofisher.com

P.M. Matricardi, MD, Assoc Prof.
Molecular Allergology and Immunomodulation Working Group, Department of Pediatric Pneumology and Immunology, Charité-Universitätsmedizin, Berlin, Germany
e-mail: paolo.matricardi@charite.de

J. Kleine-Tebbe, MD, Prof.
Allergy & Asthma Center Westend, Outpatient Clinic Hanf, Ackermann & Kleine-Tebbe, Berlin, Germany
e-mail: kleine-tebbe@allergie-experten.de

J. Kleine-Tebbe, T. Jakob (eds.), *Molecular Allergy Diagnostics*,
DOI 10.1007/978-3-319-42499-6_9

9.1 Introduction

Since Charles Blackley carried out the first in vivo test with pollen on his own skin in 1880 (Blackley 1880), the diagnosis of type I allergy has been performed using extract preparations. Almost 90 years later, shortly after the discovery of immunoglobulin E (IgE), the radioallergosorbent test (RAST) was established. This test enabled circulating specific IgE (sIgE) antibodies to be determined for the first time in vitro, using anti-IgE antibodies labeled with radioisotope (Ishizaka and Ishizaka 1967; Johansson and Bennich 1967; Wide et al. 1967). IgE binding to allergen extracts coupled to a solid phase (paper discs) was measured. The elucidation of the major birch pollen antigen Bet v 1 deoxyribonucleic acid (DNA) sequence heralded the era of molecular allergy diagnostics (Breiteneder et al. 1988). Recombinant or purified (glyco-)proteins enabled the measurement of sIgE to defined single allergens—initially in singleplex and, since 2001, also in multiplex assays (Valenta and Kraft 2001, Hiller et al. 2002) (◉ Fig. 9.1).

Multiplex assays in allergy diagnostics refer to the simultaneous determination of sIgE to different allergens or allergen extracts in a single test run. This approach has already been used in the past in the form of strip tests for allergy screening (e.g., Allergodip, Euroline, Polycheck, etc.), in order to obtain as much information as possible on the sensitization status of an allergic patient in a single test.

These strip tests are based on the "dot blot" principle, in which multiple dot-shaped or strip-shaped allergen-containing membranes serve as the solid phase. These tests enable simultaneous semiquantitative measurement of sIgE to different allergen sources; they do not, however, enable elucidation of the sensitization pattern on a molecular level, since extracts are usually used.

Definitions

Allergen (also single allergen or allergen components)	Molecule with the ability to bind sIgE or trigger sIgE production
Allergen source	Organism that expresses allergenic molecules (e.g., cat, grass pollen)
ISAC	Immuno Solid-phase Allergen Chip, multiplex tool for the determination of sIgE using microarray technology
Microarray	Term used for molecular biological test methods that allow parallel testing of multiple analytes (also known as bio- or allergen chip)
Multiplex assay	Simultaneous testing of multiple analytes in a single assay (e.g., using microarray technology)
Singleplex assay	Testing of a single analyte in a single assay
Diagnostic sensitivity	The probability that a test yields a positive result in an affected individual
Diagnostic specificity	The probability that a test yields a negative result in a healthy individual
Coefficient of variation	Measure of relative dispersion

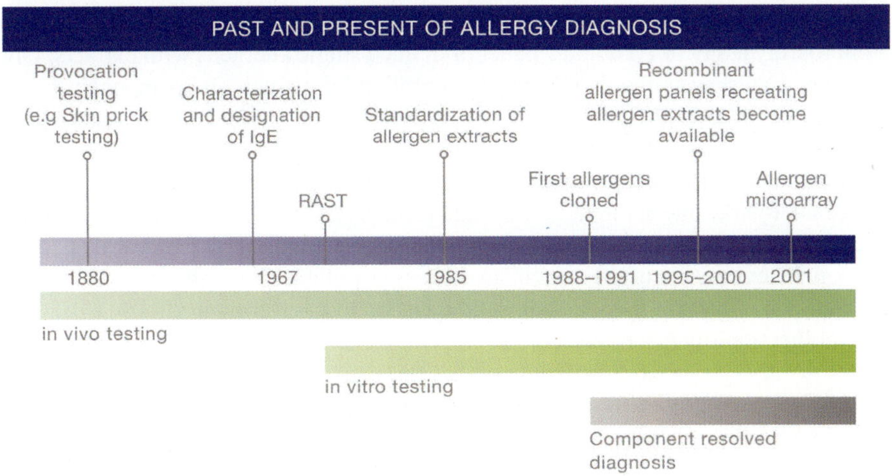

Fig. 9.1 Historical development of diagnostics in IgE-mediated allergies

Thanks to the progress made in molecular allergology and chip-based microarray technology, multiplex assays could be developed which renders the analysis of a patient's IgE profile at the level of individual molecules possible. To accomplish this, minute quantities (picogram range) of different allergens are coupled to a solid phase before these protein arrays (allergen chips) are used for simultaneous determination of allergen-specific IgE (Hiller et al. 2002). In contrast to single tests (singleplex assays) and extract-based diagnostics, allergen chips enable elucidation of an extensive sensitization profile at the individual molecule level in a single measurement. This enables a differentiated analysis of the individual IgE repertoire and reveals a patient's current sensitization status.

The present chapter first introduces the multiplex diagnostic procedure. It then goes on to discuss the advantages and limitations of this new technology for allergy diagnostics in clinical routine and in the research environment.

9.2 Molecular Allergy Diagnostics Using Multiplex Assays

Whereas singleplex assays for molecular allergy diagnostics are already used by and available from many manufacturers of diagnostic tools, there are currently only a few companies with multiplex assays for molecular allergy diagnostics at their disposal.

Of these test systems, one has established itself as the gold standard in multiplex assay molecular allergy diagnostics. This system is based on the Immuno Solid-phase Allergen Chip (ISAC), which has been available since 2001. The ISAC was initially developed and manufactured by VBC Genomics in Vienna; since 2009, it has been further developed, manufactured, and marketed by Phadia, Thermo Fisher Scientific, Uppsala, Sweden. Under the product name ImmunoCAP ISAC 112, the current version of this allergen chip enables determination of sIgE to 112 different single molecules from 51 different plant and animal allergen sources (see ◉ Table 9.1 for a detailed list of the allergens used in ISAC 112).

In addition, test systems exist that couple "classic" allergen extracts onto chips for a microarray assay or combine a panel of defined single allergens with extracts. One of these is a test system only recently CE certified for extract- and component-based diagnostics (ADAM, Microtest Diagnostics Ltd, London, UK). This fully automated test system can semiquantitatively determine sIgE to common aero- and food allergens within 4 h. The test principle is based on a protein microarray currently featuring 22 allergen extracts, three recombinant proteins (rBet v 1, rAra h 2, and rCor a 1), and one purified single allergen (nGal d 1). Since virtually no technical or clinical data on the evaluation of the system are hitherto available (Palomba et al. 2014), it is not possible at present to make any statements on test performance.

Another multiplex test system is currently being developed by Abionic. This system is also based on a fully automated microarray assay and enables measurement of sIgE reactivity to common single allergens in different screening panels, e.g., a screening panel with the food and inhalant allergens Gal d 1, Bos d 5, Ara h 2, Bet v 1, Bet v 2, Phl p 1, Phl p 5, Der p 1, Can f 1, and Fel d 1. The system is conceived as a point-of-care instrument (PoC), uses capillary blood, and—according to the manufacturer's data—enables the determination of sIgE within 20 min. There are currently no study data available on this system.

Semiquantitative multiplex testing with allergen extracts using line blot-based paper strips developed by Euroimmun has recently been complemented with allergenic molecules. Several panels are available with 6–14 purified and/or recombinant food and/or inhalant allergens, including an additional CCD marker:

A. *Peanut panel* with recombinant Ara h 1, Ara h 2, Ara h 3, Ara h 5, Ara h 6, Ara h 7, Ara h 9, and Bet v1.
B. *Cow's milk panel* with native Bos d 4, Bos d 5, Bos d 6, and Bos d 8, and cow's milk extract.
C. *Pediatric panel* with rAra h 1, rAra h 2, rAra h 3, rAra h 9, nGal d 1, nGal d 2, nGal d 3, nGal d 4, nBos d 4, nBos d 5, nBos d 6, nBos d 8, plus 2 native cow's milk extracts and rBet v 1.
D. *Pollen panel* with recombinant Bet v 1, Bet v 2, Bet v 4, Bet v 6, Phl p 1, Phl p 5, Phl p 7, Phl p 12, plus birch and timothy pollen extracts.
E. *Insect venom panel* with recombinant Api m 2, Api m 10, Ves v 1, Ves v 5, plus native bee and wasp venom extracts.

   So far no published results exist regarding technical or clinical evaluations, making it difficult to conclude on the performance characteristics of these assays.

Most recently, a multiplex test called FABER (version 244-122-122-01) was announced by MacroarrayDX for simultaneous detection of, i.e., allergen-specific IgE to 112 allergenic molecules and 112 extracts. The present custom-developed panel covers reagents allowing simultaneous antibody detection to foods from

Table 9.1 Allergen spectrum in the ImmunoCAP ISAC 112

Allergen source	Allergen	Protein family/biochemical name
Food allergens: plant		
Apple	rMal d 1	PR-10
Buckwheat	nFag e 2	2S albumin
Cashew nut	rAna o 2	Cupin
Peanut	rAra h 1	Cupin
	rAra h 2	2S albumin
	rAra h 3	Cupin
	nAra h 6	2S albumin
	rAra h 8	PR-10
	rAra h 9	nsLTP
Hazelnut	rCor a 1.0401	PR-10
	rCor a 8	nsLTP
	nCor a 9	Cupin
Kiwi	nAct d 1	Cysteine protease
	nAct d 2	Thaumatin-like protein
	nAct d 5	Kiwellin
	rAct d 8	PR-10
Brazil nut	rBer e 1	2S albumin
Peach	rPru p 1	PR-10
	rPru p 3	nsLTP
Celery	rApi g 1	PR-10
Sesame	nSes i 1	2S albumin
Soybean	rGly m 4	PR-10
	nGly m 5	Cupin
	nGly m 6	Cupin
Walnut	rJug r 1	2S albumin
	nJug r 2	Cupin
	nJug r 3	nsLTP
Wheat	rTri a 14	nsLTP
	rTri a 19	ω-5-Gliadin
	nTri a aA_TI	α-Amylase/trypsin inhibitor
Food allergens: animal		
Cod	rGad c 1	Parvalbumin
Hen's egg	nGal d 1	Ovomucoid
	nGal d 2	Ovalbumin
	nGal d 3	Conalbumin
	nGal d 5	Serum albumin

(continued)

Table 9.1 (continued)

Allergen source	Allergen	Protein family/biochemical name
Cow's milk	nBos d 4	α-Lactalbumin
	nBos d 5	β-Lactoglobulin
	nBos d 6	Serum albumin
	nBos d 8	Casein
	nBos d-lactoferrin	Transferrin
Shrimp	nPen m 1	Tropomyosin
	nPen m 2	Arginine kinase
	nPen m 4	Sarcoplasmic calcium-binding protein
Pollen allergens		
Maple-leaved plane	rPla a 1	Invertase inhibitor
	nPla a 2	Polygalacturonase
	rPla a 3	nsLTP
Arizona cypress	nCup a 1	Pectate lyase
Spreading pellitory	rPar j 2	nsLTP
Ragweed	nAmb a 1	Pectate lyase
Birch	rBet v 1	PR-10
	rBet v 2	Profilin
	rBet v 4	Polcalcin
Annual mercury	rMer a 1	Profilin
Alder	rAln g 1	PR-10
Common mugwort	nArt v 1	Defensin-like protein
	nArt v 3	nsLTP
Hazel pollen	rCor a 1.0101	PR-10
Bermuda grass	nCyn d 1	Grass group 1
Japanese cedar	nCry j 1	Pectate lyase
Timothy grass	rPhl p 1	Grass group 1
	rPhl p 2	Grass group 2/3
	nPhl p 4	Berberine bridge enzyme
	rPhl p 5	Unknown
	rPhl p 6	Unknown
	rPhl p 7	Polcalcin
	rPhl p 11	Ole e 1-related protein
	rPhl p 12	Profilin
Olive tree	rOle e 1	Olive group 1
	nOle e 7	nsLTP (putatively)
	rOle e 9	1,3-β-Glucanase
Prickly saltwort	nSal k 1	Pectin methylesterase
Ribwort plantain	rPla l 1	Ole e 1-related protein
White goosefoot	rChe a 1	Ole e 1-related protein

Table 9.1 (continued)

Allergen source	Allergen	Protein family/biochemical name
Furry animal allergens		
Dog	rCan f 1	Lipocalin
	rCan f 2	Lipocalin
	nCan f 3	Serum albumin
	rCan f 5	Arginine esterase
Cat	rFel d 1	Uteroglobin
	nFel d 2	Serum albumin
	rFel d 4	Lipocalin
Mouse	nMus m 1	Lipocalin
Horse	rEqu c 1	Lipocalin
	nEqu c 3	Serum albumin
Mite allergens		
Blomia tropicalis	rBlo t 5	Unknown
D. farinae	nDer f 1	Cysteine protease
	rDer f 2	NPC2
D. pteronyssinus	nDer p 1	Cysteine protease
	rDer p 2	NPC2
	rDer p 10	Tropomyosin
Lepidoglyphus destructor	rLep d 2	NPC2
Mold allergens		
A. alternata	rAlt a 1	Unknown
	rAlt a 6	Enolase
A. fumigatus	rAsp f 1	Mitogillin
	rAsp f 3	Peroxisomal protein
	rAsp f 6	Manganese superoxide dismutase
C. herbarum	rCla h 8	Mannitol dehydrogenase
Latex allergens		
Latex	rHev b 1	Rubber elongation factor
	rHev b 3	Small rubber particle protein
	rHev b 5	Unknown
	rHev b 6.01	Hevein precursor
	rHev b 8	Profilin
Insect venom allergens		
Common wasp	rVes v 5	Antigen 5
Honey bee	rApi m 1	Phospholipase A_2
	nApi m 4	Melittin
European paper wasp	rPol d 5	Antigen 5
Other allergens		
Pineapple	nMUXF3	Cross-reactive carbohydrate determinants (CCD)

(continued)

Table 9.1 (continued)

Allergen source	Allergen	Protein family/biochemical name
German cockroach	rBla g 1	Unknown
	rBla g 2	Aspartic protease
	rBla g 5	Glutathione S-transferase
	nBla g 7	Tropomyosin
Herring worm	rAni s 1	Unknown
	rAni s 3	Tropomyosin

nuts, seeds, and legumes ($n=46$); fruits ($n=31$); vegetables ($n=13$); milk ($n=12$); egg and fowl ($n=15$); meats ($n=6$); fish, shellfish, and mollusks ($n=17$); or inhalant allergen carriers, i.e., tree pollen ($n=13$), grass pollen ($n=8$), weed pollen ($n=8$), mites ($n=10$), epidermal and other animal proteins ($n=24$), microorganisms ($n=11$), insects ($n=7$), and additional allergen sources like insect venoms ($n=5$), parasites ($n=5$), latex ($n=10$), as well as 3 CCD-markers. The allergen reagents are (a) bound to chemically activated nanoparticles allowing individual optimization of the antigen, (b) arrayed to a solid-phase matrix, (c) to form a single-step multiplex test solution for 100 µl of serum or plasma, (d) and finally assayed and quantified by colorimetric or luminescence image capture. Up to now technical data regarding performance characteristics or clinical evaluations are not yet available.

9.3 Immuno Solid-Phase Allergen Chip (ISAC)

9.3.1 Test Procedure

The ImmunoCAP ISAC 112, a solid-phase immunoassay, comprises a polymer-coated slide with four fields, the protein microarrays (i.e., allergen chips) (◉ Fig. 9.2). One array is used per patient sample, such that four different sera can be tested with each slide. The allergens (in the picogram range) are applied in triplicates, thus enabling multiple measurements, and covalently bonded to the polymer layer. The allergen components immobilized in this way bind all allergen-specific antibodies (e.g., IgE, IgG, IgA) in the patient sample (◉ Fig. 9.3). Once the nonspecific antibodies have been washed away, a fluorescently labeled antihuman IgE antibody is added to promote complex formation. Following incubation, unbound antibodies of other isotypes (IgG, IgA, etc.) and excess unbound fluorescently labeled antihuman IgE antibodies are removed by washing. Finally, fluorescence is measured using a microarray scanner (◉ Fig. 9.4). The higher the signal, the more sIgE is present in the sample. The test results are analyzed with PC-based software, and the concentration of sIgE in the sample is calculated in the form of ISAC standard units (ISU-E). The manufacturer has adjusted the calibration curve to approximately match the units in the ImmunoCAP singleplex method (kU_A/l). The latter are derived heterologously over a total IgE standard curve, whereas ISU-E are based on calibration using the ImmunoCAP singleplex system (Phadia 250).

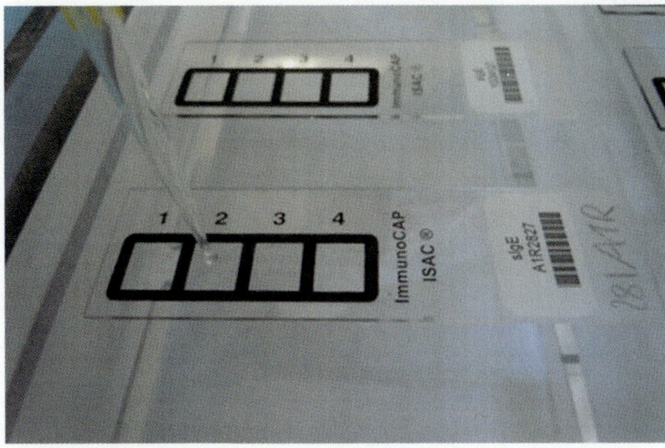

Fig. 9.2 ISAC Allergen chip: example of a commercially available multiplex assay to simultaneously measure sIgE to 112 single allergens

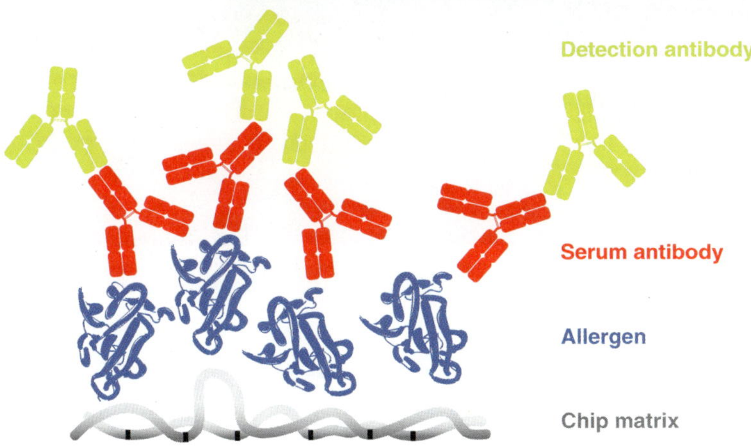

Fig. 9.3 Test principle of the ISAC allergen chip

Measurement values are reported not only quantitatively but also semiquantitatively, divided into four different categories:

1. Values <0.3 ISU-E are defined as negative.
2. Values between 0.3 and 1.0 ISU-E as low-level positive.
3. Values between 1.0 and 15.0 ISU-E as moderately high.
4. Values ≥15.0 ISU-E as very high.

Thus, test results comprise the actual measurement, plus a color-coded bar chart representation from which the approximate value of the measurement and the evaluation category can be read.

The ISAC 112 is primarily defined as a semiquantitative method, since, in the manufacturer's opinion, the miniaturization of the assay design, the shape of the calibration curve, the degree of scattering, and potential divergent values due to competitive inhibition by competing allergen-specific antibodies of other classes (see below) preclude reliable measurement of the "true" quantitative concentrations of allergen-specific IgE antibodies.

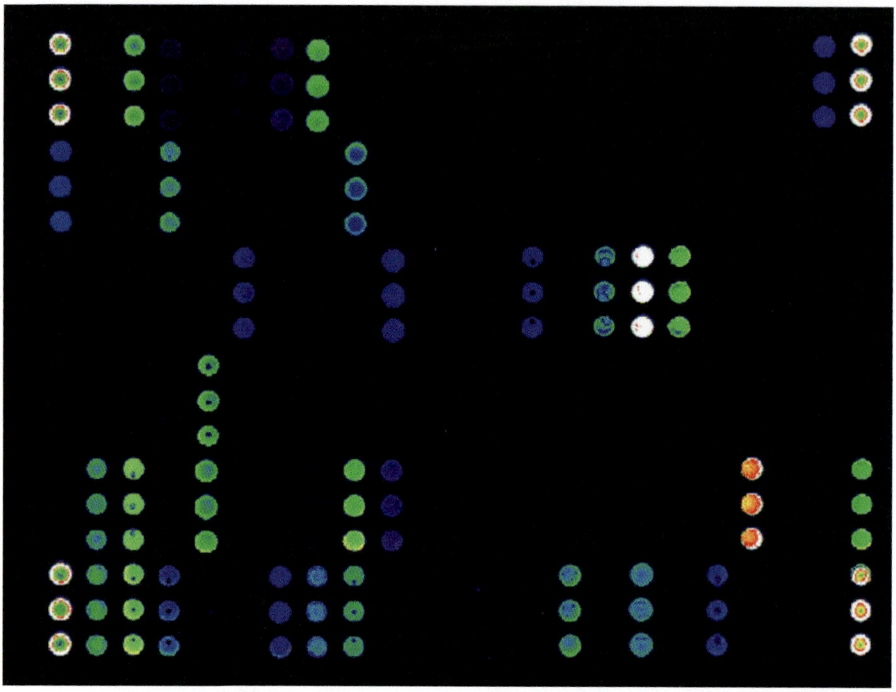

Fig. 9.4 Example of ISAC 112 microarray analysis with triplicate measurements of sIgE signals

9.3.2 Test Performance

Extensive data on test performance were collected for ISAC 112 by the manufacturer in 2011 (ImmunoCAP ISAC 112—performance characteristics, data on file, 2011) and relate to the following parameters:

- Precision (reproducibility depending on signal strength)
- Intra-assay variation coefficients (IAVC) and inter-assay variation coefficients (IEVC)
- Linearity (measurement response using diluted samples)
- Limit of detection (LoD) and limit of quantitation (LoQ)
- Matrix effects
- Total IgE interference
- Parallel comparison with singleplex tests (ImmunoCAP)

Data on precision, linearity, and LoD as well as on factors possibly causing interference in the assay are discussed in the following sections.

9.3.2.1 Intra- and Inter-Assay Variance

Data on precision were collected using sera from four multisensitized patients. The samples were measured in triplicate a total of 17 times over a 4-week period. This approach generated data on intra- and inter-assay variance for 105 of 112 allergens.

According to the manufacturer, the average coefficient of variation (CV) for all allergens tested in intra- and inter-assay comparisons is below 20 %. However, it should be noted that the CV values change depending on the test system's measurement range (0.3–1.0 ISU-E vs. 1.0–15 ISU-E vs. >15 ISU-E), with higher values reported in the lowest measurement range (◉ Fig. 9.5, ◉ Tables 9.2 and 9.3).

9.3.2.2 Linearity and Limit of Detection (LoD)

Investigations of linearity were performed using serial 1:2 dilutions on sera with high sIgE values (>5 ISU-E) to the respective allergen. In this manner, linearity curves and regression coefficients were calculated for 81 of the 112 allergens, which confirmed the linearity between measurement values and orders of dilution in wide ranges (◉ Fig. 9.6 and ◉ Table 9.4).

The LoD (▶ Chap. 7), defined as the lowest sIgE concentration that can be reliably determined, was determined for eight representative allergens (Ara h 1, Bet v 1, Der p 1, Equ c 1, Fel d 1, Gad c 1, Gal d 1, and Phl p 5) according to the global consensus on the standardization of healthcare technology guidelines (NCCLS-EP17-A). The LoD was between 0.05 and 0.28 ISU-E for the individual allergens. Based on these results, and considering the identical test conditions and known CV values in the lowest measurement range, an LoD of <0.3 ISU-E was arrived at for all 112 allergens. However, according to the manufacturer, sIgE concentrations <1 kU_A/l are

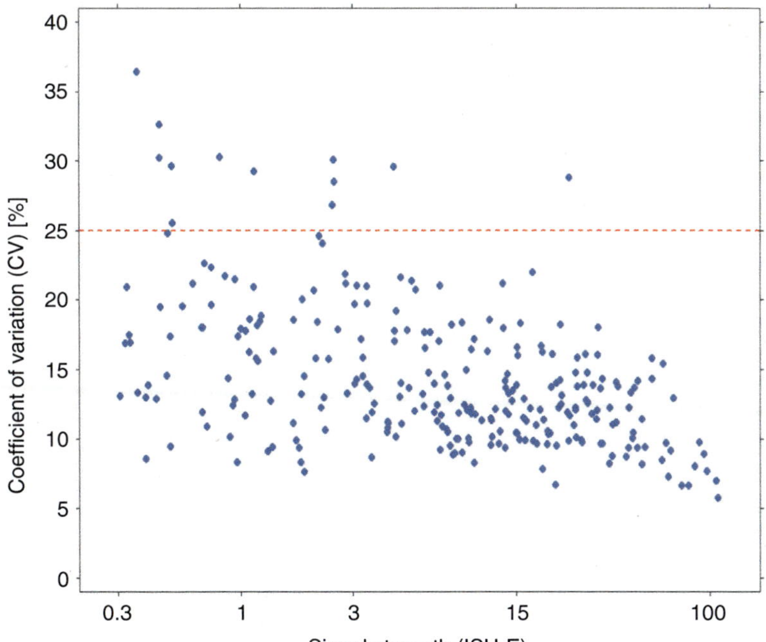

Fig. 9.5 Coefficient of variation (CV) depending on signal strength (ISU). Four serum samples covering 105 single allergens were used for calculation. Each sample was analyzed in triplicate in a total of 17 runs over a 4-week period (From "ImmunoCAP ISAC 112—performance characteristics," data on file, 2011; used with permission from Thermo Fisher Scientific)

Table 9.2 Representative examples of coefficients of variation for sIgE measurements against single allergens depending on signal strength

Sample	Allergen	Signal strength ISU-ISU-E	Mean ISU-E	CV intra-assay variance (%)	CV inter-assay variance (%)
1	Par j 2	0.33–0.98	0.32	18	9
2	Gal d 1		0.46	11	16
3	Cry j 1		0.98	12	13
4	Equ c 1	1.2–14	1.2	15	11
5	Der f 1		4.6	5	9
6	Fel d 1		14	8	9
7	Ara h 1	19–90	19	11	13
8	Phl p 5b		47	6	7
9	Bet v 1		90	7	7

CV coefficient of variation

Table 9.3 Averaged coefficient of variation for all allergens depending on signal strength

ISU-E	Class	CV intra-assay variance (%)	CV inter-assay variance (%)
0.3–1	Low	7	14
1–15	Moderate	6	10
>15	High	5	9

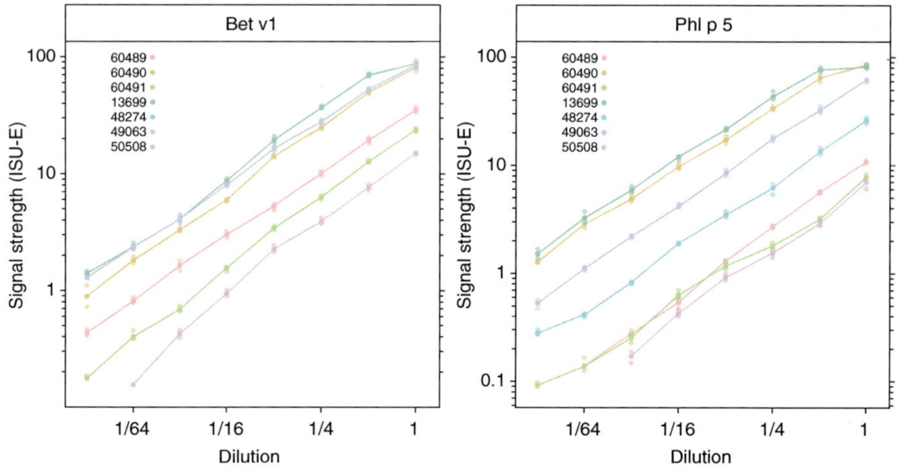

Fig. 9.6 Linearity of measurements in a dilution series using the examples of Bet v 1 and Phl p 5: serial 1:2 dilutions of seven different sera with sIgE values >5 ISU/l (From "ImmunoCAP ISAC 112—performance characteristics," data on file, 2011; used with permission from Thermo Fisher Scientific)

Table 9.4 Representative data on linearity (slope) and regression coefficient (R^2) of different allergens

Allergen	Slope	R^2
Ara h 2	1.03	0.96
Ber e 1	1.07	0.97
Bet v 1	1.16	0.95
Can f 1	1.12	0.92
Cyn d 1	1.09	0.91
Der f 2	1.01	0.99
Equ c 1	1.18	0.93
Gal d 1	1.01	0.99
Pen m 1	1.07	0.97
Phl p 1	1.12	0.97

not reliably detectable by the ISAC 112 system. Therefore, the overall sensitivity (LoD, LoQ) of ISAC 112 is to be considered lower than that of the ImmunoCAP (singleplex) method.

9.3.2.3 Sample Material and Interference

Investigations comparing sample materials were carried out on serum, citrate, heparin, and ethylenediaminetetraacetic acid (EDTA) plasma from identical donors and showed that serum, citrate, or heparin plasma from capillary or venous blood can be used. Using EDTA plasma can cause interference with Ca^{++}-binding allergens (e.g., Gad c 1, Pen m 4, or polcalcin Bet v 4 and Phl p 7) and thus lead to false-negative or false low results. When testing hemolytic or lipemic samples, neither hemolysis (up to 5 %) nor hypertriglyceridemia (triglyceride concentration up to 12 mg/ml) caused significant interference in the test system.

A factor known to influence the determination of sIgE in solid-phase assays is the level of total IgE. In order to test this influence, IgE-negative serum samples and four serum samples exhibiting sIgE to 68 of the 112 allergens were spiked with high total IgE concentrations (3,000 or 10,000 kU/l) and measured in parallel. As shown in ◉ Fig. 9.7, supplementing high concentrations of total IgE had no effect on test performance.

9.3.3 Comparison of sIgE to Single Allergens Determined in Multiplex (ISAC sIgE 112) and Singleplex Assays (ImmunoCAP)

Using 350 sera and 57 allergens that were also available as ImmunoCAP singleplex reagents, the manufacturer compared the two different measurement systems.

Depending on the frequency of sensitization, a correlation of the measured values was demonstrated for each allergen with at least five, maximally 75 sera. As shown by way of example in ◉ Fig. 9.8, a good to very good correlation of the

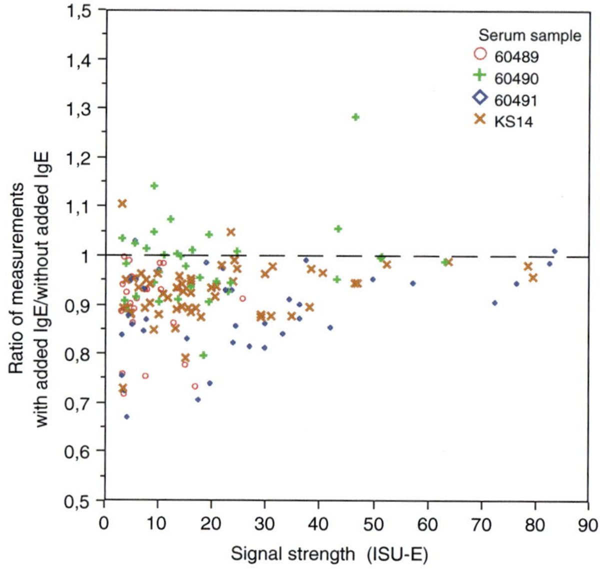

Fig. 9.7 The addition of high concentrations of IgE has no significant effect on measurements. The quotients of the measurement values obtained with and without the addition of IgE (10,000 kU/l), as measured in different serum samples, are shown (From "ImmunoCAP ISAC 112—performance characteristics," data on file, 2011; used with permission from Thermo Fisher Scientific)

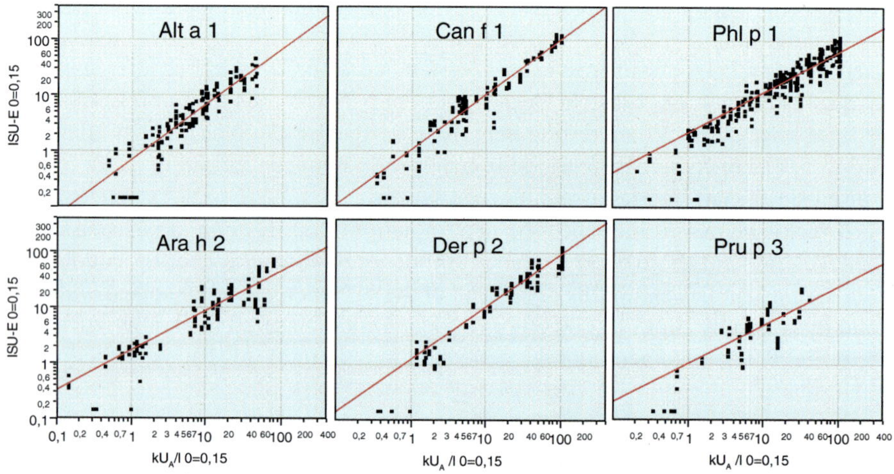

Fig. 9.8 Comparison of measurements made using the ISAC sIgE 112 (ISU-E) and ImmunoCAP (kU_A/l) systems for selected single allergens. Negative results (<0.15) are plotted as 0.15 ISU-E (From "ImmunoCAP ISAC 112—performance characteristics," data on file, 2011; used with permission from Thermo Fisher Scientific)

ISU-E values with the ImmunoCAP-derived values (kUA/l) was observed for many allergens. However, the test sensitivity of ImmunoCAP is clearly higher for some allergens (i.e., LoD is lower). Another investigation used sera from 82 patients and a total of 555 measurements of sIgE to single allergens to compare the two methods (Gadisseur et al. 2011). Using negative cutoff values of <0.3

ISU-E and <0.35 kUA/l (or <0.1 kUA/l), a concordance rate of 92.2 % (or 78.7 %) was found for the positive results. The concordance rate for the negative findings was 93.6 %.

Although excellent concordance rates were seen for most allergens, clear discrepancies were shown for isolated allergens. These included rAsp f 1 (9/14), rPup p 3 (5/13), nAna c 2 (4/11), and rApi g 1 (4/10) (Gadisseur et al. 2011). Differences in the performance of individual allergens can potentially be explained by the differing presentation of allergens on the solid phase of the assay. Compared with immobilization on the polymer coating of the glass chips, covalent binding of allergens to the cellulose matrix in the CAP system can result in different epitopes being exposed or blocked and thus to suboptimal binding of sIgE present in the sample. Additional differences between the set-ups of the two test systems can cause discrepant results in particular cases. Whereas a large excess of allergen is present in the ImmunoCAP system, thus leading to binding of all sIgE present in the sample in most cases, much less allergen is present in the ISAC assay. This can mean that not all allergen-specific IgE will find a binding partner, thus leading to lower results. In this respect, other allergen-specific antibody isotypes (particularly IgG) play a significant role, since these can also block the IgE-binding sites (IgE epitopes), resulting in lower IgE concentrations. On the other hand, the kinetics generated by the large excess of allergen in the ImmunoCAP singleplex assay allow binding of low-affinity sIgE, whereas the kinetics of ISAC 112 ensure that high-affinity sIgE is preferentially bound.

9.4 Molecular Allergy Diagnostics Using Multiplex Assays in Clinical Routine

9.4.1 Allergen Spectrum Available and Potential Advantages in Diagnostics

With 112 individual allergens from 51 allergen sources, the ImmunoCAP ISAC 112 assay currently offers the widest allergen spectrum for molecular allergy diagnostics in clinical routine. Particularly those allergens were selected that:

- Frequently cause sensitizations
- Confer an additional benefit in the interpretation of individual sensitization profiles

The current version of the allergen chip includes:

- 43 single allergens from 17 different foods
- 30 single allergens from 16 different seasonal aeroallergen sources
- 27 single allergens from 13 different perennial aeroallergen sources
- 12 additional single allergens from other allergen sources

Detailed analysis of IgE sensitizations using the allergen chip enables differentiated diagnostics, whereby the advantages of broad molecular screening are evident, even without knowledge of clinical symptoms, from a universal analytical perspective (on the test level). The following consequences or particular arguments should be considered when using these single allergens in microarray format:

A. *Increased test sensitivity* (low limit of quantitation, LoQ) achieved by using specific single allergens compared with diagnostics using allergen extracts
B. *Improved analytical specificity (selectivity)* for particular single allergens with special characteristics (e.g., IgE sensitization associated with severe reactions)
C. *Indicators of cross-reactivity* (common cause of a lack of analytical specificity of allergen extracts)
D. *Markers of primary, genuine* (possibly species-specific) *IgE sensitization*
E. Ideally, *complete representation of the individual sensitization profile* (in contrast to singleplex specific molecular IgE diagnostics)

Criterion A
Individual allergens underrepresented or lacking in an allergen extract can bind sIgE better when used in a specific manner in the microarray, thus generating positive signals and indicating sensitizations more accurately. However, the limit of quantitation (LoQ, ▶ Chap. 7) is usually lower for singleplex methods than it is in microarray, due to the large amounts of (single) allergen used. This explains the limited precision and accuracy of microarray at sIgE concentrations below 1 kUA/l. Therefore, especially sera with low total IgE (<25 kU/l) can yield false-negative values to certain single allergens in the microarray analysis; for this reason, singleplex testing is preferred (to microarray) in such constellations.

Criterion B
Increased analytical specificity is especially desirable when the specific physicochemical characteristics of the single allergens concerned are associated with particular clinical consequences (e.g., high allergen stability and/or high proportion of the total allergen source as the cause of risk-associated sensitizations, e.g., to particular foods; localization of the allergens as a means of differentiating between certain clinical presentations, e.g., sIgE to intracellular *Aspergillus* allergens in bronchopulmonary aspergillosis).

Increased analytical specificity is not an advantage per se—only when the selective information regarding the allergen in an extract is associated with a predefined (clinical) characteristic does this have a significant benefit for molecular diagnostics.

Criterion C
Single allergens improve, in particular, the allergen specificity of IgE sensitization tests. In light of this, certain conserved allergen molecules that are of similar structure, have common IgE-binding epitopes, and occur in numerous allergen sources

have proven useful as indicators for identifying potential cross-reactivity (see also ▶ Chap. 7). They form the basis for concomitant sensitizations to different allergen sources with extremely variable biological relationships.

Criterion D

Other single allergens, in contrast, yield important information regarding a genuine primary IgE sensitization on the basis of:

- Their well-defined, particular structure
- Their IgE epitopes with limited similarity in other single allergens
- Their presence in highly specific allergen sources

Single allergens reestablish the necessary analytical specificity, particularly in the case of allergen sources with known cross-reactive single allergens.

Criteria A–D are by no means mutually exclusive, since single allergens can embody several advantages. Their value in molecular diagnostics (in both single and multiplex assays) varies for each allergen molecule from case to case and must be redefined on the basis of the specific question.

Criterion E

In contrast to singleplex testing, multiplex assays ideally reveal all potential sensitizations. This discloses the entire spectrum of an individual's susceptibility to allergy, and the allergen-specific IgE repertoire can then be systematically checked for possible or absent clinical relevance. This procedure is currently also referred to as a bottom-up approach (in contrast to the top-down approach based on medical history, skin and/or IgE tests with allergen extracts, followed by specific singleplex IgE testing using single allergens).

Examples of the Advantages of Molecular Multiplex IgE Analysis

The following sections provide concrete examples of the generally formulated advantages of molecular multiplex IgE analysis.

Using molecular sensitization profiles, it is possible to differentiate, e.g., primary sensitizations (D) from cross-sensitizations (E), for instance, genuine, primary food allergies from pollen-related, secondary food allergies. These interpretations require comprehensive knowledge of the single allergens, their molecular characteristics, and their affiliation to particular protein families.

The molecular and physicochemical characteristics of single allergens represent a further level on which to base differentiation, e.g., the sensitivity or resistance of food protein to heat and peptic digestion by gastric acids. For example:

- Storage proteins (2S albumins, cupins) are characterized by their strong resistance.
- Profilins and PR-10 are characterized by high sensitivity, respectively, to heat and digestion.

The clinical relevance of the different sensitizations can be illustrated using peanut allergens as an example: sensitization to storage proteins (Ara h 2, Ara h 1, Ara h 3, and Ara h 6) is associated with a significantly increased risk of a systemic reaction following peanut consumption, whereas sensitization to the PR-10 protein from peanut (Ara h 8) is associated with only a low risk, e.g., predominantly oropharyngeal symptoms (Asarnoj et al. 2012).

◉ Table 9.1 provides a detailed list of the single allergens and their affiliation to the different protein families. Important protein families represented on the allergen chip, as well as their main characteristics, are summarized in ◉ Table 9.5.

9.4.2 Added Benefits Conferred by Molecular Allergy Diagnostics in Clinical Routine

9.4.2.1 Differentiation Between Genuine Sensitization and Cross-Reactivity with Inhalant Allergens

In pollen allergy patients exhibiting serological or skin test reactivity to various pollen species (e.g., birch, grasses, mugwort), this may indicate either a genuine sensitization to the particular type of pollen or be caused by IgE cross-reactivity to cross-reactive panallergens, such as:

- Profilins (e.g., Bet v 2, Phl p 12, Art v 4, and Amb a 8)
- Polcalcins (e.g., Bet v 4, Phl p 7, Art v 5, and Amb a 10)

Differentiation between a genuine sensitization and cross-reactivity is only possible if IgE reactivity to specific marker allergens can be demonstrated. Only then does the reactivity result from a genuine primary sensitization to the relevant allergen source. To enable such a distinction to be made, the ISAC 112 assay features numerous marker allergens from different pollen species, including:

- Bet v 1 for birch pollen
- Ole e 1 for ash pollen
- Pla a 1 for plane pollen
- Cup a 1 for cypress pollen
- Phl p 1, Phl p 2, Phl p 5, Phl p 6, and Phl p 11 for grass pollen
- Art v 1 for mugwort pollen
- Amb a 1 for ragweed
- Pla l 1 for ribwort plantain
- Che a 1 for goosefoot

At the same time, the IgE reactivity to panallergens such as profilins (Phl p 12, Bet v 2) and Polcalcins (Phl p 7, Bet v 4) can be determined in order to obtain information on potential cross-reactivity. To what extent panallergens can contribute to allergic reactions and clinical manifestations of pollen allergies is still the subject of debate. However, due to their high degree of cross-reactivity, these panallergens

Table 9.5 Cross-reactive protein families represented in ISAC 112 as well as their main characteristics

Profilins	Sensitive to heat and digestion; tolerance of cooked foods common
	Although rarely associated with clinical symptoms, can cause local and severe reactions in some patients
	Profilins are found in all pollens and plant foods
Polcalcins	Marker for cross-reactivity between different pollen species
	Polcalcins are not found in plant foods
PR-10 proteins (Bet v 1 homologs)	Generally sensitive to heat and digestion; tolerance of cooked foods common
	Generally associated with local symptoms, such as oral allergy syndrome
	Associated with allergic reactions to pollen, fruit, and vegetables
Serum albumins	Sensitive to heat and digestion
	Found in fluids and tissue, e.g., in cow's milk, blood, beef, and dander
	Cross-reactivity between serum albumins from various mammal species, e.g., between cat and dog
Nonspecific lipid transfer proteins (nsLTP)	Resistant to heat and digestion; reactions to cooked foods possible
	Often associated with systemic and severe reactions besides oral allergy syndrome
	Associated with local reactions to fruit and vegetables
	Found in some pollen species (e.g., mugwort)
Tropomyosins	Resistant to heat and digestion; reactions to cooked foods possible
	Often associated as a food allergen with systemic and severe reactions
	Proteins found in muscle fibers, responsible for cross-reactivity between invertebrates (e.g., house dust mite and shrimp)
Lipocalins	Stable proteins and important allergens in furry animals
	Allergens with different cross-reactivity between various furry animals
Storage proteins (2S albumins, cupins)	Resistant to heat and digestion; reactions to cooked foods possible
	Often associated as a food allergen with systemic and severe reactions in addition to OAS
	Found in seeds and nuts, serve as source material for growth of the new plant
Parvalbumins	Resistant to heat and digestion; reactions to cooked foods possible
	Often associated as a food allergen with systemic and severe reactions in addition to OAS
	Major allergen in fish

represent a considerable problem for the detection of allergen-specific sensitization using extract-based methods. For this reason, it is particularly important to perform sIgE diagnostics using species-specific marker allergens in polysensitized patients, alongside a consideration of the precise medical history. These tests yield information relevant to selecting the correct extract prior to commencing immunotherapy.

Diagnostic testing using the ISAC 112 multiplex platform reveals an extensive sensitization profile, including the most common marker and cross-reactive allergens, in a single measurement.

9.4.2.2 Identification of Sensitizations to Food Allergens Associated with a High Risk for Severe Allergic Reactions

IgE to food extracts can be the result of cross-reactivity with pollen-associated allergens, such as allergens of the Bet v 1 or profilin families.

Pollen allergens of the Bet v 1 family include:

- Bet v 1 (birch)
- Aln g 1 (alder)
- Cor a 1 (hazel)
- Que a 1 (oak)
- Fag s 1 (beech)

In the case of relevant sensitization to these aeroallergens, cross-reactivity with the following food allergens is common due to high sequence and structural homology:

- Pome and stone fruits and nuts (hard-shelled fruits), e.g., Act d 8 (kiwi), Cas s 1 (chestnut), Cor a 1 (hazel), Fra a 1 (strawberry), Mal d 1 (apple), Pru p 1 (peach), and Pyr c 1 (pear)
- Vegetables and legumes, e.g., Api g 1 (celery), Ara h 8 (peanut), Dau c 1 (carrot), Gly m 4 (soy), and Vig r 1 (mung bean)

Similarly, it is assumed that sensitization to pollen-mediated profilins can cause cross-reactivity with corresponding profilins in food. The pollen profilins responsible for sensitizations in areas with high grass pollen counts are mainly grass pollen profilins, such as Phl p 12 (timothy grass). Less frequently, Bet v 2 (birch) or Art v 4 (mugwort)—in other regions possibly Amb a 8 (ragweed) or Ole e 2 (olive)—can also be the cause of profilin sensitization.

In terms of food, corresponding profilins are present in fruits, e.g.:

- Ana c 1 (pineapple)
- Cit s 1 (orange)
- Cuc m 2 (melon)
- Fra a 4 (strawberry)
- Mal d 4 (apple)

As well as in legumes and vegetables:

- Ara h 5 (peanut)
- Gly m 3 (soy)
- Api g 4 (celery)

- Cap a 2 (bell pepper)
- Dau c 4 (carrot)
- Lyc e 1 (tomato)

Allergens of the Bet v 1 family and profilin family are sensitive to heat and digestion and generally only cause local oropharyngeal symptoms. Exceptions to this may be observed if large quantities of untreated, "native" allergens are consumed. In the absence of heat treatment or previous processing and denaturation of proteins, systemic reactions may occur. A classic example of this is consumption of native soy milk by individuals highly sensitized to Gly m 4.

In contrast to pollen-associated food allergies to Bet v 1 homologs or profilins, sensitization to food allergens from the storage protein families is frequently associated with a significantly increased risk for severe allergic reactions: storage proteins are extremely resistant to heat and digestion and are present in legumes and tree nuts in large quantities.

A distinction is made between different storage protein families:

- 11S globulins (legumins)
- 7S globulins (vicilins)
- 2S albumins

The following nut storage proteins are characterized:

- Hazelnut: Cor a 9, Cor a 11, and Cor a 14
- Walnut: Jug r 1, Jug r 2, and Jug r 4
- Pecan nut: Car i 1, Car i 2, and Car i 4
- Almond: Pru du 6
- Cashew: Ana o 1, Ana o 2, and Ana o 3
- Pistachio: Pis v 1, Pis v 2, Pis v 3, and Pis v 5
- Brazil nut: Ber e 1 and Ber e 2

Among the legumes:

- Peanut: Ara h 1, Ara h 2, Ara h 3, and Ara h 6
- Soy: Gly m 5, Gly m 6, and Gly m 8

The detection of sIgE to specific storage proteins serves as an indication for an increased risk of severe allergic reactions to small quantities of the allergen. IgE detections to the following allergens are particularly important:

- Ara h 2 in peanut allergy
- Cor a 9 and Cor a 14 in hazelnut allergy
- Jug r 1 and Jug r 4 in walnut allergy
- Ber e 1 in Brazil nut allergy

Similarly, the detection of sIgE to members of the lipid transfer protein (LTP) family appears to be associated with an increased risk of systemic reactions. This includes peach LTP Pru p 3—particularly in patients from Mediterranean regions that have been sensitized cutaneously by the high LTP content of the skin of ripe peaches—as well as walnut Jug r 3 and hazelnut Cor a 8. Since many of the aforementioned allergens are present on the allergen chip, the ISAC 112 multiplex diagnostic test largely reveals individual sensitization profiles and thus forms the basis for risk assessment during subsequent patient counseling.

9.4.3 Paralysis Through Analysis? Interpretation Supported by Intelligent Software and Results Evaluated by the Physician

Using ISAC 112 to simultaneously determine 112 parameters in order to generate a detailed sensitization profile presents a challenge for the physician, particularly in the case of polysensitized patients. The manufacturer's X-plain software integrated into the ISAC 112 system ensures a systematic compilation of positive results in a medical report and simplifies interpretation of the relevance of the detected sensitizations.

Section one of the medical report (▶ e.g., X-plain medical report) relates to general details about whether sensitizations to marker allergens and/or cross-allergens are present and whether IgE reactivity to allergens associated with an increased risk of systemic reactions was found.

Section two includes details on sensitizations to food allergens and aeroallergens. In addition to the IgE reactivities detected, this section provides an aid to interpretation as well as details on the particular features of specific sensitizations, such as regional variations (Ole e 1, the marker allergen for olive pollen, is considered a marker for ash sensitization in areas with high ash populations; Cry j 1, a marker allergen for the Japanese cedar, is considered a marker for sensitization to cypresses).

Section three of the medical report, which describes sensitizations to cross-reactive foods and aeroallergens, also provides interpretation aids and background information on the sensitizations detected. The medical report of a polysensitized patient in whom IgE reactivities to 70 of 112 allergen components were detected is given below by way of example.

The X-plain software can of course only deliver background information on the different allergens, and the results of the extensive sensitization test are not a substitute for an expert medical diagnosis. Therefore, all medical reports need to include a corresponding statement that the detection of IgE must always be evaluated in combination with the clinical medical history and that the computer-generated information is intended to assist the treating physician in making a clinical diagnosis and not to replace him/her.

In addition to the X-plain software developed by the manufacturer as an aid to interpretation, the "Allergenius" software-based expert system, which supports the interpretation of ISAC data according to similar principles, was also introduced recently (Melioli et al. 2014). In addition to ISAC data, data from skin prick tests and individual sIgE determinations can also be entered in the Allergenius system and included in the computer-generated report. It can be assumed that expert systems such as X-plain or Allergenius will develop rapidly and further simplify the interpretation of complex sensitization profiles in the future (Matricardi et al. 2016).

Case Study: X-Plain Medical Report

Analysis of a Polysensitized Patient in Whom IgE Reactivities to 70 of 112 Allergen Components Were Detected

General Comments

The patient is polysensitized and exhibits IgE to cross-reactive as well as species-specific allergen components. IgE to peanut Ara h 2, peanut Ara h 6, peanut Ara h 9, hazelnut Cor a 8, Brazil nut Ber e 1, sesame seed Ses i 1, walnut Jug r 3, peach Pru p 3, soybean Gly m 6, wheat Tri a 14, hazelnut Cor a 9, peanut Ara h 3, soybean Gly m 5, and cashew nut Ana o 2 are associated with systemic allergic reactions. The higher the IgE level, the greater the likelihood of clinical symptoms.

Specific Components: Foods

IgE to specific allergen components of prawn, peanut, egg, Brazil nut, sesame seed, fish, soy, kiwi, hazelnut, wheat, milk, and cashew nut were detected (listed in descending order according to titer level):

- *Hen's egg*: A high level of IgE to Gal d 1 (ovomucoid) represents a risk marker for severe clinical reactions to both raw and cooked hen's egg and increases the risk of a persistent egg allergy. IgE to egg Gal d 2 and egg Gal d 3 are associated with reactions to raw or slightly heated hen's egg.
- *Milk*: IgE to milk Bos d 4 and milk Bos d 5 are associated with reactions to fresh milk.
- *Fish*: IgE to parvalbumin (cod Gad c 1), the major allergen from fish, can cross-react with parvalbumin from other fish species. Parvalbumin content varies considerably between fish species, which could explain differences in tolerance.
- *Crustaceans*: IgE to Pen m 2 can cause cross-reactions to crustaceans (e.g., crab, lobster) and insects (e.g., cockroach). IgE to Pen m 4 can cause cross-reactivity to related crustaceans (e.g., crab, lobster).
- *Nuts and legumes*: IgE to storage proteins (peanut Ara h 2, peanut Ara h 6, Brazil nut Ber e 1, sesame seed Ses i 1, soybean Gly m 6, hazelnut Cor a 9, peanut Ara h 3, soybean Gly m 5, and cashew nut Ana o 2) are associated with a risk for systemic clinical reactions. Many storage proteins are resistant to heat and digestion and are associated with allergic reactions to cooked and uncooked foods. Cross-reactions between soybean Gly m 6, hazelnut Cor a 9, and peanut Ara h 3 are possible. Cashew nut and pistachio are closely related. Walnut and pecan nut are closely related.

- *Wheat*: IgE to wheat Tri a aA_TI are associated with reactions to wheat-based foods. IgE to Tri a aA_TI are also associated with baker's asthma.
- *Kiwi*: IgE to Act d 1, a stable allergen from kiwi, are associated with severe reactions. Kiwi allergy sufferers that are not affected by an associated pollen allergy are at high risk for systemic reactions.

Specific Components: Aeroallergens

IgE to specific allergen components from grass pollen, birch, mite, dog, cat, olive, mouse, cockroach, pellitory, cypress, Japanese cedar, and plane were detected (listed in descending order according to titer level):

- *Pollen*: IgE to timothy grass components can cross-react with related proteins from other grass species. IgE to Bermuda grass Cyn d 1 and timothy grass Phl p 1 can cross-react. An elevated IgE level points to the primary sensitizing allergen. IgE to birch Bet v 1 (PR-10 proteins) can cross-react with related tree pollen and plant foods containing PR-10 proteins. The detection of IgE to Ole e 1, the major allergen from olive pollen, suggests sensitization to ash in areas with a high ash population. IgE to Ole e 9 from olive pollen is associated with severe respiratory symptoms (in areas with high olive pollen counts). IgE to plane Pla a 2 indicate genuine sensitization to plane pollen. IgE to Cry j 1 in areas where Japanese cedar does not occur naturally are a marker for sensitization to cypress. IgE to pellitory Par j 2 are an indication of species-specific sensitization with limited cross-reactivity to LTPs of other origin (e.g., from foods). IgE to Bermuda grass Cyn d 1, timothy grass Phl p 4, cypress Cup a 1, Japanese cedar Cry j 1, and plane Pla a 2 can be partially based on cross-reactivity to the CCD components of these native purified proteins.
- *Animal dander*: Fel d 1 is the major allergen from cat epithelium and triggers primary sensitization in cat allergy. IgE to dog Can f 2 and dog Can f 1 indicate genuine sensitization to dog. IgE to mouse Mus m 1 are associated with asthma and asthma morbidity. Mus m 1 is the major allergen from mouse epithelium.
- *Mites*: IgE to house dust mite Der f 2, house dust mite Der p 2, house dust mite Der f 1, and house dust mite Der p 1, the major allergen from house dust mite, were detected. Der p 1 and Der f 1 can cross-react. Der p 2 and Der f 2 can cross-react. IgE to Lep d 2 (storage mite) show less cross-reactivity with similar house dust mite proteins. IgE to mite Blo t 2 show limited cross-reactivity to Dermatophagoides; however, co-sensitization to both allergens occurs frequently. IgE to cockroaches is associated with asthma.

Specific Components: Insect Venom

IgE to bee venom Api m 1 is detected; further diagnostic testing is indicated in the case of clinically relevant insect venom allergy. All insect venom components on the ISAC chip are CCD-free. This also applies to native bee venom component nApi m 4.

Cross-Reactive Aero- and Food Allergens

- *Serum albumin*: IgE to serum albumin can induce cross-reactivity between various animal species and cause allergic reactions following the consumption of meat and exposure to animal dander and epithelium. IgE to albumin can probably be attributed to sensitization to cow's milk, since milk contains bovine serum albumin.
- *Tropomyosin*: IgE to tropomyosins of house dust mite Der p 10, cockroach Bla g 7, prawn Pen m 1, and *Anisakis* Ani s 3 can explain allergic reactions to crustaceans (e.g., prawn, crab, escargot), mites, cockroaches, and parasites. Tropomyosin is heat-stable and can cause allergic reactions even when consumed in cooked form. Although tropomyosin is a major allergen in shrimps and other crustaceans, it is a minor allergen in mites.
- *Lipid transfer proteins (LTP)*: Even at low titers, IgEs to LTPs from foods (peanut Ara h 9, hazelnut Cor a 8, walnut Jug r 3, peach Pru p 3, and wheat Tri a 14) are risk markers for severe allergic reactions, particularly in Southern Europe. LTPs are predominantly found in the peel of fruits in the Rosaceae family as well as in nuts. These proteins are heat stable and can trigger allergic reactions even when consumed in cooked form.
- *PR-10 proteins*: In all likelihood, sensitization to PR-10 proteins was originally triggered by birch and predisposes affected individuals to allergic reactions (generally oral allergy syndrome) to fruits in the Rosaceae family as well as to hazelnuts, carrots, kiwi, and celery. Since PR-10 proteins are heat- and digestion-labile, they are generally tolerated in heated foods. A number of severe allergic reactions to Gly m 4, which occurred following the consumption of soy—often in combination with physical exertion and exposure—during the birch pollen season, have been reported

9.4.4 Special Features in Routine Use

Own experiences with the test system in routine diagnostics performed at a large outpatient allergy clinic have shown that positive sIgE values are rarely measured using ISAC 112 when total IgE concentrations are below 25 kU/l. Therefore, in our hands the test is now generally only performed when the total IgE concentration exceeds 25 kU/l (◉ Fig. 9.9).

Of the 112 allergens, six are glycosylated, i.e., have carbohydrate side chains that can bind IgE. These include walnut nJug r 2, Bermuda grass nCyn d 1, timothy

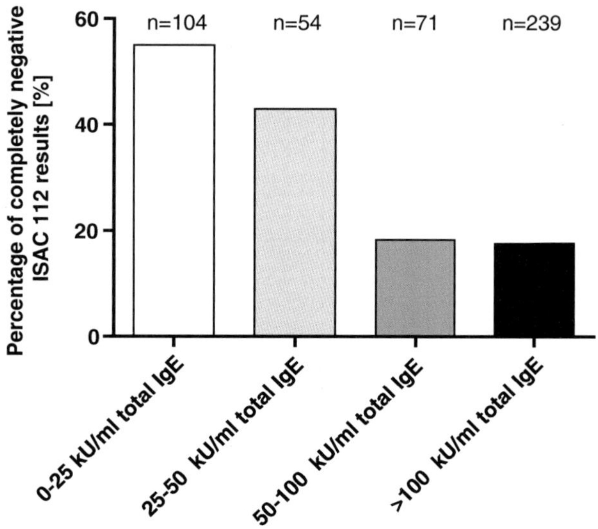

Fig. 9.9 The percentage of completely negative ISAC 112 results depending on total IgE

Table 9.6 Native glycosylated allergens bearing cross-reactive carbohydrate determinants (CCD) on the ISAC 112

Allergen source	Allergen	Protein family/biochemical name
Walnut	nJug r 2	Cupin
Bermuda grass	nCyn d 1	Grass group 1
Timothy grass	nPhl p 4	Unknown
Japanese cedar	nCry j 1	Pectate lyase
Arizona cypress	nCup a 1	Pectate lyase
Maple-leaved plane	nPla a 2	Polygalacturonase

grass nPhl p 4, Japanese cedar nCry j 1, Arizona cypress nCup a 1, and plane nPla a 2 (◉ Table 9.6). Since it is not possible to determine whether IgE to these six allergen components is directed to the protein or the carbohydrate side chain, the results need to be evaluated with caution and in the context of IgE reactivity to the CCD marker MUXF3 (van Ree et al. 2002).

9.5 Molecular Allergy Diagnostics Using Multiplex Assays in Research

9.5.1 New Insights Gained Using ISAC Technology

The small sample volumes required for multiplex assays are advantageous in the research environment, e.g., in the context of birth cohorts, since only small amounts of serum are normally available for analysis. These options made it possible to collect the following kind of data:

9.5.1.1 Diversity of Sensitization Profiles

By means of simultaneous determination of sIgE antibodies to numerous allergen molecules, patients' individual sensitization profiles can be generated with minimal effort. These profiles represent the IgE repertoire and pattern of sensitization at the molecular level and enable the great diversity of profiles in a population to be depicted. Tripodi et al. (2012) alone described 39 different profiles (sensitization patterns) in only 176 Italian, grass pollen-allergic children that were tested using eight *Phleum pratense* (timothy grass, Phl p) allergens: the spectrum extended from children who reacted to only one molecule, to children who produced antibodies to all eight allergens. A range of intermediate profiles exists between these two extremes.

9.5.1.2 Developing Sensitization Profiles

It could be shown using the ISAC method that sensitization profiles in children are simple to begin with and increase in complexity over time.

The sIgE response to the *Phleum pratense* (timothy grass) allergen molecules often develops from a simple monosensitization to a single allergen molecule into an oligomolecular sensitization, leading ultimately to a complex polymolecular pattern (Hatzler et al. 2012; Matricardi 2014). This development process usually begins with an IgE response to a initiator molecule, which, at later stages, initiates the development of antibodies to other allergen molecules. In the case of grass pollen allergy to timothy grass, this initiator molecule is usually Phl p 1, which turned out to be the protein most frequently recognized. As a result, young patients in the early stages of their sensitization often exhibit an sIgE response to only this protein. After months or years, IgE sensitizations to other timothy grass proteins can develop, commonly in a typical order: the initial sensitization to Phl p 1 is usually followed by positive reactions to Phl p 4 and Phl p 5; thereafter, IgE responses to Phl p 2, Phl p 6, and Phl p 11. Only in the clinical phase, long after all allergic symptoms had developed in these children, was it possible to detect IgE to Phl p 12 and Phl p 7–pollen panallergens with a low risk of sensitization. The time-dependent, consecutive development of allergen molecule-specific IgE sensitizations to an allergen source (grass pollen in this example) is described by the authors as "molecular spreading" (Hatzler et al. 2012).

Since the first sIgE responses to pollen are detectable years before the first symptoms occur, ISAC microarray analysis might be able to predict symptom onset on the basis of the individual sensitization profile. Indeed, approximately one-third of 3-year-old children sensitized to grass pollen develop grass pollen-associated seasonal rhinitis at the age of 12 years (Hatzler et al. 2012). Similar results were recently reported for the development of birch pollen-associated allergic rhinoconjunctivitis (Westman et al. 2015). Here again, IgE reactivity to various Bet v 1-homologous PR-10 proteins in early childhood seems to be a good predictor for the later development of a clinically manifest birch pollen allergy.

9.5.1.3 Prescribing Behavior in Allergen-Specific Immunotherapy (SIT)

Recommendations on SIT also take into consideration the efficacy of this therapy depending on how well it is adapted to the allergen sources to which the patient reacts (Zuberbier et al. 2010). SIT should be used in the case of clinical symptoms arising from IgE sensitizations to clearly definable allergen sources, including their primary major allergens, without taking cross-reactivity toward panallergens of questionable clinical relevance into consideration (Valenta 2002). The multiplex ISAC 112 system generates differentiated sensitization profiles, thus enabling "primary" genuine sensitizations to be distinguished from antibody reactions resulting from cross-reactivity. The advantage here is that it enables SIT to be individually tailored to each patient. Thus, current German language guidelines on SIT (Pfaar et al. 2014) recommend using specific single allergens in polysensitized pollen allergy patients—preferentially in singleplex rather than multiplex procedures—since generating complete sensitization profiles to answer the diagnostic questions would overshoot the target.

A multicenter Italian study (Stringari et al. 2014) has already investigated whether and how the results of molecular allergy diagnostics using singleplex assays influence physicians' prescription of SIT and decisions relating to the composition of allergen preparations for children with moderate to severe allergic rhinitis ($n = 651$). This study revealed that more SIT preparations were prescribed following molecular diagnostics: in many patients originally classified as polysensitized on the basis of skin prick tests with pollen extracts, molecular diagnostics could identify clear sensitizations to particular major allergens, the allergen sources of which would then have come into consideration for SIT. The detection of IgE to primary marker allergens thus reestablishes the analytical specificity that was lost by using allergen extracts for diagnostic purposes due to pan-pollen sensitizations. In addition, it could be shown that, in approximately 33 % of cases, SIT would have been adjusted and performed with a different composition following molecular diagnostics.

9.5.2 The Use of Individually Tailored Allergen Chips in Research

In addition to the test systems approved for sIgE routine diagnostics (e.g., ImmunoCAP ISAC 112), protein microarrays can also be developed to address specific research interests. On the basis of ISAC technology, a significantly more extensive allergen chip was developed—e.g., for birth cohort-based investigations on the mechanisms of allergy development in different regions of Europe—on which a total of 176 allergen components are represented (Lupinek et al. 2014). In a similar manner, individually designed protein microarrays can be used as allergen chips in order to answer specific diagnostic questions. Thus, customized microarrays were able to detect sIgE to various chimeric isoforms of the Api m 10 major allergen in patients allergic to bee stings (van Vaerenbergh et al. 2015). The roles of sIgE to α-, β-, or γ-gliadin in wheat-dependent exercise-induced anaphylaxis were also characterized using research microarrays (Hofmann et al. 2012), as was the relevance of the different single allergens for peanut allergy (Nicolaou et al. 2010).

A further application of array technology can be illustrated using the example of peanut allergy: rather than intact proteins, allergen peptides can also be coupled to the solid phase of the array as target structures. This type of peptide array permits the analysis of diverse linear IgE-binding sites (IgE epitopes) within an allergen (Shreffler et al. 2004) and their comparison with homologous sequences in other allergens (Rosenfeld et al. 2012).

The clear advantages of the multiplex assay for research purposes lie in the large number of detectable sensitizations, the individual composition of the allergen repertoire (personalized allergen chips), and the relatively small sample volumes required for the actual test. Particularly in the case of complex allergen sources and complicated clinical questions or in a polysensitized study population, high-definition molecular allergy diagnostics are beneficial, since the complete sensitization pattern obtained is a prerequisite for the successful interpretation of results in the context of the patient's clinical medical history.

9.6 Summary and Perspectives

The ISAC 112 microarray platform currently available enables the analysis of specific IgE to as many single allergens as possible in a single assay, using a small amount of serum (◉ Table 9.7). Strictly speaking, the assay represents 112 immunoassays, the corresponding allergen components of which are derived from natural or recombinant sources and have been individually evaluated for their suitability. This relates to allergen-dependent test parameters, such as LoD, linearity, precision,

Table 9.7 Advantages and disadvantages of test methods using the example of ImmunoCAP technology

Method	Advantages	Disadvantages
sIgE determination in ISAC multiplex assay	30 µl serum or plasma 112 allergen components No interference with high tIgE	Manual methods Less sensitive Higher coefficient of variation
sIgE determination in singleplex assay, e.g., ImmunoCAP	Automated Quantitative High test sensitivity Low coefficient of variation Well suited to monitoring/follow-up	40 µl serum/plasma per analysis Low-affinity antibodies are also detected (virtually no clinical relevance)
Skin prick test (SPT)	High test sensitivity Simple and quick to perform	Manual One allergen per test Only extracts available

Adapted from Canonica et al. (2013)

effect of total IgE, IgE inhibition, matrix effects, and comparability with established methods for detecting specific IgE to define single allergens.

The analytical advantages of molecular diagnostics using single allergens also apply to multiplex analysis:

1. Increased test sensitivity (lower LoD) by using specific (e.g., allergens underrepresented or lacking in the allergen extract) single allergens
2. Increased analytical specificity (selectivity) for single allergens with defined clinical characteristics (e.g., risk association, disease association)
3. Defined single allergens (e.g., panallergens) as markers for cross-reactivity
4. Single allergens (e.g., species-specific marker allergens) as indicators of a primary, genuine IgE sensitization to the associated allergen source

The additional advantage of multiplex analysis is that it generates an extensive (ideally complete) IgE sensitization profile (complete allergen-specific IgE repertoire).

Since the reliability and accuracy of the current microarray test decrease significantly at sIgE concentrations below 1 kU/l, singleplex methods are—where possible—to be preferred over multiplex assays in the case of low serum total IgE (<25 kU/l) or only slightly increased sIgE values ($0.1 < sIgE < 1.0\ kU_A/l$).

A number of important allergen components, particularly in the area of food allergens (e.g., additional storage proteins; missing, potentially important pollen allergens; mold allergens; animal allergens) are lacking. Other allergen components currently featured on the allergen chip would be better dispensed with, since they lead more to confusion than to clarification. These include insect venom allergens, since analysis of specific IgE to these allergens is only indicated on the basis of clear signs of an anaphylactic reaction to insect stings in the patient's medical history, and not as a screening test. Due to the high prevalence of insect venom sensitization in approximately 25 % of the population, nonspecific screening would generate an abundance of clinically irrelevant results and serve to unsettle patients and their physicians. On the basis of the appropriate indication, sensitization to single insect venom allergens can be detected using singleplex methods. Alternatively, specific multiplex analysis with all available insect venom allergens—a test currently under development and known as the insect venom allergen chip—would be useful. In this regard, it is conceivable that a range of microarray formats will be available in the future, which, depending on the clinical question, will cover different allergen spectra, such as food allergies, inhalant allergies, insect venom allergies, and medication allergies. In light of the fact that there are probably over 3000 single allergens, it can be expected that the rapid developments in miniaturization and automation will fuel many more innovations in the field of multiplex allergy diagnostics.

Conclusions

The ISAC 112 microarray platform currently available represents an important step in the further development of in vitro allergy diagnostics in that it enables the analysis of specific IgE to as many single allergens as possible in a single assay, using a small amount of serum. The advantages of molecular allergy diagnostics (greater test sensitivity, increased analytical specificity, and the ability to identify risk, primary, and cross-sensitizations) are broadened by the comprehensive generation of virtually complete sensitization profiles.

Positive IgE microarray results indicate sIgE sensitizations to the relevant single allergens—sensitizations that are only clinically relevant in the presence of corresponding symptoms following exposure to the associated allergen source. Clinical relevance needs to be investigated for each allergen source or single allergen separately, possibly by means of a targeted follow-up patient history or, where possible, by means of challenge testing with the relevant allergen source. Conversely, IgE sensitizations detected on the microchip in the absence of clinical information on physical symptoms, allergic reactions, or individual diseases in the affected individual are of limited value: neither the level of sIgE nor the extent or pattern of IgE sensitizations to single allergens reveals anything about their potential clinical relevance. The IgE sensitizations detected can only be conclusively interpreted in combination with knowledge of the clinical symptoms. This remains the task of the physician and cannot be substituted even by detailed information on sIgE to all conceivable single allergens.

References

Asarnoj A, Nilsson C, Lidholm J, et al. Peanut component Ara h 8 sensitization and tolerance to peanut. J Allergy Clin Immunol. 2012;130:468–72.

Blackley CH. Hay fever; its causes, treatment, and effective prevention. London: Ballière; 1880.

Breiteneder H, Hassfeld W, Pettenburger K, et al. Isolation and characterization of messenger RNA from male inflorescences and pollen of the white birch (Betula verrucosa). Int Arch Allergy Appl Immunol. 1988;87:19–24.

Canonica GW, Ansotegui IJ, Pawankar R, et al. A WAO – ARIA – GA2LEN consensus document on molecular-based allergy diagnostics. World Allergy Organ J. 2013;136:17–34.

Gadisseur R, Chapelle JP, Cavalier E. A new tool in the field of in-vitro diagnosis of allergy: preliminary results in the comparison of ImmunoCAP 250 with the ImmunoCAP ISAC. Clin Chem Lab Med. 2011;49:277–80.

Hatzler L, Panetta V, Lau S, et al. Molecular spreading and predictive value of preclinical IgE response to Phleum pratense in children with hay fever. J Allergy Clin Immunol. 2012;130:894–901.

Hiller R, Laffer S, Harwanegg C, et al. Microarrayed allergen molecules: diagnostic gatekeepers for allergy treatment. FASEB. 2002;J16:414–6.

Hofmann SC, Fischer J, Eriksson C, et al. IgE detection to α/β/γ-gliadin and its clinical relevance in wheat-dependent exercise-induced anaphylaxis. Allergy. 2012;67:1457–60.

Ishizaka K, Ishizaka T. Identification of gamma-E antibodies as a carrier of reaginic antibody. J Immunol. 1967;99:1187–98.

Johansson SGO, Bennich H. Immunological studies of an atypical (myeloma) immunoglobulin. Immunology. 1967;13:381–94.

Lupinek C, Wollmann E, Baar A, et al. Advances in allergen-microarray technology for diagnosis and monitoring of allergy: the MeDALL allergen-chip. Methods. 2014;66:106–19.

Matricardi PM. Allergen-specific immunoprophylaxis: toward secondary prevention of allergic rhinitis? Pediatr Allergy Immunol. 2014;25:15–8.

Matricardi PM, Kleine-Tebbe J, Hoffmann HJ et al. EAACI molecular allergology user's guide. Pediatr Allergy Immunol. 2016;27:(suppl 23):1–250.

Melioli G, Spenser C, Reggiardo G, et al. Allergenius, an expert system for the interpretation of allergen microarray results. World Allergy Organ J. 2014;7:15.

Nicolaou N, Poorafshar M, Murray C, et al. Allergy or tolerance in children sensitized to peanut: prevalence and differentiation using component-resolved diagnostics. J Allergy Clin Immunol. 2010;125:191–7.

Palomba A, Maccari M, Baldracchini F, et al. Evaluation of a new microarray based system for allergy testing. EAACI, Copenhagen, Abstract # 18; 2014.

Pfaar O, Bachert C, Bufe A, et al. Guideline on allergen-specific immunotherapy in IgE-mediated allergic diseases—S2k Guideline of the German Society for Allergology and Clinical Immunology (DGAKI), the Society for Pediatric Allergy and Environmental Medicine (GPA), the Medical Association of German Allergologists (AeDA), the Austrian Society for Allergy and Immunology (ÖGAI), the Swiss Society for Allergy and Immunology (SGAI), the German Society of Dermatology (DDG), the German Society of Oto-Rhino-Laryngology, Head and Neck Surgery (DGHNO-KHC), the German Society of Pediatrics and Adolescent Medicine (DGKJ), the Society for Pediatric Pneumology (GPP), the German Respiratory Society (DGP), the German Association of ENT Surgeons (BV-HNO), the Professional Federation of Paediatricians and Youth Doctors (BVKJ), the Federal Association of Pulmonologists (BDP) and the German Dermatologists Association (BVDD). Allergo J Int. 2014;23:282–319. doi:10.1007/s40629-014-0032-2.

Rosenfeld L, Shreffler W, Bardina L, et al. Walnut allergy in peanut-allergic patients: significance of sequential epitopes of walnut homologous to linear epitopes of Ara h 1, 2 and 3 in relation to clinical reactivity. Int Arch Allergy Immunol. 2012;157:238–45.

Shreffler WG, Beyer K, Chu TH, et al. Microarray immunoassay: association of clinical history, in vitro IgE function, and heterogeneity of allergenic peanut epitopes. J Allergy Clin Immunol. 2004;113:776–82.

Stringari G, Tripodi S, Caffarelli C, et al; Italian Pediatric Allergy Network (I-PAN). The effect of component-resolved diagnosis on specific immunotherapy prescription in children with hay fever. J Allergy Clin Immunol. 2014;134:75–81.

Thermo Fisher Scientific. ImmunoCAP ISAC 112—performance characteristics, data on file, Oct 2011. Uppsala: Thermo Fisher Scientific; 2011.

Tripodi S, Frediani T, Lucarelli S, et al. Molecular profiles of IgE to Phleum pratense in children with grass pollen allergy: implications for specific immunotherapy. J Allergy Clin Immunol. 2012;129:834–9.

Valenta R. The future of antigen-specific immunotherapy of allergy. Nat Rev Immunol. 2002;2:446–53.

Valenta R, Kraft D. Recombinant allergen molecules: tools to study effector cell activation. Immunol Rev. 2001;179:119–27.

van Ree R. Carbohydrate epitopes and their relevance for the diagnosis and treatment of allergic diseases. Int Arch Allergy Immunol. 2002;129:189–97.

van Vaerenbergh M, De Smet L, Rafei-Shamsabadi D, et al. IgE recognition of chimeric isoforms of the honeybee (Apis mellifera) venom allergen Api m 10 evaluated by protein array technology. Mol Immunol. 2015;63:449–55.

Westman M, Lupinek C, Bousquet J, et al; Mechanisms for the Development of Allergies (MeDALL) Consortium. Early childhood IgE reactivity to pathogenesis-related class 10 proteins predicts allergic rhinitis in adolescence. J Allergy Clin Immunol. 2015;135:1199–206.

Wide L, Bennich H, Johansson SG. Diagnosis of allergy by an in vitro test for allergen antibodies. Lancet. 1967;II:1105–7.

Zuberbier T, Bachert C, Bousquet PJ, et al. GA^2 LEN/EAACI pocket guide for allergen-specific immunotherapy for allergic rhinitis and asthma. Allergy. 2010;65:1525–30.

Part III

Marker Allergens

Marker Allergens and Panallergens in Tree and Grass Pollen Allergy

10

K. Gangl, V. Niederberger, J. M. Davies, R. Valenta, and A. Nandy

Abbreviations

CCD	Cross-reactive carbohydrate determinants
cDNA	Complementary deoxyribonucleic acid
CRD	Component resolved diagnostics
Fab	Antigen-binding fragment
IgE	Immunoglobulin E
LTP	Lipid transfer protein
nsLTP	Nonspecific lipid transfer protein
OAS	Oral allergy syndrome
PR-10	Pathogenesis-related proteins

The present chapter is based on and modified from an article by the authors published in 2015 in *Allergo Journal International* (Gangl K, Niederberger V, Valenta R, Nandy A: Marker allergens and pan allergens in tree and grass pollen allergy. Allergo J Int 2015, 24:158–169).
The authors gratefully thank Greg Plunkett PhD, ALK Inc. Headquarters and Analytical Laboratories, Round Rock, TX, USA, for reviewing the manuscript and for his editorial assistance and helpful suggestions including a North American perspective.

K. Gangl, MD (✉) • V. Niederberger, MD, Prof.
Department of Otorhinolaryngology, Medical University of Vienna, Vienna, Austria
e-mail: katharina.gangl@meduniwien.ac.at; verena.niederberger@meduniwien.ac.at

J.M. Davies, PhD, Prof.
Centre for Children's Health Research, Institute of Health and Biomedical Innovation, Queensland University of Technology, South Brisbane, QLD, Australia
e-mail: j36.davies@qut.edu.au

R. Valenta, MD, Prof.
Center for Pathophysiology, Infectiology and Immunology, Medical University of Vienna, Vienna, Austria
e-mail: rudolf.valenta@meduniwien.ac.at

A. Nandy, PhD
Business Unit Allergy, Research & Development,
Allergopharma GmbH and Co. KG, Reinbek, Germany
e-mail: andreas.nandy@allergopharma.com

J. Kleine-Tebbe, T. Jakob (eds.), *Molecular Allergy Diagnostics*,
DOI 10.1007/978-3-319-42499-6_10

10.1 Introduction

Many allergens from botanically related sources share structural similarities resulting in IgE cross-reactivity. As a consequence, allergens sharing similar structures are often also related on an immunological level, and patients sensitized to one specific allergen may show clinical or *in vitro* reactivity to structurally similar allergenic proteins of other allergen sources. Different IgE sensitization profiles can be identified in allergic patients according to reactivity to certain allergens. These allergens are defined as marker allergens (Kazemi-Shirazi et al. 2002; Suphioglu 2000; Valenta et al. 2007).

Today, genuine allergic sensitization can be differentiated from cross-reactivity using modern allergen component resolved diagnostics (CRD) (Valenta et al. 1999; Hiller et al. 2002; Lupinek et al. 2014). In grass and tree pollen allergy, CRD can identify the appropriate immunotherapy in poly-sensitized patients. Since specific immunotherapy is time-consuming (taking up to several years) and burdensome, early identification of patients suffering from genuine sensitization to grass or tree pollen who should benefit from a specific immunotherapy is important for clinical management of patients.

Allergens that pinpoint genuine sensitization and may be defined as marker allergens for specific tree and grass pollen allergies, will be described in this article.

10.2 Allergen Sources in Trees and Grasses

Tree and grass pollen from wind-pollinated plants are a frequent source of allergens. Between 12 and 17 % of the general population in Europe suffer from pollen allergy with almost 10 % suffering from tree pollen allergy (Blomme et al. 2013; Wüthrich et al. 1995). After hydration, tree and grass pollen rapidly release large amounts of allergens, i.e., defined IgE-binding proteins and glycoproteins. Upon contact with the mucosal surfaces of the respiratory tract, these allergens trigger allergic symptoms in susceptible patients (Grote et al. 2001; Vrtala et al. 1993).

10.2.1 Grasses

Most allergenic grasses belong to a botanical family of grasses called Poaceae, which is mainly found in temperate climate zones. As examples, timothy grass (*Phleum pratense*), perennial ryegrass (*Lolium perenne*), orchard grass (*Dactylis glomerata*), and Kentucky bluegrass (*Poa pratensis*) belong to the Pooideae subfamily and are closely related. Other grasses, such as Bermuda grass (*Cynodon dactylon*), Rhodes grass (*Chloris gayana*), love grass (*Eragrostis tenella*), rice (*Oryza sativa*), common reed (*Phragmites communis*), Bahia grass (*Paspalum notatum*), Johnson grass (*Sorghum halepense*), corn (*Zea mays*), and buffel grass

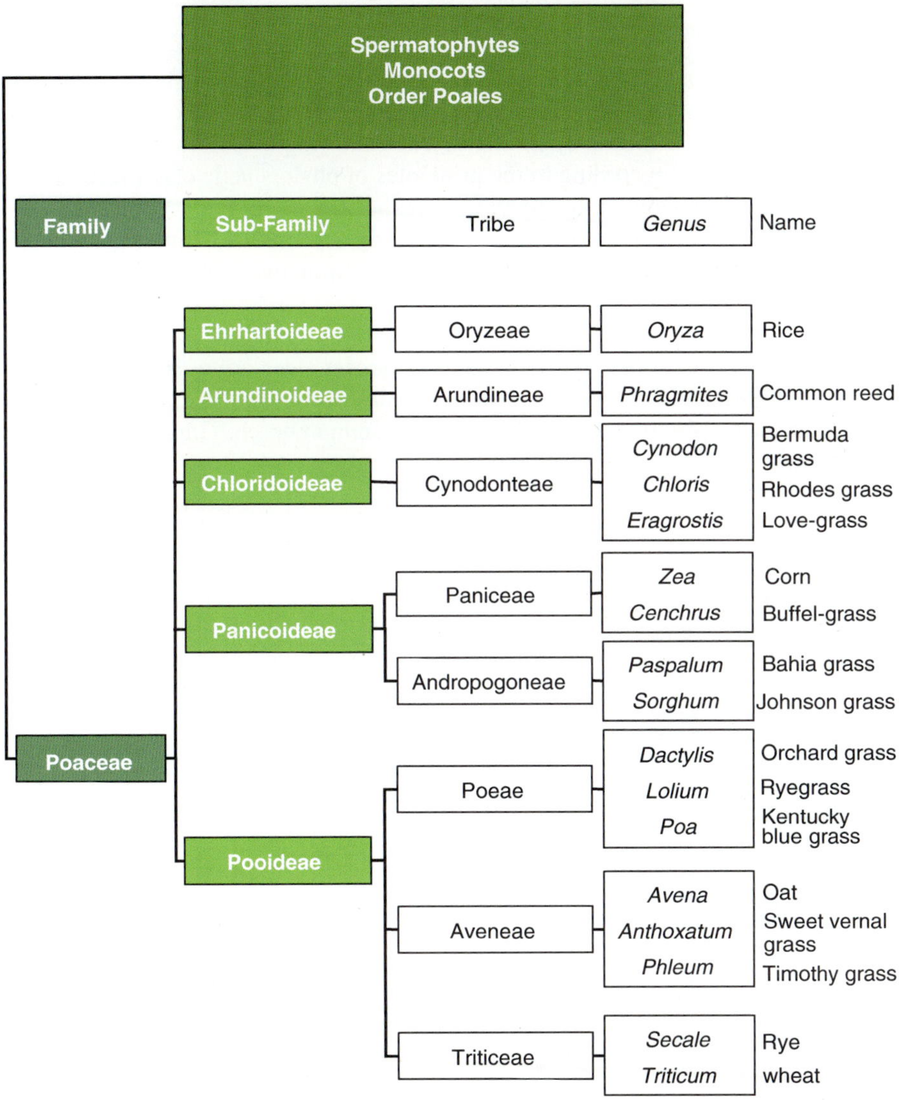

Fig. 10.1 Phylogenetic botanical relationship between important allergenic grasses (Adapted from Simon et al. (2011))

(*Cenchrus ciliaris*), belong to the Chloridoideae, Ehrhartoideae, Arundinoideae, and Panicoideae subfamilies, respectively, found in subtropical and tropical climate zones (Andersson and Lidholm 2003; Hejl et al. 2009; Johansen et al. 2009; Simon et al. 2011; Davies 2014). An overview of the botanical relationship between grasses is shown in ◉ Fig. 10.1.

10.2.2 Trees

Unlike grass pollen, allergenic tree pollen originates from different botanical groups of spermatophytes occurring in different geographical regions (Mothes et al. 2004; Swoboda et al. 2008; Marth et al. 2014). The following overview and ◉ Fig. 10.2 have been compiled according to the principles of phylogenetic classification (The Angiosperm Phylogeny Group 2009; Christenhusz et al. 2011).

The majority of trees are flowering plants (angiosperms). An important group of cross-reactive allergenic tree pollen originates from two families of the order Fagales:

- The Betulaceae family (birch, *Betula verrucosa*; alder, *Alnus glutinosa*; hazelnut, *Corylus avellana*; and hornbeam, *Carpinus betulus*)
- The Fagaceae family (oak, *Quercus alba*; common beech, *Fagus sylvatica*; and chestnut, *Castanea sativa*)

These trees are mainly found in temperate climate zones of Northern Europe, North America, and other continents (Wuthrich et al. 1995; Mothes et al. 2004; Asam et al. 2015).

Trees of the family Oleaceae (order Lamiales) are the source of a second important group of cross-reactive allergenic pollen. They are endemic all over Europe, but

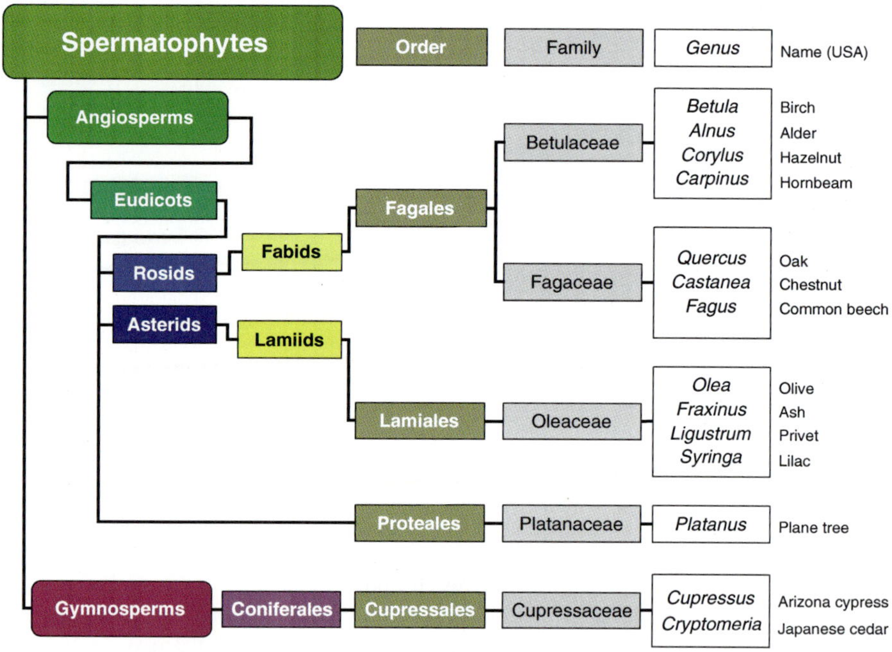

Fig. 10.2 Phylogenetic botanical relationship between important allergenic trees (Adapted from The Angiosperm Phylogeny Group (2009) and Christenhusz et al. (2011))

are also found in North America and other continents (Marth et al. 2014; Asam et al. 2015). The olive tree (*Olea europaea*) is the most widely spread species, especially in the Mediterranean region (Bousquet et al. 1984), but *Olea* ssp. is also found in other continents in areas with a Mediterranean climate, e.g., the Southwestern USA. Other allergenic members of the Oleaceae family are privet (*Ligustrum vulgare*), lilac (*Syringa vulgaris*), and ash trees (*Fraxinus excelsior*).

In some areas of the Mediterranean, different species of plane tree (order Proteales, family Platanaceae) represent a locally important source of allergens originating from angiosperms. Plane trees are also increasingly planted for ornamental purposes in many regions of Europe and North America and may cause allergic symptoms there (Asam et al. 2015).

Another important source of cross-reactive allergenic pollen originates from the botanical group of gymnosperms. The most important trees belong to the order of Cupressales (family Cupressaceae), such as the Arizona cypress (*Cupressus arizonica*), mountain cedar (*Juniperus ashei*), and the Japanese cedar (*Cryptomeria japonica*) (Swoboda et al. 2008; Di Felice et al. 2001; Marth et al. 2014). While the Arizona cypress has been widely exported from its native southwest of North America to Europe, and is frequently found in regions around the Mediterranean, the mountain cedar is of particular importance in southwestern North America, especially in Texas.

10.3 Important Grass Pollen Allergens

◉ Table 10.1 gives an overview of the most important grass pollen allergens.

10.3.1 Allergens Found in all Poaceae Grasses

10.3.1.1 Marker Allergen for all Poaceae Grasses: Group 1 (Phl p 1)

Group-1 allergens have been isolated and/or cloned from more than 20 Poaceae species (Andersson and Lidholm 2003; Griffith et al. 1991; Johnson and Marsh 1965; Laffer et al. 1994a; Perez et al. 1990). Phl p 1 is the group-1 allergen of timothy grass. It has a sequence identity of between 85 and 95 % with other members of the Pooideae subfamily. Most amino acid substitutions found in isoforms and in group-1 allergens of other Pooideae species (e.g., Hol l 1, Poa p 1, und Lol p 1) do not significantly alter allergenicity of the molecule (Andersson and Lidholm 2003; Johansen et al. 2009; Laffer et al. 1994a, b). Most IgE epitopes of Phl p 1 cluster at the c-terminus (Flicker et al. 2006), and grass pollen-specific IgE antibodies have been shown to bind with high density to the Phl p 1 molecule (Madritsch et al. 2015).

Up to 90% of all grass pollen allergic patients show IgE reactivity to group-1 allergens of other grass species (Andersson and Lidholm 2003; Johansen et al. 2009; Laffer et al. 1994a, 1996; Van Ree et al. 1992). Phl p 1 is the most important group-1 allergen and represents an important cross-reactive major allergen.

Table 10.1 Important grass pollen allergens (Example: Timothy grass)

Protein	Significance	Example	Molecular weight (kDa)
Marker allergens for grass pollen			
Group-1 grass pollen allergen Glycosylated, β-expansin	Major allergen, all grasses	Phl p 1	31–35
Group-5 grass pollen allergen Unknown function	Major allergen, subfamiliy of Pooideae	Phl p 5	27–33
Other important allergens			
Allergens in all grasses			
Group-13 grass pollen allergen Glycosylated, polygalacturonase	Grass pollen specific	Phl p 13	~55
Allergens in some grasses			
Group-2 grass pollen allergen Expansin-related protein	Grass pollen specific	Phl p 2	10–12
Group-6 grass pollen allergen P-particle-associated-protein	Grass pollen specific	Phl p 6	~13
Group-11 grass pollen allergen Glycosylated, Ole-e-1-like protein	Little cross-reactivity	Phl p 11	~20
Allergens, not specific for grasses			
Polcalcin 2 EF-hand	Panallergen, cross-reactivity between different plant pollen	Phl p 7	~9
Profilin	Panallergen, cross-reactivity between many plant pollen, plant-derived food, and latex	Phl p 12	~14
Berberine bridge enzyme Glycosylated	Panallergen, clinically reduced relevance	Phl p 4	50–67

Cross-reactivity of group-1 allergens has been demonstrated in many studies with natural extracts of different Pooideae species and other Poaceae subfamilies (Johansen et al. 2009; Laffer et al. 1994b; Van Ree et al. 1992). Purified recombinant Phl p 1 inhibited binding of patient sera to natural extracts of eight different grasses (timothy grass, *Phleum pratense*; sweet vernal grass, *Anthoxanthum odoratum*; oat, *Avena sativa*; Bermuda grass, *Cynodon dactylon*; perennial ryegrass, *Lolium perenne*; common reed, *Phragmites communis*; Kentucky bluegrass, *Poa pratensis*; and rye, *Secale cereale*) inducing an average inhibition of 76 % (Laffer et al. 1996). Monoclonal antibodies raised against Phl p 1 and defining four distinct epitopes as well as recombinant human Phl p 1-specific IgE-Fabs (antigen-binding fragments) recognize and bind to a panel of natural group-1 allergens of different Pooideae grasses (Flicker et al. 2006; Duffort et al. 2008).

Sequence homologies and cross-reactivity between Phl p 1 and group-1 allergens of subtropical grasses such as Bermuda grass (*Cynodon dactylon*; 67–70 % sequence identity) or Bahia grass (*Paspalum notatum*) are less pronounced (Andersson and Lidholm 2003; Johansen et al. 2009; Davies 2014; Timbrell et al. 2014). There is no complete cross inhibition between group-1 allergens of grasses originating in temperate climate zones and group-1 allergens of grasses originating in subtropical climate zones, especially with patient sera from subtropical climate zones (overview presented in Davies (2014)). However, there are indications that these species-specific IgE epitopes are not protein epitopes but carbohydrate epitopes without clinical relevance (Cabauatan et al. 2014).

Phl p 1 is the most important marker allergen for genuine sensitization to grasses belonging to all subfamilies of Poaceae for the following reasons:

- Approximately 90 % of grass pollen allergic patient sera contain specific IgE against Phl p 1.
- Group-1 allergens have been found in all Poaceae grasses, but not in other taxonomically unrelated plants.
- There is widespread cross-reactivity between group-1 allergens from different grass species (Niederberger et al. 1998a).

10.3.1.2 Group 13

The group-13 grass pollen allergen, a 55-kDa protein, has also been described in all grasses examined to date (Suck et al. 2000). Although over 50 % of grass pollen allergic patients display IgE reactivity against Phl p 13, it has only little clinical relevance as it showed only low allergenic reactivity in clinical and *in vitro* studies (Westritschnig et al. 2008).

10.3.2 Allergens Found Only in Pooideae Grasses

10.3.2.1 Marker Allergen for Pooideae: Group 5 (Phl p 5)

Group-5 allergens are marker allergens for Pooideae grasses. Homologous allergens have been found in all grasses of the Pooideae subfamily, such as timothy grass (*Phleum pratense*), rye (*Secale cereale*), Kentucky bluegrass (*Poa pratense*), and perennial ryegrass (*Lolium perenne*). Group-5 allergens are not found in grasses belonging to the Panicoideae, Chloridoideae, Ehrhartoideae, or Arundinoideae subfamilies, which are mainly distributed in the southern hemisphere and are highly prevalent in tropical and subtropical climate zones (Davies 2014). Group-5 allergens are not found in corn (*Zea mays*), Bermuda grass (*Cynodon dactylon*), or rice (*Oryza sativa*), for example (Niederberger et al. 1998a).

Phl p 5, one of the best characterized group-5 allergens, is one of several allergens to occur in different isoallergenic forms as Phl p 5a (i.e., Phl p 5.01) and Phl p 5b (i.e., Phl p 5.02). The overall sequence identity between Phl p 5a and Phl p 5b is approximately 65 % but is higher (70–77 %) in important parts of the molecule. Multiple independent IgE epitopes have been identified on both isoforms of Phl p 5 (Levin et al. 2014).

Between 65 and 85 % of grass pollen allergic patients in temperate climate zones display IgE reactivity to group-5 allergens, and the clinical allergenic activity of Phl p 5a is very high (Andersson and Lidholm 2003; Westritschnig et al. 2008; Flicker et al. 2000; Vrtala et al. 1993).

Most patients display extensive IgE cross-reactivity to the Phl p 5 isoallergens as well as to different group-5 allergens from Pooideae grasses (Andersson and Lidholm 2003; Niederberger et al. 1998a; van Ree 2002).

Phl p 5 is therefore an important marker allergen for sensitization to grasses of the Pooideae subfamily.

10.3.2.2 Other Pooideae-Specific Allergens

Group-2/group-3 and group-6 allergens are also only found in the pollen of Pooideae grasses. In some populations more than 50 % of grass pollen allergic patients display IgE reactivity to these molecules, yet the overall rate of patient sensitization is not high enough to give them the status of marker allergens (for an overview, see Andersson and Lidholm 2003; Gangl et al. 2013). Although patient IgE titers against group-2/group-3 allergens are often rather low, Phl p 2 shows high allergenic activity in skin tests (Westritschnig et al. 2008). The allergenic activity of Phl p 6 has not been tested yet in clinical studies.

Group-11 allergens are not very important in the clinic. Although few patients react with these allergens, they have been found in *Phleum pratense* and *Lolium perenne* (Marknell DeWitt et al. 2002), and homologs from other plants, e.g., olive (Ole e 1), corn (Zea m 13), and tomato, have been identified. Cross-reactivity between homologs from taxonomically unrelated allergen sources is very limited.

10.3.3 Allergens from Tropical and Subtropical Grasses

Subtropical grasses of the Panicoideae (e.g., *Paspalum notatum* (Bahia grass), *Sorghum halepense* (Johnson grass), *Imperata cylindrica* (cogon grass), *Cenchrus* sp. (buffel grass)) and Chloridoideae (e.g., *Cynodon dactylon* (Bermuda grass), *Eragrostis* sp. (e.g., Boer love), *Chloris gayana* (Rhodes grass)) subfamilies are abundant in regions adjacent to the equator (Esch 2004; Seidel et al. 2008) and appear to be clinically important for pollen allergy in subtropical regions of Africa, Asia, Central America, and southern parts of the USA (e.g., Florida, Texas) (Prescott and Potter 2001; Liang et al. 2010; Sam et al. 1998; Phillips et al. 1989; Calabria and Dice 2007). Allergens of Panicoideae (Pas n 1 and Pas n 13 of Bahia grass pollen and Sor h 1, Sor h 2, Sor h 13, and Sor h 23 of Johnson grass) and Chloridoideae (Cyn d 1, Cyn d 4, and Cyn d 22) species have potential to serve as diagnostic markers, but studies in relevant patient populations with recombinant allergens devoid of CCD are needed to determine the clinical relevance (Cabauatan et al. 2014; Davies et al. 2011; Davies 2014; Campbell et al. 2015). Notably, studies from Zimbawe show that tropical grasses are more prevalent than temperate grasses (Westritschnig et al. 2003).

Subjects with and without allergic symptoms from the Philippines contained IgE antibodies against tropical grasses and were mainly sensitized against carbohydrate epitopes which did not induce basophil activation. In this study it is likely that sensitization to tropical grasses is of low clinical relevance, but this needs to be investigated in other populations (Cabauatan et al. 2014). Recombinant Pas n 1 of Bahia grass pollen activated basophils of grass pollen allergic patients indicating clinically relevant sensitization in the Australian population exposed to and allergic to Bahia grass pollen (Davies et al. 2008).

10.3.4 Marker Allergens for Grass Pollen Allergy: Summary

Group-1 and group-5 allergens account for 60–80 % of grass pollen allergic patient IgE in different populations from different geographic areas (Laffer et al. 1996). Extensive cross inhibition of IgE binding of patients to nine different grass pollen extracts (sweet vernal grass, *Anthoxanthum odoratum*; oat, *Avena sativa*; Bermuda grass, *Cynodon dactylon*; perennial ryegrass, *Lolium perenne*; common reed, *Phragmites australis*; Kentucky bluegrass, *Poa pratensis*; rye, *Secale cereale*; wheat, *Triticum sativum*; and corn, *Zea mays*) was achieved with a small panel of purified, recombinant, grass pollen allergens (Phl p 1, Phl p 2, and Phl p 5) and profilin (Bet v 2) (Niederberger et al. 1998a). In a clinical vaccination study involving 64 subjects, patients were successfully treated with a mixture of recombinant Phl p 1, Phl p 2, Phl p 5a + b, and Phl p 6 (Jutel et al. 2005). A proof of principle was thus established that successful therapy of temperate grass pollen allergy in patients from Europe is possible using a combination of distinct grass pollen-specific and clinically important allergens. Recently, a novel recombinant hypoallergenic grass pollen allergy vaccine based on allergen peptides derived from the abovementioned grass pollen allergens has been developed for safe immunotherapy of grass pollen allergy (Focke-Tejkl et al. 2015) and, in clinical trials, has been shown to be hypoallergenic (Niederberger et al. 2015) as well as clinically effective for treatment (Zieglmayer et al. 2016; Cornelius et al. 2016; Gerlich and Glebe 2016).

> Group-1 and group-5 allergens, such as Phl p 1 and Phl p 5, are the most suitable marker allergens for diagnosis of grass pollen allergy in temperate climate zones.

10.3.5 Carbohydrate Sensitivity in Grass Pollen Allergic Patients

Phl p 1, Phl p 4, Phl p 11, Phl p 13 and their subtropical orthologs (e.g., Cyn d 1, Cyn d 4, and Pas n 13) are glycoproteins carrying cross-reactive carbohydrate determinants (CCD). Using CCD-free recombinant allergens in allergen CRD has the advantage that only functional IgE (i.e., capable of IgE aggregation) directed against protein epitopes is detected. For instance, up to 85 % of grass pollen allergic patients have detectable group-4 allergen-specific IgE. Group-4 allergens are glycoproteins with a molecular weight of 50–67 kDa. However, specific IgE in patient sera is often rather low, and despite *in vitro* reactivity, no clinical reactivity has been described (Andersson and Lidholm 2003; Westritschnig et al. 2008; Niederberger et al. 2001; Zafred et al. 2013). In tropical regions, IgE cross-reactivity is based nearly exclusively on CCD of these glycoproteins (Cabauatan et al. 2014), and in temperate climate zones, the frequency of sensitization seen in patient sera is less than 60 % if recombinant Phl p 4 is used for diagnosis (Tripodi et al. 2012).

Phl p 4 homologous proteins are found in *Ambrosia* sp. and birch pollen, as well as in peanut, apple, celery, and carrot, but clinical significance remains unclear (Grote et al. 2002).

10.4 Important Tree Pollen Allergens

◉ Table 10.2 gives an overview of the most important tree pollen allergens.

10.4.1 Allergens of Trees of the Order Fagales

10.4.1.1 Marker Allergen for Fagales: Bet v 1

The complementary deoxyribonucleic acid (cDNA) of Bet v 1, the major allergen of birch, was isolated in 1989 (Breiteneder et al. 1989), the 17-kDa protein allergen was produced using recombinant gene technology, and IgE reactivity in up to 95 % of birch pollen allergic patients was detected (Valenta et al. 1991b; Menz et al. 1996).

The major allergens of other tree pollen in the order of Fagales from the families of Betulaceae, (alder, *Alnus glutinosa*, Aln g 1; hornbeam, *Carpinus betulus*, Car p 1; hazelnut, *Corylus avellana*, Cor a 1) and Fagaceae (oak, *Quercus alba*, Que a 1; chestnut, *Castanea sativa*, Cas s 1; common beech, *Fagus sylvatica*, Fag s 1) all show pronounced cross-reactivities and sequence homologies within the group and to Bet v 1 (Mothes et al. 2004; Valenta et al. 1991b; Ipsen and Hansen 1991; Marth et al. 2014). Together, they form a group known as pathogenesis-related proteins (PR-10). Recombinant Bet v 1 inhibits IgE reactivity of patient sera with other tree pollen of the Fagales order (Niederberger et al. 1998b). A great number of proteins from different plant foods (nuts, vegetables and spices) display homology and cross-reactivity to Bet v 1, e.g., apple (*Malus domestica*, Mal d 1), hazelnut (*Corylus avellana*, Cor a 1), sweet cherry (*Prunus avium*, Pru av 1), apricot (*Prunus armeniaca*, Pru ar 1), peach (*Prunus persica*, Pru p 1), pear (*Pyrus communis*, Pyr c 1), carrot (*Daucus carota*, Dau c 1), celery (*Apium graveolens*, Api g 1), and soybean (*Glycine max*, Gly m 4) (Mothes et al. 2004; Swoboda et al. 2008; Heiss et al. 1996; Kazemi-Shirazi et al. 2000), and are responsible for birch pollen-related oral allergy syndrome (see Chap. 2).

Table 10.2 Important tree pollen allergens

Pollen	Example	Molecular weight (kDa)	Allergen	Protein
Fagales, e.g., birch	Bet v 1	~17	Marker allergen, major allergen, cross-reactivity with Fagales tree pollen; oral allergy syndrome	PR-10 protein
	Bet v 2	~15	Panallergen, cross-reactivity between plant pollen, plant-derived food, and latex	Profilin
	Bet v 3	~24	Panallergen, cross-reactivity between different plant pollen	Polcalcin family (3 EF-hand)
	Bet v 4	7–9	Panallergen, cross-reactivity between different plant pollen	Polcalcin family (2 EF-hand)
	Bet v 6	~33	Minor allergen	Isoflavone reductase
	Bet v 7	~18	Minor allergen	Cyclophilin
	Bet v 8	~66	–	Pectinesterase
Lamiales, e.g., olive tree	Ole e 1	~16	Marker allergen, major allergen, cross-reactivity between Lamiales tree pollen	Ole-e-1-like protein family, glycosylated
	Ole e 2	15–18	Panallergen, cross-reactivity between plant pollen, plant-derived food, and latex	Profilin
	Ole e 3	~9	Panallergen, cross-reactivity between different plant pollen	Polcalcin family (2 EF-hand)
	Ole e 5	~16	Minor allergen	Superoxide dismutase
	Ole e 6	~6–10	Minor allergen	–
	Ole e 7	~10	Minor allergen, limited cross-reactivity to other nsLTP	Nonspecific lipid transfer protein (nsLTP)
	Ole e 8	~21	Panallergen, cross-reactivity between different plant pollen	Polcalcin family (4 EF-hand)
	Ole e 9	~46	Minor allergen, pollen-fruit-latex syndrome	β-1,8-glucanase
	Ole e 10	~11	Minor allergen, pollen-fruit-latex syndrome	X8-domain protein, glycosyl hydrolase
	Ole e 11	39.4	Minor allergen	Pectin methyl-esterase
Platanaceae, e.g., plane tree	Pla a 1	~18	Marker allergen, major allergen	Invertase inhibitor
	Pla a 2	~43	–	Polygalacturonase
Cupressales, e.g., Arizona cypress, Japanese cedar	Cry j 1/ Cup a 1	41–45	Marker allergen, major allergen	Pectate lyase, glycosylated

Due to the high number of IgE-binding epitopes, Bet v 1 is thought to be the original sensitizing protein in clinically manifest allergy to Fagales pollen or in oral allergy syndrome (Kazemi-Shirazi et al. 2002; Swoboda et al. 2008; Moverare et al. 2002). In birch pollen allergic patients, exposure to birch pollen primarily increased Bet v 1-specific IgE without increasing IgE to other birch pollen allergens such as Bet v 2 (Birkner et al. 1990). Allergy patients in Central Africa reacting with natural birch pollen extracts did not display IgE antibodies against Bet v 1 but against other birch pollen allergens (Westritschnig et al. 2003; Odongo et al. 2015).

Several studies have shown that subcutaneous immunotherapy with birch pollen extract alone is equally effective as therapy with a mixture of different Fagales tree pollen extracts in tree pollen allergic patients (Henzgen et al. 1989; Petersen et al. 1988). Allergy diagnosis (skin test, specific IgE) with recombinant Bet v 1 is as effective in detecting birch pollen allergic patients as diagnosis using natural birch pollen extracts (Tresch et al. 2003).

> As a consequence of these in vitro and in vivo data, Bet v 1 represents the marker allergen for sensitization to Fagales tree pollen and indicates the possibility of an associated oral allergy syndrome.

10.4.1.2 Other Fagales-Specific Minor Allergens

Bet v 6 (formerly known as Bet v 5), an isoflavone reductase, is a minor allergen which is cross-reactive with pollen and proteins from several edible plants (fruits, vegetables, and spices); Bet v 7 is a cyclophilin. Both are recognized by less than 20 % of birch pollen allergic patients. Bet v 8 is a pectinesterase with a clinical significance that has yet to be determined (for an overview, see (Mothes et al. 2004; Marth et al. 2014) and Table 10.2).

10.4.2 Allergens of Trees of the Order Lamiales

10.4.2.1 Marker Allergen for Lamiales: Ole e 1

Ole e 1, the most important olive pollen allergen, exists in a non-glycosylated (19 kDa) and a glycosylated (21 kDa) form and is recognized by more than 70 % of olive pollen allergic patients (Villalba et al. 1993). It displays substantial sequence homologies with other members of the Ole-e-1-like protein family. This protein family derives from pollen of other Oleaceae species (for an overview, see Rodriguez et al. 2007) such as:

- Ash (*Fraxinus excelsior*, Fra e 1)
- Privet (*Ligustrum vulgare*, Lig v 1)
- Lilac (*Syringa vulgaris*, Syr v 1)

Moreover this protein family comprises Pla l 1 from plantain (*Plantago lanceolata*, family of Plantaginaceae) as well as allergens from taxonomically unrelated species such as Lol p 11 from *Lolium perenne* (perennial ryegrass), Phl p 11 from *Phleum pratense* (timothy grass), and Che a 1 from *Chenopodium album* (white goosefoot).

There is extensive cross-reactivity between Ole e 1 homologous allergens of the Oleaceae (Overview in Valenta et al. 2007). IgE from sera of two different groups of European patients either sensitized to olive or ash pollen was inhibited from binding to extracts of different Oleaceae pollen by Ole e 1. Birch pollen, grass pollen, and weed pollen extracts did not inhibit patient IgE binding to Ole e 1 (Palomares et al. 2006) showing the existence of specific epitopes for Oleaceae pollen in Ole e 1.

In patients from regions without local sources of olive pollen such as Austria, Germany, or Northern Italy, specific IgE against Ole e 1 indicates a sensitization to ash pollen (*Fraxinus excelsior*, Fra e 1) (Asero 2011; Niederberger et al. 2002). This is relevant in patients showing clinical symptoms during the birch pollen season, but who are not sensitized to birch or any other member of the Fagales order (Palomares et al. 2006).

> Ole e 1 is the marker allergen for sensitization to olive pollen and is important in this respect in the Mediterranean region. In regions without olive pollen, Ole e 1 can be used as a marker allergen for sensitization to ash pollen.

The group-11 grass pollen allergens Phl p 11 and Lol p 11 are members of the Ole-e-1-like protein family due to structural homologies and sequence homologies (e.g., approximately 30 % sequence identity between Ole e 1 and Phl p 11). However, they do not share any IgE epitopes with Ole e 1, and no significant cross-reactivity was detected between Ole e 1 and Phl p 11 or Lol p 11 (Palomares et al. 2006).

10.4.2.2 Other Lamiales-Specific Allergens

Other specific minor allergens of olive pollen have been described (for an overview, see (Rodriguez et al. 2007) and ◉ Table 10.2). Ole e 7 is a member of the nonspecific lipid transfer protein (nsLTP) family. Sensitization to Ole e 7 is associated with a tendency for severe allergic reactions; however, cross-reactivity with other nonspecific LTP seems to be limited (Tordesillas et al. 2011). In some regions of southern Spain, an elevated prevalence of sensitization against Ole e 7 and Ole e 9 was seen, and in some regions, up to 40 % of Ole-e-1-negative allergic patients are sensitized to Ole e 7 (Barber et al. 2007). Ole e 9 und Ole e 10 are also possibly associated with cross-reactivity to birch, tomato, potato, bell pepper, banana, and latex (Palomares et al. 2005; Quiralte et al. 2007).

10.4.3 Allergens of Trees of the Order Proteales

Tree pollen from trees of the Platanaceae family, genus Platanus, comprising about ten species (e.g., London plane tree, *Platanus acerifolia*), are highly cross-reactive and induce severe symptoms in a small number of sensitized patients. In regions with many plane trees, such as Spain, peaks of allergy symptoms are seen during the wind pollination season (Varela et al. 1997). Pla a 1 from the London plane tree, an invertase inhibitor, is recognized by up to 90 % of all plane tree allergic patients and is therefore considered a major allergen of plane trees (Asturias et al. 2002). Pla a 1 is used as a marker allergen for plane tree allergy (◉ Table 10.2); however, the allergen Pla a 2, a polygalacturonase, may also be important in this respect (Asturias et al. 2002, 2006).

10.4.4 Allergens of Trees of the Order Cupressales

Pollen from trees of the Cupressaceae family (e.g., Arizona cypress, *Cupressus arizonica*; Japanese cedar, *Cryptomeria japonica*; mountain cedar, *Juniperus ashei)* are highly cross-reactive (for an overview, see Di Felice et al. 2001; Marth et al. 2014). The prevalence of allergy to different Cupressaceae pollen has increased in Central Europe, even though Cupressaceae trees are distributed mainly in the Mediterranean region (Panzner et al. 2014). It is possible that allergy to Cupressales pollen was underestimated for a long time, because the flowering season is in winter (January to March/April), and clinical symptoms of allergy to Cupressales may have been mistaken for the common cold or thought to have been caused by perennial allergens such as from house dust mite (D'Amato et al. 2007).

Cry j 1 (from Japanese cedar) is a 40-kDa protein and was the first Cupressaceae allergen to be described (Yasueda et al. 1983). Cry j 1 displays high sequence homology and IgE cross-reactivity with other Cupressaceae allergens such as Cup a 1 from the Arizona cypress (Aceituno et al. 2000) and Jun a 1 from the mountain cedar (Midoro-Horiuti et al. 1999). These allergens are glycosylated pectate lyases. Although the major allergen of ragweed (*Ambrosia artemisiifolia*, Amb a 1) is also a pectate lyase, there is only very limited cross-reactivity with the above mentioned allergens (Pichler et al. 2015). Cup a 1 and Cry j 1 are used as marker allergens for Cupressales allergy.

10.5 Panallergens: Markers for Cross-Reactivity

Panallergens are found in grass and tree pollen as well as in many other botanically unrelated plants. They belong either to the polcalcin (calcium-binding allergens carrying two, three, or four binding sites for calcium, so-called EF-hands) or profilin protein families. Amino acid sequences of both protein families are highly conserved regardless of the taxonomical relationship of allergenic plant species leading to extensive immunological cross-reactivity. Therefore, they are considered marker allergens for cross-reactivity in the diagnosis of grass and tree pollen allergy (see Chap. 3).

10.5.1 Polcalcins

Members of the polcalcin protein family (approximately 9-kDa proteins) from tree and grass pollen include:

- 2-EF-hand-proteins Bet v 4, Aln g 4, Ole e 3, Cyn d 7, Phl p 7, Cyn d 7
- 3-EF-hand-protein Bet v 3
- 4-EF-hand-protein Ole e 8

Polcalcins have only been found in the pollen of trees, grasses, and weeds. Almost 10 % of grass pollen allergic patients in temperate regions have specific IgE to Phl p 7, but in sensitized patients, Phl p 7 displays a high allergenic activity (see Chap. 3) (Kazemi-Shirazi et al. 2002; Niederberger et al. 1999).

10.5.2 Profilins

Profilin (Bet v 2, 15 kDa) was first identified in birch pollen (Valenta et al. 1991a) and has since been found in the pollen of many grasses (e.g., Phl p 12, Cyn d 12), trees (e.g., Ole e 2), and weeds, but also in plant-derived food and latex (for an overview. see Kazemi-Shirazi et al. 2002; Radauer et al. 2006). The amount of specific patient IgE varies according to geographical region and allergen source and is found in approximately 10–30 % of pollen allergic patients.

10.5.3 Panallergens: Summary

Cross-inhibition experiments between polcalcins from different sources and between profilins from different sources have confirmed extensive cross-reactivity of allergens within these two protein families; the highest IgE reactivity is observed with the grass pollen allergens, i.e., Phl p 7 for the polcalcins and Phl p 12 for profilins (Tinghino et al. 2002; Radauer et al. 2006).

> Phl p 7 and Phl p 12 are considered marker allergens for cross-reactivity, and the presence of specific IgE to either of these allergens in patient sera may explain clinical symptoms upon exposure to a range of different allergen sources. Sensitization to either of these panallergens, Phl p 7 or Phl p 12, may result in apparent polysensitization presenting as multiple positive skin tests to pollen extracts and potential symptoms with unrelated allergen sources.

In patients with grass pollen allergy, sensitizations to Phl p 7 and Phl p 12 are often seen in later stages of allergic disease after sensitization to Phl p 1 and Phl p 5 (Hatzler et al. 2012) and may be considered as markers for clinically manifest grass pollen allergy.

10.6 Conclusions for Clinical Routine Work

Structured Approach to Routine Clinical Work

Diagnostic tests with marker allergens, Phl p 1/Phl p 5 (marker for grass pollen), Bet v 1 (marker for beech and birch trees as well as other Fagales trees), Ole e 1 (marker for olive trees and other Oleaceae trees including ash), Pla a 1 (marker for plane trees), and Cup a 1/Cry j 1 (marker for cypress trees), and with the panallergens (e.g., timothy grass, polcalcin/profilin), Phl p 7/Phl p 12 (indicators for cross-reactivity), establish a patient allergen-specific sensitization profile to tree and grass pollen allergens.

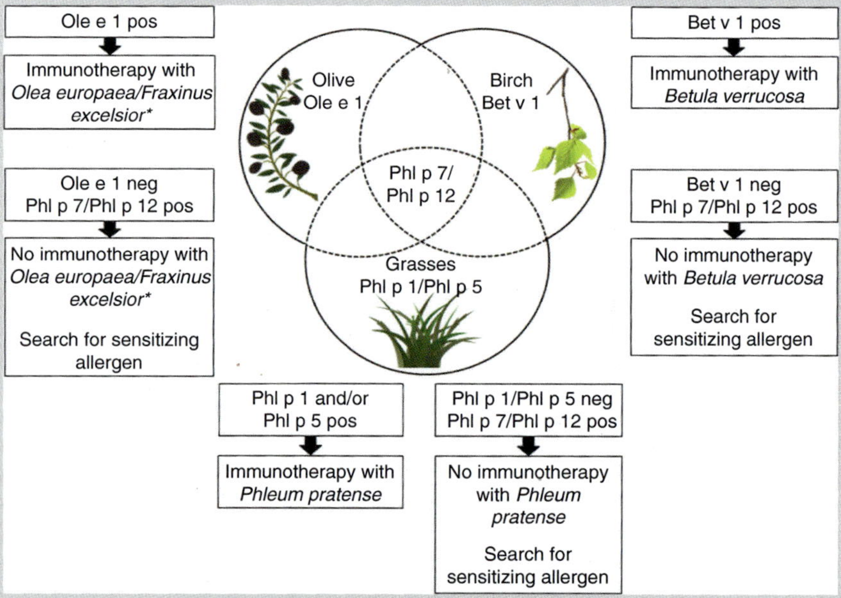

Fig. 10.3 Proposal for a structured diagnostic procedure in clinical routine work using important marker allergens: Phl p 1, Phl p 5, Phl p 7, Phl p 12, Ole e 1, Fra e 1*, and Bet v 1. *if available and in regions without distribution of *Olea europaea*

Genuine sensitization to grass pollen in Europe is reliably diagnosed with a combination of the major grass pollen allergens Phl p 1 and Phl p 5 (◉ Fig. 10.3). If sensitization to Phl p 1 without IgE reactivity to Phl p 5 (and in addition, no reactivity to Phl p 2/Phl p 3 and Phl p 6) is found, this may be due to sensitization to one of the tropical/subtropical grass subfamilies.

Specific IgE to Bet v 1 characterizes sensitization to Fagales trees (birch, alder, hornbeam, hazelnut, common beech, oak, chestnut) and possible related oropharyngeal symptoms (oral allergy syndrome) due to reactions with cross-reactive plant-derived foods (e.g., apple, hazelnut, pear, sweet cherry, peach, carrot, celery, soybean) (see Chap. 2).

Ole e 1 is the major allergen in olive pollen. It displays extensive sequence identity and cross-reactivity with other major allergens of the Oleaceae family such as ash, privet, and lilac. In the Mediterranean region, genuine sensitization to olive pollen is diagnosed with Ole e 1; in more temperate climate zones such as Central Europe, Ole e 1 can be used to prove sensitization to ash pollen and to distinguish it from the clinical symptoms of birch pollen allergy occurring in the same season.

Sensitization to tree pollen of the Platanaceae family is diagnosed with Pla a 1 (possibly including Pla a 2), sensitization to pollen of trees of the Cupressaceae family with Cup a 1/Cry j 1.

Association of the abovementioned marker allergens with specific clinically relevant sensitization profiles was confirmed in clinical studies (Canis et al. 2011; Jahn-Schmid et al. 2003; Twardosz-Kropfmuller et al. 2010; Moreno et al. 2014; Darsow et al. 2014).

If no clear-cut sensitization to one of the abovementioned marker allergens can be detected, the following rules apply:

- Low or no IgE reactivity to genuine marker allergens indicates that a patient is not sensitized to the corresponding allergen source. An allergen extract from this source is not suitable for specific immunotherapy.
- Exclusive sensitization to the panallergens profilin and polcalcin (e.g., Phl p 7 and Phl p 12 from timothy grass pollen) is very rare. This sensitization profile often cannot be attributed to one specific allergen source. Patients therefore are not suited for specific immunotherapy.
- The presence of specific IgE to profilin and/or polcalcin by nature of their cross-reactivity rules out further diagnosis with natural (pollen) extracts, as sensitization to panallergens abolishes analytical specificity (selectivity) of natural extracts.

In these cases, allergy CRD together with a detailed patient history should be used to reach a therapeutic decision. This will ensure that the correct decision for or against specific immunotherapy and its correct composition is taken (Douladiris et al. 2013; Letrán et al. 2013).

Conclusions

Detection of specific IgE using component resolved diagnostics (CRD) identifies the underlying allergen source in suspected cases of tree and grass pollen allergy. Suitable marker allergens can be used to distinguish genuine sensitization to tree or grass pollen from cross-reactivity to pollen panallergens (e.g., profilin and polcalcins) and to overcome the lack of analytical specificity of natural allergen extracts. In allergic patients suspected of polysensitization who react with a variety of pollen extracts, CRD allows specific allergen diagnosis regardless of the confounding effect of panallergenic cross-reactivity and prescription of tailored, specific immunotherapy.

Allergens defined as marker allergens for tree and grass pollen allergy are:

- Bet v 1 (birch pollen major allergen) for birch, beech, and other trees from the Fagales order
- Ole e 1 (olive tree major allergen) for olive and other trees including ash from the Oleaceae family
- Pla a 1 (major allergen of the London plane) for plane trees
- Cry j 1 (major allergen of the Japanese cedar)
- Cup a 1 (major allergen of the Arizona cypress) for cypress trees
- Jun a 1 (major allergen of mountain cedar) for juniper trees
- Phl p 1 (timothy grass group-1 major allergen) for most grasses including rye (*Secale* sp.)
- Phl p 5 (timothy grass group-5 major allergen) for "temperate climate" grasses (*Pooideae*)

Grass and tree pollen allergens with serological and clinical cross-reactivity to a great number of allergen sources are also identified as possible confounding factors in allergen-specific diagnosis with natural extracts. Structured diagnostic procedures for clinical routine work are needed to improve the appropriate selection of allergen sources for AIT.

References

Aceituno E, Del Pozo V, Minguez A, Arrieta I, Cortegano I, Cardaba B, Gallardo S, Rojo M, Palomino P, Lahoz C. Molecular cloning of major allergen from Cupressus arizonica pollen: Cup a 1. Clin Exp Allergy. 2000;30:1750–8.

Andersson K, Lidholm J. Characteristics and immunobiology of grass pollen allergens. Int Arch Allergy Immunol. 2003;130:87–107. doi:69013.

Asam C, Hofer H, Wolf M, Aglas L, Wallner M. Tree pollen allergens – an update from a molecular perspective. Allergy. 2015;70:1201–11.

Asero R. Analysis of hypersensitivity to oleaceae pollen in an olive-free and ash-free area by commercial pollen extracts and recombinant allergens. Eur Ann Allergy Clin Immunol. 2011;43:77–80.

Asturias JA, Ibarrola I, Amat P, Tella R, Malet A, Cistero-Bahima A, Enrique E, Malek T, Martinez A. Purified allergens vs. complete extract in the diagnosis of plane tree pollen allergy. Clin Exp Allergy. 2006;36:1505–12.

Asturias JA, Ibarrola I, Bartolome B, Ojeda I, Malet A, Martinez A. Purification and characterization of Pla a 1, a major allergen from Platanus acerifolia pollen. Allergy. 2002;57:221–7.

Barber D, Moreno C, Ledesma A, Serrano P, Galan A, Villalba M, Guerra F, Lombardero M, Rodriguez R. Degree of olive pollen exposure and sensitization patterns. Clinical implications. J Investig Allergol Clin Immunol. 2007;17 Suppl 1:11–6.

Birkner T, Rumpold H, Jarolim E, Ebner H, Breitenbach M, Skvaril F, Scheiner O, Kraft D. Evaluation of immunotherapy-induced changes in specific IgE, IgG and IgG subclasses in birch pollen allergic patients by means of immunoblotting. Correlation with clinical response. Allergy. 1990;45:418–26.

Blomme K, Tomassen P, Lapeere H, Huvenne W, Bonny M, Acke F, Bachert C, Gevaert P. Prevalence of allergic sensitization versus allergic rhinitis symptoms in an unselected population. Int Arch Allergy Immunol. 2013;160:200–7.

Bousquet J, Cour P, Guerin B, Michel FB. Allergy in the Mediterranean area. I. Pollen counts and pollinosis of Montpellier. Clin Allergy. 1984;14:249–58.

Breiteneder H, Pettenburger K, Bito A, Valenta R, Kraft D, Rumpold H, Scheiner O, Breitenbach M. The gene coding for the major birch pollen allergen Bet v 1, is highly homologous to a pea disease resistance response gene. Embo J. 1989;8:1935–8.

Cabauatan CR, Lupinek C, Scheiblhofer S, Weiss R, Focke-Tejkl M, Bhalla PL, Singh MB, Knight PA, van Hage M, Ramos JD, Valenta R. Allergen microarray detects high prevalence of asymptomatic IgE sensitizations to tropical pollen-derived carbohydrates. J Allergy Clin Immunol. 2014;133:910–4.

Calabria CW, Dice J. Aeroallergen sensitization rates in military children with rhinitis symptoms. Ann Allergy Asthma Immunol. 2007;99:161–9.

Campbell BC, Gilding EK, Timbrell V, Guru P, Loo D, Zennaro D, Mari A, Solley G, Hill MM, Godwin ID, Davies JM. Total transcriptome, proteome, and allergome of Johnson grass pollen, which is important for allergic rhinitis in subtropical regions. J Allergy Clin Immunol. 2015;135:133–42.

Canis M, Groger M, Becker S, Klemens C, Kramer MF. Recombinant marker allergens in diagnosis of patients with allergic rhinoconjunctivitis to tree and grass pollens. Am J Rhinol Allergy. 2011;25:36–9.

Christenhusz MJM, Reveal JL, Farjon A, Gardner MF, Mill RR, Chase MW. A new classification and linear sequence of extant gymnosperms. Phytotaxa. 2011;19:55–70.

Cornelius C, Schöneweis K, Georgi F, Weber M, Niederberger V, Zieglmayer P, Niespodziana K, Trauner M, Hofer H, Urban S, Valenta R. Immunotherapy With the PreS-based Grass Pollen Allergy Vaccine BM32 Induces Antibody Responses Protecting Against Hepatitis B Infection. EBioMedicine. 2016;11:58–67.

D'Amato G, Cecchi L, Bonini S, Nunes C, Annesi-Maesano I, Behrendt H, Liccardi G, Popov T, van Cauwenberge P. Allergenic pollen and pollen allergy in Europe. Allergy. 2007;62:976–90.

Darsow U, Brockow K, Pfab F, Jakob T, Petersson CJ, Borres MP, Ring J, Behrendt H, Huss-Marp J. Allergens. Heterogeneity of molecular sensitization profiles in grass pollen allergy – implications for immunotherapy? Clin Exp Allergy. 2014;44:778–86.

Davies JM, Mittag D, Dang TD, Symons K, Voskamp A, Rolland JM, O'Hehir RE. Molecular cloning, expression and immunological characterisation of Pas n 1, the major allergen of Bahia grass Paspalum notatum pollen. Mol Immunol. 2008;46:286–93.

Davies JM, Voskamp A, Dang TD, Pettit B, Loo D, Petersen A, Hill MM, Upham JW, Rolland JM, O'Hehir RE. The dominant 55kDa allergen of the subtropical Bahia grass (Paspalum notatum) pollen is a group 13 pollen allergen, Pas n 13. Mol Immunol. 2011;48:931–40.

Davies JM. Grass pollen allergens globally: the contribution of subtropical grasses to burden of allergic respiratory diseases. Clin Exp Allergy. 2014;44:790–801.

Di Felice G, Barletta B, Tinghino R, Pini C. Cupressaceae pollinosis: identification, purification and cloning of relevant allergens. Int Arch Allergy Immunol. 2001;125:280–9.

Douladiris N, Savvatianos S, Roumpedaki I, Skevaki C, Mitsias D, Papadopoulos NG. A molecular diagnostic algorithm to guide pollen immunotherapy in southern Europe: towards component-resolved management of allergic diseases. Int Arch Allergy Immunol. 2013;162:163–72.

Duffort O, Quintana J, Ipsen H, Barber D, Polo F. Antigenic similarity among group 1 allergens from grasses and quantitation ELISA using monoclonal antibodies to Phl p 1. Int Arch Allergy Immunol. 2008;145:283–90.

Flicker S, Steinberger P, Ball T, Krauth MT, Verdino P, Valent P, Almo S, Valenta R. Spatial clustering of the IgE epitopes on the major timothy grass pollen allergen Phl p 1: importance for allergenic activity. J Allergy Clin Immunol. 2006;117:1336–43.

Esch RE. Grass pollen allergens. Clin Allergy Immunol. 2004;18:185–205.

Flicker S, Vrtala S, Steinberger P, Vangelista L, Bufe A, Petersen A, Ghannadan M, Sperr WR, Valent P, Norderhaug L, Bohle B, Stockinger H, Suphioglu C, Ong EK, Kraft D, Valenta R. A human monoclonal IgE antibody defines a highly allergenic fragment of the major timothy grass pollen allergen, Phl p 5: molecular, immunological, and structural characterization of the epitope-containing domain. J Immunol. 2000;165:3849–59.

Focke-Tejkl M, Weber M, Niespodziana K, Neubauer A, Huber H, Henning R, Stegfellner G, Maderegger B, Hauer M, Stolz F, Niederberger V, Marth K, Eckl-Dorna J, Weiss R, Thalhamer J, Blatt K, Valent P, Valenta R. Development and characterization of a recombinant, hypoallergenic, peptide-based vaccine for grass pollen allergy. J Allergy Clin Immunol. 135:1207–7. e1201–11.

Gangl K, Niederberger V, Valenta R. Multiple grass mixes as opposed to single grasses for allergen immunotherapy in allergic rhinitis. Clin Exp Allergy. 2013;43:1202–16.

Gerlich WH, Glebe D. Development of an Allergy Immunotherapy Leads to a New Type of Hepatitis B Vaccine. EBioMedicine. 2016;11:5–6.

Griffith IJ, Smith PM, Pollock J, Theerakulpisut P, Avjioglu A, Davies S, Hough T, Singh MB, Simpson RJ, Ward LD, et al. Cloning and sequencing of Lol pI, the major allergenic protein of rye-grass pollen. FEBS Lett. 1991;279:210–5.

Grote M, Stumvoll S, Reichelt R, Lidholm J, Rudolf V. Identification of an allergen related to Phl p 4, a major timothy grass pollen allergen, in pollens, vegetables, and fruits by immunogold electron microscopy. Biol Chem. 2002;383:1441–5.

Grote M, Vrtala S, Niederberger V, Wiermann R, Valenta R, Reichelt R. Release of allergen-bearing cytoplasm from hydrated pollen: a mechanism common to a variety of grass (Poaceae) species revealed by electron microscopy. J Allergy Clin Immunol. 2001;108:109–15.

Hatzler L, Panetta V, Lau S, Wagner P, Bergmann RL, Illi S, Bergmann KE, Keil T, Hofmaier S, Rohrbach A, Bauer CP, Hoffman U, Forster J, Zepp F, Schuster A, Wahn U, Matricardi PM. Molecular spreading and predictive value of preclinical IgE response to Phleum pratense in children with hay fever. J Allergy Clin Immunol. 2012;130:894–901.

Heiss S, Fischer S, Muller WD, Weber B, Hirschwehr R, Spitzauer S, Kraft D, Valenta R. Identification of a 60 kd cross-reactive allergen in pollen and plant-derived food. J Allergy Clin Immunol. 1996;98:938–47.

Hejl C, Wurtzen PA, Kleine-Tebbe J, Johansen N, Broge L, Ipsen H. Phleum pratense alone is sufficient for allergen-specific immunotherapy against allergy to Pooideae grass pollens. Clin Exp Allergy. 2009;39:752–9. .

Henzgen M, Wenz W, Strumpfel R. Experiences with desensitization of early spring pollen allergy using 2 tree pollen extracts. Z Gesamte Inn Med. 1989;44:691–3.

Hiller R, Laffer S, Harwanegg C, Huber M, Schmidt WM, Twardosz A, Barletta B, Becker WM, Blaser K, Breiteneder H, Chapman M, Crameri R, Duchene M, Ferreira F, Fiebig H, Hoffmann-Sommergruber K, King TP, Kleber-Janke T, Kurup VP, Lehrer SB, Lidholm J, Muller U, Pini C, Reese G, Scheiner O, Scheynius A, Shen HD, Spitzauer S, Suck R, Swoboda I, Thomas W, Tinghino R, Van Hage-Hamsten M, Virtanen T, Kraft D, Muller MW, Valenta R. Microarrayed allergen molecules: diagnostic gatekeepers for allergy treatment. Faseb J. 2002;16:414–6.

Ipsen H, Hansen OC. The NH2-terminal amino acid sequence of the immunochemically partial identical major allergens of Alder (Alnus glutinosa) Aln g I, birch (Betula verrucosa) Bet v I, hornbeam (Carpinus betulus) Car b I and oak (Quercus alba) Que a I pollens. Mol Immunol. 1991;28:1279–88.

Jahn-Schmid B, Harwanegg C, Hiller R, Bohle B, Ebner C, Scheiner O, Mueller MW. Allergen microarray: comparison of microarray using recombinant allergens with conventional diagnostic methods to detect allergen-specific serum immunoglobulin E. Clin Exp Allergy. 2003;33: 1443–9.

Johansen N, Weber RW, Ipsen H, Barber D, Broge L, Hejl C. Extensive IgE cross-reactivity towards the Pooideae grasses substantiated for a large number of grass-pollen-sensitized subjects. Int Arch Allergy Immunol. 2009;150:325–34.

Johnson P, Marsh DG. 'Isoallergens' from rye grass pollen. Nature. 1965;206:935–7.

Jutel M, Jaeger L, Suck R, Meyer H, Fiebig H, Cromwell O. Allergen-specific immunotherapy with recombinant grass pollen allergens. J Allergy Clin Immunol. 2005;116:608–13.

Kazemi-Shirazi L, Niederberger V, Linhart B, Lidholm J, Kraft D, Valenta R. Recombinant marker allergens: diagnostic gatekeepers for the treatment of allergy. Int Arch Allergy Immunol. 2002;127:259–68.

Kazemi-Shirazi L, Pauli G, Purohit A, Spitzauer S, Froschl R, Hoffmann-Sommergruber K, Breiteneder H, Scheiner O, Kraft D, Valenta R. Quantitative IgE inhibition experiments with purified recombinant allergens indicate pollen-derived allergens as the sensitizing agents responsible for many forms of plant food allergy. J Allergy Clin Immunol. 2000;105:116–25.

Laffer S, Duchene M, Reimitzer I, Susani M, Mannhalter C, Kraft D, Valenta R. Common IgE-epitopes of recombinant Phl p I, the major timothy grass pollen allergen and natural group I grass pollen isoallergens. Mol Immunol. 1996;33:417–26.

Laffer S, Valenta R, Vrtala S, Susani M, van Ree R, Kraft D, Scheiner O, Duchene M. Complementary DNA cloning of the major allergen Phl p I from timothy grass (Phleum pratense); recombinant Phl p I inhibits IgE binding to group I allergens from eight different grass species. J Allergy Clin Immunol. 1994a;94:689–98.

Laffer S, Vrtala S, Duchene M, van Ree R, Kraft D, Scheiner O, Valenta R. IgE-binding capacity of recombinant timothy grass (Phleum pratense) pollen allergens. J Allergy Clin Immunol. 1994b;94:88–94.

Letrán A, Espinazo M, Moreno F. Measurement of IgE to pollen allergen components is helpful in selecting patients for immunotherapy. Ann Allergy Asthma Immunol. 2013;111:295–7.

Levin M, Rotthus S, Wendel S, Najafi N, Kallstrom E, Focke-Tejkl M, Valenta R, Flicker S, Ohlin M. Multiple independent IgE epitopes on the highly allergenic grass pollen allergen Phl p 5. Clin Exp Allergy. 2014;44:1409–19.

Liang KL, Su MC, Shiao JY, Wu SH, Li YH, Jiang RS. Role of pollen allergy in Taiwanese patients with allergic rhinitis. J Formosan Med Assoc. 2010;109:879–85.

Lupinek C, Wollmann E, Baar A, Banerjee S, Breiteneder H, Broecker BM, Bublin M, Curin M, Flicker S, Garmatiuk T, Hochwallner H, Mittermann I, Pahr S, Resch Y, Roux KH, Srinivasan B, Stentzel S, Vrtala S, Willison LN, Wickman M, Lodrup-Carlsen KC, Anto JM, Bousquet J, Bachert C, Ebner D, Schlederer T, Harwanegg C, Valenta R. Advances in allergen-microarray technology for diagnosis and monitoring of allergy: the MeDALL allergen-chip. Methods. 2014;66:106–19.

Madritsch C, Gadermaier E, Roder UW, Lupinek C, Valenta R, Flicker S. High-density IgE recognition of the major grass pollen allergen Phl p 1 revealed with single-chain IgE antibody fragments obtained by combinatorial cloning. J Immunol. 2015;194:2069–78.

Marknell DeWitt A, Niederberger V, Lehtonen P, Spitzauer S, Sperr WR, Valent P, Valenta R, Lidholm J. Molecular and immunological characterization of a novel timothy grass (Phleum pratense) pollen allergen, Phl p 11. Clin Exp Allergy. 2002;32:1329–40.

Marth K, Garmatiuk T, Swoboda I, Valenta R. Tree pollen allergens. In: Lockey RF, Ledford DK, editors. Allergens and allergen immunotherapy. 5th ed. London: CRC Press; 2014. p. 113–32.

Menz G, Dolecek C, Schonheit-Kenn U, Ferreira F, Moser M, Schneider T, Suter M, Boltz-Nitulescu G, Ebner C, Kraft D, Valenta R. Serological and skin-test diagnosis of birch pollen allergy with recombinant Bet v I, the major birch pollen allergen. Clin Exp Allergy. 1996;26:50–60.

Midoro-Horiuti T, Goldblum RM, Kurosky A, Goetz DW, Brooks EG. Isolation and characterization of the mountain Cedar (Juniperus *ashei)* pollen major allergen, Jun a 1. J Allergy Clin Immunol. 1999;104:608–12.

Moreno C, Justicia JL, Quiralte J, Moreno-Ancillo A, Iglesias-Cadarso A, Torrecillas M, Labarta N, Garcia MA, Davila I. Olive, grass or both? Molecular diagnosis for the allergen immunotherapy selection in polysensitized pollinic patients. Allergy. 2014;69:1357–63.

Mothes N, Horak F, Valenta R. Transition from a botanical to a molecular classification in tree pollen allergy: implications for diagnosis and therapy. Int Arch Allergy Immunol. 2004;135:357–73.

Moverare R, Westritschnig K, Svensson M, Hayek B, Bende M, Pauli G, Sorva R, Haahtela T, Valenta R, Elfman L. Different IgE reactivity profiles in birch pollen-sensitive patients from six European populations revealed by recombinant allergens: an imprint of local sensitization. Int Arch Allergy Immunol. 2002;128:325–35.

Niederberger V, Hayek B, Vrtala S, Laffer S, Twardosz A, Vangelista L, Sperr WR, Valent P, Rumpold H, Kraft D, Ehrenberger K, Valenta R, Spitzauer S. Calcium-dependent immunoglobulin E recognition of the apo- and calcium-bound form of a cross-reactive two EF-hand timothy grass pollen allergen, Phl p 7. Faseb J. 1999;13:843–56.

Niederberger V, Laffer S, Froschl R, Kraft D, Rumpold H, Kapiotis S, Valenta R, Spitzauer S. IgE antibodies to recombinant pollen allergens (Phl p 1, Phl p 2, Phl p 5, and Bet v 2) account for a high percentage of grass pollen-specific IgE. J Allergy Clin Immunol. 1998a;101:258–64.

Niederberger V, Pauli G, Gronlund H, Froschl R, Rumpold H, Kraft D, Valenta R, Spitzauer S. Recombinant birch pollen allergens (rBet v 1 and rBet v 2) contain most of the IgE epitopes present in birch, alder, hornbeam, hazel, and oak pollen: a quantitative IgE inhibition study with sera from different populations. J Allergy Clin Immunol. 1998b;102:579–91.

Niederberger V, Purohit A, Oster JP, Spitzauer S, Valenta R, Pauli G. The allergen profile of ash (Fraxinus excelsior) pollen: cross-reactivity with allergens from various plant species. Clin Exp Allergy. 2002;32:933–41.

Niederberger V, Stubner P, Spitzauer S, Kraft D, Valenta R, Ehrenberger K, Horak F. Skin test results but not serology reflect immediate type respiratory sensitivity: a study performed with recombinant allergen molecules. J Invest Dermatol. 2001;117:848–51.

Niederberger V, Marth K, Eckl-Dorna J, Focke-Tejkl M, Weber M, Hemmer W, Berger U, Neubauer A, Stolz F, Henning R, Valenta R. Skin test evaluation of a novel peptide carrier-based vaccine, BM32, in grass pollen-allergic patients. J Allergy Clin Immunol. 2015;136:1101-3.e8.

Odongo L, Mulyowa G, Goebeler M, Trautmann A. Bet v 1- and Bet v 2-Associated Plant Food Sensitization in Uganda and Germany: differences and similarities. Int Arch Allergy Immunol. 2015;167:264–9.

Palomares O, Swoboda I, Villalba M, Balic N, Spitzauer S, Rodriguez R, Valenta R. The major allergen of olive pollen Ole e 1 is a diagnostic marker for sensitization to Oleaceae. Int Arch Allergy Immunol. 2006;141:110–8.

Palomares O, Villalba M, Quiralte J, Polo F, Rodriguez R. 1,3-beta-glucanases as candidates in latex-pollen-vegetable food cross-reactivity. Clin Exp Allergy. 2005;35:345–51.

Panzner P, Vachova M, Vitovcova P, Brodska P, Vlas T. A comprehensive analysis of middle-European molecular sensitization profiles to pollen allergens. Int Arch Allergy Immunol. 2014;164:74–82. .

Perez M, Ishioka GY, Walker LE, Chesnut RW. cDNA cloning and immunological characterization of the rye grass allergen Lol p I. J Biol Chem. 1990;265:16210–5.

Petersen BN, Janniche H, Munch EP, Wihl JA, Bowadt H, Ipsen H, Lowenstein H. Immunotherapy with partially purified and standardized tree pollen extracts. I. Clinical results from a three-year double-blind study of patients treated with pollen extracts either of birch or combinations of alder, birch and hazel. Allergy. 1988;43:353–62.

Phillips JW, Bucholtz GA, Fernandez-Caldas E, Bukantz SC, Lockey RF. Bahia grass pollen, a significant aeroallergen: evidence for the lack of clinical cross-reactivity with timothy grass pollen. Ann Allergy. 1989;63:503–7.

Pichler U, Hauser M, Wolf M, Bernardi ML, Gadermaier G, Weiss R, Ebner C, Yokoi H, Takai T, Didierlaurent A, Rafaiani C, Briza P, Mari A, Behrendt H, Wallner M, Ferreira F. Pectate lyase pollen allergens: sensitization profiles and cross-reactivity pattern. PLoS One. 2015;10, e0120038.

Prescott RA, Potter PC. Allergenicity and cross-reactivity of buffalo grass (Stenotaphrum secundatum). South African Med J. 2001;91:237–43.

Quiralte J, Palacios L, Rodriguez R, Cardaba B, Arias de Saavedra JM, Villalba M, Florido JF, Lahoz C. Modelling diseases: the allergens of Olea europaea pollen. J Investig Allergol Clin Immunol. 2007;17 Suppl 1:24–30.

Radauer C, Willerroider M, Fuchs H, Hoffmann-Sommergruber K, Thalhamer J, Ferreira F, Scheiner O, Breiteneder H. Cross-reactive and species-specific immunoglobulin E epitopes of plant profilins: an experimental and structure-based analysis. Clin Exp Allergy. 2006;36:920–9.

Rodriguez R, Villalba M, Batanero E, Palomares O, Quiralte J, Salamanca G, Sirvent S, Castro L, Prado N. Olive pollen recombinant allergens: value in diagnosis and immunotherapy. J Investig Allergol Clin Immunol. 2007;17 Suppl 1:4–10.

Sam CK, Kesavan P, Liam CK, Soon SC, Lim AL, Ong EK. A study of pollen prevalence in relation to pollen allergy in Malaysian asthmatics. Asian Pac J Allergy Immunol. 1998;16:1–4.
Seidel DJ, Fu Q, Randel WJ, Riechler TJ. Widening of the tropical belt in a changing climate. Nat Geosci. 2008;1:21–4.
Simon BK, Clayton W, Harman K, Vorontsova M, Brake I, Healy D, Alfonso Y. 2011. Last accessed 22 Sept 2014.
Suck R, Hagen S, Cromwell O, Fiebig H. The high molecular mass allergen fraction of timothy grass pollen (Phleum pratense) between 50-60 kDa is comprised of two major allergens: Phl p 4 and Phl p 13. Clin Exp Allergy. 2000;30:1395–402.
Suphioglu C. What are the important allergens in grass pollen that are linked to human allergic disease? Clin Exp Allergy. 2000;30:1335–41.
Swoboda I, Twaroch T, Valenta R, Grote M. Tree pollen allergens. Clin Allergy Immunol. 2008;21:87–105.
The Angiosperm Phylogeny Group. An update of the Angiosperm Phylogeny Group classification for the orders and families of flowering plants: APG III. Botanical J Linnean Soc. 2009;161:105–21.
Timbrell VL, Riebelt L, Simmonds C, Solley G, Smith WB, McLean-Tooke A, van Nunen S, Smith PK, Upham JW, Langguth D, Davies JM. An immunodiagnostic assay for quantitation of specific IgE to the major pollen allergen component, Pas n 1, of the subtropical Bahia grass. Int Arch Allergy Immunol. 2014;165:219–28.
Tinghino R, Twardosz A, Barletta B, Puggioni EM, Iacovacci P, Butteroni C, Afferni C, Mari A, Hayek B, Di Felice G, Focke M, Westritschnig K, Valenta R, Pini C. Molecular, structural, and immunologic relationships between different families of recombinant calcium-binding pollen allergens. J Allergy Clin Immunol. 2002;109:314–20.
Tordesillas L, Sirvent S, Diaz-Perales A, Villalba M, Cuesta-Herranz J, Rodriguez R, Salcedo G. Plant lipid transfer protein allergens: no cross-reactivity between those from foods and olive and Parietaria pollen. Int Arch Allergy Immunol. 2011;156:291–6.
Tresch S, Holzmann D, Baumann S, Blaser K, Wuthrich B, Crameri R, Schmid-Grendelmeier P. In vitro and in vivo allergenicity of recombinant Bet v 1 compared to the reactivity of natural birch pollen extract. Clin Exp Allergy. 2003;33:1153–8.
Tripodi S, Frediani T, Lucarelli S, Macri F, Pingitore G, Di Rienzo BA, Dondi A, Pansa P, Ragusa G, Asero R, Faggian D, Plebani M, Matricardi PM. Molecular profiles of IgE to Phleum pratense in children with grass pollen allergy: implications for specific immunotherapy. J Allergy Clin Immunol. 2012;129:834–9.e838.
Twardosz-Kropfmuller A, Singh MB, Niederberger V, Horak F, Kraft D, Spitzauer S, Valenta R, Swoboda I. Association of allergic patients' phenotypes with IgE reactivity to recombinant pollen marker allergens. Allergy. 2010;65:296–303.
Valenta R, Duchene M, Pettenburger K, Sillaber C, Valent P, Bettelheim P, Breitenbach M, Rumpold H, Kraft D, Scheiner O. Identification of profilin as a novel pollen allergen; IgE autoreactivity in sensitized individuals. Science. 1991a;253:557–60.
Valenta R, Duchene M, Vrtala S, Birkner T, Ebner C, Hirschwehr R, Breitenbach M, Rumpold H, Scheiner O, Kraft D. Recombinant allergens for immunoblot diagnosis of tree-pollen allergy. J Allergy Clin Immunol. 1991b;88:889–94.
Valenta R, Lidholm J, Niederberger V, Hayek B, Kraft D, Grönlund H. The recombinant allergen-based concept of component-resolved diagnostics and immunotherapy (CRD and CRIT). Clin Exp Allergy. 1999;29:896–904.
Valenta R, Twaroch T, Swoboda I. Component-resolved diagnosis to optimize allergen-specific immunotherapy in the Mediterranean area. J Investig Allergol Clin Immunol. 2007;17 Suppl 1:36–40.
van Ree R. Isoallergens: a clinically relevant phenomenon or just a product of cloning? Clin Exp Allergy. 2002;32:975–8.
Van Ree R, Driessen MN, Van Leeuwen WA, Stapel SO, Aalberse RC. Variability of crossreactivity of IgE antibodies to group I and V allergens in eight grass pollen species. Clin Exp Allergy. 1992;22:611–7.

Varela S, Subiza J, Subiza JL, Rodriguez R, Garcia B, Jerez M, Jimenez JA, Panzani R. Platanus pollen as an important cause of pollinosis. J Allergy Clin Immunol. 1997;100:748–54.

Villalba M, Batanero E, Lopez-Otin C, Sanchez LM, Monsalve RI, Gonzalez de la Pena MA, Lahoz C, Rodriguez R. The amino acid sequence of Ole e I, the major allergen from olive tree (Olea europaea) pollen. Eur J Biochem. 1993;216:863–9.

Vrtala S, Sperr WR, Reimitzer I, van Ree R, Laffer S, Muller WD, Valent P, Lechner K, Rumpold H, Kraft D, et al. cDNA cloning of a major allergen from timothy grass (Phleum pratense) pollen; characterization of the recombinant Phl pV allergen. J Immunol. 1993;151:4773–81.

Westritschnig K, Horak F, Swoboda I, Balic N, Spitzauer S, Kundi M, Fiebig H, Suck R, Cromwell O, Valenta R. Different allergenic activity of grass pollen allergens revealed by skin testing. Eur J Clin Invest. 2008;38:260–7.

Westritschnig K, Sibanda E, Thomas W, Auer H, Aspock H, Pittner G, Vrtala S, Spitzauer S, Kraft D, Valenta R. Analysis of the sensitization profile towards allergens in central Africa. Clin Exp Allergy. 2003;33:22–7.

Wuthrich B, Schindler C, Leuenberger P, Ackermann-Liebrich U. Prevalence of atopy and pollinosis in the adult population of Switzerland (SAPALDIA study). Swiss Study on Air Pollution and Lung Diseases in Adults. Int Arch Allergy Immunol. 1995;106:149–56.

Yasueda H, Yui Y, Shimizu T, Shida T. Isolation and partial characterization of the major allergen from Japanese cedar (Cryptomeria japonica) pollen. J Allergy Clin Immunol. 1983;71:77–86.

Zafred D, Nandy A, Pump L, Kahlert H, Keller W. Crystal structure and immunologic characterization of the major grass pollen allergen Phl p 4. J Allergy Clin Immunol. 2013;132:696–703. e610.

Zieglmayer P, Focke-Tejkl M, Schmutz R, Lemell P, Zieglmayer R, Weber M, Kiss R, Blatt K, Valent P, Stolz F, Huber H, Neubauer A, Knoll A, Horak F, Henning R, Valenta R. Mechanisms, safety and efficacy of a B cell epitope-based vaccine for immunotherapy of grass pollen allergy. EBioMedicine. 2016;11:43–57.

Marker Allergens of Weed Pollen: Basic Considerations and Diagnostic Benefits in Routine Clinical Practice

11

G. Gadermaier, T. Stemeseder, W. Hemmer, and T. Hawranek

11.1 Introduction

Plants typically referred to as weeds are heterogeneous and do not correspond to any particular botanical group of plants. The term Kraut evolved from the Old High German term "krut," which simply defined usable plants. Now the term kraut usually refers to a herb and unkraut, a weed. The English term weeds refers to plants growing where they are not desired (by random seed dispersal), although many are used as food or for medicinal purposes by various cultures. Weeds are conceptually distinct from herbaceous plants. The latter group comprises non-ligneous plants with succulent, green stems that completely die off after the vegetation period. Thus, grasses, which may produce allergenic pollen, are not considered weeds.

Pollen of weeds mediating IgE-related allergies are found in the plant families of Asteraceae, Plantaginaceae, Urticaceae, Amaranthaceae, and Euphorbiaceae

This contribution is based on a review article that was published in 2014 in *Allergo Journal International* (Stemeseder T et al. Marker allergens of weed pollen – basic considerations and diagnostic benefits in the clinical routine. Allergo J Int 2014; 23:274–80) and has now been modified and updated as a book chapter.
The authors gratefully thank Dr. Steve Love, PhD, Laguna Niguel, CA, USA, for reading the manuscript, helpful suggestions, and editorial assistance with the English translation.

G. Gadermaier, PhD, Prof. (✉) • T. Stemeseder
Department of Molecular Biology, University of Salzburg, Salzburg, Austria
e-mail: gabriele.gadermaier@sbg.ac.at; teresa.stemeseder@sbg.ac.at

W. Hemmer, PhD, Assoc Prof.
FAZ – Floridsdorf Allergy Center, Vienna, Austria
e-mail: hemmer@faz.at

T. Hawranek, MD
Department of Dermatology, Paracelsus Private Medical University Salzburg, Salzburg, Austria
e-mail: t.hawranek@salk.at

J. Kleine-Tebbe, T. Jakob (eds.), *Molecular Allergy Diagnostics*,
DOI 10.1007/978-3-319-42499-6_11

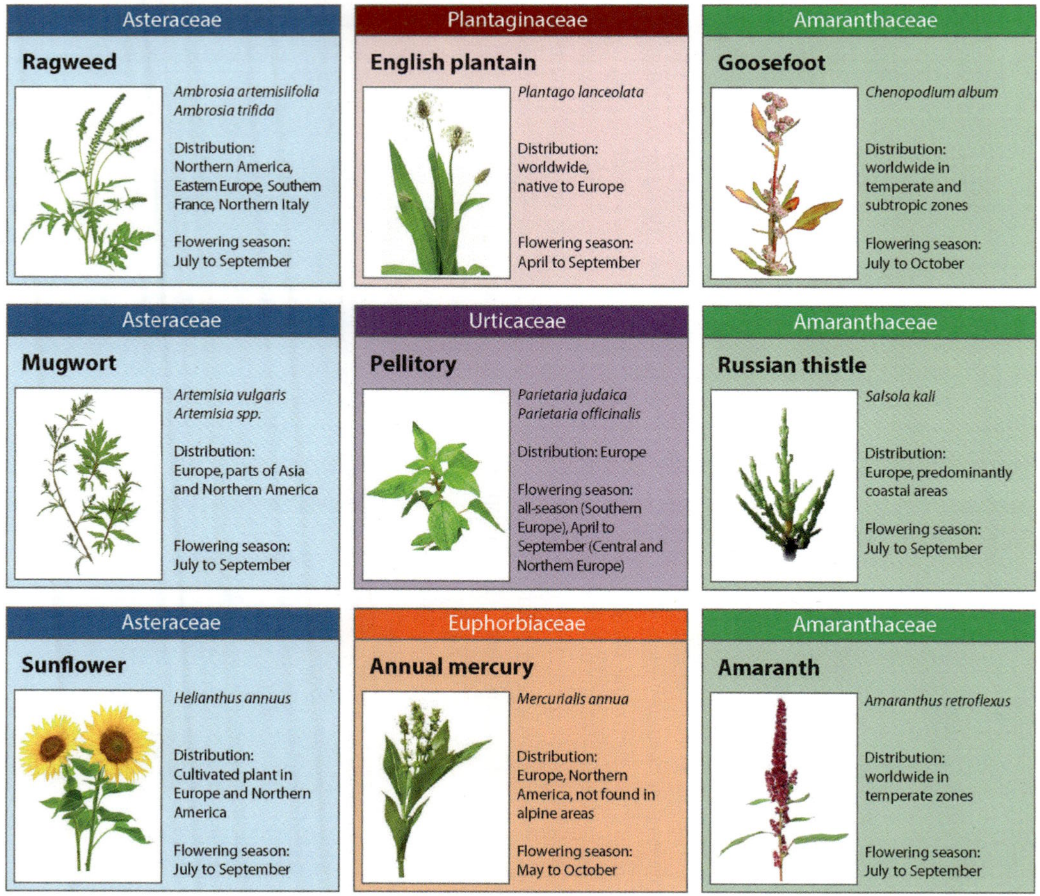

Fig. 11.1 Allergenic weeds in Europe (Reproduced from Stemeseder et al. 2014. Source: © Ragweed, Elenathewise; English plantain, Schlierner; Goosefoot, tosoth; Mugwort, Joachim Opelka; Pellitory, MIMOHE; Russian thistle, petepahham; Sunflower, ksena32; Annual mercury, Alois; Amaranth, Alois/(9×) fotolia.com)

(⊙ Fig. 11.1). Common ragweed has been unintentionally introduced from the United States and is now persistent predominantly in Southern and Eastern Europe. Due to climatic changes, ragweed already shows a prolonged flowering season (Ziska et al. 2011). The botanically related plant mugwort, which has many common local names in the United States, grows in the entire Northern hemisphere and is a relevant source of allergens in Europe as well as in Asia (Smith et al. 2014). Pellitory is predominantly found in Mediterranean coastal regions and has a particularly long flowering period. Although English plantain (introduced from Europe into the United States) flowers at the same time as grasses, it is a weed and presents a distinct allergen repertoire (Gadermaier et al. 2014a). In distinct geographical regions, other weeds such as goosefoot, Russian thistle (Russian tumbleweed), and annual mercury can contribute to high local exposure and sensitization rates.

11.2 Allergen Nomenclature

To date, 36 molecules originating from pollen of 12 different weeds have been officially acknowledged as allergens (www.allergen.org). ⊙ Table 11.1 presents an overview on the clinically most relevant weeds and their respective allergens. A comprehensive list of known weed pollen allergens can be found in Gadermaier et al. (2014b) (see also Matricardi et al. 2016), and the recently identified ragweed Amb a 11 is described by Bouley, Groeme (Bouley et al. 2015). As weeds belong to diverse botanical families, they present different allergen panels with major allergens from various protein families. To date, 35 weed allergens have been purified from pollen and/or have been recombinantly produced. Among these, all relevant molecules are also commercially available for clinical diagnosis (⊙ Table 11.1). Highest IgE reactivity can be found in allergens from the protein families of pectate lyases, defensin-like proteins, nonspecific lipid transfer proteins (nsLTP) and Ole e 1-like proteins.

11.3 Structure and Biological Function of Relevant Protein Families

11.3.1 Pectate Lyases

The allergenic pectate lyases from ragweed and mugwort, Amb a 1 and Art v 6, are, in contrast to homologous representatives from cedar and cypress, not glycosylated. Pectate lyases have a characteristic tunnellike three-dimensional fold (Wopfner et al. 2009). This structure consists of parallel β-sheets stacked on one another and forming a cavity. The natural and the recombinant protein can be cleaved into two proteolytic subunits (Wopfner et al. 2009). Pectate lyases play a role as enzymes in the maturation and rotting process of plant tissue. In pollen they are expressed in the late developmental phase, as they enable growth and emergence of the pollen tube by loosening the cell wall.

Table 11.1 Relevant allergens in weed pollen

	Pectate lyases	Defensin-like protein (PR-12)	nsLTP (PR-14)	Ole e 1-like proteins	Profilins	Polcalcins	Pectin methyl-esterase	Cysteine proteases
Ragweed *Ambrosia artemisiifolia*	**Amb a 1**[a,b]	Amb a 4	Amb a 6		Amb a 8	Amb a 9 Amb a 10		**Amb a 11**
Mugwort *Artemisia vulgaris*	Art v 6	**Art v 1**[a,b]	Art v 3[a,b]		Art v 4	Art v 5		
Sunflower *Helianthus annuus*		Hel a 1 (tentatively SF 18)			Hel a 2			
English plantain Plantago lanceolata				**Pla l 1**[a, b]	Pla l 2			
Pellitory *Parietaria judaica*			**Par j 1** **Par j 2**[a,b]		Par j 3	Par j 4		
Goosefoot *Chenopodium album*				**Che a 1**[b]	Che a 2	Che a 3		
Russian thistle *Salsola kali*				Sal k 5	Sal k 4		**Sal k 1**[a,b]	
Amaranth *Amaranthus retroflexus*					Ama r 2			
Annual mercury *Mercurialis annua*					**Mer a 1**[b]			

[a]ImmunoCAP allergens, Thermo Scientific
[b]ImmunoCAP ISAC, Thermo Scientific
Bold: major allergens

11.3.2 Defensin-Like Proteins

Allergenic molecules consisting of a fusion of a defensin-like and a proline-rich domain have to date only been identified in the family of Asteraceae. Art v 1 from mugwort pollen has the highest allergologic relevance. Further, Amb a 4 from ragweed, SF18 from sunflower pollen, and the recently cloned Par h 1 from feverfew play a role in allergy (Gruber et al. 2009; Pablos et al. 2015). The compact defensin domain is stabilized by four disulfide bridges and has a typical alpha/beta motif (Razzera et al. 2010). The C-terminal region is relatively flexible and the majority of prolines are hydroxylated and carry diverse plant-specific O-glycans (Himly et al. 2003). Defensin-like proteins are frequently found in peripheral cell layers. This suggests a role in the first line of defense and, thus, they were grouped into the pathogenesis-related (PR)-12 protein family. The function can be explained by the formation of protein pores in invasive microbial membranes or by charge-induced permeability of these membranes (Marmiroli and Maestri 2014). However, an antibacterial or antifungal mode of action has not been proven for allergenic defensin-like proteins.

11.3.3 Nonspecific Lipid Transfer Proteins

Nonspecific lipid transfer proteins (nsLTP) are members of the prolamin superfamily and are small, basic proteins with a compact, alpha-helical structure. Despite considerable variability in the primary sequence, they present a highly conserved, disulfide bond-stabilized three-dimensional fold. This compact structure confers the particularly high proteolytic and thermal resistance of the molecule. High concentrations of nsLTP can be found in peripheral cell layers. The hydrophobic cavity accommodates various fatty acids and, thus, facilitates the binding and transport of phospholipids. However, the role in plant defense against fungi and bacteria (PR-14 proteins) might be biologically more relevant; nsLTP expression was shown to be induced by stress and injury (Egger et al. 2010).

11.3.4 Ole e 1-Like Proteins

Proteins assigned to the Ole e 1-like family share a short, consensus sequence, while the remainder of the primary sequence varies considerably among family members. Representatives of this family typically contain one N-glycosylation site and proteins are usually partially glycosylated (Gadermaier et al. 2014a). Recent X-ray crystallographic analysis of recombinant Pla l 1 revealed a structure composed mainly of beta sheets stabilized by three disulfide bridges (PDB ID: 4Z8W). The biological function of Ole e 1-like proteins is to date unknown, but structurally similar proteins were found to play a role in cell wall membrane anchoring.

11.4 Clinical Relevance of Allergens

11.4.1 Pectate Lyases

Amb a 1 is the dominant allergen in pollen of ragweed, with a sensitization frequency of >95 %. The homologous molecule Art v 6 plays, however, only a minor role in mugwort pollen allergy. Both molecules present partial antibody cross-reactivity and Amb a 1 encompasses a larger amount of IgE and T-cell epitopes (Jahn-Schmid et al. 2012). The recently identified ragweed allergen Amb a 11 has physicochemical properties similar to Amb a 1 but has been classified into the protein family of cysteine proteases (Bouley et al. 2015). With a sensitization rate of 66 %, it represents an additional major allergen from *Ambrosia*. In comparison to Amb a 1, the novel allergen Amb a 11 exhibits a lower allergenicity, and isolated monosensitization seems to be rare.

11.4.2 Defensin-Like Proteins

Sensitization to Art v 1 from mugwort pollen ranges from 60 to 95 %, rendering it the most important as well as best studied allergen in this protein family. The vast majority of conformational IgE-binding epitopes are localized on the defensin domain, while the C-terminal region containing the glycan moiety has only minor clinical relevance (Razzera et al. 2010; Dedic et al. 2009). Art v 1 possesses one dominant T-cell epitope associated with the HLA class II histocompatibility antigen DRB1*01 expression, a restriction which is, to date, a unique feature for allergens (Jahn-Schmid et al. 2005). Homologous allergens are present in the pollen of ragweed (Amb a 4), feverfew (Par h 1), and sunflower (SF18) (Gruber et al. 2009; Pablos et al. 2015; Leonard et al. 2010).

11.4.3 Nonspecific Lipid Transfer Proteins (nsLTP)

Allergenic members of this protein family are found predominantly in food plants (e.g., Pru p 3 from peach), while expression in pollen is restricted to weeds, olive, and plane trees. Par j 1 and Par j 2 (48–50 % sequence identity) demonstrate a sensitization frequency of 95 % and 83 %, respectively, and represent the major allergens of pellitory pollen (Costa et al. 1994; Stumvoll et al. 2003). In contrast to other allergenic nsLTP, they both have a higher molecular mass and do not show IgE cross-reactivity with other representatives of this protein family (Tordesillas et al. 2011). Art v 3, the nsLTP from mugwort pollen, was shown to trigger respiratory symptoms in sensitized patients (Sanchez-Lopez et al. 2014). However, clinically irrelevant Art v 3 reactivity due to primary Pru p 3 sensitization is frequently noted, while on the other hand, Art v 3 can in some cases also lead to food allergic reactions against peaches (Egger et al. 2010; Gao et al. 2013).

11.4.4 Ole e 1-Like Proteins

Ole e 1-like proteins represent major allergens in pollen of English plantain (Pla l 1) and goosefoot (Che a 1). As the primary sequence of Ole e 1-like proteins varies considerably among members, IgE cross-reactivity is mostly confined to botanical closely related molecules (Calabozo et al. 2003).

11.5 Sensitization Frequencies

The clinical relevance of weed pollen sensitization is clearly dependent on geographic regions and, hence, pollen exposure. Sensitization to *Ambrosia spp.* in the general population is high in Northern America (8.7–15.3 %), while in the European population, skin prick test reactivity is typically less frequent (Bousquet et al. 2007; Chan-Yeung et al. 2010). A study, conducted in Germany, evaluating 1,039 randomly selected adults showed a sensitization rate of 0.7 % against Amb a 1 and 4.4 % against Art v 1 (Boehme et al. 2013). Geographical differences were also found in a comparative study with mugwort-positive patients from Northern and Southern Europe and North America. Similarly distributed sensitization rates against Art v 1 and Amb a 1 were observed in patients from Northern (84 % and 20 %) and Southern Europe (74 % and 16 %), respectively (Moverare et al. 2011). A different sensitization pattern was found in North America; 46 % of patients were reactive to Art v 1, while 68 % were positive to Amb a 1 (Moverare et al. 2011). A study on pollen-allergic patients from Spain revealed a sensitization frequency of 13 % for Art v 1 (Barber et al. 2009).

The high frequency of true mugwort pollen sensitization (68 % reactive to Art v 1, 8 % reactive to Amb a 1) was also found in another study investigating weed pollen-allergic patients from Germany (Canis et al. 2012). Mugwort and ragweed are, e.g., both important causes of weed pollen allergy in eastern Austria. In western Austria, however, they demonstrate only minor relevance due to the different climatic conditions in mountainous areas. In this region, pollen of English plantain is the major weed pollen allergen. In China, sensitization to mugwort among asthma and/or rhinitis patients is 11 %, while reactivity to ragweed is 4–7 % (Li et al. 2009). Sensitization to Amb a 1 is typically less frequent and uncommon in the absence of Art v 1 reactivity which indicates primary sensitization to *Artemisia* species in this population (Hao et al. 2013).

A recent epidemiologic study investigated IgE sensitization to 112 different allergens among 501 randomly selected 13–2-year-old school children from Salzburg (Western Austria) using the ImmunoCAP ISAC (Stemeseder et al. 2016). Thirty-eight percent of sensitized subjects were reactive to weed pollen allergens, while the overall atopy rate was 54 %. Highest prevalence to weed pollen sensitization was found against Pla l 1 (10 %), which confirms the importance of English plantain as a relevant allergen source. Other weed pollen sensitizations were against Art v 1 (7 %), Mer a 1 (6 %), Che a 1 (5 %), Amb a 1 (1 %), and Sal k 1 (0.4 %). None of the study participants showed IgE reactivity against Par j 2. Among pollen-allergic patients in Spain, genuine plantain allergy determined by Pla l 1-positive reactions are considered the second cause of pollinosis in some northern areas and are frequently associated with grass sensitization (Barber et al. 2009; Couto and Miranda 2011).

Allergic reactions to *Parietaria* allergens are almost exclusively reported in the southern European population, while sensitization in the non-Mediterranean population is low presumably due to limited pollen exposure (Bousquet et al. 2007; D'Amato et al. 2007; Cuesta-Herranz et al. 2010). In some coastal areas in southern Europe, sensitization rates to Par j 2 may reach 60–90 % among pollen-sensitized individuals (Gadermaier et al. 2014b; Moverare et al. 2011). Pollen of *Chenopodium spp.*, *Amaranthus spp., and Salsola spp.* are typically found in desert and semidesert areas of the Middle East with local sensitization frequencies up to 70 % among pollen-allergic patients (Villalba et al. 2014). More recently, these weeds also account for adverse reactions in southern Spain with, e.g., up to 80 % IgE reactivity to Sal k 1 among patients suffering from seasonal allergies (Barber et al. 2008, 2009). In some areas of Spain, reactivity to *Mercurialis annua* ranges from 28 to 56 % (Gadermaier et al. 2014b).

11.6 Cross-Reactive Versus Marker Allergens

Marker allergens have been identified for all relevant weed pollen; they also constitute the major allergens of respective pollen sources. These comprise Amb a 1 (ragweed), Art v 1 (mugwort), Pla l 1 (English plantain), Par j 2 (pellitory), Che a 1 (goosefoot), and Sal k 1 (Russian thistle) (⊙ Table 11.1). Although Pla l 1 demonstrates moderate sequence identity with Che a 1 and Ole e 1, IgE cross-reactivity seems to be low (Calabozo et al. 2003). Recent data of the authors' group showed no correlation in reactivity to Pla l 1 and other Ole e 1-like allergens.

Analogous to tree and grass pollen, weed pollen also contains the IgE cross-reactive panallergens, profilin and polcalcin (⦿ Table 11.1). Their relevance as sensitizers is highly dependent on local pollen exposure (Orovitg et al. 2011). In regions with high pollen exposure, panallergen sensitization can be due to primary weed pollen sensitization; in regions with low or no exposure reactivity, it is usually due to profilin or polcalcin from other pollen sources (Stumvoll et al. 2003; Asero et al. 2008). An intermediate position is attributed to nsLTPs. Par j 2 from pellitory is not cross-reactive with other nsLTPs and thus represents a valid and specific marker allergen (Stumvoll et al. 2003; Tordesillas et al. 2011). But this is not the case for the IgE cross-reactive minor allergen from mugwort, Art v 3. Clinically manifested mugwort pollen allergy is almost exclusively associated with sensitization to Art v 1.

In pollen of mugwort and ragweed, homologs of the major allergens Art v 1 and Amb a 1 exist and show moderate cross-reactivity. The defensin-like domain of Amb a 4 from ragweed presents 69 % sequence identity with Art v 1, and partial IgE cross-reactivity was demonstrated (Leonard et al. 2010). Inhibition experiments indicate primary sensitization with Art v 1, while genuine sensitization to Amb a 4 is less common and predominately observed in high ragweed-exposed cohorts (Pablos et al. 2015; Oberhuber et al. 2008). IgE cross-reactivity was also observed between Amb a 1 and Art v 6 (65 % sequence identity). Sixty-three percent of Amb a 1-positive patients suffering from late summer pollinosis demonstrated in vitro reactivity to Art v 6. T-cell stimulation and inhibition experiments in a limited number of patients point at a frequent primary sensitization to Amb a 1. However, in rare cases, primary sensitization with Art v 6 and cross-reactivity to Amb a 1 seems to exist (Jahn-Schmid et al. 2012).

In summary, the above-described IgE cross-reactivities are a plausible explanation for the frequently observed double sensitizations to mugwort and ragweed in routine extract diagnostics. Studies have demonstrated the strong primary sensitizing capacities of Art v 1 and Amb a 1, while genuine sensitization with the cross-reactive homologs Amb a 4 and Art v 6 seems to be less common. Thus, Art v 1 and Amb a 1 can be considered genuine marker allergens for mugwort and ragweed pollen allergy, respectively, in the vast majority of cases. To what extent genuine mugwort and ragweed pollen allergy is diagnosed inappropriately needs to be further investigated. Whether double sensitizations to mugwort and ragweed pollen are due to co- or cross-reactivity depends primarily on pollen exposure and the patient population (Canis et al. 2012; Oberhuber et al. 2008; Asero et al. 2006, 2014).

Food plant allergies related to weed pollen sensitization are predominantly observed in patients allergic to mugwort and ragweed pollen. So far, members of the profilin and nsLTP family, as well as high molecular weight (glycan) components, were suggested as causative cross-reactive allergens (Egger et al. 2006; Gadermaier et al. 2011).

Due to IgE cross-reactivity, weed pollen allergies might lead to type 2 food allergies ("pollen-food syndrome"). Typical examples are the celery-mugwort-spice syndrome, the ragweed-melon-banana syndrome, or the mugwort-peach association.

11.7 Allergy Diagnosis

According to the current GA²LEN recommendations for harmonization of skin prick tests in Europe, mugwort, ragweed, and pellitory pollen are included in routine diagnostics, while plantain, goosefoot, and Russian thistle are not (Heinzerling et al. 2009). Since the clinical relevance of certain weeds has considerable geographic variability, local modifications in diagnostics are considered useful and necessary. Weed pollen sensitization is commonly observed in polysensitized patients, while monosensitization is rather infrequent. Thus, molecule-based allergy diagnostics is a valuable tool and should be used for discrimination when practical.

To date, virtually all major allergens of weed pollen are commercially available for component-resolved diagnosis (⊙ Table 11.1). Che a 1 is presently the only exception, being available only on the ImmunoCAP ISAC and not as a single agent for ImmunoCAP testing. Components are available either as recombinant molecules (rPla l 1, rChe a 1, rPar j 2) or as CCD (N-glycan)-free, natural molecules (nArt v 1, nAmb a 1). In the case of Sal k 1, false-positive results due to the partial N-glycan moiety might be observed. Specific diagnosis of IgE antibodies against profilins and polcalcins from weed pollen is currently available for the profilin of annual mercury (Mer a 1). Due to the high IgE cross-reactivity with grass and birch pollen profilin, interpretation of these results is difficult.

11.8 Added Value of Molecular Allergy Diagnostics

Molecule-based allergy diagnostics is particularly advantageous in cases of weed pollen sensitization, as patients are frequently polysensitized, and the clinical history does not provide unequivocal answers – possibly due to overlapping flowering seasons.

In clinical practice, Art v 1 and Amb a 1 are particularly useful as specific marker allergens for mugwort and ragweed pollen allergy, as identification of the responsible weed is difficult to assess using extract-based diagnostics (⊙ Fig. 11.2). Although a misleading diagnosis due to cross-reactivity (Art v 1 – Amb a 4 and Amb a 1 – Art v 6) cannot entirely be ruled out, the primary sensitizer is correctly identified for the vast majority of patients. Thus, unnecessary (double) immunotherapies can efficiently be avoided. Although Art v 3 does not constitute a marker for mugwort pollen allergy, it is considered a useful diagnostic option for patients suffering from mugwort pollen-associated food allergies (e.g., celery allergy) (Egger et al. 2010; Gadermaier et al. 2011).

To date, limited data are available suggesting Pla l 1 as useful allergen for the diagnosis of English plantain allergy in Central Europe (Gadermaier et al. 2014a). However, lack of IgE cross-reactivity with Che a 1 and Ole e 1 indicates that non-glycosylated recombinant Pla l 1 is a highly specific marker for genuine English plantain allergy (Calabozo et al. 2003; Matricardi et al. 2016).

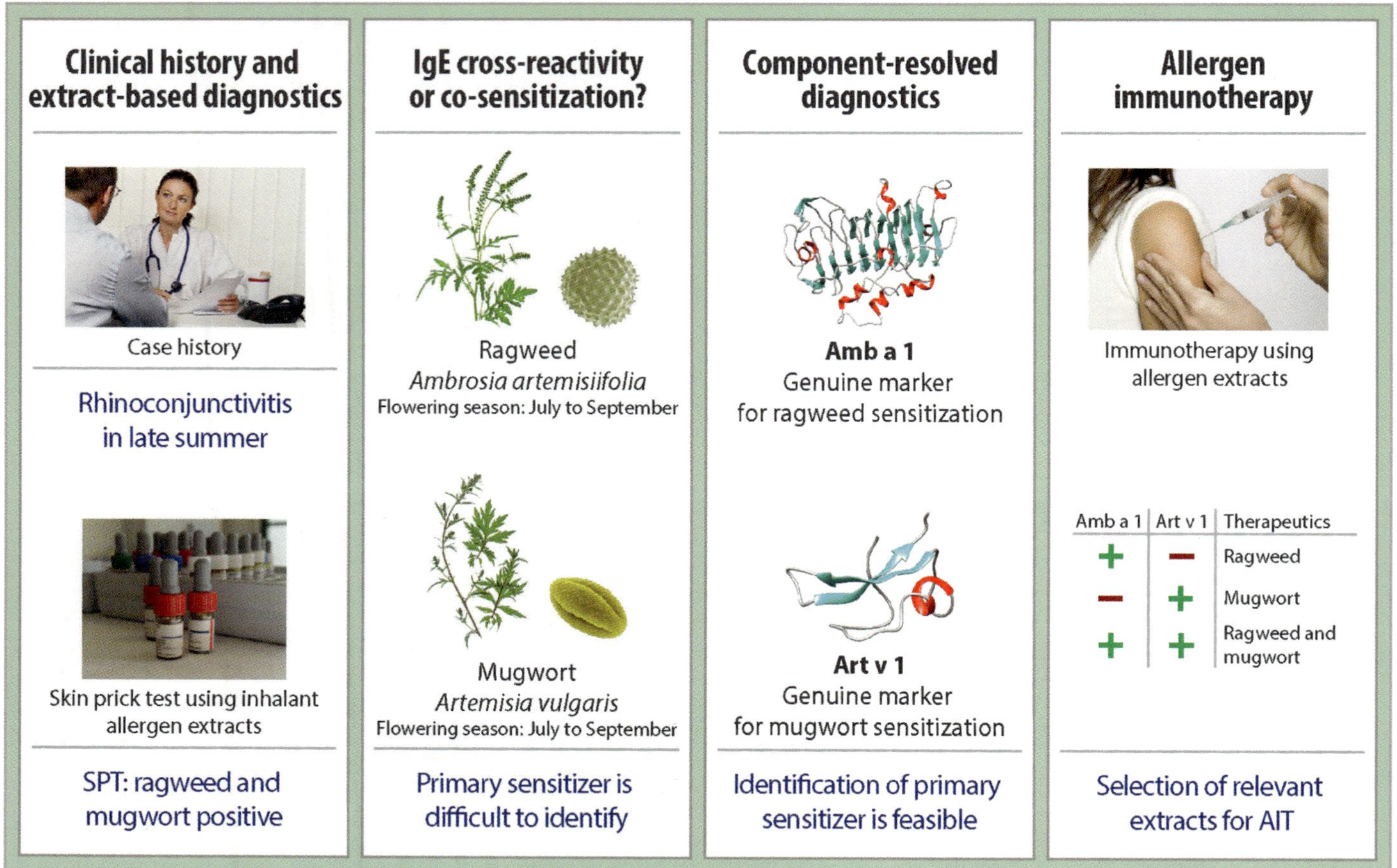

Fig. 11.2 Added value of molecular diagnostics for allergen immunotherapy selection using ragweed and mugwort as examples; depictions of molecules prepared with UCSF Chimera (Reproduced from Stemeseder et al. 2014. Source: © Ragweed, Elenathewise; Mugwort, Joachim Opelka; Case history, G. Sanders; Immunotherapy, A. Gregor/(4x) fotolia.com; Prick test and molecular structures, G. Gadermaier; http://swissmodel.expasy.org/; www.cgl.ucsf.edu/chimera/download.html)

Par j 2 and Sal k 1 play an important role for IgE detection in the Mediterranean population. Notably, Par j 2 from the Mediterranean wall pellitory should theoretically be able to detect genuine sensitization against *Parietaria officinalis*, an indigenous weed in Central and Northern Europe (Matricardi et al. 2016). However, this weed does not seem to be a relevant allergen in Central Europe (Heinzerling et al. 2009). Even though goosefoot is ubiquitous in Central Europe, the relevance as an allergen elicitor has been little investigated in this population and seems to be low. The use of Che a 1 as indicator of a genuine goosefoot pollen allergy is limited, since the efficacy of the respective immunotherapeutic agent has not been verified.

11.9 Therapeutic Recommendations

Identification of the primary sensitizer is usually supported using marker allergens specific for weed pollen (⊙ Fig. 11.2) (more examples in Matricardi et al. 2016). In difficult or doubtful cases of polysensitization, allergen extracts of plants triggering the most profound symptoms are typically selected for therapy. Presently, a limited availability of weed pollen extracts for subcutaneous immunotherapy exists. Due to regulatory considerations and enhanced standardization for allergen products together with economic considerations, several providers (particularly in Germany) already have or are planning to withdraw their weed pollen extracts from the market. For one company selling in Austria, weed pollen extracts only constitute 0.9 % of the total annual turnover. On the other hand, the same provider specified figures of 25.1 % for Greece and 73.7 % for Hungary for the same products. One might speculate that the sales discrepancies for these products might be due to fewer regulatory restrictions and much greater demand. However, regulatory and insurance considerations, e.g., in the United States are in constant flux and might also affect usage of such products. On average, the European market for weed pollen allergens constitutes only 2.6 % of the market share.

Currently, five single extracts and nine combination products (mugwort, pellitory, and English plantain pollen) for subcutaneous immunization are available and registered in Central Europe (Paul-Ehrlich-Institut, www.pei.de). In the United States, various standardized subcutaneous weed pollen solutions and, a tablet for sublingual immunotherapy of ragweed pollen allergy have been brought to market.

11.10 Perspectives

The use of purified allergen molecules as patient-specific immunotherapy has been investigated in several clinical studies. The efficacy of natural, recombinant, or hypoallergenic allergen molecules has already been demonstrated in clinical trials of birch and grass pollen-allergic patients (Wallner et al. 2013). Hypoallergenic derivatives of allergenic molecules from weeds, i.e., ragweed, mugwort, and pellitory pollen, have been engineered. These molecules demonstrate lower IgE-binding capacity and, thus, potentially less side effects for therapeutic applications (Gadermaier et al. 2014b). Clinical investigations of these hypoallergenic weed pollen molecules are, however, not yet available. The efficacy and safety of an Amb a 1 T-cell epitope-based peptide for immunotherapy has been demonstrated in 275 ragweed-allergic patients (Hafner et al. 2012).

11.11 Conclusions for Routine Clinical Practice

Overlapping flowering periods, polysensitization, and geographic differences all affect the clinical relevance of allergenic weeds and can complicate the vaccine choice for allergen immunotherapy. Plant-specific marker allergens are available for all relevant weed pollen to support the laboratory diagnosis of clinically relevant sensitizations. Based on the results of molecular diagnostics in conjunction with the patient's history, appropriate extracts can be selected for allergen immunotherapy.

Acknowledgments Austrian Federal Ministry of Science, Research and Economy and Austrian National Federation for Research, Technology and Development

References

Asero R, et al. Artemisia and Ambrosia hypersensitivity: co-sensitization or co-recognition? Clin Exp Allergy. 2006;36:658–65.

Asero R, Monsalve R, Barber D. Profilin sensitization detected in the office by skin prick test: a study of prevalence and clinical relevance of profilin as a plant food allergen. Clin Exp Allergy. 2008;38:1033–7.

Asero R, et al. Concomitant sensitization to ragweed and mugwort pollen: who is who in clinical allergy? Ann Allergy Asthma Immunol. 2014;113:307–13.

Barber D, et al. Understanding patient sensitization profiles in complex pollen areas: a molecular epidemiological study. Allergy. 2008;63:1550–8.

Barber D, et al. Component-resolved diagnosis of pollen allergy based on skin testing with profilin, polcalcin and lipid transfer protein pan-allergens. Clin Exp Allergy. 2009;39:1764–73.

Boehme MW, et al. Respiratory symptoms and sensitization to airborne pollen of ragweed and mugwort of adults in Southwest Germany. Dtsch Med Wochenschr. 2013;138:1651–8.

Bouley J, et al. Identification of the cysteine protease Amb a 11 as a novel major allergen from short ragweed. J Allergy Clin Immunol. 2015;136:1055–64.

Bousquet PJ, et al. Geographical variation in the prevalence of positive skin tests to environmental aeroallergens in the European Community Respiratory Health Survey I. Allergy. 2007;62: 301–9.

Calabozo B, et al. Cloning and expression of biologically active Plantago lanceolata pollen allergen Pla l 1 in the yeast Pichia pastoris. Biochem J. 2003;372(Pt 3):889–96.

Canis M, et al. IgE reactivity patterns in patients with allergic rhinoconjunctivitis to ragweed and mugwort pollens. Am J Rhinol Allergy. 2012;26:31–5.

Chan-Yeung M, et al. Geographical variations in the prevalence of atopic sensitization in six study sites across Canada. Allergy. 2010;65:1404–13.

Costa MA, et al. cDNA cloning, expression and primary structure of Par jI, a major allergen of Parietaria judaica pollen. FEBS Lett. 1994;341:182–6.

Couto M, Miranda M. Proposed GA2LEN standardized allergen battery: what about regional sensitization differences? J Investig Allergol Clin Immunol. 2011;21:491–2.
Cuesta-Herranz J, et al. Differences among pollen-allergic patients with and without plant food allergy. Int Arch Allergy Immunol. 2010;153:182–92.
D'Amato G, et al. Allergenic pollen and pollen allergy in Europe. Allergy. 2007;62:976–90.
Dedic A, et al. Immune recognition of novel isoforms and domains of the mugwort pollen major allergen Art v 1. Mol Immunol. 2009;46:416–21.
Egger M, et al. Pollen-food syndromes associated with weed pollinosis: an update from the molecular point of view. Allergy. 2006;61:461–76.
Egger M, et al. The role of lipid transfer proteins in allergic diseases. Curr Allergy Asthma Rep. 2010;10:326–35.
Gadermaier G, et al. Sensitization prevalence, antibody cross-reactivity and immunogenic peptide profile of Api g 2, the non-specific lipid transfer protein 1 of celery. PLoS One. 2011;6:e24150.
Gadermaier G, et al. Plantago lanceolata: an important trigger of summer pollinosis with limited IgE cross-reactivity. J Allergy Clin Immunol. 2014a;134:472–5.
Gadermaier G, Hauser M, Ferreira F. Allergens of weed pollen: an overview on recombinant and natural molecules. Methods. 2014b;66:55–66.
Gao ZS, et al. Peach allergy in China: a dominant role for mugwort pollen lipid transfer protein as a primary sensitizer. J Allergy Clin Immunol. 2013;131:224–6.e1-3.
Gruber P, et al. Role of the polypeptide backbone and post-translational modifications in cross-reactivity of Art v 1, the major mugwort pollen allergen. Biol Chem. 2009;390(5–6):445–51.
Hafner RP, et al. Validation of peptide immunotherapy as a new approach in the treatment of rhinoconjunctivitis: the clinical benefits of treatment with Amb a 1 derived T cell epitopes. J Allergy Clin Immunol. 2012;129:AB368.
Hao GD, et al. Prevalence of sensitization to weed pollens of Humulus scandens, Artemisia vulgaris, and Ambrosia artemisiifolia in northern China. J Zhejiang Univ Sci B. 2013;14:240–6.
Heinzerling LM, et al. GA(2)LEN skin test study I: GA(2)LEN harmonization of skin prick testing: novel sensitization patterns for inhalant allergens in Europe. Allergy. 2009;64:1498–506.
Himly M, et al. Art v 1, the major allergen of mugwort pollen, is a modular glycoprotein with a defensin-like and a hydroxyproline-rich domain. FASEB J. 2003;17:106–8.
Jahn-Schmid B, et al. Antigen presentation of the immunodominant T-cell epitope of the major mugwort pollen allergen, Art v 1, is associated with the expression of HLA-DRB1 *01. J Allergy Clin Immunol. 2005;115:399–404.
Jahn-Schmid B, et al. Humoral and cellular cross-reactivity between Amb a 1, the major ragweed pollen allergen, and its mugwort homolog Art v 6. J Immunol. 2012;188:1559–67.
Leonard R, et al. A new allergen from ragweed (Ambrosia artemisiifolia) with homology to art v 1 from mugwort. J Biol Chem. 2010;285:27192–200.
Li J, et al. A multicentre study assessing the prevalence of sensitizations in patients with asthma and/or rhinitis in China. Allergy. 2009;64:1083–92.
Marmiroli N, Maestri E. Plant peptides in defense and signaling. Peptides. 2014;56C:30–44.
Matricardi PM, Kleine-Tebbe J, Hoffmann HJ, Valenta R, Hilger C, Hofmaier S, Aalberse RC, Agache I, Asero R, Ballmer-Weber B, Barber D, Beyer K, Biedermann T, Biló MB, Blank S, Bohle B, Bosshard PP, Breiteneder H, Brough HA, Caraballo L, Caubet JC, Crameri R, Davies JM, Douladiris N, Ebisawa M, Eigenmann PA, Fernandez-Rivas M, Ferreira F, Gadermaier G, Glatz M, Hamilton RG, Hawranek T, Hellings P, Hoffmann-Sommergruber K, Jakob T, Jappe U, Jutel M, Kamath SD, Knol EF, Korosec P, Kuehn A, Lack G, Lopata AL, Mäkelä M, Morisset M, Niederberger V, Nowak-Wezgrzyn AH, Papadopoulos NG, Pastorello EA, Pauli G, Platts-Mills T, Posa D, Poulsen LK, Raulf M, Sastre J, Scala E, Schmid JM, Schmid-Grendelmeier P, van Hage M, van Ree R, Vieths S, Weber R, Wickman M, Muraro A, Ollert M. EAACI molecular allergology user's guide. Pediatr Allergy Immunol. 2016;27(Suppl23):1–250.
Moverare R, et al. Mugwort-sensitized individuals from North Europe, South Europe and North America show different IgE reactivity patterns. Int Arch Allergy Immunol. 2011;154:164–72.

Oberhuber C, et al. Prevalence of IgE-binding to Art v 1, Art v 4 and Amb a 1 in mugwort-allergic patients. Int Arch Allergy Immunol. 2008;145:94–101.
Orovitg A, et al. Enhanced diagnosis of pollen allergy using specific immunoglobulin E determination to detect major allergens and panallergens. J Investig Allergol Clin Immunol. 2011;21:253–9.
Pablos I, et al. Allergenic members of the defensin-like protein family share structural features but show distinct immunological properties. In: European Academy of Allergy and Clinical Immunology Congress 2015. Barcelona; 2015.
Razzera G, et al. Mapping the interactions between a major pollen allergen and human IgE antibodies. Structure. 2010;18:1011–21.
Sanchez-Lopez J, et al. Role of Art v 3 in pollinosis of patients allergic to Pru p 3. J Allergy Clin Immunol. 2014;133:1018–25.e3.
Smith M, et al. Geographic and temporal variations in pollen exposure across Europe. Allergy. 2014;69:913–23.
Stemeseder T, et al. Cross-sectional study on allergic sensitization of Austrian adolescents using molecule-based IgE profiling. Allergy. 2016. doi: 10.1111/all.13071.
Stemeseder T, Hemmer W, Hawranek T, Gadermaier G. Marker allergens of weed pollen - basic considerations and diagnostic benefits in the clinical routine: Part 16 of the Series Molecular Allergology. Allergo J Int. 2014;23:274–280.
Stumvoll S, et al. Identification of cross-reactive and genuine Parietaria judaica pollen allergens. J Allergy Clin Immunol. 2003;111:974–9.
Tordesillas L, et al. Plant lipid transfer protein allergens: no cross-reactivity between those from foods and olive and Parietaria pollen. Int Arch Allergy Immunol. 2011;156:291–6.
Villalba M, et al. Amaranthaceae pollens: review of an emerging allergy in the mediterranean area. J Investig Allergol Clin Immunol. 2014;24:371–81; quiz 2 p preceding 382.
Wallner M, Pichler U, Ferreira F. Recombinant allergens for pollen immunotherapy. Immunotherapy. 2013;5:1323–38.
Wopfner N, et al. The alpha and beta subchain of Amb a 1, the major ragweed-pollen allergen show divergent reactivity at the IgE and T-cell level. Mol Immunol. 2009;46:2090–7.
Ziska L, et al. Recent warming by latitude associated with increased length of ragweed pollen season in central North America. Proc Natl Acad Sci U S A. 2011;108:4248–51.

Molecular Diagnostics for Peanut Allergy 12

L. Lange, K. Beyer, and J. Kleine-Tebbe

12.1 The Peanut's Role as an Allergen

Peanut belongs to the family of legumes and is the most common cause of food-induced anaphylactic reactions. Being responible for the largest percentage of deaths among food allergens (Pumphrey 2000), peanuts are the most important primary food allergen. Following peanut provocations, respiratory difficulties are common (Ahrens et al. 2012). The stable nature of peanut allergens, as well as the relatively high proportion of total protein amount, contributes to the enormous health threat peanuts can pose. Peanut contains a high protein percentage of 24–29 % (Koppelman et al. 2001),

This chapter is based on a publication (Lange K, Beyer K, Kleine-Tebbe J: Benefits and limitations of molecular diagnostics in peanut allergy. Allergo J 2014; 23: 158–163) submitted in the *Allergo Journal International* 2014, which the authors have now updated and revised.
The authors gratefully thank Prof. Anna Nowak-Wegrzyn, MD, Icahn School of Medicine at Mount Sinai, Jaffe Food Allergy Institute, New York, NY, USA, for reviewing the manuscript and providing expert editorial assistance and helpful suggestions regarding this chapter. A special thanks goes to Prof. Bodo Niggemann (Department of Pediatric Pneumology and Immunology, University Children's Hospital, Campus Rudolf Virchow, Charité Medical University, Berlin, Germany) for his advice during the development of the presented flowcharts for the diagnostic work-up of peanut-allergic subjects.

L. Lange, MD, Assoc Prof. (✉)
St. Marien Hospital, Bonn, Germany

Department of Pediatrics, St. Marien-Hospital, Bonn, Germany
e-mail: Lars.Lange@marien-hospital-bonn.de

K. Beyer, MD, Prof.
Department of Pediatric Pneumology and Immunology, Charité-Universitätsmedizin, Berlin, Germany
e-mail: kirsten.beyer@charite.de

J. Kleine-Tebbe, MD, Prof.
Allergy & Asthma Center Westend, Outpatient Clinic Hanf, Ackermann & Kleine-Tebbe, Berlin, Germany
e-mail: kleine-tebbe@allergie-experten.de

J. Kleine-Tebbe, T. Jakob (eds.), *Molecular Allergy Diagnostics*,
DOI 10.1007/978-3-319-42499-6_12

mostly storage proteins, which leads to the low threshold for reactions in peanut allergy sufferers. Even extremely small peanut quantities (1.6 mg peanut protein) cause allergic reactions in 5 % of peanut-allergic individuals (Blom et al. 2013).

Epidemiology
In the USA and Great Britain, between 1 and 2 % of infants and young children have been diagnosed with a peanut allergy (Nicolaou and Custovic 2011), and in Australia the percentage lies at 3 %. In Germany, peanut allergy seems to be slightly less common. Nevertheless, 10.6 % of German children and teenagers have an elevated peanut-specific IgE (Schmitz et al. 2013). A multicenter and multinational study concerning the prevalence of sensitizations to food allergens among adults in Europe (EuroPrevall) showed a high variability (Burney et al. 2014). Using extract-based diagnostics, the sensitization rates varied between 0.5 % in Reykjavik, 5 % in Zürich, 1.6 % in Utrecht, and 7.2 % in Madrid. The analysis of the prevalence of peanut storage proteins sensitization rates, which is typical of childhood peanut allergy (Ballmer-Weber et al. 2015), significantly altered the picture: no sensitizations were recorded in Sofia and Lodz, 0.1 % in Utrecht, 0.4 % in Zürich, and 0.5 % in Madrid.

The high sensitization rates to peanut extract in different parts of Europe are caused by cross-reactions through:

- Birch Bet v t-homolog PR-10-proteins (Ara h 8)
- Lipid transfer proteins (Ara h 9) for patients in the Mediterranean region
- Profilins (Ara h 5)
- Carbohydrate determinant-(CCD-) carrying glycoproteins for patients with primary sensitizations to birch pollen (PR-10-proteins), peach-LTP (Pru p 3), or grass pollen (profilins and CCDs)

Peanut's Role in the Food Industry
In Europe and North America, peanuts are mostly consumed roasted, e.g., still in their shell, salted and peeled, or processed into peanut butter or peanut puffs. As a nonrefined product, peanut oil may contain relevant quantities of the peanut allergen and may cause allergic reactions. In Asian regions, raw peanuts are mostly consumed as an ingredient in cooked dishes. The allergenicity of raw peanuts decreases through a long cooking process. In contrast, roasting at very high temperatures facilitates the formation of compact, globular protein aggregates, which can augment the allergenicity of Ara h 1 and 2 (Vissers et al. 2011).

12.2 Individual Peanut Allergens

The clinical reactions are determined by the characteristics of the individual proteins (◉ Figs. 12.1 and 12.2, ◉ Table 12.1), especially when the sensitization encompasses a single allergen family. In addition, primary and secondary

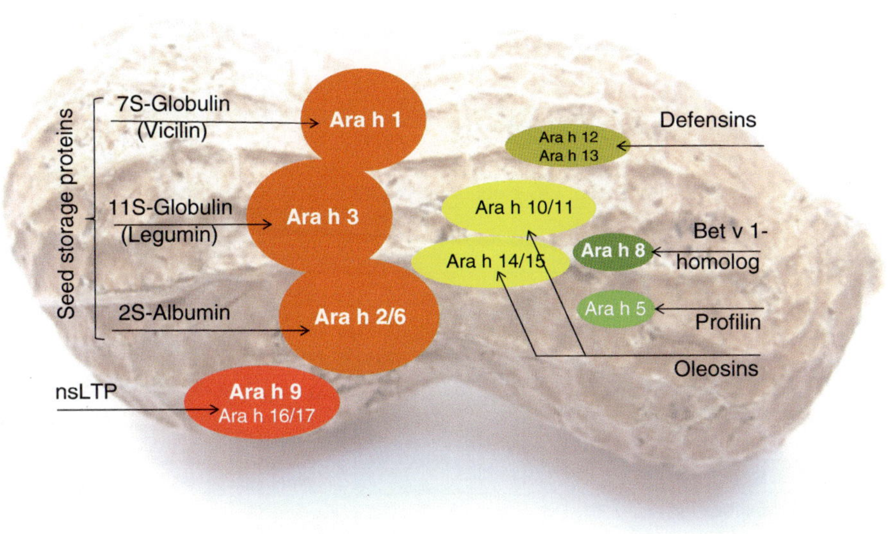

Fig. 12.1 Currently identified peanut allergens. The *ellipse* sizes roughly indicate their percentage of the total protein (***Fettdruck***: available for specific IgE diagnostic)

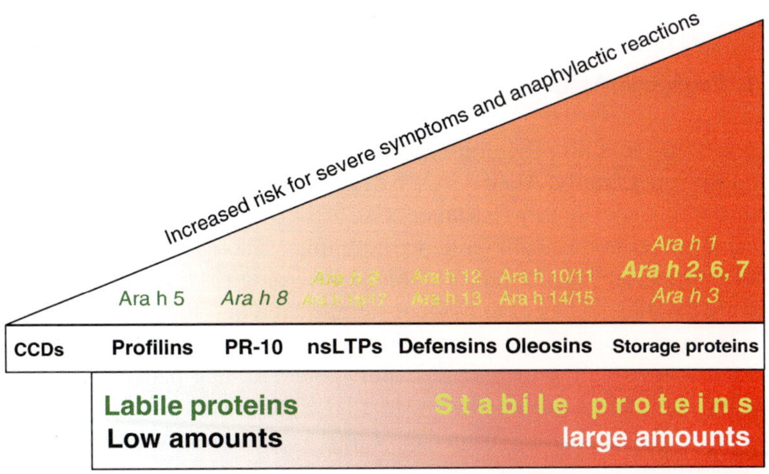

Fig. 12.2 Peanut allergens and their role in determining clinical symptoms according to the "risk ramp". While allergens which are unstable and occur in smaller quantities (left) tend to induce no or mild oropharyngeal symptoms, IgE sensitizations to those which are stable and occur abundantly (right) are more commonly associated with severe allergic symptoms

allergens are differentiated: the primary (class I) food allergens induce sensitization via the cutaneous or gastrointestinal route, whereas the secondary (class II) food allergens mainly cross-react to structurally similar epitopes, e.g., following predominantly an inhalant sensitization.

Table 12.1 Peanut allergens (www.allergen.org, 03-04-2016)

Allergen	Biochemical name	MW	Heat stability
Ara h 1	Cupin (vicillin-type, 7S globulin)	64	Yes
Ara h 2	Conglutin (2S albumin)	17	Yes
Ara h 3	Cupin (legumin-type, 11S globulin, glycinin)	60, 37 (fragment)	Yes
Ara h 5	Profilin	15	No
Ara h 6	Conglutin (2S albumin)	15	Yes
Ara h 7	Conglutin (2S albumin)	15	Yes
Ara h 8	Pathogenesis-related protein, PR-10, Bet v 1 family member	17	No
Ara h 9	Nonspecific lipid transfer protein type 1	9.8	Yes
Ara h 10	Oleosin	16	Yes
Ara h 11	Oleosin	14	Yes
Ara h 12	Defensins	8	
Ara h 13	Defensins	8	
Ara h 14	Oleosin	17.5	Yes
Ara h 15	Oleosin	17	Yes
Ara h 16	Nonspecific lipid transfer protein 2	8.5	Yes
Ara h 17	Nonspecific lipid transfer protein 1	11	Yes

12.2.1 Primary Major Allergens: Storage Proteins

Ara h 1 is a 7S-globulin of vicilin-type and Ara h 3 a 11S-globulin, both members of the cupin-super family. Ara h 2, Ara h 6, and Ara h 7 are 2S-albumins and belong to the prolamin-super family (Radauer et al. 2012). As opposed to Ara h 7, Ara h 2 and Ara h 6 possess significant sequence homology. Though they belong to different protein families, Ara h 1, 2, and 3 exhibit high serological cross-reactivity and thus complicate the diagnostics of individual storage proteins (Bublin et al. 2013).

The storage proteins are the major allergens in primary peanut allergy. Sensitization to storage proteins are mainly found among patients who have suffered from a childhood peanut allergy. In a large, multicenter study including both children and adults (Ballmer-Weber et al. 2015), IgE specific to storage proteins was found exclusively in patients whose allergy had developed before the age of 14. Specific IgE against Ara h 2 and Ara h 6 was present in 76–96 % of children suffering from peanut allergy in the USA, Central and Northern Europe, but only in 42 % in Spain. For Ara h 1, the rate falls between 63 and 80 %. For Ara h 3 the rate is lower, and for Ara h 7 it merely adds up to 43 % (Codreanu et al. 2011; Vereda et al. 2011), defining it as a minor allergen.

12.2.2 Primary Minor Allergens: Oleosins

Oleosins are considered structure proteins of plant cells and function as potential allergens in legumes, seeds, and tree nuts. Their three-part form, similar to that of a hair needle, with ambiphilic (both hydro- and lipophilic) ends and an extended hydrophobic domain, situated in the oil-matrix, contributes to the formation and stability of oil particles (oleosomes) and prevents the clotting of individual lipid drops. Several purified, native, or recombinant oleosin-isoforms of the peanut 14 (Ara h 11), 16 (Ara h 10), and 18 kDa are available. It has been shown that they can interact with one another in order to create oligomers, which are larger complexes (Cabanos et al. 2011).

Sensitization to oleosins probably only affects a minority of peanut allergy sufferers, but exact statistics are not known. As watery extract fluids of the nut contain little to no oleosins, this diagnostic gap complicates the identification of the affected patients (Aalberse et al. 2013).

Both storage proteins and oleosins are highly resistant to heat and digestion and thus relevant as primary food allergens (◉ Fig. 12.2).

12.2.3 Secondary Allergens: nsLTPs and Cross-Reactive Aeroallergens

Ara h 9, a nonspecific lipid transfer protein (nsLTP), is known as a secondary food allergen, especially in Mediterranean countries. The (secondary) sensitization/cross-reaction is most likely caused by other nsLTPs. Probably Pru p 3 in the peach fruit initiates the sensitization through skin contact. nsLTPs are also heat and digestion resistant; therefore, the affected patients may develop systemic symptoms (Petersen and Scheurer 2011).

Sensitizations to the Bet v t-homolog PR-10-protein Ara h 8, the profilin Ara h 5 and glycoproteins (CCD) are usually interlinked with cross-reactivity to pollen allergens. The sensitization rates vary depending on the regional pollen exposure. The birch tree predominance induces a distinct north–south pattern for cross-reactivity to Ara h 8; in regions with stronger grass, pollen exposure increased cross-reactive IgE against Ara h 5, and CCD-containing peanut extracts can be expected. The corresponding proteins are sensitive to heat and digestion, therefore since raw peanuts are generally not consumed, the pollen-associated peanut allergies only rarely account for symptoms, which are predominantly local oropharyngeal in nature.

12.3 Clinical Data Concerning Molecular *Diagnostics*

Peanut is the most commonly researched food allergen in clinical studies concerning the relevance of molecular allergy diagnostics. To date, studies attempted a better clinical interpretation of the specific serum-IgE-concentration against single allergens, specifically:

- A stronger association between specific IgE-sensitization profiles and clinical allergic reactions (risk rate for clinical/systemic reactions, odds ratio, OR)
- An increased diagnostic sensitivity and/or specificity (as shown in receiver operating characteristics-curves, ROC-curves)

- More accurate predictions ("predictive value") and calculable cutoff values/decision points for a positive (facilitated by the "positive prediction value", PPV) or negative prediction (facilitated by the "negative prediction value", NPV) of clinical reactions

In an earlier study, sensitization to one of the storage proteins Ara h 1–3 among children led highly significantly more often to systemic and severe clinical symptoms compared to sensitization to only Ara h 8 but to none of the storage proteins (Asarnoj et al. 2010). In a subsequent study encompassing 144 children and adolescents, it was found that a sensitization to only Ara h 8 without IgE against Ara h 1–3 always indicates tolerance to peanut. In only one child with systemic symptoms during the provocation, sensitization to Ara h 6 without IgE against Ara h 1–3 could be identified in the post hoc analysis of the sensitization spectrum (Asarnoj et al. 2012a). Several case reports in literature show patients with systemic reactions after contact with peanut and a sensitization to Ara h 6 without detectable IgE against Ara h 1, and 3 (Asarnoj et al. 2012b). In one rare observation, a 16-year-old female patient, who was mono-sensitized to Ara h 8, developed an anaphylactic reaction after consuming a large amount of peanuts (Glaumann et al. 2013).

An Australian study evaluated the benefits of measuring specific IgE against Ara h 2 among infants with a positive prick test against peanut to predict a clinical allergy. A model calculation in which only children with Ara h 2-specific IgE between 0.1 and 1 kU_A/l were admitted for the provocation test and children with Ara h 2-specific IgE >1 kU_A/l were considered allergic, the necessity for an additional provocation test for 95 children could be minimized to 44 children and therefore be reduced by half. The rate of false-negative results, regarding the Ara h 2-specific IgE diagnostics, amounted to 5 %, the rate of false-positive results to 3 % (Dang et al. 2012). Nineteen out of 100 children, who are identified as allergic, had IgE levels against Ara h 2 lower than 0.35 kU_A/l. Five of these did not have detectable antibodies against Ara h 1 or 3, none against Ara h 8 or 9.

Numerous different studies analyzed the diagnostic sensitivity and specificity of various IgE levels against Ara h 2 for the prediction of an allergic reaction. Eller and Bindslev-Jensen (2013) calculated a diagnostic specificity of 100 % and a sensitivity of 70 % for a cutoff value of 1.63 kU_A/l among 205 Danish patients aged 1–26; Nicolaou et al. (2011) determined a sensitivity of 93 % and a specificity of 100 % for a cutoff of 0.55 kU_A/l among 81 British children. In a French study, only 7 out of 166 peanut-allergic children and adolescent were not sensitized to Ara h 2. For a cutoff value of 0.23 kU_A/l, a diagnostic sensitivity of 93 % and a specificity of 96 % were calculated. The analysis of Ara h 6-specific IgE provided added value (Codreanu et al. 2011).

One of the largest cohort studies (210 children suspected to be peanut allergic) took place in Germany and examined patients using standardized peanut provocations (Beyer et al. 2015). During this study, probability curves (◉ Fig. 12.3) for a

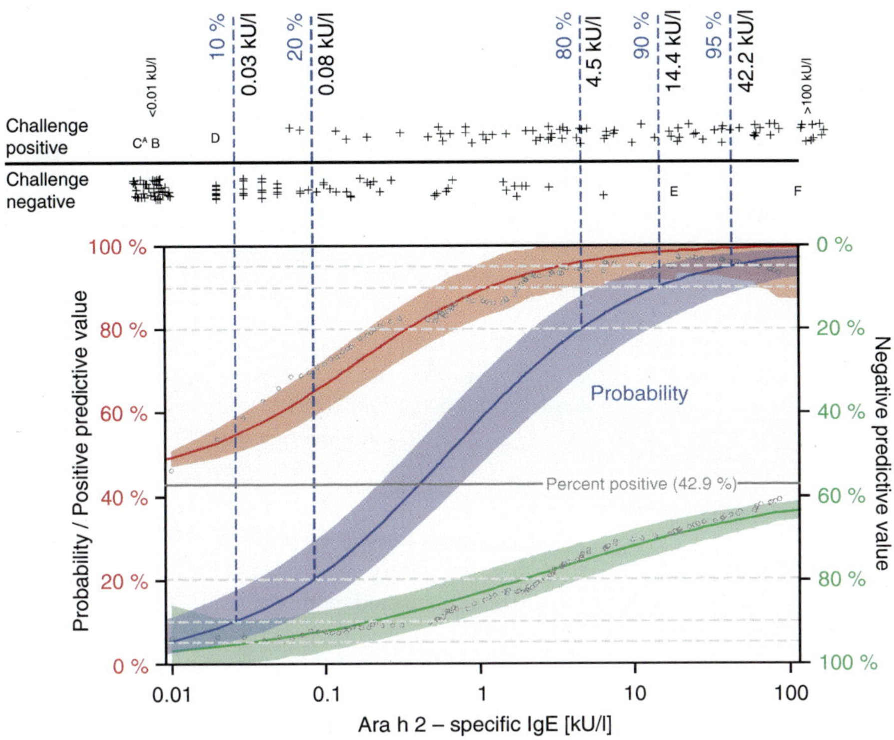

Fig. 12.3 Results concerning probability for a positive peanut food challenge by Ara h 2-specific IgE. Sigmoidal calculated probability for a positive peanut challenge resulting from Ara h 2-specific IgE concentration (*blue line* and band). Estimated IgE levels at given probabilities (5, 10, 20 % and 80, 90, 95 %) above figure (*dashed lines*). Estimated positive (*left axis, red line,* and band) and negative (*right axis, green line*, and band) predictive value, and real cases (*gray dots*). Actual IgE levels by challenge outcome above figure (*plus sign*). *Letters* indicate positive challenge outcomes (*A–D*) with Ara h 2-specific IgE <0.03 kU_A/l (below the 10 % probability) and negative challenges (*E, F*) with Ara h 2-specific IgE >14.4 kU_A/l (levels above 90 % probability (Adapted from Beyer et al. 2015)

clinically relevant allergy to Ara h 2 were first calculated. The cutoff value for a 95 % prediction of peanut allergy using Ara h 2-specific IgE amounted to 42 kU_A/l (ImmunoCAP Singleplex, ThermoFisher). This high value resulted from unselected inclusion of children, leading to the participation of patients with higher Ara h 2-specific IgE levels. Two of these children were tolerant to peanut during the provocation despite their high Ara h 2-specific IgE levels (18 kU_A/l and >100 kU_A/l, respectively). In contrast, 4 patients without sensitizations to Ara h 1–3 showed clinical symptoms, presumably due to clinically relevant sensitizations to other single allergens not identified. Specific IgE to Ara h 6 was not tested.

Take-Home Message of the Multicenter Peanut Study (Beyer et al. 2015)

- Ara h 2-specific IgE currently shows the best association with systemic reactions to peanut in the context of oral provocation.
- In order to predict a positive provocation with a 95 % probability, the Ara h 2-specific IgE must have a value >42.2 kU_A/l – an uncommon constellation and thus only useful in similarly extreme cases.
- In order to predict a negative provocation a 90 % probability, the Ara h 2-specific IgE must have a value <0.03 kU_A/l – apart from deviating individual cases.
- Due to exceptions, a definite 100 % prediction via Ara h 2-specific IgE is not possible. Therefore, the clinical relevance of allergen-specific IgE levels (e.g., against single allergens of legumes) must be determined by the attending physician.

It was previously reported that young children (below 24 months of age) with a sensitization to peanut recognize predominantly seed-storage proteins particularly Ara h 1 (Trendelenburg et al. 2014). Identified with the slightly less sensitive Microarray-System ISAC (ThermoFisher), these IgE sensitizations were partly also clinically relevant, though specific IgE against Ara h 2 was not determined. In addition, the benefits of analyzing IgE levels against the three storage proteins (Ara h 1–3) in adult patients, who probably developed their allergy in childhood years, could be shown among 74 Swedish patients (Movérare et al. 2011).

On the other hand, a subproject of the EuroPREVALL study throughout Europe identified adults, whose peanut allergy had only manifested itself from an age of 14 or older, who did not show sensitizations against Ara h 1–3 or Ara h 6 (Ballmer-Weber et al. 2015). The majority of these adults had strikingly low titers of specific IgE to the total extract of the peanut. These patients were often sensitized against the nsLTP Ara h 9 in Southern Europe. Several patients did not show specific IgE to any of the tested components. The reason for this could be sensitization against oleosins (Ara h 10 and 11); however, their potential relevance can only be assumed, as they have until now not been available for IgE diagnostics.

These data show that in general, patients from Middle Europe, who developed their peanut allergy up to adolescence, probably do not have a clinically relevant allergy, if they lack IgE against storage proteins Ara h 1–3 and Ara h 6.

Due to varying prediction values and the fact that some relevant peanut allergens are still unavailable for diagnostic purposes, the determination of the anaphylaxis risk is not possible solely through the determination of IgE against Ara h 2.

Confounding factors such as age, underlying medical conditions, total IgE, or sensitization to other allergens inevitably are disregarded during cohort analyses, which may lead to enormous deviations and in turn, create false-positive results.

This was once again demonstrated in a Berlin study, during which all children with suspected peanut allergy were challenged with peanut, regardless of their level of peanut-specific IgE. Twenty-seven percent of the children with detectable levels of specific IgE against Ara h 2 were tolerant and partially showed high levels of Ara h 2-specific IgE (Lopes de Oliveira et al. 2013).

In Southern Europe, specific IgE against the lipid transfer protein Ara h 9 is also considered to possess a predictive value for a systemic allergic reaction (Krause et al. 2009). The majority of patients in these regions are not sensitized against Ara h 2, but against Ara h 9 (Vereda et al. 2011).

12.4 Diagnostics with Peanut Allergens

12.4.1 Available Single Allergens

Specific IgE antibodies can be determined against the crude peanut extract, the storage proteins Ara h 1, h 2, h 3, and h 6, against the nsLTP Ara h 9, and against the PR-10-protein Ara h 8 (◉ Fig. 12.2).

12.4.2 Potential Benefits of Molecular Diagnostics with Peanut Allergens

When IgE sensitization is identified through the determination of single peanut allergens, the test properties are altered (without necessarily impacting on the clinical relevance of the test results) (Matricardi et al. 2016). Furthermore, it allows the detection of marker allergens and may provide indications of primary sensitization:

- The assay sensitivity is improved through the introduction of underrepresented or absent peanut allergens (lower "limit of quantitation", LoQ).
  Examples: Ara h 8, Ara h 10/11 (the latter ones not yet available for diagnostics).
- The analytical specificity (selectivity) of the determination of IgE is augmented through the determination of single allergens in comparison to whole extract diagnostics. This is especially appropriate for risk associated peanut allergens, which are rather interlinked with clinical reactions (Ara h 2), as well as for low risk peanut proteins, which are connected to serological, yet clinically irrelevant cross-reactions (Ara h 8).
- Markers for general cross-reactions connected with peanut allergens include in particular Ara h 8 (Bet v 1-associated cross-reactivity), Ara h 5 (profilin-associated cross-reactivity), MUXF3 (CCD-induced cross-reactivity). They are responsible for the unsatisfactory specificity of peanut extracts regarding the detection of differentiated IgE sensitization.
- Peanut allergens (Ara h 1, 2, or 3) do serve as an indicator for a primary, species-specific sensitization, which developed in childhood years, so long as the specific IgE against corresponding storage proteins (2S-albumins, 7S- and 11S-globulins) of other legumes (e.g., soy) or other nuts (tree nuts, drupes, and capsule fruits) or seeds is considerably lower. A number of storage proteins for specific IgE

diagnostics are still missing, which would be necessary in order to systematically differentiate dominant, primary sensitizations from serological cross-reactions.

12.4.3 Procedure for Diagnosing Peanut Allergy in Childhood (<14 Years)

Various diagnostic questions arise depending on medical history and preliminary findings:

A. Desire for exclusion of peanut allergy (e.g., among patients with atopic dermatitis or other food allergies), prior to the consumption of peanut-containing products (◉ Fig. 12.4)
B. Incidental finding of a sensitization (e.g., raised IgE against peanut in the panel- or screening test) (◉ Fig. 12.5)
C. Allergic reaction following peanut contact or consumption (◉ Fig. 12.6)

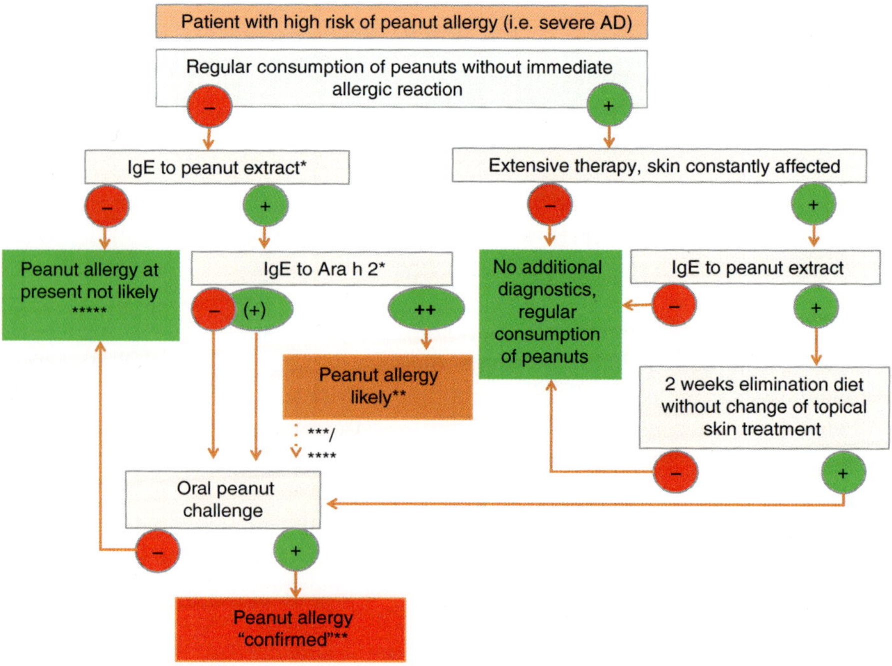

Fig. 12.4 Model of a diagnostic algorithm for excluding the possibility of peanut allergy when suspected. * Consider tests in parallel, ** prescribe emergency kit/drugs, *** consider oral challenge test to confirm the diagnosis, **** oral challenge test at appropriate intervals to detect tolerance development, ***** in case of sensitization without clinical symptoms regular consumption of peanut products 3×/week recommended

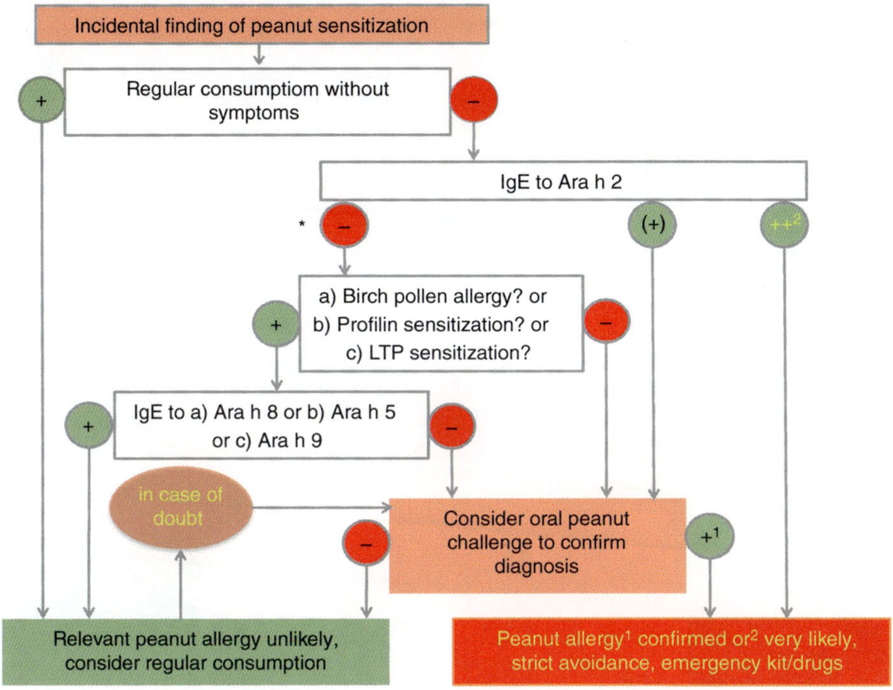

Fig. 12.5 Model of a diagnostic algorithm for sensitizations detected by chance (* For maximum diagnostic reliability IgE against Ara h 1, 3, 6 should be considered)

Ad A

IgE against whole peanut extract is well suited as a screening parameter (especially for exclusion) of peanut allergy: undetectable peanut-IgE has a high negative predictive value (rare exception: relevant sensitizations against oleosins Ara h 10/11). A positive IgE result is only clinically relevant if the symptoms correspond (low diagnostic specificity). In the case of negative-specific IgE, an additional prick test (e.g., prick-to-prick test with native peanut) serves as a sensitization verification or exclusion criteria. If positive, an oral provocation should be considered.

Ad B

In clinical practice, positive IgE results against peanut may be recorded accidentally. A stepwise approach (◉ Fig. 12.4) takes into account potential consequences and the cost-benefit ratio of diagnostics. The most important initial question is concerned with the regular (e.g., more than once a month) and recent (e.g., within the period of the last 6 weeks) consumption of a relevant quantity of peanut.

Ad C

The determination of IgE level against Ara h 2 is an important parameter in patients suspected to have a primary peanut allergy, which developed in

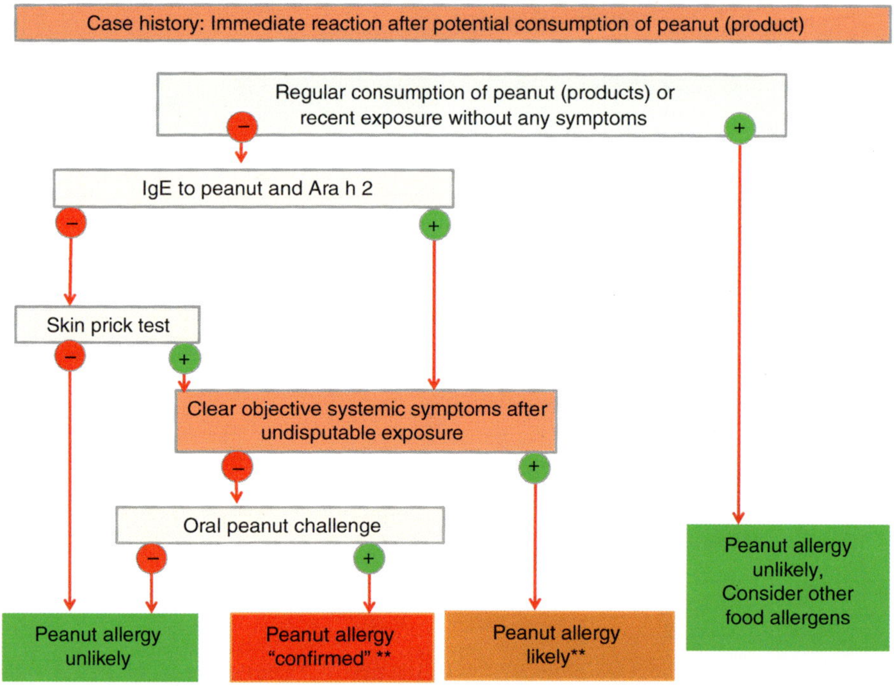

Fig. 12.6 Diagnostic algorithm for immediate type reactions following peanut consumption "** prescribe emergency kit/drugs"

childhood years. A clinically relevant allergy is probable in the case of significantly raised specific IgE and positive patient history of immediate allergic reactions following peanut consumption. However, the published data are heterogeneous and the calculated cutoffs (between 1 and 42 kU_A/l for Ara h 2-specific IgE) resulted in different diagnostic sensitivities and specificities in the examined patient populations. Nevertheless, probability curves were now calculated for a clinically relevant allergy against Ara h 2. The specific IgE against Ara h 6 may be a similarly relevant parameter; however, there is insufficient data available in comparison to Ara h 2.

12.4.4 Common Peanut Cross-Reactions Regarding Birch Pollen Sensitization

If birch pollen–associated sensitization is suspected, determining the IgE levels against Ara h 8 and Ara h 2 is useful. If Ara h2 is negative and Ara h 8 positive, this indicates a Bet v 1-related cross-reactivity with low clinical relevance. Cross-reactions induced by CCD or profilins may present further reasons for positive IgE results.

12.4.5 Less Common Sensitization Patterns in Peanut Allergy

Evidence of sensitization against Ara h 1 and 3 is often not necessary, as a high cross-reactivity exists between the storage proteins (Bublin et al. 2013) and mono-sensitization against Ara h 1 and/or 3 is rare. In cases where undetectable or low IgE against Ara h 2 raise doubt, a double-blind oral provocation with peanut can provide clarity to the diagnosis. If IgE is undetectable to all of the storage proteins, the possibility of a clinically relevant peanut allergy is relatively unlikely, yet cannot be excluded if clinical symptoms suggest otherwise. A diagnostic gap is present among infants (Trendelenburg 2014) and adults who developed their allergy after adolescence and in regard to oleosins Ara 10/11. Furthermore, IgE levels of patients from Mediterranean regions should additionally be tested against the nsLTP Ara h 9.

12.5 Cross-Reactive Allergens

Clinically relevant cross-reactions are predominantly induced through storage proteins. Reactions are possible to legumes, such as lupines and lentils, but also to nuts, such as hazelnuts, walnuts, or seeds, such as sesame. Serological cross-reactions must be critically evaluated in order to prove clinical relevance. For instance, the detection of IgE antibodies to soybean is mostly irrelevant for peanut allergy sufferers.

12.6 Conclusions: Relevance in Daily Clinical Practice

Molecular allergy diagnostics (Matricardi et al. 2016) has considerable significance in the diagnostic procedure of peanut allergy:

- Numerous sensitizations against peanut extracts in our latitudes evolve from pollen-associated cross-reactions, which can be differentiated with IgE measurement against available marker allergens (e.g., Bet v 1-homologs Ara h 8, CCD MUXF3, Profilin Phl p 12).
- The corresponding clinical reactions are often mild and mostly limited to local reactions of mouth- and throat regions.
- For peanut allergy sufferers from the Mediterranean regions, Ara h 9 is included in IgE diagnostics as nsLTP can be associated with systemic reactions.
- Considerably raised specific IgE against stable storage proteins like Ara h 2 (and probably Ara h 6) are often associated with systemic reactions and a clinically relevant peanut allergy.
- In patients with reliable systemic reactions to peanut and sensitization especially to Ara h 2, a further oral food allergen provocation is not necessary.
- Storage proteins are most likely not the responsible major allergens, if the peanut allergy only develops in adult years.

- If uncertain, the clinical diagnosis of peanut allergy can be verified by an oral provocation due to the following reasons:
  - Some patients with Ara h 2-specific IgE may be tolerant and some affected individuals may react systemically despite lacking Ara h 2-specific IgE for peanut.
  - Not all relevant peanut allergens are available for diagnostics.
  - Traceable specific IgE concentrations correspond to a sensitization (allergic disposition), which is only clinically relevant in connection with the corresponding symptoms.

References

Aalberse JA, Meijer Y, Derksen N, van der Palen-Merkus T, Knol E, Aalberse RC. Moving from peanut extract to peanut components: towards validation of component-resolved IgE tests. Allergy. 2013;68:748–56.

Ahrens B, Niggemann B, Wahn U, Beyer K. Organ-specific symptoms during oral food challenge in children with food allergy. J Allergy Clin Immunol. 2012;130:549–51.

Asarnoj A, Movérare R, Ostblom E, Poorafshar M, Lilja G, Hedlin G, van Hage M, Ahlstedt S, Wickman M. IgE to peanut allergen components: relation to peanut symptoms and pollen sensitization in 8-year-olds. Allergy. 2010;65:1189–95.

Asarnoj A, Nilsson C, Lidholm J, Glaumann S, Östblom E, Hedlin G, van Hage M, Lilja G, Wickman M. Peanut component Ara h 8 sensitization and tolerance to peanut. J Allergy Clin Immunol. 2012a;130:468–72.

Asarnoj A, Glaumann S, Elfström L, Lilja G, Lidholm J, Nilsson C, Wickman M. Anaphylaxis to peanut in a patient predominantly sensitized to Ara h 6. Int Arch Allergy Immunol. 2012b;159:209–12.

Ballmer-Weber BK, Lidholm J, Fernández-Rivas M, Seneviratne S, Hanschmann KM, Vogel L, Bures P, Fritsche P, Summers C, Knulst AC, Le TM, Reig I, Papadopoulos NG, Sinaniotis A, Belohlavkova S, Popov T, Kralimarkova T, de Blay F, Purohit A, Clausen M, Jedrzejczak-Czechowcz M, Kowalski ML, Asero R, Dubakiene R, Barreales L, Clare Mills EN, van Ree R, Vieths S. IgE recognition patterns in peanut allergy are age dependent: perspectives of the EuroPrevall study. Allergy. 2015;70:391–407.

Beyer K, Grabenhenrich L, Beder A, Kalb B, Ziegert M, Finger A, Harandi N, Schlags R, Gappa M, Puzzo L, Röblitz H, Millner-Uhlemann M, Büsing S, Ott H, Lange L, Niggemann B. Predictive values of component-specific IgE for the outcome of peanut and hazelnut food challenges in children. Allergy. 2015;70:90–9.

Blom WM, Vlieg-Boerstra BJ, Kruizinga AG, van der Heide S, Houben GF, Dubois AE. Threshold dose distributions for 5 major allergenic foods in children. J Allergy Clin Immunol. 2013;131:172–9.

Bublin M, Kostadinova M, Radauer C, Hafner C, Szépfalusi Z, Varga EM, Maleki SJ, Hoffmann-Sommergruber K, Breiteneder H. IgE cross-reactivity between the major peanut allergen Ara h 2 and the nonhomologous allergens Ara h 1 and Ara h 3. J Allergy Clin Immunol. 2013;132:118–24.

Burney PG, Potts J, Kummeling I, Mills EN, Clausen M, Dubakiene R, Barreales L, Fernandez-Perez C, Fernandez-Rivas M, Le TM, Knulst AC, Kowalski ML, Lidholm J, Ballmer-Weber BK, Braun-Fahlander C, Mustakov T, Kralimarkova T, Popov T, Sakellariou A, Papadopoulos NG, Versteeg SA, Zuidmeer L, Akkerdaas JH, Hoffmann-Sommergruber K, Van Ree R. The prevalence and distribution of food sensitization in European adults. Allergy. 2014; 69:365–71.

Cabanos C, Katayama H, Tanaka A, Utsumi S, Maruyama N. Expression and purification of peanut oleosins in insect cells. Protein J. 2011;30:457–63.

Codreanu F, Collignon O, Roitel O, Thouvenot B, Sauvage C, Vilain AC, Cousin MO, Decoster A, Renaudin JM, Astier C, Monnez JM, Vallois P, Morisset M, Moneret-Vautrin DA, Brulliard M, Ogier V, Castelain MC, Kanny G, Bihain BE, Jacquenet S. A novel immunoassay using recombinant allergens simplifies peanut allergy diagnosis. Int Arch Allergy Immunol. 2011;154:216–26.

Dang TD, Tang M, Choo S, Licciardi PV, Koplin JJ, Martin PE, Tan T, Gurrin LC, Ponsonby AL, Tey D, Robinson M, Dharmage SC, Allen KJ, HealthNuts Study. Increasing the accuracy of peanut allergy diagnosis by using Ara h 2. J Allergy Clin Immunol. 2012;129:1056–63.

Eller E, Bindslev-Jensen C. Clinical value of component-resolved diagnostics in peanut-allergic patients. Allergy. 2013;68:190–4.

Glaumann S, Nopp A, Johansson SG, Borres MP, Lilja G, Nilsson C. Anaphylaxis to peanuts in a 16-year-old girl with birch pollen allergy and with monosensitization to Ara h 8. J Allergy Clin Immunol Pract. 2013;1:698–9.

Koppelman SJ, Vlooswijk RA, Knippels LM, Hessing M, Knol EF, van Reijsen FC, Bruijnzeel-Koomen CA. Quantification of major peanut allergens Ara h 1 and Ara h 2 in the peanut varieties Runner, Spanish, Virginia, and Valencia, bred in different parts of the world. Allergy. 2001;56:132–7.

Krause S, Reese G, Randow S, Zennaro D, Quaratino D, Palazzo P, Ciardiello MA, Petersen A, Becker WM, Mari A. Lipid transfer protein (Ara h 9) as a new peanut allergen relevant for a Mediterranean allergic population. J Allergy Clin Immunol. 2009;124:771–8.

Lopes de Oliveira LC, Aderholz M, Brill M, Schulz G, Rolinck-Werninghaus C, Mills ENC, Naspitz CK, Niggemann B, Wahn U, Beyer K. The value of specific IgE to peanut and its component Ara h 2 in the diagnosis of peanut allergy. J Allergy Clin Immunol Pract. 2013;1:394–8.

Matricardi PM, Kleine-Tebbe J, Hoffmann HJ, Valenta R, Hilger C, Hofmaier S, Aalberse RC, Agache I, Asero R, Ballmer-Weber B, Barber D, Beyer K, Biedermann T, Biló MB, Blank S, Bohle B, Bosshard PP, Breiteneder H, Brough HA, Caraballo L, Caubet JC, Crameri R, Davies JM, Douladiris N, Ebisawa M, Eigenmann PA, Fernandez-Rivas M, Ferreira F, Gadermaier G, Glatz M, Hamilton RG, Hawranek T, Hellings P, Hoffmann-Sommergruber K, Jakob T, Jappe U, Jutel M, Kamath SD, Knol EF, Korosec P, Kuehn A, Lack G, Lopata AL, Mäkelä M, Morisset M, Niederberger V, Nowak-Wezgrzyn AH, Papadopoulos NG, Pastorello EA, Pauli G, Platts-Mills T, Posa D, Poulsen LK, Raulf M, Sastre J, Scala E, Schmid JM, Schmid-Grendelmeier P, van Hage M, van Ree R, Vieths S, Weber R, Wickman M, Muraro A, Ollert M. EAACI molecular allergology user's guide. Pediatr Allergy Immunol. 2016;27 Suppl 23:1–250.

Movérare R, Ahlstedt S, Bengtsson U, Borres MP, van Hage M, Poorafshar M, Sjölander S, Akerström J, van Odijk J. Evaluation of IgE antibodies to recombinant peanut allergens in patients with reported reactions to peanut. Int Arch Allergy Immunol. 2011;156:282–90.

Nicolaou N, Custovic A. Molecular diagnosis of peanut and legume allergy. Curr Opin Allergy Clin Immunol. 2011;11:222–8.

Nicolaou N, Murray C, Belgrave D, Poorafshar M, Simpson A, Custovic A. Quantification of specific IgE to whole peanut extract and peanut components in prediction of peanut allergy. J Allergy Clin Immunol. 2011;127:684–5.

Petersen A, Scheurer S. Stabile pflanzliche Nahrungsmittelallergene: Lipid-Transfer-Proteine. Allergo J. 2011;20:384–6.

Pumphrey RS. Lessons for management of anaphylaxis from a study of fatal reactions. Clin Exp Allergy. 2000;30:1144–50.

Radauer C, Kleine-Tebbe J, Beyer K. Stabile pflanzliche Nahrungsmittelallergene: Speicherproteine. Allergo J. 2012;21:8888–92.

Schmitz R, Ellert U, Kalcklösch M, Damm S, Thamm M. Patterns of sensitization to inhalant and food allergens – findings from the German Health Interview and Examination Survey for Children and Adolescents (KiGGS). Int Arch Allergy Immunol. 2013;162:263–70.

Trendelenburg V, Rohrbach A, Schulz G, Schwarz V, Beyer K. Molecular sIgE profiles in infants and young children with peanut sensitization and dermatitis. Allergo J Int. 2014;23:152–7.

Vereda A, van Hage M, Ahlstedt S, Ibañez MD, Cuesta-Herranz J, van Odijk J, Wickman M, Sampson HA. Peanut allergy: clinical and immunologic differences among patients from 3 different geographic regions. J Allergy Clin Immunol. 2011;127:603–7.

Vissers YM, Blanc F, Skov PS, Johnson PE, Rigby NM, Przybylski-Nicaise L, Bernard H, Wal JM, Ballmer-Weber B, Zuidmeer-Jongejan L, Szépfalusi Z, Ruinemans-Koerts J, Jansen AP, Savelkoul HF, Wichers HJ, Mackie AR, Mills CE, Adel-Patient K. Effect of heating and glycation on the allergenicity of 2S albumins (Ara h 2/6) from peanut. PLoS One. 2011;6:e23998.

Molecular Diagnostics for Tree Nut Allergy

13

L. Lange, K. Beyer, and J. Kleine-Tebbe

13.1 Allergen Determination

The general term nuts includes various seeds, which belong to different botanical species. The following nuts require declaration (◉ Fig. 13.1):

- Tree nuts (hazelnut, walnut, macadamia nut, pecan nut)
- Drupes (almond, pistachio, cashew)
- Capsule fruit (Brazil nut)

Despite different botanical backgrounds, serological and clinical cross-reactions occur between the individual nuts. Their cross-reactions are caused by plant allergen families, which are present in the majority of seeds (hazelnut, e.g., ◉ Fig. 13.2).

The following chapter is based on a publication (Lange K, Beyer K, Kleine-Tebbe J: Molekulare Diagnostik bei Allergie gegen Schalenfrüchten. Allergo J 2012; 21: 398–402) submitted in the *Allergo Journal International* 2012, which the authors have now updated and revised.
The authors gratefully thank Prof. Robert A. Wood, MD, Pediatric Allergy and Immunology, Johns Hopkins University School of Medicine, Baltimore, MD, USA, for reviewing the manuscript, expert editorial assistance, and helpful suggestions regarding this chapter.

L. Lange, MD, Assoc Prof. (✉)
St. Marien Hospital, Bonn, Germany

Department of Pediatrics, St. Marien-Hospital, Bonn, Germany
e-mail: lars.lange@marien-hospital-bonn.de

K. Beyer, MD, Prof.
Department of Pediatric Pneumology and Immunology, Charité-Universitätsmedizin, Berlin, Germany

J. Kleine-Tebbe, MD, Prof.
Allergy & Asthma Center Westend, Outpatient Clinic Hanf, Ackermann & Kleine-Tebbe, Berlin, Germany
e-mail: kleine-tebbe@allergie-experten.de

J. Kleine-Tebbe, T. Jakob (eds.), *Molecular Allergy Diagnostics*,
DOI 10.1007/978-3-319-42499-6_13

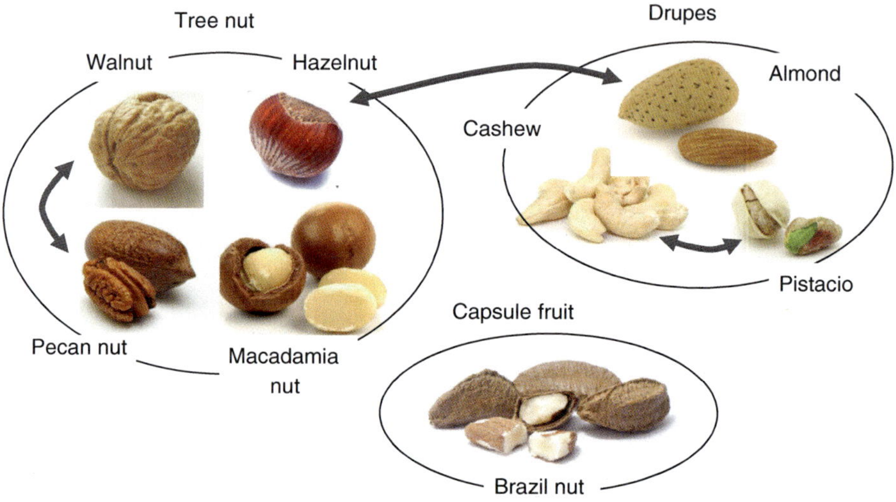

Fig. 13.1 Nuts, their botanic relations and cross-reactions. The cross-reactions (*arrows*) to extracts of nuts, drupes, and capsule fruits do not remain limited to their botanical classification. They lead back to storage proteins, which occur in various representatives (◉ Table 13.1)

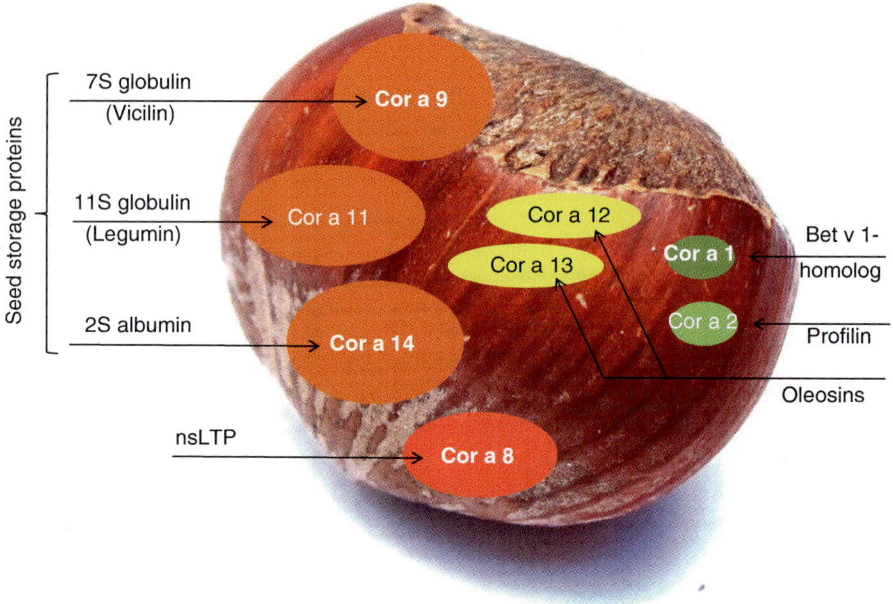

Fig. 13.2 Allergens of the hazelnut and their protein families. The protein content (between 12 and 18/100 g hazelnut) mainly consists of storage proteins (*brown*). Lipid transfer proteins (LTP, *red*), with IgE sensitizations present mostly in Mediterranean countries, may also cause systemic reactions. Bet v 1-homologs Cor a 1 and hazelnut profilin are probably only present in small quantities – common cause of local reactions to hazelnut, which are rarely life threatening

As their function suggests, storage proteins have the largest percentage of total protein. The best described and most clinically relevant are:

- 2S albumins (Cor a 14, Jug r 1, Ana o 3, Ber e 1)
- 7S globulins (Jug r 2)
- 11S globulins (Cor a 9) (Radauer et al. 2012) (▶ Chap. 5)

Sensitization to Bet v 1-homolog stress-induced ("pathogenesis-related") PR-10-proteins are common in Northern and Central Europe (Kleine-Tebbe et al. 2010) (▶ Chap. 2).

In Southern Europe, however, the triggering allergens are often nonspecific lipid transfer proteins (nsLTP, PR-14-proteins): Cor a 8 and Jug r 3 (Petersen and Scheurer 2011) (▶ Chap. 4).

Other allergens in nuts, such as profilins (e.g., Cor a 2, Pru du 4), are most often related to serological cross-reactivity without clinical relevance (Hauser et al. 2012) (▶ Chap. 3).

Some allergen families have until now only been described in specific nuts, for example:

- Thaumatin in almonds (Pru du 2)
- Ribosomal protein P2 in almonds (Pru du 5) (Costa et al. 2012)
- Legumin-like protein in walnuts (Jug r 4)
- Superoxide dismutase in pistachio (Pis v 4)

Recent studies additionally suggest that water-insoluble proteins, oleosins, may be clinically relevant, for example, among hazelnut allergy sufferers (Cor a 12, Cor a 13) (Zuidmeer-Jongejan et al. 2014). Oleosins account for 10–20 % of the protein content of hazelnuts.

13.2 Structure, Function, and Role of Allergens

Clinical reactions can often be traced to characteristics of individual proteins. This is especially the case, when the sensitization is restricted to one allergen family.

Storage proteins are heat and mostly digestion resistant (Costa et al. 2014; Radauer et al. 2012) and constitute a significant portion of the total protein in tree nuts (e.g., approximately 87 % of total protein in hazelnut) (▶ Chap. 5). Small quantities are often capable of triggering clinically relevant reactions.

Within the group of storage proteins, 2S albumins seem to have an especially significant role (e.g., Cor a 14). Evidence for this is available primarily for peanut, but also increasingly for the 2S albumin Cor a 14 in hazelnut (Beyer et al. 2015). Among peanut allergy sufferers, a sensitization to Ara h 2 is the best indicator of a clinically relevant allergy (▶ Chap. 11).

The allergenicity of storage proteins cannot be reduced through processing methods, such as cooking or heating. It is also not denatured through digestion. It has been shown that the process of roasting even increases the allergenicity of peanut. The threat of developing anaphylaxis against the nut is therefore especially high among patients with a clinically relevant allergy to storage proteins. As lipid transfer proteins or thaumatins are also heat and digestion resistant to a certain degree, this is partially true for patients with allergies against these proteins as well.

Bet v 1-homologous PR-10-proteins, on the other hand, are for the largest part heat and digestion labile. Among patients with a birch pollen-associated nut allergy, symptoms are therefore often limited to the oropharyngeal cavity. After consumption of moderate allergen quantities, systemic reactions are only described in rare cases. Processing methods (e.g., roasting, baking, cooking) clearly lower allergenicity levels (Worm et al. 2009). *Profilins* likely play an even smaller role clinically.

The role of *oleosins* is currently not fully clarified. Due to their structure, they belong to the hydrophobic proteins, which are both heat and digestion resistant. It was recently shown that a relevant number of hazelnut-allergic subjects are sensitized to oleosins (Zuidmeer-Jongejan et al. 2014). Some patients were sensitized exclusively to oleosins. This finding was notable, as oleosins are not present in aqueous allergen extracts. Therefore, false-negative results may be seen with prick test extracts. During the retrospective analysis of a larger pool of patients, a higher rate of severe reactions was found in the group of sensitized patients, which suggests an important clinical relevance of sensitization to oleosins.

13.3 Sensitization Frequencies

There are few population-based studies concerning nut allergy prevalence for Central Europe. Nuts present the second most frequent trigger of food-related anaphylaxis. Hazelnut is most common, followed by cashew, almond, and walnut (Hompes et al. 2010). The frequencies vary from country to country, depending on consumer habits.

Anaphylactic reactions to nuts also play an important role among adults. Data regarding the sensitization rates in various European countries has recently been published (Burney et al. 2014). Large differences in sensitization rates for hazelnut based on allergen extracts were shown across Europe, with a rate of 17.8 % in Zurich, 12 % in Utrecht, and 1.3 % in Reykjavik, and for walnut 7.7 % in Madrid and 0.1 % in Reykjavik. However, when the sensitization rates to primary allergens – in this case to nsLTPs and storage proteins – were analyzed, a different picture emerged. For hazelnut, the highest sensitization rate was shown against Cor a 8, Cor a 9, and Cor a 11 in Sofia with 3 % and the lowest with 0 % in Utrecht. For walnut, Jug r 2 and Jug r 4 were analyzed during the study, which showed very few sensitizations (between 0 und 0.4 %).

13.4 Serological Cross-Reactions

Pistachio, cashew, walnut and pecan nut, as well as almond and hazelnut, show distinctive serological cross-reactions (Maloney et al. 2008). Groups with increased serological cross-reactions have also been shown with walnut, pecan nut, and hazelnut, as well as with hazelnut, cashew, pistachio, Brazil nut, and almond (Goetz et al. 2005). It remains unclear which allergen family these cross-reactions stem from and how high the degree of sequence homology is between the different nuts. Until now only some publications exist on this topic: Botanically related types show high homology (96 %), for example, Jug r 1 in walnut and Jug n 1 in pecan nut; for less related types, such as Jug r 1 and Cor a 14 – both at least classified as nuts – the homology was lower (57 %) (Costa et al. 2014). On the other hand, a comparatively high cross-reactivity between Ara h 2, the 2S albumin in peanut, and Jug r 2, the vicilin in walnut, was shown, though the sequence homology was low (Maleki et al. 2011). In a further examination, common IgE-binding epitopes of the vicilins in peanut (Ara h 1), hazelnut (Cor a 11), walnut (Jug r 2), and cashew (Ana o 1) were identified.

The rate of sensitizations to more than one nut increases with age and reaches up to 83 % in 12- and 13-year-olds (Clark and Ewan 2005). Up to 86 % of patients demonstrate serological cross-reactivity between tree nuts and peanuts, as representatives of legumes (Maloney et al. 2008).

Provisional data demonstrates that these observations in cohorts without considerable Bet v 1-associated cross-reactions evidently lead back to storage proteins.

The rate of clinically relevant allergies to several different tree nuts increases with age, from 2 % among 2-year-olds to 47 % among 14-year-olds. Twenty-one to fifty percent of peanut-allergic children are also allergic to tree nuts (De Knop et al. 2011).

13.5 Diagnostics: Available Single Allergens

13.5.1 Hazelnut

Currently the amount of single allergens available for serological diagnostics is still limited. The majority of single components are available for diagnostics of hazelnut:

Cor a 1 (Bet v 1-homolog) (◉ Fig. 13.3a), Cor a 8 (nsLTP) (◉ Fig. 13.3b), Cor a 9 (11S globulin), and Cor a 14 (2S albumin) (◉ Fig. 13.3c).

Potential Benefits of Molecular Diagnostics with Hazelnut Allergens

When IgE sensitization is identified through the implementation of single hazelnut allergens, the test properties differ from the use of whole extracts (without regard to the clinical relevance). Furthermore, it allows the detection of marker allergens and may provide indications of primary sensitization:

- The test sensitivity could be increased through underrepresented or absent hazelnut allergens ("Limit of Quantitation," LoQ).
  Examples: Cor a 12/13 (not yet available for diagnostics).
- The analytical specificity (selectivity) of the determination of IgE is augmented through the implementation of single allergens in comparison to extract diagnostics. This is especially appropriate for risk-associated hazelnut allergens, which are

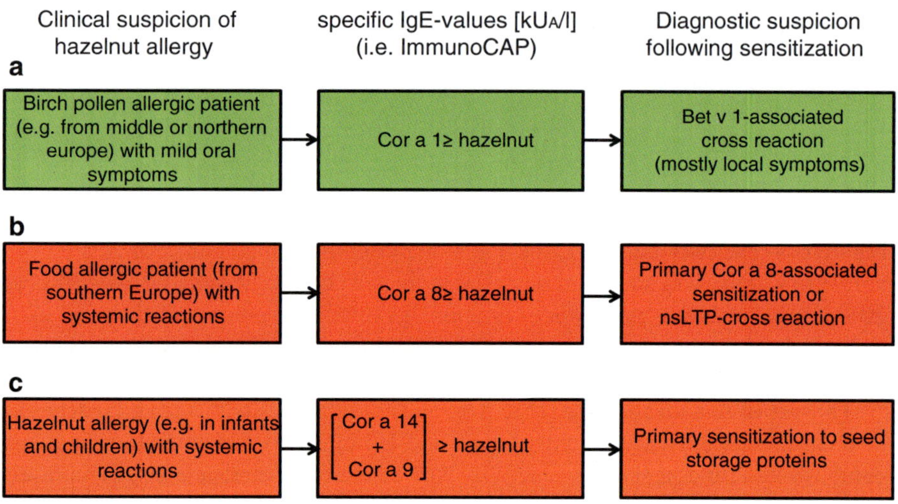

Fig. 13.3 Typical patterns of nut allergies, using the example of the hazelnut: (**a**) Birch pollen-associated, Bet v 1-linked cross-reaction. (**b**) LTP-linked sensitization/cross-reaction. (**c**) Direct indicator of sensitization/cross-reaction to storage proteins

rather associated with clinical reactions (Cor a 8 for LTP syndrome, Cor a 9, Cor a 14), as well as for low-risk hazelnut proteins, which are associated with serological, yet clinically irrelevant cross-reactions (Cor a 1).

- Hazelnut allergens (Cor a 9, Cor a 14) can serve as indicators for a primary, species-specific sensitization, if the specific IgE corresponding to storage proteins (2S-albmunins, 7S and 11S globulins) of other nuts (tree nuts, drupes, and capsule fruits), legumes (e.g., peanut, soy), or seeds is considerably lower. A number of storage proteins for specific IgE diagnostics are still missing, which would be necessary in order to systematically differentiate dominant, primary sensitizations from serological cross-reactions.

Results of Clinical Studies on Molecular Hazelnut Diagnostics

A sensitization to Cor a 8, Cor a 9, or Cor a 14 can therefore indicate a primary hazelnut allergy or a serological cross-reaction to nsLTPs or storage proteins. A nsLTP-sensitization is more common among patients in Mediterranean regions than among those in Central Europe (◉ Fig. 13.3b). Sensitizations to Cor a 8 were, however, shown among children in the Netherlands; they increase with age and are associated with systemic symptoms (De Knop et al. 2011; Flinterman et al. 2008), yet a sensitization to Cor a 8 in Central Europe is generally rare (Masthoff et al. 2013; Beyer et al. 2015).

Better data are available regarding sensitization to Cor a 9 and Cor a 14. Sensitization to Cor a 9 is already present among young infants (Beyer et al. 2002; Verweij et al. 2011). A study with adults and children showed that sensitization to Cor a 9 and Cor a 14 allows the prediction of an objective allergic reaction, especially in childhood years (Masthoff et al. 2013). This is also the case for adults; however, sensitizations to Cor a 9 and Cor a 14 are far less common than among children.

In Germany, a large multicenter study among children with suspected hazelnut allergy who underwent oral hazelnut provocations was conducted and sensitization patterns were documented. Cor a 14-specific IgE evidently allowed the best prediction of a clinically relevant food allergy (◉ Figs. 13.4), even better than specific IgE against Cor a 9. Only 2 of 44 children with clinical relevant hazelnut allergy did not show sensitization to Cor a 14. A positive prediction value for a clinically relevant hazelnut allergy of 90 % was calculated for a Cor a 14-specific IgE concentration of 48 kU/l. Therefore, as with peanut allergy, the possibility of predicting clinical relevance only through the analysis of molecular sensitization patterns is limited.

Clinical Implication of the Multicenter Hazelnut Study (Beyer et al. 2015)

- Cor a 14-specific IgE currently shows the best association with systemic reactions to hazelnut during oral hazelnut provocation.
- In order to predict clinical reaction with a 90 % probability, the Cor a 14-specific IgE must have a value of >47.8 kU_A/l – an uncommon constellation and thus only useful in similarly extreme cases.
- In order to predict clinical tolerance with a 95 % probability, the Cor a 14-specific IgE must have a value of <0.02 kU_A/l – apart from few individual cases.
- Due to exceptions, a definite 100 % prediction based on Cor a 14-specific IgE is not possible. Therefore, the clinical relevance of allergen-specific IgE levels (e.g., against single allergens of legumes) must be assessed on an individual patient basis.

On the other hand, it was shown that the prediction of clinical tolerance among children is possible through the specific IgE to hazelnut extract and Cor a 1. This is assured in the case of sensitization exclusively to the PR-10-protein Cor a 1: If the IgE concentration to Cor a 1 in comparison to hazelnut total extract is greater, this suggests a monosensitization to the Bet v 1-homolog hazelnut allergen (Lange et al. 2015).

Especially among adults, sensitization patterns to single hazelnut allergens are relatively diverse and depend on environmental influences, such as birch pollen exposure (Hansen et al. 2009). A definite classification of individual allergens for the prediction of systemic reactions is usually not possible. The involvement of currently available hazelnut allergens can be depicted as a whole through a "risk ramp" (◉ Fig. 13.5).

13.5.2 Walnut

Jug r 1 (2S albumin), Jug r 2 (7S globulin), and Jug r 3 (nsLTP) are major allergens of the walnut (Costa et al. 2014) and can be associated with storage proteins or lipid transfer proteins in the case of corresponding IgE sensitization (Magnusson et al.

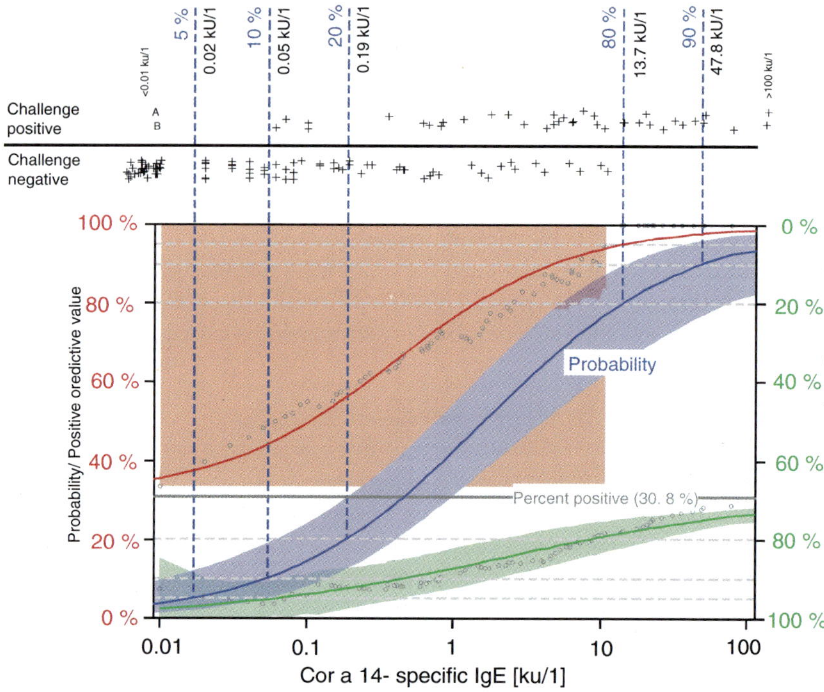

Figs. 13.4 Results concerning the probability of a positive hazelnut food challenge, by Cor a 14-specific IgE. The calculated probability for a positive hazelnut challenge resulting from Cor a 14-specific serum IgE concentration (*blue line and band*). Estimated IgE levels at given probabilities (5, 10, 20 % and 80, 90, 95 %) above figure (*dashed lines*). Estimated positive (*left axis, red line*, and band) and negative (*right axis, green line*, and band) predictive value and real cases (*gray dots*). Actual IgE levels by challenge outcome above figure (*plus sign*). *Capital letters* mark unexpected positive peanut provocations among exceptions (individual cases *A* and *B*) despite low Cor a 14-specific IgE concentration of <0.02 kU_A/l (in the <5 % probability range) (Adapted from Beyer et al. 2015)

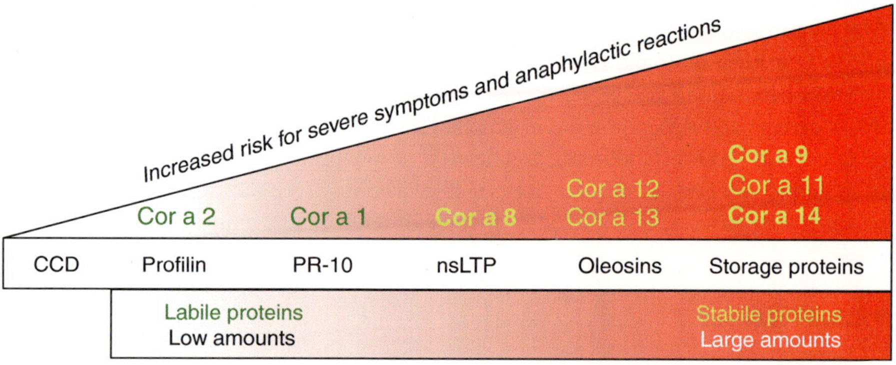

Fig. 13.5 Hazelnut allergens and their role in determining clinical symptoms according to the "risk ramp." While allergens which are unstable and occur in smaller quantities (*left*) tend to induce primarily oropharyngeal symptoms, IgE sensitizations to those which are stable and occur abundantly (*right*) are more commonly associated with severe allergic symptoms

2012). Patients who have shown systemic symptoms in their medical history are more often sensitized to storage proteins, especially Jug r 1 (Ciprandi et al. 2014); however, data from larger studies is not available.

13.5.3 Other Nuts

Ana o 2 (11S globulin) and Ana o 3 (2S albumin) are storage proteins of the cashew. Sensitization to Ana o 3 seems to be a valuable tool for the diagnosis of cashew allergy. This was shown in a study in Greek children (Savvatianos et al. 2015). In a German multicenter study on the same topic, all cashew-allergic children were sensitized to Ana o 3 (Lange et al. 2016). No patient without Ana o 3-sensitization was allergic. It was possible to calculate a 95 % probability for a positive cashew challenge of 2.0 kU/l for Ana o 3 compared to cashew extract of 28.9 kU/l. In receiver operation curves, Ana o 3 discriminated between allergic and tolerant children with an area under the curve of 0.94. All in all the diagnostic accuracy was comparable to Ara h 2 for peanut allergy.

Ber e 1 (2S albumin) is a storage protein of the Brazil nut. Though this presumption lacks clinical data, it can be assumed a sensitization to these allergens is associated with the occurrence of systemic reactions.

Not Yet Available Single Allergens

A sensitization to Cor a 11, the vicilin of the hazelnut, was found most often among toddlers, who developed systemic symptoms hazelnut allergens after consumption, according to a study from Belgium (Verweij et al. 2011). A much larger amount of patients was additionally sensitized to Cor a 9, possibly an indicator of serological cross-reactions, leading the clinical prediction value of a sensitization to Cor a 11 to remain unclear.

13.6 Clinical Value of Molecular Diagnostics

The clinical value of molecular diagnostics (Matricardi et al. 2016) regarding nut allergies is limited. Hazelnut is the only nut that has been researched more extensively. In the diagnostics of hazelnut allergy, the distinct role of one single allergen regarding its clinical relevance – as for Ara h 2 in peanut allergy – is not evident.

Since hazelnut, in comparison with peanut, is not only consumed roasted, there are cases of patients, especially in adult years, where a sensitization to the PR-10-protein is associated with severe allergic reactions (Le et al. 2013). This sensitization is probably not accompanied by severe systemic symptoms among children (Lange et al. 2015).

High-titer IgE levels to storage proteins Cor a 9 and especially Cor a 14 are overall the best predictors of primary hazelnut allergy, as well as partly of the risk of anaphylactic reactions.

13.7 Perspectives

Many allergens in nuts and seeds have already been identified (◉ Table 13.1). In the following years, they will become more increasingly available for molecular diagnostics (Matricardi et al. 2016). The implementation of single allergens from nuts for determination of specific IgE potentially:

- Increases the test sensitivity (lower "Limit of Quantitation," LoQ)
- Improves the analytical specificity (selectivity) compared to extract diagnostics (see also ▶ Chaps. 5 and 7)
- Facilitates detection of marker allergens for serological cross-reactions (e.g., for Bet v 1 homolog profilin-, or CCD-linked cross-reactivity)
- Allows identification of primary, genuine nut allergies

To what extent these results can reflect or predict clinical cross-reactions or the severity of reactions depends on the outcome of clinical studies, which have until now only been completed for several single allergens (e.g., Ara h 2, Cor a 14, Ana o 3).

13.8 Conclusions: Relevance in Daily Clinical Practice

Though many nut allergens have been identified, their clinical usage for molecular diagnostics remains limited as many of them are still commercially unavailable and clinical data are still missing. Using the example of hazelnut allergy, molecular diagnostics can be used to better define the probability of true allergy in patients testing positive to crude hazelnut extracts. IgE tests will detect or exclude the possibility of sensitizations/cross-reactions:

- Against Cor a 1 in the case of an (exclusive) cross-reaction to Bet v 1-proteins (specific IgE against Cor a 1≥ specific IgE against undiluted hazelnut extract/hazelnut total extract); in Central and Northern Europe more commonly due to large numbers of birch pollen allergy sufferers; relatively low threatening potential (Lange et al. 2015).
- Against Cor a 8, a stable hazelnut-LTP, in Central and Northern Europe, much rarer than in Mediterranean regions and more often associated with systemic reactions.
- Against storage proteins: high specific IgE concentrations against Cor a 9 and especially Cor a 14 indicate a sensitization to storage proteins, in Northern and Central Europe, the most important triggers of primary hazelnut allergy, presumably acquired during childhood, with potentially severe reactions.
- Definite predictions of systemic reactions are not possible, resulting in the necessity of thorough patient history and oral provocation testing if a nut allergy is suspected.

Table 13.1 Nuts, their allergens and botanical families

		Storage proteins			"Pathogenesis-related" (PR)-proteins			
		11S globulins (Legumine)	7S globulins (Viciline)	2S albumins	Bet v 1-homolog (PR-10)	nsLTP (PR-14)	Oleosins	Profilin
Nuts	Hazelnut (*Corylus avellana*)	Cor a 9[a,b]	Cor a 11	Cor a 14[b]	Cor a 1[a,b,c]	Cor a 8[a,b]	Cor a 12 Cor a 13	Cor a 2
	Walnut (*Juglans regia*)	Jug r 4	Jug r 2[a]	Jug r 1[a,b]		Jug r 3[a,b]		Jug r 5
	Pecan nut (*Carya illinoensis*)	Car i 4	Car i 2	Car i 1				
Drupes	Almond (*Prunus amygdalus*)	Pru du 6			Pru du 1	Pru du 3		Pru du 4
	Cashew (*Anacardium occidentale*)	Ana o 2[a]	Ana o 1	Ana o 3[b]				
	Pistachio (*Pistacia vera*)	Pis v 2 Pis v 5	Pis v 3	Pis v 1				
Capsule fruits	Brazil nut (*Bertholletia excelsa*)	Ber e 2		Ber e 1[a,b]				

Currently available for allergen-specific IgE diagnostics in different test systems:
[a]ImmunoCAP ISAC
[b]ImmunoCAP
[c]ALLERG-O-LIQ

References

Beyer K, Grishina G, Bardina L, Grishin A, Sampson HA. Identification of an 11S globulin as a major hazelnut food allergen in hazelnut induced systemic reactions. J Allergy Clin Immunol. 2002;110:517–23.

Beyer K, Grabenhenrich L, Beder A, Kalb B, Ziegert M, Finger A, Harandi N, Schlags R, Gappa M, Puzzo L, Röblitz H, Millner-Uhlemann M, Büsing S, Ott H, Lange L, Niggemann B. Predictive values of component-specific IgE for the outcome of peanut and hazelnut food challenges in children. Allergy. 2015;70:90–9.

Burney PG, Potts J, Kummeling I, Mills EN, Clausen M, Dubakiene R, Barreales L, Fernandez-Perez C, Fernandez-Rivas M, Le TM, Knulst AC, Kowalski ML, Lidholm J, Ballmer-Weber BK, Braun-Fahlander C, Mustakov T, Kralimarkova T, Popov T, Sakellariou A, Papadopoulos NG, Versteeg SA, Zuidmeer L, Akkerdaas JH, Hoffmann-Sommergruber K, Van Ree R. The prevalence and distribution of food sensitization in European adults. Allergy. 2014;69:365–71.

Ciprandi G, Pistorio A, Silvestri M, Rossi GA, Tosca MA. Walnut anaphylaxis: the usefulness of molecular-based allergy diagnostics. Immunol Lett. 2014;161:138–9.

Clark AT, Ewan PW. The development and progression of allergy to multiple nuts at different ages. Pediatr Allergy Immunol. 2005;16:507–11.

Costa J, Mafra I, Carrapatoso I, Oliveira MB. Almond allergens: molecular characterization, detection and clinical relevance. J Agric Food Chem. 2012;60:1337–49.

Costa J, Carrapatoso I, Oliveira M, Mafra I. Walnut allergens: molecular characterisation, detection and clinical relevance. Clin Exp Allergy. 2014;44:319–41.

De Knop KJ, Verweij MM, Grimmelikhuijsen M, Philipse E, Hagendorens MM, Bridts CH, De Clerck LS, Stevens WJ, Ebo DG. Age-related sensitization profiles for hazelnut (Corylus avellana) in a birch-endemic region. Pediatr Allergy Immunol. 2011;22:e139–49.

Flinterman AE, Akkerdaas JA, den Hartog Jager CF, Rigby NM, Fernandez-Rivas M, Hoekstra MO, Bruijnzeel-Koomen CA, Knulst AC, van Ree R, Pasmans SG. Lipid transfer protein–linked hazelnut allergy in children from a non-Mediterranean birch-endemic area. J Allergy Clin Immunol. 2008;121:423–8.

Goetz D, Whisman B, Goetz A. Cross-reactivity among edible nuts: double immunodiffusion, crossed immunoelectrophoresis, and human specific IgE serologic surveys. Ann Allergy Asthma Immunol. 2005;95:45–52.

Hansen KS, Ballmer-Weber BK, Sastre J, Lidholm J, Andersson K, Oberhofer H, Lluch-Bernal M, Ostling J, Mattsson L, Schocker F, Vieths S, Poulsen LK. Component-resolved in vitro diagnosis of hazelnut allergy in Europe. J Allergy Clin Immunol. 2009;123:1134–41.

Hauser M, Wallner M, Ferreira F, Mahler V, Kleine-Tebbe J. Das Konzept der Pollen-Panallergene: Profiline und Calcium-bindende Proteine(Polcalcine). Allergo J. 2012;21:291–3.

Hompes S, Scherer K, Köhli A, Rueff F, Mahler V, Lange L, Treudler R, Rietschel E, Szépfalusi Z, Lang R, Rabe U, Reese T, Beyer K, Schwerk N, Worm M. Nahrungsmittelanaphylaxie: Daten aus dem Anaphylaxie-Register. Allergo J. 2010;19:234–42.

Kleine-Tebbe J, et al. Bet v 1 und Homologe – Verursacher der Baumpollenallergie und birkenpollenassozierter Kreuzreaktionen. Allergo J. 2010;19:462–3.

Lange L, Finger A, Buderus S, Ott H. The ratio between Cor a 1- and hazelnut-specific IgE predicts negative challenge outcome in children. Pediatr Allergy Immunol Pulmonol. 2015;28:7–12.

Lange L, Lasota L, Finger A, Vlajnic D, Büsing S, Meister J, Broekaert I, Pfannenstiel C, Friedrichs F, Price M, Trendelenburg V, Beyer K, Niggemann B. Ana o 3-specific IgE is a good predictor for clinical relevant cashew allergy in children. Submitted to Allergy. 2016. doi:10.1111/all.13050.

Le TM, van Hoffen E, Lebens AF, Bruijnzeel-Koomen CA, Knulst AC. Anaphylactic versus mild reactions to hazelnut and apple in a birch-endemic area: different sensitization profiles? Int Arch Allergy Immunol. 2013;160:56–62.

Magnusson U, Mattsson L, Marknell DeWitt Å, Everberg H, Vieths S, Lidholm J. Analysis of component-resolved sensitisation among walnut-sensitised subjects. Abstract 204; EAACI-Kongress 2012. 2012.

Maleki SJ, Teuber SS, Cheng H, Chen D, Comstock SS, Ruan S, Schein CH. Computationally predicted IgE epitopes of walnut allergens contribute to cross-reactivity with peanuts. Allergy. 2011;66:1522–9.

Maloney JM, Rudengren M, Ahlstedt S, Bock SA, Sampson HA. The use of serum-specific IgE measurements for the diagnosis of peanut, tree nut, and seed allergy. J Allergy Clin Immunol. 2008;122:145–51.

Masthoff LJ, Mattsson L, Zuidmeer-Jongejan L, Lidholm J, Andersson K, Akkerdaas JH, Versteeg SA, Garino C, Meijer Y, Kentie P, Versluis A, den Hartog Jager CF, Bruijnzeel-Koomen CA, Knulst AC, van Ree R, van Hoffen E, Pasmans SG. Sensitization to Cor a 9 and Cor a 14 is highly specific for a hazelnut allergy with objective symptoms in Dutch children and adults. J Allergy Clin Immunol. 2013;132:393–9.

Matricardi PM, Kleine-Tebbe J, Hoffmann HJ, Valenta R, Hilger C, Hofmaier S, Aalberse RC, Agache I, Asero R, Ballmer-Weber B, Barber D, Beyer K, Biedermann T, Biló MB, Blank S, Bohle B, Bosshard PP, Breiteneder H, Brough HA, Caraballo L, Caubet JC, Crameri R, Davies JM, Douladiris N, Ebisawa M, Eigenmann PA, Fernandez-Rivas M, Ferreira F, Gadermaier G, Glatz M, Hamilton RG, Hawranek T, Hellings P, Hoffmann-Sommergruber K, Jakob T, Jappe U, Jutel M, Kamath SD, Knol EF, Korosec P, Kuehn A, Lack G, Lopata AL, Mäkelä M, Morisset M, Niederberger V, Nowak-Wezgrzyn AH, Papadopoulos NG, Pastorello EA, Pauli G, Platts-Mills T, Posa D, Poulsen LK, Raulf M, Sastre J, Scala E, Schmid JM, Schmid-Grendelmeier P, van Hage M, van Ree R, Vieths S, Weber R, Wickman M, Muraro A, Ollert M. EAACI molecular allergology user's guide. Pediatr Allergy Immunol. 2016;27(Suppl23):1–250.

Petersen A, Scheurer S. Stabile pflanzliche Nahrungsmittelallergene: Lipid-Transfer-Proteine. Allergo J. 2011;20:384–6.

Radauer C, Kleine-Tebbe J, Beyer K. Stabile pflanzliche Nahrungsmittelallergene: Speicherproteine. Allergo J. 2012;21:8888–92.

Savvatianos S, Konstantinopoulos AP, Borgå Å, Stavroulakis G, Lidholm J, Borres MP, Manousakis E, Papadopoulos NG. Sensitization to cashew nut 2S albumin, Ana o 3, is highly predictive of cashew and pistachio allergy in Greek children. J Allergy Clin Immunol. 2015;136:192–4.

Verweij MM, Hagendorens MM, De Knop KJ, Bridts CH, De Clerck LS, Stevens WJ, Ebo DG. Young infants with atopic dermatitis can display sensitization to Cor a 9, an 11S legumin-like seed-storage protein from hazelnut (Corylus avellana). Pediatr Allergy Immunol. 2011;22:196–201.

Worm M, Hompes S, Fiedler EM, Illner AK, Zuberbier T, Vieths S. Impact of native, heat-processed and encapsulated hazelnuts on the allergic response in hazelnut-allergic patients. Clin Exp Allergy. 2009;39:159–66.

Zuidmeer-Jongejan L, Fernandez-Rivas M, Winter M, Akkerdas JH, Summers C, Lebens A, Knulst AC, Schilte P, Briza P, Gademaier G, van Ree R. Oil body-associated hazelnut allergens including oleosins are underrepresented in diagnostic extracts but associated with severe symptoms. Clin Transl Allergy. 2014;4:4.

14 Molecular Diagnostics of Allergy to Fruits and Vegetables

B.K. Ballmer-Weber and K. Hoffmann-Sommergruber

14.1 Introduction

Apart from tree nuts and legumes, fruits and vegetables are the most common triggers of food allergies in adulthood. In a 2011 review (Ballmer-Weber and Hoffmann-Sommergruber 2011), the most important research findings from 2009 to 2010 on molecular diagnostics in allergies to fruits and vegetables were collated. The following chapter is based on this summary and also includes new data on this subject.

This contribution is based on a publication by the authors that appeared in the *Allergo Journal International* in 2014 (Ballmer-Weber BK, Hoffmann-Sommergruber K: Update: molecular diagnostics of allergies to vegetables and fruits. Allergo J Int 2014; 23: 24–34), which has been updated and expanded as a chapter for this book.
The authors gratefully thank Jan B. Bernhisel-Broadbent, MD (Granger Asthma & Allergy, Murray, UT); Kate Broadbent, PhD, Salt Lake City, UT; and Kenneth R. Broadbent, MD (Wasatch Pediatrics at St. Marks) Salt Lake City, UT, USA, for carefully reviewing the manuscript, helpful suggestions, and editorial assistance with the English translation

B.K. Ballmer-Weber, MD, Prof. (✉)
Center of Dermatology and Allergology, Kantonsspital Luzern, Lucerne, Switzerland

Department of Dermatology, University Hospital Zürich, Zurich, Switzerland
e-mail: barbara.ballmer@usz.ch

K. Hoffmann-Sommergruber, PhD, Prof.
Department of Pathophysiology and Allergy Research, Medical University of Vienna, Vienna, Austria

J. Kleine-Tebbe, T. Jakob (eds.), *Molecular Allergy Diagnostics*,
DOI 10.1007/978-3-319-42499-6_14

14.2 Epidemiology of Fruit and Vegetable Allergy

Most research on the prevalence of food allergy has provided information based on regional data. Unfortunately, Pan-European findings on type and frequency of food allergy from the multicenter cross-sectional study within the EuroPrevall project have still not yet been released (Kummeling et al. 2009). Two investigations on sensitization to food in Europe have, however, been published. The first of these, dating from 2010, was carried out as part of the European Community Respiratory Health Survey. Sera from 4,522 European adults and 13 countries were analyzed (Burney et al. 2010). In another study, also published by Burney et al. (2014), sera from 2,335 European subjects recruited within the EuroPrevall project were tested for sensitization to foods, in part with use of an allergen microarray.

The most common allergic sensitizations are to foods of plant origin.

It is important to note that we are dealing here with sensitization and not with confirmed allergy. In these two studies, the highest rates of sensitization to vegetables were to carrot at 3.6 and 5.0 %, to celery at 3.5 and 6.3 %, and to tomato at 3.3 and 4.9 %, respectively (Burney et al. 2010, 2014). The highest sensitization rates to fruits were to peach at 5.4 and 7.9 %, to apple at 4.2 and 6.6 %, and to kiwi fruit at 3.5 and 5.2 %, respectively (Burney et al. 2010, 2014).

A meta-analysis from 2008 looking at the frequency of food allergies to foods of plant origin covered 36 studies, including more than 250,000 children and adults. It should be mentioned that in only six investigations was food allergy confirmed by oral provocation. Within these studies, the prevalence rate calculated for vegetable allergies was 1.4 % and that for fruit allergies was 0.1–4.3 % (Zuidmeer et al. 2008).

14.3 Potential Benefits of Molecular Diagnostics in Food Allergy

Depending on the sensitization pathway, allergies to foods of plant origin are acquired either primarily, i.e., directly via the gastrointestinal tract or presumably through the skin, or secondarily as a consequence of cross-sensitization, generally after primary sensitization to inhalant allergens (Steckelbroeck et al. 2008).

Allergens able to induce primary food allergy tend to be resistant to proteolytic digestion and also to degradation during the extraction process.

These allergens are, therefore, often well represented in diagnostic extracts and frequently associated with high sensitivity of extract-based diagnostics in primary food allergy (Lidholm et al. 2006). Clinically, these proteins tend to trigger more severe reactions than the more labile allergens that lead to secondary sensitization (Ballmer-Weber and Hoffmann-Sommergruber 2011). The latter have a tendency to degrade during the extraction process, hence the lower sensitivity of extract-based diagnostics in secondary food allergy (Lidholm et al. 2006).

Identification of individual allergenic molecules from a given food is an important step toward improvement of in vitro diagnostics (Matricardi et al. 2016).

In past years, numerous allergenic components have been identified, characterized, and in some cases produced using recombinant technology. The observation

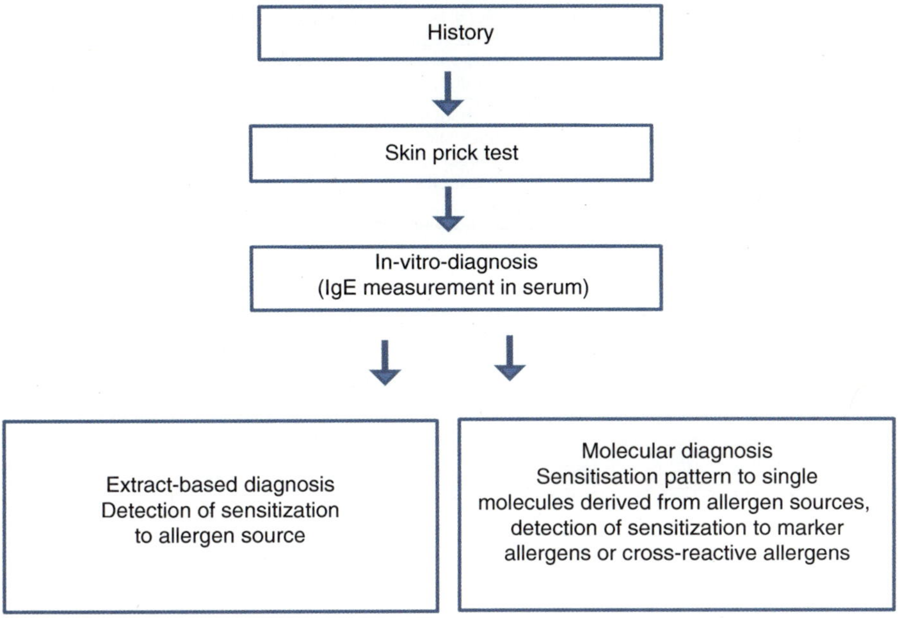

Fig. 14.1 Flowchart for diagnosing possible fruit and vegetable allergies

that the severity of a clinical reaction depends partly on the sensitization pattern will open up new diagnostic avenues in the future. Molecular, allergen-specific diagnostics (Matricardi et al. 2016) will enhance test sensitivity, especially in secondary food allergy, and also provide scope for drawing up a patient-specific risk profile with regard to severity of the clinical reaction (Fig. 14.1).

14.4 Allergies to Fruits and Vegetables: The Most Important Allergen Families

According to Jenkins et al. (2005), over 65 % of food allergens of plant origin belong to only four protein families: the prolamins, the Bet v 1 family, the cupins, and the profilins.

◉ Figure 14.2 The most important allergen families of plant origin involved in fruit and vegetable allergy

Some of the allergens described have already been incorporated into routine diagnostic practice. The following ImmunoCAP tests are available for in vitro diagnostics in fruit and vegetable allergy:

- From peach: Pru p 1 (Bet v 1 homolog), Pru p 3 (nonspecific lipid transfer protein, nsLTP), and Pru p 4 (profilin)
- From apple: Mal d 1 (Bet v 1 homolog) and Mal d 3 (nsLTP)
- From celery root: Api g 1.01 (Bet v 1 homolog)
- From kiwi fruit: Act d 8 (Bet v 1 homolog)

	nsLTP	**Profilin**	**Bet v 1-homologs (PR-10 family)**	**Thaumatin-like protein (TLP)**	**Endochitinase**	**β-1,3-glucanase**
Function	Pathogen resistance, lipid transfer	Actin binding, regulatory function	Pathogen resistance, steroid transporter	Pathogen resistance	Pathogen resistance, chitin degradation	Pathogen resistance
Mol.mass [kDa]	7–9	14	17	20–25	25–35	25–35
Number of food allergens	30	25	18	9	8	5
Abundance	In all plant foods	In all plant foods	In all plant foods	Kiwi, citrus, stone fruits, grapes, tomato	Banana, avocado, tomato	Banana, avocado, tomato
Structure	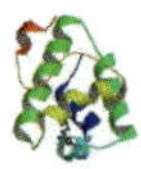	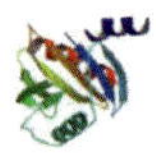	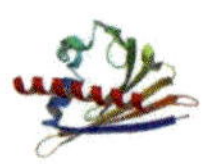	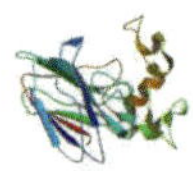	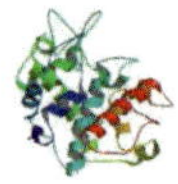	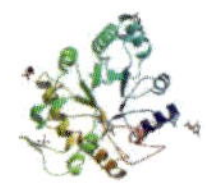
	PDB: 2B5S	PDB: 1CQA	PDB: 2BKO	PDB: 2AHN	PDB: 2BAA	PDB: 1Q9B

Fig. 14.2 Overview of the most important protein families for fruit and vegetable allergies, arranged by prevalence (Number of allergens: Allfam database, www.meduniwien.ac.at/allergens/allfam/)

ImmunoCAP ISAC microarray testing is also available for the following additional allergens:

- From kiwi fruit: Act d 1 (cysteine protease), Act d 2 (thaumatin-like protein), and Act d 5 (kiwellin)
- From carrot: Dau c 1 (Bet v 1 homolog)

14.5 Molecular Diagnostics in Vegetable Allergy

The only studies to date on the use of molecular diagnostics (Matricardi et al. 2016) in vegetable allergy that include patients with confirmed food allergy, based on positive, double-blind, placebo-controlled oral provocation challenges, are for celery root and carrot allergy. The role of molecular diagnostics is discussed below in relation to tomato allergy, as well.

14.5.1 Celery Root Allergy

Celery root (celeriac) belongs to the Apiaceae family. Allergy to this vegetable is acquired as a result of primary sensitization to birch and/or mugwort pollen.

To date, there are no case reports of primary, pollen-independent allergy to celery root.

There are a multitude of clinical manifestations of celery root allergy, ranging from banal contact urticaria of the oral mucosa, known as oral allergy syndrome, to life-threatening anaphylactic reactions (Ballmer-Weber et al. 2000).

Two isoforms of the Bet v 1 homologous allergen Api g 1 have been identified in celery root (Hoffmann-Sommergruber et al. 2000). In addition to the profilin Api g 4 (Scheurer et al. 2000), Api g 5, occurring as a mixture of two proteins with a molecular mass of 53 and 57 kDa, has been described. The latter belong to the flavoprotein family. As revealed by mass spectrometry analysis, the protein core of Api g 5 carries at least three N-glycans of the MMXF and MUXF type. Removal of the carbohydrate structures results in loss of IgE binding to Api g 5. This suggests that IgE binding to Api g 5 is directed toward the carbohydrate structure (Bublin et al. 2003).

The largest study to date on molecular diagnostics in celery root allergy was published by Bauermeister et al. (2009). Sera from 24 patients with positive provocation to celery root were tested for sensitization to Api g 1 (Bet v 1 homolog), Api g 4 (profilin), and Api g 5 (glycoprotein from the flavoprotein family). The sensitivity of extract-based diagnostics was 67 %. Even the sole addition of Api g 1 led to an increase in sensitivity to 75 %. Inclusion of Api g 4 resulted in further increase in sensitivity to 88 %, whereas inclusion of Api g 5 did not further enhance sensitivity. None of these allergens appeared suitable as a marker for severe allergy to celery root. Particularly severe clinical reactions to celery root have been reported in mugwort-associated celery root allergy. Overall, 12 % of the subjects in the research by Bauermeister et al., including in particular those sensitized to mugwort pollen, did not exhibit any sensitization to the three tested allergens. This suggests the presence of an additional, as-yet-unidentified allergen in severe celery root allergy.

Gadermaier et al. (2011) have identified and characterized Api g 2, a lipid transfer protein (nsLTP type 1) from celery stalks. The authors showed that the LTP from celery stalk is thermostable and acid resistant, as are other previously identified LTPs. Sera from 786 patients from Italy were analyzed using an ImmunoCAP ISAC microarray test. Of these, 32 sera displayed sensitization to the LTP from celery stalk. However, only approximately one-third of these persons had a history of celery stalk allergy, suggesting clinically nonrelevant sensitization to celery stalk LTP in over two-thirds of cases. Only one individual had a history of anaphylactic reaction after consumption of stalk celery. A related protein from celery root has recently been identified: Api g 6, which belongs to the nsLTP type 2 protein family (Vejvar et al. 2013). Sensitization to Api g 6 was detected in 12 of 37 sera of individuals with celery root allergy. The study's authors demonstrated that only limited IgE cross-reactivity exists between Api g 2 and Api g 6.

The clinical relevance of Api g 2 and Api g 6 in persons with celery root allergy awaits further clarification.

14.5.2 Carrot Allergy

The majority of patients with carrot allergy (Apiaceae family) are also sensitive to birch or mugwort pollen.

The clinical manifestation of carrot allergy tends to be milder than that of celery root allergy.

Nevertheless, up to 50 % of carrot-allergic patients develop a systemic reaction (Ballmer-Weber et al. 2001). Two Bet v 1 homologous allergens have been identified in carrot, the isoforms Dau c 1.0104 and Dau c 1.0201, as has the profilin Dau c 4 (Ballmer-Weber et al. 2005; Hoffmann-Sommergruber et al. 1999). An isoflavone reductase-like protein, corresponding to Bet v 6 in birch pollen, has also been found in carrot (Karamloo et al. 2001). Furthermore, Japanese investigators report cyclophilin as an IgE-binding allergen in this vegetable (Fujita et al. 2001).

A study published in 2012 included 49 carrot-allergic individuals from three geographical regions of Europe (Denmark, Switzerland, and Spain. Their sera were analyzed for IgE binding to carrot extract using ImmunoCAP, as was IgE binding to the recombinant carrot allergens Dau c 1.0104, Dau c 1.0201, Dau c 4, the recently characterized isoflavone reductase-like proteins rDau c IFR 1, rDau c IFR 2, and the cyclophilin from carrot rDau c Cyc (Ballmer-Weber et al. 2012). The name Dau c 5 has been proposed for the isoflavone reductase-like protein in carrot.

The sensitivity of the extract-based test was 82 %. Addition of the recombinant allergens led to a slight improvement in test sensitivity to 90 %. The Dau c 1 isoforms were major allergens for those subjects in Switzerland and Denmark with carrot allergy. For the subjects in Spain, the major allergen was the profilin, Dau c 4. Sensitization to carrot cyclophilin was found in only one individual. This allergen appears to be of little relevance in the European population. In contrast, 6 % of subjects were sensitized to Dau c IFR 1 and 22 % to Dau c IFR 2.

In an earlier study, we were unable to detect carrot LTP (cloned from genomic material) in the edible parts of carrot (Ballmer-Weber et al. 2005). LTP is unlikely to be a problem for persons with carrot allergy.

A link between severity of allergic reaction and the pattern of sensitization to the various carrot allergens could not be established.

14.5.3 Tomato Allergy

Consumption of tomatoes (Solanaceae family) is increasing globally. In a German study, 9 % of patients, most of them birch pollen sensitized, reported allergic reactions upon ingestion of tomato (Foetisch et al. 2001). To date, according to the IUIS Allergen Nomenclature Sub-Committee (▶ www.allergen.org), five tomato allergens have been officially accepted:

- Sola l 1 (previously Lyc e 1, profilin, 14 kDa)
- Sola l 2 (previously Lyc e 2, β-fructofuronidase, 50 kDa)
- Sola l 3 (previously Lyc e 3, nsLTP, 6 kDa)
- Sola l 4 (previously Lyc e 4, intracellular pathogenesis-related protein TSI-11 of the Bet v 1 family)
- Sola l 5 (cylophilin)
- Sola l 6 (nsLTP type 2, 7 kDa)
- Sola l 7 (nsLTP type 1, 12.5 kDa)

Sola l 4 and Sola l 1 are potential cross-reactive allergens between tomatoes and birch pollen. The expression of Sola l 1 and Sola l 3 has recently been suppressed in transgenic tomatoes. This led to a marked reduction in the allergenicity of tomato, confirming the clinical relevance of these two allergens (Le et al. 2010).

In an investigation in Spain, only 16 % of patients with sensitization to tomato actually experienced clinical symptoms on ingestion of this food. These results suggest that tomato sensitization frequently remains clinically silent. Most of those included in the study were sensitized to mugwort or plane tree pollen, a possible indication of cross-sensitizing allergens in these pollens and in tomatoes (Larramendi et al. 2008).

Further tomato allergens have been identified in an immunoblot study: LTP and β-fructofuronidase, an osmotin-like protein (thaumatin-like protein), an endochitinase precursor, and a pectinesterase-I precursor. Patients with monosensitization to LTPs had a history of severe reactions upon ingestion of tomato (Pravettoni et al. 2009). Recently, two additional nsLTP proteins have been identified; a type 2 nsLTP, Sola l 6 (Giangrieco et al. 2015), and Sola l 7, a member of the type 1 protein family. In addition, two storage proteins, a legumin and a vicilin, have been identified as allergens in tomato seeds (Bassler et al. 2009). Some tomato allergens (e.g., chitinase and glucanase) have also been described in connection with sensitization to natural rubber latex.

The tomato is a complex allergenic food. Future studies will reveal which allergens need to be considered in component-resolved diagnostics.

14.6 Molecular Diagnostics in Fruit Allergy

In regard to food allergy to fruits, the abovementioned meta-analysis by Zuidmeer et al. (2008) provides prevalence data of 0.1–4.3 % and refers to studies with positive food provocation. In contrast, the prevalence of subjectively experienced fruit allergy was found to be 0.1–3.5 % in adults and up to 11.5 % in children. The main causes of fruit allergies are reported as being apple and citrus fruits (orange and lemon). In research by Burney et al. (2010, 2014), "the most frequent sensitization rates found among fruits were to peach (5.4–8.0 %), apple (4.2–6.5 %), kiwi fruit (3.6–5.2 %), banana (2.5–3.8 %) and melon (1.6–3.1 %)."

Because of the comparatively high prevalence rates for apple and peach allergy, allergen-specific diagnostics and food provocation procedures for these fruits have been refined and improved in recent years (Fernandez-Rivas et al. 2003, 2006; Gonzalez-Mancebo et al. 2008). In both of these fruits of the Rosaceae family, the most important allergens have been identified and can be used for component-resolved diagnostics.

This is not yet the case with kiwi fruit. It is only recently that allergy to this fruit has been investigated more closely, the spectrum of kiwi fruit allergens characterized, and the sensitization pattern compared with reference to clinical relevance (Bublin et al. 2010, 2011; Palacin et al. 2008).

14.6.1 Kiwi Fruit Allergy

Kiwi fruit is regarded today as one of the most important causes of fruit allergy and is a prime example of the development of allergies to novel foods. In the 1980s, kiwi fruit was imported to Europe as an exotic fruit and its consumption was promoted as a rich source of vitamin C. Several years later, the first reports emerged of the occurrence of allergic symptoms after consumption of kiwi fruit. Now, according to studies from Finland, Sweden, and France, kiwi fruit is among the top ten causative agents of food allergy (Eriksson et al. 2003; Mattila et al. 2003; Rance et al. 2005).

With regard to sensitization, primary and secondary possibilities are again distinguished:

- In the case of monosensitization, allergic symptoms are induced only by consumption of kiwi fruit.
- Where there is preexisting sensitization to birch pollen, grass pollen, or natural rubber latex, cross-reaction may also result in allergic reaction to kiwi fruit (Brehler et al. 1997; Gall et al. 1994; Palacin et al. 2008).

Allergic symptoms can range from mild, local manifestations to severe, generalized systemic reactions.

Currently, 13 different allergens have been identified from green kiwi fruit (*Actinidia deliciosa*) and are listed in the official IUIS database of allergen nomenclature (www.allergen.org; Table 14.1).

- Actinidin, Act d 1 (30 kDa), the major allergen of kiwi fruit, is a papain-like cysteine protease concentrated in ripe fruits (up to 50 % of the soluble protein fraction) (Aleman et al. 2004; Palacin et al. 2008; Pastorello et al. 1998). Act d 1 is a highly active protease that contributes to the rapid degradation of other proteins in the total extract. This enzymatic activity is, at least in part, responsible for the marked differences in quality among kiwi fruit extracts for skin prick tests. The IgE-binding activity of active Act d 1 has been sufficiently investigated. However, inactivated Act d 1 is still capable of binding to specific IgE antibodies even after enzymatic treatment, thermal treatment, and alteration of the pH environment (Grozdanovic et al. 2012).
- Another important kiwi fruit allergen is Act d 2, a member of the family of thaumatin-like proteins (Gavrovic-Jankulovic et al. 2002).
- Act d 3 (40 kDa) is a glycosylated protein with high sensitization potential. Its function in the plant is still unknown (Palacin et al. 2008).
- Phytocystatin, Act d 4 (11 kDa), is an inhibitor of cysteine protease (Gavrovic-Jankulovic et al. 2002).
- Act d 5 (kiwellin) is a protein of the cell wall that contributes to the fruit's ripening process (Tamburrini et al. 2005). In a study, Tuppo et al. (2008) showed that the enzymatic activity of Act d 1 results in two domains of Act d 5 being formed: the C-terminal fragment, KiTH (20 kDa), and a peptide of 39 amino acids, kissper, which is involved in the formation of ion channels and of pores in cell

membranes (Tuppo et al. 2008). IgE-binding activity was demonstrated for both fragments.
- Two further allergens subsequently identified were Act d 6 (18 kDa), an inhibitor of pectin methylesterase, and Act d 7 (50 kDa), a pectin methylesterase (Ciardiello et al. 2008).
- Homologs to the pollen allergens Bet v 1 and profilin have also been identified in the green kiwi fruit and received the allergen names Act d 8 (Bet v 1 homologs; 17 kDa) and Act d 9 (profilin, 14 kDa). These two allergens are responsible for cross-reactivity with pollen (Bublin et al. 2010; Oberhuber et al. 2008).
- The lipid transfer protein (LTP) from kiwi fruit was given the allergen designation Act d 10 and has structural elements characteristic of all members of the LTP protein family. Despite this, the sequence homology to other LTPs, such as Pru p 3 from peach, is relatively low, so the risk of cross-reactivity is limited (Bernardi et al. 2011).
- Act d 11 (17 kDa) belongs to the family of major latex proteins, or ripening-related proteins, and is a member of the Bet v 1 superfamily. This protein has low sequence homology to Act d 8; its concentration in the fruit is dependent on the fruit's ripening process, and its production can be enhanced by storage conditions such as ethylene treatment (D'Avino et al. 2011).
- Finally, the allergens most recently identified from kiwi fruit are Act d 12, a member of the 11S globulin family, and Act d 13, a 2S albumin (D'Avino et al. 2011) (www.allergen.org). Both proteins are found in the seeds of kiwi fruit.

Bublin et al. tested sera from 30 kiwi fruit-allergic patients as to their specific IgE reactivity pattern. The criterion for inclusion in the study was positive food provocation with kiwi fruit. Sera were tested for the kiwi fruit allergens Act d 1–5 and Act d 8–9, using an ImmunoCAP system. Combined, the sensitivity of these tests with individual molecular allergens reached 77 %. By comparison, the sensitivity of the test with total extract was just 17 % (Bublin et al. 2010). Analysis of the results obtained with Act d 1–5 reveals that the test's sensitivity was 40 % and its specificity 90 %. Additionally, this study showed that sensitization to Act d 1 correlates significantly with monosensitization to kiwi fruit, whereas sensitization to Act d 8 and Act d 9 is specific to those with pollen-kiwi fruit allergies.

Research in Spain, by Palacin et al. (2008), used Act d 1, Act d 2, and Act d 3 for in vitro and in vivo skin prick testing (SPT) in 90 individuals with kiwi fruit allergy. More than half of the tested sera (60 %) had specific IgE antibodies toward all three allergens and positive reactions in SPT (50 %). Sensitization to Act d 1 and Act d 3 was significantly correlated with anaphylactic reactions. In a follow-up study by Bublin et al. (2011), Act d 1–9, Act d 11, and Pru p 3 (LTP from peach) were attached to microarrays using chip technology, and 237 sera of subjects with kiwi fruit allergy were tested. This testing revealed a sensitivity of 66 % and a specificity of 56 %. In this test, too, Act d 1 was a marker allergen for kiwi fruit monosensitization. Sensitization to Act d 6 was not established in any of the sera. Act d 2, Act d 8, and Act d 11 contributed to enhancement of the test's specificity, whereas Act d 7

Table 14.1 Allergens from carrot, celery, tomato, kiwi fruit, and peach according to IUIS Allergen Nomenclature Sub-Committee (www.allergen.org)

Allergens	Molecular mass	Biochemical name	Remarks[a]
Carrot			
Dau c 1	16 kDa	Pathogenesis-related protein PR-10	Primarily intraoral symptoms but also potential for systemic reactions
Dau c 4	14 kDa	Profilin	
Dau c 5	33 kDa	Isoflavone reductase-like protein	
Celery			
Api g 1[b,c]	15 kDa	Pathogenesis-related protein PR-10	Primarily intraoral symptoms but also potential for systemic reactions
Api g 2	9 kDa	Lipid transfer protein	Previously detected only in celery stalks
Api g 3		Chlorophyll a-/chlorophyll b-binding protein	Not yet investigated
Api g 4	14 kDa	Profilin	
Api g 5	58 kDa	FAD-containing oxidase	
Api g 6	7 kDa	Lipid transfer protein type 2	
Tomato			
Sola l 1	14 kDa	Profilin	
Sola l 2	50 kDa	β-fructofuronidase	
Sola l 3	6 kDa	Lipid transfer protein	
Sola l 4	18 kDa	Intracellular pathogenesis-related protein TSI-1	
Sola l 5	19 kDa	Cyclophilin	
Sola l 6	7 kDa	Lipid transfer protein type 2	
Sola l 7	13 kDa	Lipid transfer protein type 1	
Kiwi fruit			
Act d 1[c]	30 kDa	Cysteine protease (Actinidin)	Marker for primary kiwi fruit allergy, potential for systemic reactions
Act d 2[c]	24 kDa	Thaumatin-like protein	
Act d 3	40 kDa		
Act d 4	11 kDa	Phytocystatin	
Act d 5[2]	26 kDa	Kiwellin	
Act d 6	18 kDa	Pectin methylesterase inhibitor	Not yet investigated
Act d 7	50 kDa	Pectin methylesterase	Not yet investigated
Act d 8[b,c]	17 kDa	Pathogenesis-related protein PR-10	Primarily intraoral symptoms
Act d 9	14 kDa	Profilin	

Table 14.1 (continued)

Allergens	Molecular mass	Biochemical name	Remarks[a]
Act d 10	10 kDa	Lipid transfer protein	
Act d 11	17 kDa	Major latex protein	Not yet investigated
Act d 12	50 kDa	11S globulin	
Act d 13	11 kDa	2S albumin	
Peach			
Pru p 1[b,c]	18 kDa	Pathogenesis-related protein PR-10	Primarily intraoral symptoms
Pru p 2	25–28 kDa	Thaumatin-like protein	
Pru p 3[b,c]	10 kDa	Lipid transfer protein	Risk marker for systemic reactions
Pru p 4[b]	14 kDa	Profilin	
Pru p 7	7 kDa	Gibberellin-regulated protein	Not yet investigated

[a]With the exception of the allergens described, the rest have particularly high potential for intraoral symptoms
[b]Available for IgE diagnostics: ImmunoCAP (ThermoFisher)
[c]Available for IgE diagnostics: ISAC (ThermoFisher, Microarray)

and Act d 9 reduced its specificity. Hev b 11, a chitinase from natural rubber latex, was identified as a cross-reactive component in patients with kiwi fruit-latex allergy.

Although there are currently 11 different kiwi fruit allergens available for refined in vitro diagnostics, the panel of allergens in the kiwi fruit appears to be not yet complete, as studies performed so far continue to yield identified sera that did not react with any of the tested components (Bublin et al. 2011).

In kiwi fruit allergy, component-resolved diagnostics allows a distinction to be made between pollen-associated and clinically severe primary allergy to the fruit. However, the current allergy panel for green kiwi fruit appears to be incomplete.

Following the commercial success of green kiwi fruit (*Actinidia deliciosa* cv. Hayward), 1999 saw the start of imports of golden kiwi fruit (*Actinidia chinensis* cv. Hort16A) to Europe. Shortly after the introduction of this new species of the fruit, it became apparent that most kiwi fruit-allergic patients exhibited considerably milder symptoms with golden kiwi fruit than with its green counterpart. This appears to be due to the amount of Act d 1 being 50 times lower in the golden kiwi fruit (Bublin et al. 2004). In a study by Le et al. (2011), six different kiwi fruit cultivars already available in Europe or soon to be introduced to the market were tested for allergen content on kiwi fruit-allergic subjects in the Netherlands and Switzerland, using prick-to-prick tests and provocation. In addition to the golden kiwi fruit, a second kiwi fruit variety, Summer 3373, was identified as a variant with reduced allergen content.

Different species and varieties of kiwi fruit differ considerably in allergen content.

14.6.2 Peach Allergy

In Mediterranean countries, peach (*Prunus persica*) is the most frequent cause of food allergy of plant origin (Asero et al. 2009; Cuesta-Herranz et al. 2010). Of these patients, 80 % are sensitized to Pru p 3, an LTP mainly concentrated in the fruit's skin (Fernandez-Rivas et al. 2003; Sanchez-Monge et al. 1999). The structure, with four disulfide bridges and hence characteristic of nsLTPs, is important for the allergenic effect of the protein. As Toda et al. (2011) were able to show, after reduction and alkylation of Pru p 3 the allergenic properties are considerably reduced, and enzymatic degradation of the protein is accelerated. Homologs of the pollen allergens Pru p 1 (Bet v 1 homolog) and Pru p 4 (profilin) have also been identified (Gaier et al. 2008; Rodriguez-Perez et al. 2003).

Palacin et al. identified thaumatin-like proteins (TLPs, Pru p 2) from peach as allergens of high relevance for the Spanish population (Palacin et al. 2010). These proteins (20–25 kDa) also have a characteristic three-dimensional structure that is stabilized by eight disulfide bridges and exhibits relatively high resistance toward enzymatic degradation. In the plant, TLPs, which belong to the family of pathogenesis-related proteins, are active in defense against pathogens. TLPs were first reported as allergens in the genus *Capsicum* (peppers) and cherry (Jensen-Jarolim et al. 1998; Inschlag et al. 1998). Allergens from this protein family have now been identified in a number of fruits, vegetables, spices, and pollens and have been described as panallergens. However, their clinical relevance in food allergies is not yet fully known and the general rate of sensitization to them in foods tested is below 50 %.

Recently, a new allergen from peach was included in the allergen database. Named Pru p 7, (6.9 kDa), it is a gibberellin-related protein and has induced a positive skin test in 14 of 33 peach-allergic patients (▶ www.allergen.org).

Pru p 3 is listed as a risk marker for systemic reactions to peach. Pru p 1, by contrast, generally causes intraoral symptoms.

Pru p 3 has been regarded as a genuine food allergen with primary sensitization activity. However, case reports are consistently being published that describe cosensitization with LTPs from cypress pollen (Sanchez-Lopez et al. 2011). In a study in southern France, however, these cosensitizations between Pru p 3 and pollen allergens from cypress were not demonstrated (Caimmi et al. 2013). Cross-reactivity between Pru p 3 and Art v 3, the LTP from mugwort, is found, this being the case where exposure levels to mugwort pollen are high. In an investigation from China including 24 patients with allergy to peach and to mugwort pollen, the authors detected cross-reactivity between Pru p 3 and Art v 3. They assumed that primary sensitization to peach involves mugwort pollen (Gao et al. 2013). The authors explain their conclusions in terms of primary pollen allergy prior to onset of the fruit allergy and high exposure to mugwort pollen. This exposure is not prevalent in all regions of Europe.

A further Spanish study investigated sera of 45 individuals with peach allergy using ImmunoCAP ISAC microarray technology. These subjects were sensitized to LTP and had no specific IgE antibodies to Bet v 1-homologs or profilin (Pascal et al. 2012). The patients developed symptoms upon consumption of peach, as well as a number of other foods (lettuce, walnut, hazelnut, peanut, and green beans).

Symptoms ranged from local reactions (oral allergy syndrome, OAS) to generalized symptoms (anaphylaxis). Some individuals reported that cofactors (concomitant use of nonsteroidal anti-inflammatory drugs (NSAIDs), sports-related exertion) induced or aggravated their symptoms.

A recent study by Palacin et al. (2010) found a sensitization rate of 77 % for Pru p 2 in a group of patients in Spain. In a follow-up investigation, sera of 212 subjects with fruit allergy and 111 with pollen allergy were tested for sensitization to 16 TLPs using a microarray system (Palacin et al. 2012). This Spanish multicenter study compared rates of sensitization from different geographic regions and investigated possible cosensitization to TLPs from pollen. Specific IgE antibodies to Pru p 2 (isoform Pru p 2.0201) were found in the sera, with levels varying by geographical region from 18 % (Alicante) to 70 % (Canary Islands). However, most sera were from individuals with pollen allergy who showed no clinical reactions to foods of plant origin. It has long been thought that a close relationship exists between sensitization to TLPs from pollen and fruits. In the study patient population, a close correlation between Pru p 2 and the TLP from plane tree pollen was demonstrated, primarily in persons with fruit allergy. It is not yet known whether this cosensitization is uniquely relevant to peach-allergic subjects or whether it merely represents a common sensitization pattern.

The molecular basis of pollen-peach cross-reactivity has not yet been identified.

14.6.3 Latex-Fruit Syndrome and the Relevance of the Hevein-Like Domain

In 30–70 % of natural rubber latex-allergic patients, food allergy also occurs. These individuals suffer from latex-fruit syndrome, in which the main causes of allergic symptoms involve banana, kiwi fruit, sweet chestnut, and avocado. Cross-reactivity is chiefly attributed to the major latex allergen, hevein (Hev b 6), and the hevein-like domains (*HLDs*) of the class I chitinases that are present in natural rubber latex (Hev b 11) and various fruits. In a study, Radauer et al. tested the relevance of hevein and HLDs in subjects with natural rubber latex allergy ($n=59$) and in a retrospective investigation of patients with various fruit and vegetable allergies ($n=16{,}408$). The sera were tested in vitro for specific IgE reactions to Hev b 6, Hev b 11, and the HLDs from banana and avocado (Radauer et al. 2011). In accordance with the results of other studies, hevein was identified as the sensitizing allergen for HLD sensitization in various fruits.

No significant correlation has yet been found between sensitization to hevein or HLDs and the occurrence of latex-fruit syndrome.

14.7 Summary and Outlook

In recent years, an increasing number of studies have been carried out in patient groups with food allergies verified by double-blind, placebo-controlled food challenge (DBPCFC), employing molecular diagnostics (Matricardi et al. 2016) to investigate their sensitization patterns. Research conducted on carrot, celery root, and kiwi fruit provides good examples of these. With illustrative reference to kiwi fruit allergy, a marker allergen, Actinidin (Act d 1), has been identified for monosensitization. Act d 1 is the marker allergen that points to more severe symptoms. By contrast, Act d 8 and Act d 9 constitute markers of cross-sensitization to pollen allergies. However, current allergen panels contain gaps that need to be filled through further research. In celery root allergy, for example, the marker allergen for the important celery-mugwort syndrome has not yet been identified. Further, screening of sera can be employed to ascertain the relevance of individual allergens for particular patient groups and defined geographical regions and hence to distinguish between major, intermediate, and minor allergens.

14.8 Conclusion: Potential for Routine Clinical Practice

The pilot studies cited in this chapter have shown how component-resolved analysis of sera can be used to enhance both the sensitivity and specificity of diagnostic tests in patients with food allergy to fruits and vegetables. It is evident that this approach needs to be adopted individually for the most important allergenic foods. Component-resolved diagnostics help to identify marker allergens and determine the potential extent of any cross-reactivity with clinical relevance. This provides definite advantages to patients with food allergies, with respect to both their specific diagnoses and their management, allowing more precisely informed dietary recommendations to avoid allergy-triggering foods while also reducing unnecessary exclusion diets.

References

Aleman A, Sastre J, Quirce S, de las Heras M, Carnes J, Fernandez-Caldas E, Pastor C, Blazquez AB, Vivanco F, Cuesta-Herranz J. Allergy to kiwi: a double-blind, placebo-controlled food challenge study in patients from a birch-free area. J Allergy Clin Immunol. 2004;113:543–50.

Asero R, Antonicelli L, Arena A, Bommarito L, Caruso B, Crivellaro M, De Carli M, Della Torre E, Della Torre F, Heffler E, Lodi Rizzini F, Longo R, Manzotti G, Marcotulli M, Melchiorre A, Minale P, Morandi P, Moreni B, Moschella A, Murzilli F, Nebiolo F, Poppa M, Randazzo S, Rossi G, Senna GE. EpidemAAITO: features of food allergy in Italian adults attending allergy clinics: a multi-centre study. Clin Exp Allergy. 2009;39:547–55.

Ballmer-Weber BK, Vieths S, Luttkopf D, Heuschmann P, Wuthrich B. Celery allergy confirmed by double-blind, placebo-controlled food challenge: a clinical study in 32 subjects with a history of adverse reactions to celery root. J Allergy Clin Immunol. 2000;106:373–8.

Ballmer-Weber BK, Wuthrich B, Wangorsch A, Fotisch K, Altmann F, Vieths S. Carrot allergy: double-blinded, placebo-controlled food challenge and identification of allergens. J Allergy Clin Immunol. 2001;108:301–7.

Ballmer-Weber BK, Wangorsch A, Bohle B, Kaul S, Kundig T, Fotisch K, van Ree R, Vieths S. Component-resolved in vitro diagnosis in carrot allergy: does the use of recombinant carrot allergens improve the reliability of the diagnostic procedure? Clin Exp Allergy. 2005;35:970–8.

Ballmer-Weber BK, Hoffmann-Sommergruber K. Molecular diagnosis of fruit and vegetable allergy. Curr Opin Allergy Clin Immunol. 2011;11:229–35.

Ballmer-Weber BK, Skamstrup Hansen K, Sastre J, Andersson K, Batscher I, Ostling J, Dahl L, Hanschmann KM, Holzhauser T, Poulsen LK, Lidholm J, Vieths S. Component-resolved in vitro diagnosis of carrot allergy in three different regions of Europe. Allergy. 2012;67:758–66.

Bassler OY, Weiss J, Wienkoop S, Lehmann K, Scheler C, Dolle S, Schwarz D, Franken P, George E, Worm M, Weckwerth W. Evidence for novel tomato seed allergens: IgE-reactive legumin and vicilin proteins identified by multidimensional protein fractionation-mass spectrometry and in silico epitope modeling. J Proteome Res. 2009;8:1111–22.

Bauermeister K, Ballmer-Weber BK, Bublin M, Fritsche P, Hanschmann KM, Hoffmann-Sommergruber K, Lidholm J, Oberhuber C, Randow S, Holzhauser T, Vieths S. Assessment of component-resolved in vitro diagnosis of celeriac allergy. J Allergy Clin Immunol. 2009;124:1273–81.

Bernardi ML, Giangrieco I, Camardella L, Ferrara R, Palazzo P, Panico MR, Crescenzo R, Carratore V, Zennaro D, Liso M, Santoro M, Zuzzi S, Tamburrini M, Ciardiello MA, Mari A. Allergenic lipid transfer proteins from plant-derived foods do not immunologically and clinically behave homogeneously: the kiwifruit LTP as a model. PLoS One. 2011;6:e27856.

Brehler R, Theissen U, Mohr C, Luger T. "Latex-fruit syndrome": frequency of cross-reacting IgE antibodies. Allergy. 1997;52:404–10.

Bublin M, Radauer C, Wilson IB, Kraft D, Scheiner O, Breiteneder H, Hoffmann-Sommergruber K. Cross-reactive N-glycans of Api g 5, a high molecular weight glycoprotein allergen from celery, are required for immunoglobulin E binding and activation of effector cells from allergic patients. FASEB J. 2003;17:1697–9.

Bublin M, Mari A, Ebner C, Knulst A, Scheiner O, Hoffmann-Sommergruber K, Breiteneder H, Radauer C. IgE sensitization profiles toward green and gold kiwifruits differ among patients allergic to kiwifruit from 3 European countries. J Allergy Clin Immunol. 2004;114:1169–75.

Bublin M, Pfister M, Radauer C, Oberhuber C, Bulley S, Dewitt AM, Lidholm J, Reese G, Vieths S, Breiteneder H, Hoffmann-Sommergruber K, Ballmer-Weber BK. Component-resolved diagnosis of kiwifruit allergy with purified natural and recombinant kiwifruit allergens. J Allergy Clin Immunol. 2010;125:687–94.

Bublin M, Dennstedt S, Buchegger M, Antonietta Ciardiello M, Bernardi ML, Tuppo L, Harwanegg C, Hafner C, Ebner C, Ballmer-Weber BK, Knulst A, Hoffmann-Sommergruber K, Radauer C, Mari A, Breiteneder H. The performance of a component-based allergen microarray for the diagnosis of kiwifruit allergy. Clin Exp Allergy. 2011;41:129–36.

Burney P, Summers C, Chinn S, Hooper R, van Ree R, Lidholm J. Prevalence and distribution of sensitization to foods in the European Community Respiratory Health Survey: a EuroPrevall analysis. Allergy. 2010;65:1182–8.

Burney PG, Potts J, Kummeling I, Mills EN, Clausen M, Dubakiene R, Barreales L, Fernandez-Perez C, Fernandez-Rivas M, Le TM, Knulst AC, Kowalski ML, Lidholm J, Ballmer-Weber BK, Braun-Fahlander C, Mustakov T, Kralimarkova T, Popov T, Sakellariou A, Papadopoulos NG, Versteeg SA, Zuidmeer L, Akkerdaas JH, Hoffmann-Sommergruber K, van Ree R. The prevalence and distribution of food sensitization in European adults. Allergy. 2014;69:365–71.

Caimmi D, Barber D, Hoffmann-Sommergruber K, Amrane H, Bousquet PJ, Dhivert-Donnadieu H, Demoly P. Understanding the molecular sensitization for Cypress pollen and peach in the Languedoc-Roussillon area. Allergy. 2013;68:249–51.

Ciardiello MA, D'Avino R, Amoresano A, Tuppo L, Carpentieri A, Carratore V, Tamburrini M, Giovane A, Pucci P, Camardella L. The peculiar structural features of kiwi fruit pectin methylesterase: amino acid sequence, oligosaccharides structure, and modeling of the interaction with its natural proteinaceous inhibitor. Proteins. 2008;71:195–206.

Cuesta-Herranz J, Barber D, Blanco C, Cistero-Bahima A, Crespo JF, Fernandez-Rivas M, Fernandez-Sanchez J, Florido JF, Ibanez MD, Rodriguez R, Salcedo G, Garcia BE, Lombardero M, Quiralte J, Rodriguez J, Sanchez-Monge R, Vereda A, Villalba M, Alonso

Diaz de Durana MD, Basagana M, Carrillo T, Fernandez-Nieto M, Tabar AI. Differences among pollen-allergic patients with and without plant food allergy. Int Arch Allergy Immunol. 2010;153:182–92.

D'Avino R, Bernardi ML, Wallner M, Palazzo P, Camardella L, Tuppo L, Alessandri C, Breiteneder H, Ferreira F, Ciardiello MA, Mari A. Kiwifruit Act d 11 is the first member of the ripening-related protein family identified as an allergen. Allergy. 2011;66:870–7.

Eriksson N, Werner S, Foucard T, Möller C, Berg T, Kiviloog J. Self-reportend hypersensitivity to exotic fruit in brich pollen-allergic patients. Allergol Int. 2003;52:199–206.

Fernandez-Rivas M, Gonzalez-Mancebo E, Rodriguez-Perez R, Benito C, Sanchez-Monge R, Salcedo G, Alonso MD, Rosado A, Tejedor MA, Vila C, Casas ML. Clinically relevant peach allergy is related to peach lipid transfer protein, Pru p 3, in the Spanish population. J Allergy Clin Immunol. 2003;112:789–95.

Fernandez-Rivas M, Bolhaar S, Gonzalez-Mancebo E, Asero R, van Leeuwen A, Bohle B, Ma Y, Ebner C, Rigby N, Sancho AI, Miles S, Zuidmeer L, Knulst A, Breiteneder H, Mills C, Hoffmann-Sommergruber K, van Ree R. Apple allergy across Europe: how allergen sensitization profiles determine the clinical expression of allergies to plant foods. J Allergy Clin Immunol. 2006;118:481–8.

Foetisch K, Son DY, Altmann F, Aulepp H, Conti A, Haustein D, Vieths S. Tomato (*Lycopersicon esculentum*) allergens in pollen-allergic patients. Eur Food Res Technol. 2001;213:259–66.

Fujita C, Moriyama T, Ogawa T. Identification of cyclophilin as an IgE-binding protein from carrots. Int Arch Allergy Immunol. 2001;125:44–50.

Gadermaier G, Hauser M, Egger M, Ferrara R, Briza P, Santos KS, Zennaro D, Girbl T, Zuidmeer-Jongejan L, Mari A, Ferreira F. Sensitization prevalence, antibody cross-reactivity and immunogenic peptide profile of Api g 2, the non-specific lipid transfer protein 1 of celery. PLoS One. 2011;6:e24150.

Gaier S, Marsh J, Oberhuber C, Rigby NM, Lovegrove A, Alessandri S, Briza P, Radauer C, Zuidmeer L, van Ree R, Hemmer W, Sancho AI, Mills C, Hoffmann-Sommergruber K, Shewry PR. Purification and structural stability of the peach allergens Pru p 1 and Pru p 3. Mol Nutr Food Res. 2008;52 Suppl 2:S220–9.

Gall H, Kalveram KJ, Forck G, Sterry W. Kiwi fruit allergy: a new birch pollen-associated food allergy. J Allergy Clin Immunol. 1994;94:70–6.

Gao ZS, Yang ZW, Wu SD, Wang HY, Liu ML, Mao WL, Wang J, Gadermaier G, Ferreira F, Zheng M, van Ree R. Peach allergy in China: a dominant role for mugwort pollen lipid transfer protein as a primary sensitizer. J Allergy Clin Immunol. 2013;131(224–226):e221–3.

Gavrovic-Jankulovic M, cIrkovic T, Vuckovic O, Atanaskovic-Markovic M, Petersen A, Gojgic G, Burazer L, Jankov RM. Isolation and biochemical characterization of a thaumatin-like kiwi allergen. J Allergy Clin Immunol. 2002;110:805–10.

Giangrieco I, Alessandri C, Rafaiani C, Santoro M, Zuzzi S, Tuppo L, Tamburrini M, D'Avino R, Ciardiello MA, Mari A. Structural features, IgE binding and preliminary clinical findings of the 7 kDa lipid transfer protein from tomato seeds. Mol Immunol. 2015;66:154–63.

Gonzalez-Mancebo E, Fernandez-Rivas M. Outcome and safety of double-blind, placebo-controlled food challenges in 111 patients sensitized to lipid transfer proteins. J Allergy Clin Immunol. 2008;121:1507–8.

Grozdanovic M, Popovic M, Polovic N, Burazer L, Vuckovic O, Atanaskovic-Markovic M, Lindner B, Petersen A, Gavrovic-Jankulovic M. Evaluation of IgE reactivity of active and thermally inactivated actinidin, a biomarker of kiwifruit allergy. Food Chem Toxicol. 2012;50:1013–8.

Hoffmann-Sommergruber K, O'Riordain G, Ahorn H, Ebner C, Laimer Da Camara Machado M, Puhringer H, Scheiner O, Breiteneder H. Molecular characterization of Dau c 1, the Bet v 1 homologous protein from carrot and its cross-reactivity with Bet v 1 and Api g 1. Clin Exp Allergy. 1999;29:840–7.

Hoffmann-Sommergruber K, Ferris R, Pec M, Radauer C, O'Riordain G, Laimer Da Camara Machado M, Scheiner O, Breiteneder H. Characterization of Api g 1.0201, a new member of the Api g 1 family of celery allergens. Int Arch Allergy Immunol. 2000;122:115–23.

Inschlag C, Hoffmann-Sommergruber K, O'Riordain G, Ahorn H, Ebner C, Scheiner O, Breiteneder H. Biochemical characterization of Pru a 2, a 23-kD thaumatin-like protein representing a potential major allergen in cherry *(Prunus avium)*. Int Arch Allergy Immunol. 1998;116:22–8.

Jenkins JA, Griffiths-Jones S, Shewry PR, Breiteneder H, Mills EN. Structural relatedness of plant food allergens with specific reference to cross-reactive allergens: an in silico analysis. J Allergy Clin Immunol. 2005;115:163–70.

Jensen-Jarolim E, Santner B, Leitner A, Grimm R, Scheiner O, Ebner C, Breiteneder H. Bell peppers (*Capsicum annuum*) express allergens (profilin, pathogenesis-related protein P23 and Bet v 1) depending on the horticultural strain. Int Arch Allergy Immunol. 1998;116:103–9.

Karamloo F, Wangorsch A, Kasahara H, Davin LB, Haustein D, Lewis NG, Vieths S. Phenylcoumaran benzylic ether and isoflavonoid reductases are a new class of cross-reactive allergens in birch pollen, fruits and vegetables. Eur J Biochem. 2001;268:5310–20.

Kummeling I, Mills EN, Clausen M, Dubakiene R, Perez CF, Fernandez-Rivas M, Knulst AC, Kowalski ML, Lidholm J, Le TM, Metzler C, Mustakov T, Popov T, Potts J, van Ree R, Sakellariou A, Tondury B, Tzannis K, Burney P. The EuroPrevall surveys on the prevalence of food allergies in children and adults: background and study methodology. Allergy. 2009;64:1493–7.

Larramendi CH, Ferrer A, Huertas AJ, Garcia-Abujeta JL, Andreu C, Tella R, Cerda MT, Bartra J, Lavin JR, Pagan JA, Lopez-Matas MA, Fernandez-Caldas E, Carnes J. Sensitization to tomato peel and pulp extracts in the Mediterranean Coast of Spain: prevalence and co-sensitization with aeroallergens. Clin Exp Allergy. 2008;38:169–77.

Le LQ, Mahler V, Scheurer S, Foetisch K, Braun Y, Weigand D, Enrique E, Lidholm J, Paulus KE, Sonnewald S, Vieths S, Sonnewald U. Yeast profilin complements profilin deficiency in transgenic tomato fruits and allows development of hypoallergenic tomato fruits. FASEB J. 2010;24:4939–47.

Le TM, Fritsche P, Bublin M, Oberhuber C, Bulley S, van Hoffen E, Ballmer-Weber BK, Knulst AC, Hoffmann-Sommergruber K. Differences in the allergenicity of 6 different kiwifruit cultivars analyzed by prick-to-prick testing, open food challenges, and ELISA. J Allergy Clin Immunol. 2011;127:677–9.

Lidholm J, Ballmer-Weber BK, Mari A, Vieths S. Component-resolved diagnostics in food allergy. Curr Opin Allergy Clin Immunol. 2006;6:234–40.

Matricardi PM, Kleine-Tebbe J, Hoffmann HJ, Valenta R, Hilger C, Hofmaier S, Aalberse RC, Agache I, Asero R, Ballmer-Weber B, Barber D, Beyer K, Biedermann T, Biló MB, Blank S, Bohle B, Bosshard PP, Breiteneder H, Brough HA, Caraballo L, Caubet JC, Crameri R, Davies JM, Douladiris N, Ebisawa M, Eigenmann PA, Fernandez-Rivas M, Ferreira F, Gadermaier G, Glatz M, Hamilton RG, Hawranek T, Hellings P, Hoffmann-Sommergruber K, Jakob T, Jappe U, Jutel M, Kamath SD, Knol EF, Korosec P, Kuehn A, Lack G, Lopata AL, Mäkelä M, Morisset M, Niederberger V, Nowak-Wezgrzyn AH, Papadopoulos NG, Pastorello EA, Pauli G, Platts-Mills T, Posa D, Poulsen LK, Raulf M, Sastre J, Scala E, Schmid JM, Schmid-Grendelmeier P, van Hage M, van Ree R, Vieths S, Weber R, Wickman M, Muraro A, Ollert M. EAACI molecular allergology user's guide. Pediatr Allergy Immunol. 2016;27 Suppl 23:1–250.

Mattila L, Kilpelainen M, Terho EO, Koskenvuo M, Helenius H, Kalimo K. Food hypersensitivity among Finnish university students: association with atopic diseases. Clin Exp Allergy. 2003;33:600–6.

Oberhuber C, Bulley SM, Ballmer-Weber BK, Bublin M, Gaier S, DeWitt AM, Briza P, Hofstetter G, Lidholm J, Vieths S, Hoffmann-Sommergruber K. Characterization of Bet v 1-related allergens from kiwifruit relevant for patients with combined kiwifruit and birch pollen allergy. Mol Nutr Food Res. 2008;52 Suppl 2:S230–40.

Palacin A, Rodriguez J, Blanco C, Lopez-Torrejon G, Sanchez-Monge R, Varela J, Jimenez MA, Cumplido J, Carrillo T, Crespo JF, Salcedo G. Immunoglobulin E recognition patterns to purified Kiwifruit (*Actinidinia deliciosa*) allergens in patients sensitized to Kiwi with different clinical symptoms. Clin Exp Allergy. 2008;38:1220–8.

Palacin A, Tordesillas L, Gamboa P, Sanchez-Monge R, Cuesta-Herranz J, Sanz ML, Barber D, Salcedo G, Diaz-Perales A. Characterization of peach thaumatin-like proteins and their identification as major peach allergens. Clin Exp Allergy. 2010;40:1422–30.

Palacin A, Rivas LA, Gomez-Casado C, Aguirre J, Tordesillas L, Bartra J, Blanco C, Carrillo T, Cuesta-Herranz J, Bonny JA, Flores E, Garcia-Alvarez-Eire MG, Garcia-Nunez I, Fernandez FJ, Gamboa P, Munoz R, Sanchez-Monge R, Torres M, Losada SV, Villalba M, Vega F, Parro V, Blanca M, Salcedo G, Diaz-Perales A. The involvement of thaumatin-like proteins in plant food cross-reactivity: a multicenter study using a specific protein microarray. PLoS One. 2012;7:e44088.

Pascal M, Munoz-Cano R, Reina Z, Palacin A, Vilella R, Picado C, Juan M, Sanchez-Lopez J, Rueda M, Salcedo G, Valero A, Yague J, Bartra J. Lipid transfer protein syndrome: clinical pattern, cofactor effect and profile of molecular sensitization to plant-foods and pollens. Clin Exp Allergy. 2012;42:1529–39.

Pastorello EA, Conti A, Pravettoni V, Farioli L, Rivolta F, Ansaloni R, Ispano M, Incorvaia C, Giuffrida MG, Ortolani C. Identification of actinidin as the major allergen of kiwi fruit. J Allergy Clin Immunol. 1998;101:531–7.

Pravettoni V, Primavesi L, Farioli L, Brenna OV, Pompei C, Conti A, Scibilia J, Piantanida M, Mascheri A, Pastorello EA. Tomato allergy: detection of IgE-binding lipid transfer proteins in tomato derivatives and in fresh tomato peel, pulp, and seeds. J Agric Food Chem. 2009;57:10749–54.

Radauer C, Adhami F, Furtler I, Wagner S, Allwardt D, Scala E, Ebner C, Hafner C, Hemmer W, Mari A, Breiteneder H. Latex-allergic patients sensitized to the major allergen hevein and hevein-like domains of class I chitinases show no increased frequency of latex-associated plant food allergy. Mol Immunol. 2011;48:600–9.

Radauer C, Nandy A, Ferreira F, Goodman RE, Larsen JN, Lidholm J, Pomes A, Raulf-Heimsoth M, Rozynek P, Thomas WR, Breiteneder H. Update of the WHO/IUIS Allergen Nomenclature Database based on analysis of allergen sequences. Allergy. 2014;69:413–9.

Rance F, Grandmottet X, Grandjean H. Prevalence and main characteristics of schoolchildren diagnosed with food allergies in France. Clin Exp Allergy. 2005;35:167–72.

Rodriguez-Perez R, Fernandez-Rivas M, Gonzalez-Mancebo E, Sanchez-Monge R, Diaz-Perales A, Salcedo G. Peach profilin: cloning, heterologous expression and cross-reactivity with Bet v 2. Allergy. 2003;58:635–40.

Sanchez-Lopez J, Asturias JA, Enrique E, Suarez-Cervera M, Bartra J. Cupressus arizonica pollen: a new pollen involved in the lipid transfer protein syndrome? J Investig Allergol Clin Immunol. 2011;21:522–6.

Sanchez-Monge R, Lombardero M, Garcia-Selles FJ, Barber D, Salcedo G. Lipid-transfer proteins are relevant allergens in fruit allergy. J Allergy Clin Immunol. 1999;103(3 Pt 1):514–9.

Scheurer S, Wangorsch A, Haustein D, Vieths S. Cloning of the minor allergen Api g 4 profilin from celery (*Apium graveolens*) and its cross-reactivity with birch pollen profilin Bet v 2. Clin Exp Allergy. 2000;30:962–71.

Steckelbroeck S, Ballmer-Weber BK, Vieths S. Potential, pitfalls, and prospects of food allergy diagnostics with recombinant allergens or synthetic sequential epitopes. J Allergy Clin Immunol. 2008;121:1323–30.

Tamburrini M, Cerasuolo I, Carratore V, Stanziola AA, Zofra S, Romano L, Camardella L, Ciardiello MA. Kiwellin, a novel protein from kiwi fruit. Purification, biochemical characterization and identification as an allergen*. Protein J. 2005;24:423–9.

Toda M, Reese G, Gadermaier G, Schulten V, Lauer I, Egger M, Briza P, Randow S, Wolfheimer S, Kigongo V, Del Mar San Miguel Moncin M, Fotisch K, Bohle B, Vieths S, Scheurer S. Protein unfolding strongly modulates the allergenicity and immunogenicity of Pru p 3, the major peach allergen. J Allergy Clin Immunol. 2011;128:1022–30.

Tuppo L, Giangrieco I, Palazzo P, Bernardi ML, Scala E, Carratore V, Tamburrini M, Mari A, Ciardiello MA. Kiwellin, a modular protein from green and gold kiwi fruits: evidence of in vivo and in vitro processing and IgE binding. J Agric Food Chem. 2008;56:3812–7.

Vejvar E, Himly M, Briza P, Eichhorn S, Ebner C, Hemmer W, Ferreira F, Gadermaier G. Allergenic relevance of nonspecific lipid transfer proteins 2: identification and characterization of Api g 6 from celery tuber as representative of a novel IgE-binding protein family. Mol Nutr Food Res. 2013;57:2061–70.

Zuidmeer L, Goldhahn K, Rona RJ, Gislason D, Madsen C, Summers C, Sodergren E, Dahlstrom J, Lindner T, Sigurdardottir ST, McBride D, Keil T. The prevalence of plant food allergies: a systematic review. J Allergy Clin Immunol. 2008;121:1210–8.

Cow's Milk and Hen's Egg Allergy: What Do Molecular-Based Allergy Diagnostics Have to Offer?

15

I. Reese and L. Lange

15.1 Introduction

Cow's milk and hen's egg (referred to as milk and egg below) are basic foodstuffs in countries with a Western lifestyle. They provide not only numerous macro- and micronutrients. For example, meeting daily calcium requirements, without dairy products, is challenging. However, milk and egg are major elicitors of allergic, sometimes even anaphylactic, reactions in early childhood (Grabenhenrich et al. 2016). In the case of allergy, all foodstuffs containing the respective allergen need to be strictly avoided and replaced with nutritionally adequate substitutes. This type of time-consuming management is only justified in cases where the diagnosis "food allergy" can be made unequivocally. The present chapter discusses the relevance of molecular-based methods in allergy diagnostics and whether, based on this, avoidance of the foods in raw and/or processed form is necessary.

The present chapter is based on, and modified from, an article by the authors that appeared in 2015 in *Allergo Journal International* (Reese I, Lange L. Cow's milk and hen's egg allergy: what do molecular-based allergy diagnostics have to offer? Allergo J Int. 2015;24:312–9).
The authors gratefully thank Dr. Steve Love, PhD, Laguna Niguel, CA, USA, for reading the manuscript, helpful suggestions, and editorial assistance with the English translation.

I. Reese, Dr. oec troph. (✉)
Nutrition Counseling and Therapy with Special Focus on Allergology,
Munich, Germany
e-mail: info@ernaehrung-allergologie.de

L. Lange, MD, Assoc Prof.
St. Marien Hospital, Bonn, Germany

Department of Pediatrics, St. Marien-Hospital, Bonn, Germany

J. Kleine-Tebbe, T. Jakob (eds.), *Molecular Allergy Diagnostics*,
DOI 10.1007/978-3-319-42499-6_15

Sensitization to milk and/or egg is common in early childhood and may be uncovered in testing for general food intolerance. The relevant food only needs to be avoided if symptoms occur. From a treatment perspective, not only allergen avoidance but also appropriate substitution is necessary to ensure a balanced diet in such cases.

15.2 Allergen Nomenclature

Numerous allergens have been identified both in cow's milk and in hen's egg (◉ Tables 15.1 and 15.2) (◉ Figs. 15.1 and 15.2), only a few of which are clinically relevant.

Cow's milk consists of a casein fraction (80 %) and a whey protein fraction (20 %). The latter is removed during cheese manufacture; thus, "Quark" (a German milk product) and cheese contain primarily casein. Individuals allergic to milk are often simultaneously sensitized to several milk allergens; these include primarily casein (Bos d 8) and β-lactoglobulin (Bos d 5), with significantly lower incidence for α-lactalbumin (Bos d 4) and bovine serum albumin (Bos d 6). The casein fraction is made up of four proteins: αS1-casein (Bos d 9), αS2-casein (Bos d 10), β-casein (Bos d 11), and k-casein (Bos d 12) (Hochwallner et al. 2014).

A large number of sensitizations in hen's egg allergy are due to allergens in egg white, in particular ovomucoid (Gal d 1) and ovalbumin (Gal d 2). However, due to

Table 15.1 Important cow's milk allergens

Biochemical name	Allergen name[a]	Concentration (g/l)	Prevalence of sensitization (%)	Thermal stability	Proteolytic stability
α-Lactalbumin	**Bos d 4**[b,c]	1–1.5	0–67	(+)	
β-Lactoglobulin	**Bos d 5**[b,c]	3–4	13–62	–	+
Bovine serum albumin	**Bos d 6**[b,c]	0.1–0.4	0–76	–	
Immunoglobulins	Bos d 7	0.6–1.0	12–36	(+)	
Casein, whole	**Bos d 8**[b,c]	30		+	–
αS1-Casein	Bos d 9	12–15	65–100	+	–
αS2-Casein	Bos d 10	3–4		+	–
β-Casein	Bos d 11	9–11	35–44	+	–
k-Casein	Bos d 12	3–4	35–41	+	–

Modified according to Hochwallner et al. 2014, Jäger et al. 2008
+ high, (+) somewhat, – not at all
[a]Boldface: available for in vitro diagnostics
[b]ImmunoCAP
[c]ImmunoCAP ISAC

Table 15.2 Important hen's egg allergens

Biochemical name	Allergen name[a]	Fraction of whole egg white/egg yolk protein (%)	Thermal stability	Proteolytic stability
Egg white				
Ovomucoid (egg white)	**Gal d 1**[b,c]	11	+	–
Ovalbumin	**Gal d 2**[b,c]	54	–	+
Ovotransferrin (conalbumin)	**Gal d 3**[b,c]	12	–	
Lysozyme	**Gal d 4**[b,c]	3.5	–	?
Serum albumin	**Gal d 5**[c]			
Egg yolk				
α-Livetin	**Gal d 5**[c]	~10		
YGP-42, vitellogenin	Gal d 6			

Modified from Benede et al. (2015), Jäger et al. (2008)
+ stable, – unstable, ? not known.<blank=??>
[a]Boldface: available for in vitro diagnostics
[b]ImmunoCAP
[c]ImmunoCAP ISAC

its widespread use as a bacteriolytic preservative, the minor allergen lysozyme (Gal d 4) is also relevant in nutritional therapy (Benede et al. 2015). In contrast to the classic egg allergy in early childhood, which is to allergens in egg white, the "bird-egg syndrome" described in adulthood is apparently attributable to allergens such as α-livetin (Gal d 5) from egg yolk (Szepfalusi et al. 1994).

Numerous allergens, of which only a handful is clinically relevant, have been identified in cow's milk and hen's egg.

15.3 Properties of the Most Relevant Allergens

15.3.1 Cow's Milk

Casein serves to store and transport calcium and phosphate in milk. It is heat stable and breaks down only at relatively high temperatures. Since caseins are in no way species-specific and are highly conserved from an evolutionary perspective, there is high cross-reactivity with caseins from other animal species. The casein fraction in cow's milk is approximately 30 g/l and consists of 32 % αS1-casein (Bos d 9), 10 % αS2-casein (Bos d 10), 28 % β-casein (Bos d 11), and 10 % k-casein (Bos d 12) (Hochwallner et al. 2014). Reports of tolerance to goat's milk in cow's milk allergy are attributed to the different composition of the casein fraction in goat's milk, as

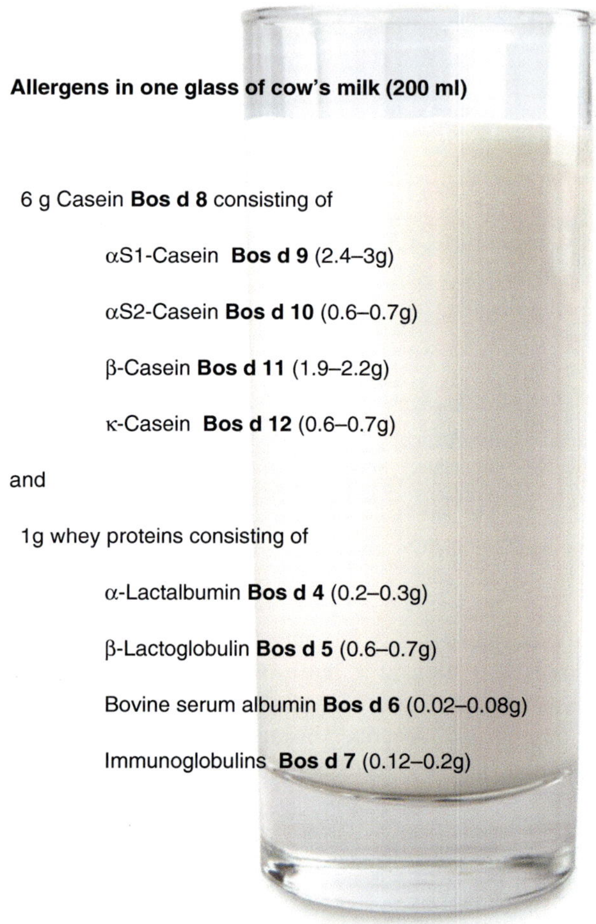

Fig. 15.1 Allergens in a glass of milk (200 ml)

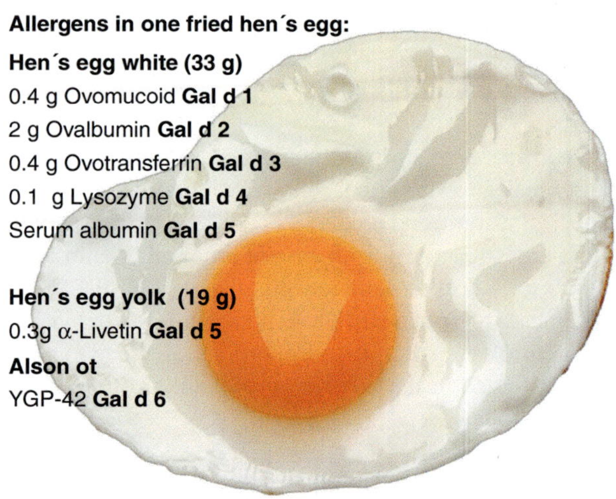

Fig. 15.2 Allergens in a fried egg

well as to β-casein's (Bos d 11) lack of cross-reactivity (Hazebrouck et al. 2014). β-Casein makes up approximately 60 % of the casein fraction in goat's milk. Despite a 91 % sequence homology with β-casein (Bos d 11) from cow, β-casein (Cap h 5) from goat is not (always) recognized as an allergen.

Whey proteins make up 5 g/l of cow's milk, the most important being β-lactoglobulin (Bos d 5) at 3–4 g/l and α-lactalbumin (Bos d 4) at 1–1.5 g/l. Cow's milk contains 0.1–0.4 g/l bovine serum albumin (Bos d 6) and 0.6–1 g/l immunoglobulins (Hochwallner et al. 2014). Whey proteins are even more heat stable than casein. β-Lactoglobulin is the major whey protein in mammalian milk; only in human and rodent milk is it not found. Disulfide bridges confer high proteolytic stability (Hochwallner et al. 2014). Heat treatment improves digestibility, while at the same time reducing allergenicity (Benede et al. 2015). α-Lactalbumin (Bos d 5), a calcium-binding whey protein, plays an important role in the production of lactose. As a subunit of lactose synthase, it was previously considered heat labile (Jäger et al. 2008); however, Hochwallner and coworkers (2010) were able to demonstrate good thermostability, which they attributed to its calcium-binding properties.

Although cross-reactions to bovine meat are rare, the majority of children with bovine meat allergy have a clinically relevant concomitant cow's milk allergy. This is attributed to a clinically relevant allergy to bovine serum albumin (Bos d 6), as this allergen is present in both foods in adequate concentrations (Martelli et al. 2002; Werfel et al. 1997).

> Casein, the most common cow's milk allergen, is largely heat stable and responsible for high serological and clinical cross-reactivity to milk from other mammals.

15.3.2 Hen's Egg

The most important allergens from hen's egg are ovomucoid (Gal d 1), comprising 11 % of egg white proteins, and ovalbumin (Gal d 2), which accounts for 54 % of the total protein.

Ovomucoid (Gal d 1) is a highly soluble glycoprotein that remains in solution and antigenic after boiling for 1 h (Benede et al. 2015; Kato et al. 2000). Its stability is attributed primarily to nine disulfide bridges. When processed together with wheat flour and heated, however, irreversible denaturation takes places, and allergenicity is reduced (Kato et al. 2001). Heating at 180 °C for as little as 10 min results in the formation of insoluble polymerization products (Benede et al. 2015). In processed foods (e.g., muffins), this is referred to as a matrix effect. Furthermore, heat treatment reduces the immunoglobulin E (IgE)-binding capacity of Gal d 1. Although it accounts for only 11 % of egg white protein, it is considered a major allergen in hen's egg (Benede et al. 2015; Benhamou et al. 2010).

Ovalbumin (Gal d 2) is a phosphoglycoprotein that makes up 54 % of egg white protein (Benede et al. 2015; Jäger et al. 2008). It contains only one disulfide bridge and is significantly more heat labile than is Gal d 1. On the other hand, it is partially resistant to pepsin.

Lysozyme (Gal d 4) makes up only 3.5 % of egg white and has four disulfide bridges (Benede et al. 2015). Sensitivity to proteases is controversial (Benede et al. 2015). Although only around 30 % of individuals allergic to egg are sensitized to Gal d 4, lysozyme is relevant due to its widespread use as a bacteriolytic additive (e.g., in cheese) (Marseglia et al. 2013).

Heat-stable ovomucoid is a major allergen in hen's egg. IgE sensitizations to lysozyme may be responsible for reactions following the consumption of products treated with bacteriolytic lysozymes but which do not contain hen's egg itself.

15.3.3 Special Case: Cow's Milk and Hen's Egg in Baked Foods

In 2008, the working group of Nowak-Wegrzyn reported that the majority of children allergic to cow's milk or hen's egg (75 % and 68 %, respectively) tolerated milk or hen's egg in baked goods without any allergic reaction (Lemon-Mule et al. 2008; Nowak-Wegrzyn et al. 2008). The tolerance to these baked products can be attributed to extensive heating or, in eggs, at least to some extent, to the matrix effects described above (Miceli Sopo et al. 2016). Since tolerance of milk and egg in baked products, especially when consumed regularly, leads to a favorable prognosis of the relevant allergy (Kim et al. 2011; Peters et al. 2014), it is assumed that, although allergen recognition still takes place after heating, it is not sufficient to trigger clinical reactions (Benede et al. 2015; Martos et al. 2011).

Hen's egg and cow's milk are often tolerated in baked goods even by individuals with clinically relevant allergy and evidently have a favorable prognosis if consumed regularly.

15.4 Prevalence, Distribution, and Prognosis of Sensitization

Cow's milk and hen's egg allergies are among the most frequent early childhood allergies in Europe and the USA. A meta-analysis by Rona and coworkers (2007) revealed that the self-reported prevalence of cow's milk allergy varied between 1.2 and 17 % and between 0.2 and 7 % for hen's egg allergy. The prevalence of IgE sensitization varied between 2 and 9 % for milk and from less than 1–9 % for egg. In contrast, the prevalence determined by oral challenge was from 0 to 3 % for milk and 0 to 1.7 % for egg.

The latest analyses of the EuroPrevall cohort of 9336 children from nine European countries that were observed for a 2-year period confirms that milk and egg allergy are rarer than previously assumed (Schoemaker et al. 2015; Xepapadaki et al. 2016): milk allergy was confirmed by double-blind, placebo-controlled food challenge in 55 of 358 suspected diagnoses and egg allergy 86 of 298 suspected diagnoses. However, only 172 children with suspected egg allergy were challenged. This puts the incidence of milk allergy proven by provocation at 0.54 % and the incidence of egg allergy proven by challenge at 0.84 %. The adjusted mean incidence of egg allergy was 1.23 % considering possible egg-allergic children within the non-challenged group. However, for both food allergies, there were considerable international differences. While the incidence of milk allergy in the Netherlands and Great Britain was 1 %, less than 0.3 % were affected in Lithuania, Germany, and Greece. No milk-specific IgE was detected in almost 25 % of the children. For egg allergy, the incidence ranged from 2.2 % in Great Britain to 0.07 % in Greece. One year after initial diagnosis, 69 % of milk-allergic individuals tolerated milk and half of the egg-allergic children tolerated egg. Upon reevaluation, milk was tolerated by all subjects with non-IgE-mediated and by 57 % with IgE-mediated milk allergy.

Proven prevalence rates of clinically relevant milk or egg allergy are significantly lower than are self-assessed prevalence rates. Current data from the EuroPrevall cohort indicate significant international differences.

15.4.1 Prognosis

With regard to prognosis, a recent North American prospective study of 293 milk-allergic children revealed that approximately 50 % were no longer allergic by 5 years of age. Moreover, milk-specific IgE of <2 kU_A/l, small skin prick test wheal (<5 mm), and no, or only mild, atopic dermatitis had a favorable effect on prognosis (Wood et al. 2013).

In a German cohort, on the other hand, atopic dermatitis was not a predictor for the persistence of allergy (Ahrens et al. 2012). According to Ahrens and coworkers (2012), cow's milk-specific IgE is a suitable prognostic marker for cow's milk allergy. In their study, analysis of specific IgE (sIgE) to β-lactoglobulin, α-lactalbumin, or casein provided no additional information.

On average, egg allergy persists longer than milk allergy. An additional prospective study conducted by the same North American working group on 213 allergic individuals demonstrated that just under 50 % had become tolerant only after 74 months (Sicherer et al. 2014). Low baseline IgE to hen's egg (<2 kU_A/l) and small skin prick test wheal (<5 mm) were likewise associated with tolerance development. Although the presence of atopic dermatitis had no prognostic value in terms of tolerance in egg-allergic individuals, allergic skin reactions were indeed of prognostic value compared with extracutaneous systemic reactions. Of 24 children that tolerated egg in baked goods, 17 (70 %) exhibited significantly better tolerance development.

In an Australian prospective cohort of 5276 infants, 66 of the 140 (47 %) hen's egg-allergic infants had already developed tolerance by the age of 2 years

(Peters et al. 2014). However, a significantly higher percentage of infants (80 %) tolerated egg in baked form in this study. Tolerance was considerably rarer in infants that did not tolerate egg in baked form compared with those that tolerated baked egg from the outset (13 % vs. 56 %). Moreover, the likelihood of developing complete tolerance increased if baked egg was consumed regularly. Besides allergy to egg in baked goods, both high baseline (>1.7 kU_A/l) and persistently high hen's egg-specific IgE, as well as larger skin prick test wheal (>4 mm) at baseline and during the study course, predicted persistent hen's egg allergy.

> Overall, 50 % of cow's milk- or hen's egg-allergic children develop tolerance by the ages of 5 or 6 years. A small skin prick test wheal and low milk- or egg-specific IgE at diagnosis lead to a more favorable prognosis.

15.5 Diagnostic Methods

15.5.1 Assessing Clinical Relevance

Current German (AWMF S2-type, http://www.awmf.org/en/awmf.html) guidelines on the management of IgE-mediated food allergy emphasize that a clinically relevant allergy can only be conclusively diagnosed "in conjunction with patient history and/or food challenge" (Worm et al. 2015).

The guidelines state the following on diagnostic methods in cow's milk allergy: "Complex sensitization patterns to predominantly stable cow milk proteins and the fact that these are well represented in cow milk extracts are rationales to use the total extract for diagnostic purposes."

Measuring single allergens to hen's egg-specific IgE likewise confers little or no additional benefit in the evaluation of clinically relevant sensitization (Alvaro et al. 2014; Benhamou Senouf et al. 2015). However, a distinction must be made in the assessment of clinical relevance between those patients that do not tolerate egg either in cooked or raw form and those that react only to raw hen's egg. In order to make a differential assessment of this kind, sera from 44 children were analyzed: an egg-specific IgE cutoff value of 1.6 kU_A/l permitted discrimination between children that were only allergic to raw egg, yet tolerated cooked egg, and those who were egg intolerant. However, a distinction between children that did not tolerate egg either in raw or cooked form and egg-tolerant children was only possible with an egg-specific IgE cutoff value of 4.1 kU_A/l (Benhamou Senouf et al. 2015). For better interpretation, the authors recommend combining IgE testing with single allergen measurements—in native and denatured form where possible.

Single allergen measurements can help clarify whether cooked egg is tolerated, since ovalbumin (Gal d 2) is significantly more heat labile than ovomucoid (Gal d 1) (Benhamou Senouf et al. 2015; Alessandri et al. 2012; Vazquez-Ortiz et al. 2014; Haneda et al. 2012; Urisu et al. 1997). An investigation by Alessandri and coworkers (2012) revealed that 44 of 47 Gal d 1-negative patients tolerated cooked egg. Haneda and coworkers (2012) found that the probability of not reacting to cooked egg was 88 % if no IgE to Gal d 1 was detected. Urisu et al. (1997) showed that egg-allergic individuals that had an allergic reaction to cooked egg tolerated cooked egg if Gal d 1 had been previously depleted. In their patients, Vazquez-Ortiz and coworkers (2014) found that a Gal d 1 IgE level of 3.7 kU/l predicted an allergic reaction to cooked egg with a 92 % probability. The study by Benhamou Senouf et al. (2015) also showed that the mean Gal d 1-specific IgE level was <0.35 kU_A/l in hen's egg-intolerant children and 0.67 kU_A/l in children that tolerated cooked egg. For the latter, however, in one child a level of 8.56 kU_A/l was found.

A meta-analysis on the predictive value of skin testing and IgE tests on the prognosis of a food allergy concluded the following (Peters et al. 2013): although casein and lactalbumin have proved to be good prognostic parameters for persistent cow's milk allergy, their reliability is only comparable with that of milk-specific IgE. Thus, determining single allergens is of almost no benefit in routine clinical practice. From the authors' point of view, measuring sIgE to Gal d 1 might be helpful in identifying children with persistent hen's egg allergy.

15.5.2 Assessing Tolerance in Baked Goods

The reliability of single allergen measurements in predicting tolerance to baked milk or baked egg products was comparable to milk- or egg-specific IgE (Lemon-Mule et al. 2008; Nowak-Wegrzyn et al. 2008). There were no significant differences for egg between groups on the basis of Gal d 1-specific IgE levels. Only for values above 50 kU_A/l was it possible to predict a reaction to baked egg products. Nor could any other values be found that were predictive of challenge outcome in individuals allergic to egg—not even a history of anaphylaxis proved to be predictive. The unpredictability of challenge outcome was confirmed by other working groups (Turner et al. 2013, 2014). For milk, on the other hand, the authors recommended two values as decision-making criteria: a level of <5 kU_A/l cow's milk-specific IgE predicted tolerance to heated/baked milk with a 90 % probability. On the other hand, the probability of a reaction to baked milk products was 85 % at a milk-specific IgE level of >35 kU_A/l. No children with milk-specific IgE level of <0.35 kU_A/l or a skin prick test wheal <than 5 mm reacted to milk.

Milk- or egg-specific IgE is sufficient for the diagnosis of the respective allergy, as well as to assess tolerance in baked form. Low or undetectable Gal d 1 increases the likelihood of tolerance to cooked egg. A definitive conclusion on clinical relevance can only be drawn in conjunction with patient history and/or oral food challenge.

15.6 Additional Benefits Conferred by Molecular-Based Allergy Diagnostics

Currently, molecular-based allergy diagnostics yields no advantage—either in terms of diagnosing cow's milk or hen's egg allergy or of predicting whether the allergen will be tolerated in baked form—over classic measurements of milk- or egg-specific IgE using extracts. Measuring Gal d 1 sIgE can help clarify whether cooked egg will be tolerated. However, double-blind, placebo-controlled challenge testing remains the diagnostic gold standard. Although molecular-based allergy diagnostics confers no benefit in terms of prognosis of milk allergy, it may have some utility in the prognosis of egg allergy (Peters et al. 2013).

Measuring sIgE to lysozyme (Gal d 4), an enzyme used as a preservative in cheese, may be of therapeutic relevance. A study of 54 hen's egg-allergic children aged 2–13 years found sensitization to Gal d 4 in 21 by means of blood tests—skin tests were negative in all patients. Oral challenge results with cheese, prepared with or without lysozyme resulted in six severe and three mild reactions in Gal d 4-sensitized children following consumption of lysozyme-containing cheese. None of the children reacted to cheese with no lysozyme content. Severe reactions were associated with a Gal d 4 SIgE level >7 kU_A/l. Three non-sensitized children reacted with mild oral symptoms to lysozyme-containing and two to non-lysozyme-containing cheese. These reactions were attributed to the presence of histamine.

> Molecular-based allergy diagnostics confer no additional benefit over standard methods in milk allergy. They may be helpful in egg allergy to assess whether cooked egg will be tolerated and whether lysozyme-treated products should be avoided.

15.7 Treatment and Recommendations

In the case of proven milk or egg allergy, strict avoidance of these triggers is indicated (Worm et al. 2015). Since milk and egg are used in numerous processed foods, strict avoidance is only possible with a basic knowledge, as well as continual updating on the constituents of these foods. In order to achieve such elaborate management while at the same time ensuring a balanced diet, counseling by a qualified nutritionist is essential. Particularly in cases where milk and milk products must be avoided, the risk of inadequate calcium intake, especially in children, needs to be borne in mind (Nachshon et al. 2014).

Given that milk and egg in baked products are both well tolerated by the majority of children, testing for this type of tolerance is recommended. Tolerance to milk and egg in baked form not only has advantages in terms of food allergy management, it also has a favorable effect on prognosis if these foods are consumed regularly (Kim et al. 2011; Peters et al. 2014). Although open food challenge with these allergens in baked form is possible, challenge should always be performed under medical supervision, given that severe allergic reactions have been described, particularly for hen's egg (Lemon-Mule et al. 2008; Turner et al. 2013).

15.8 Conclusions for Clinical Practice

Determining IgE to single allergens confers no benefit in the diagnostic workup of cow's milk and hen's egg allergy in routine clinical practice compared with the determination of milk- and egg-specific IgE using extracts. It is important, in the interests of young allergic individuals, to unequivocally identify or exclude a clinically relevant allergy. Thereby, the effort and limitations associated with an elimination diet can be restricted to those cases where it is necessary. In terms of ascertaining whether cooked egg is tolerated, measuring sIgE to ovomucoid (Gal d 1) can be useful. Measuring sIgE to Gal d 4 can help to assess whether lysozyme-containing cheese products should be avoided. Early nutrition counseling and supervision substantially reduces the risk of malnutrition. If milk and/or egg are tolerated in baked products, their regular consumption has a favorable prognosis.

References

Ahrens B, Lopes de Oliveira LC, Grabenhenrich L, Schulz G, Niggemann B, Wahn U, et al. Individual cow's milk allergens as prognostic markers for tolerance development? Clin Exp Allergy. 2012;42:1630–7.

Alessandri C, Zennaro D, Scala E, Ferrara R, Bernardi ML, Santoro M, et al. Ovomucoid (Gal d 1) specific IgE detected by microarray system predict tolerability to boiled hen's egg and an increased risk to progress to multiple environmental allergen sensitisation. Clin Exp Allergy. 2012;42:441–50.

Alvaro M, Garcia-Paba MB, Giner MT, Piquer M, Dominguez O, Lozano J, et al. Tolerance to egg proteins in egg-sensitized infants without previous consumption. Allergy. 2014;69:1350–6.

Benede S, Lopez-Exposito I, Molina E, Lopez-Fandino R. Egg proteins as allergens and the effects of the food matrix and processing. Food Funct. 2015;6:694–713.

Benhamou Senouf AH, Borres MP, Eigenmann PA. Native and denatured egg white protein IgE tests discriminate hen's egg allergic from egg-tolerant children. Pediatr Allergy Immunol. 2015;26:12–7.

Benhamou AH, Caubet JC, Eigenmann PA, Nowak-Wegrzyn A, Marcos CP, Reche M, et al. State of the art and new horizons in the diagnosis and management of egg allergy. Allergy. 2010;65:283–9.

Grabenhenrich LB, Dolle S, Moneret-Vautrin A, Kohli A, Lange L, Spindler T, et al. Anaphylaxis in children and adolescents: the European Anaphylaxis Registry. J Allergy Clin Immunol. 2016;137:1128–37.e1.

Haneda Y, Kando N, Yasui M, Kobayashi T, Maeda T, Hino A, et al. Ovomucoids IgE is a better marker than egg white-specific IgE to diagnose boiled egg allergy. J Allergy Clin Immunol. 2012;129:1681–2.

Hazebrouck S, Ah-Leung S, Bidat E, Paty E, Drumare MF, Tilleul S, et al. Goat's milk allergy without cow's milk allergy: suppression of non-cross-reactive epitopes on caprine beta-casein. Clin Exp Allergy. 2014;44:602–10.

Hochwallner H, Schulmeister U, Swoboda I, Focke-Tejkl M, Civaj V, Balic N, et al. Visualization of clustered IgE epitopes on alpha-lactalbumin. J Allergy Clin Immunol. 2010;125:1279–1285.e9.

Hochwallner H, Schulmeister U, Swoboda I, Spitzauer S, Valenta R. Cow's milk allergy: from allergens to new forms of diagnosis, therapy and prevention. Methods. 2014;66:22–33.

Jäger L, Wüthrich B, Ballmer-Weber B, V S. Nahrungsmittelallergien und -intoleranzen. 3rd ed. München: Urban & Fischer; 2008.

Kato Y, Watanabe H, Matsuda T. Ovomucoid rendered insoluble by heating with wheat gluten but not with milk casein. Biosci Biotechnol Biochem. 2000;64:198–201.

Kato Y, Oozawa E, Matsuda T. Decrease in antigenic and allergenic potentials of ovomucoid by heating in the presence of wheat flour: dependence on wheat variety and intermolecular disulfide bridges. J Agric Food Chem. 2001;49:3661–5.

Kim JS, Nowak-Wegrzyn A, Sicherer SH, Noone S, Moshier EL, Sampson HA. Dietary baked milk accelerates the resolution of cow's milk allergy in children. J Allergy Clin Immunol. 2011;128:125–31.

Lemon-Mule H, Sampson HA, Sicherer SH, Shreffler WG, Noone S, Nowak-Wegrzyn A. Immunologic changes in children with egg allergy ingesting extensively heated egg. J Allergy Clin Immunol. 2008;122:977–83.

Marseglia A, Castellazzi AM, Valsecchi C, Licari A, Piva G, Rossi F, et al. Outcome of oral provocation test in egg-sensitive children receiving semi-fat hard cheese Grana Padano PDO (protected designation of origin) containing, or not, lysozyme. Eur J Nutr. 2013;52:877–83.

Martelli A, De Chiara A, Corvo M, Restani P, Fiocchi A. Beef allergy in children with cow's milk allergy; cow's milk allergy in children with beef allergy. Ann Allergy Asthma Immunol. 2002;89:38–43.

Martos G, Lopez-Exposito I, Bencharitiwong R, Berin MC, Nowak-Wegrzyn A. Mechanisms underlying differential food allergy response to heated egg. J Allergy Clin Immunol. 2011;127:990–7.

Miceli Sopo S, Greco M, Cuomo B, Bianchi A, Liotti L, Monaco S, et al. Matrix effect on baked egg tolerance in children with IgE-mediated hen's egg allergy. Pediatr Allergy Immunol. 2016;27(5):465–70.

Nachshon L, Goldberg MR, Schwartz N, Sinai T, Amitzur-Levy R, Elizur A, et al. Decreased bone mineral density in young adult IgE-mediated cow's milk-allergic patients. J Allergy Clin Immunol. 2014;134:1108–13.

Nowak-Wegrzyn A, Bloom KA, Sicherer SH, Shreffler WG, Noone S, Wanich N, et al. Tolerance to extensively heated milk in children with cow's milk allergy. J Allergy Clin Immunol. 2008;122:342–7.

Peters RL, Gurrin LC, Dharmage SC, Koplin JJ, Allen KJ. The natural history of IgE-mediated food allergy: can skin prick tests and serum-specific IgE predict the resolution of food allergy? Int J Environ Res Public Health. 2013;10:5039–61.

Peters RL, Dharmage SC, Gurrin LC, Koplin JJ, Ponsonby AL, Lowe AJ, et al. The natural history and clinical predictors of egg allergy in the first 2 years of life: a prospective, population-based cohort study. J Allergy Clin Immunol. 2014;133:485–91.

Rona RJ, Keil T, Summers C, Gislason D, Zuidmeer L, Sodergren E, et al. The prevalence of food allergy: a meta-analysis. J Allergy Clin Immunol. 2007;120:638–46.

Schoemaker AA, Sprikkelman AB, Grimshaw KE, Roberts G, Grabenhenrich L, Rosenfeld L, et al. Incidence and natural history of challenge-proven cow's milk allergy in European children - EuroPrevall birth cohort. Allergy. 2015;70(8):963–72.

Sicherer SH, Wood RA, Vickery BP, Jones SM, Liu AH, Fleischer DM, et al. The natural history of egg allergy in an observational cohort. J Allergy Clin Immunol. 2014;133:492–9.

Szepfalusi Z, Ebner C, Pandjaitan R, Orlicek F, Scheiner O, Boltz-Nitulescu G, et al. Egg yolk alpha-livetin (chicken serum albumin) is a cross-reactive allergen in the bird-egg syndrome. J Allergy Clin Immunol. 1994;93:932–42.

Turner PJ, Mehr S, Joshi P, Tan J, Wong M, Kakakios A, et al. Safety of food challenges to extensively heated egg in egg-allergic children: a prospective cohort study. Pediatr Allergy Immunol. 2013;24:450–5.

Turner PJ, Kumar K, Fox AT. Skin testing with raw egg does not predict tolerance to baked egg in egg-allergic children. Pediatr Allergy Immunol. 2014;25:657–61.

Urisu A, Ando H, Morita Y, Wada E, Yasaki T, Yamada K, et al. Allergenic activity of heated and ovomucoid-depleted egg white. J Allergy Clin Immunol. 1997;100:171–6.

Vazquez-Ortiz M, Pascal M, Jimenez-Feijoo R, Lozano J, Giner MT, Alsina L, et al. Ovalbumin-specific IgE/IgG4 ratio might improve the prediction of cooked and uncooked egg tolerance development in egg-allergic children. Clin Exp Allergy. 2014;44:579–88.

Werfel SJ, Cooke SK, Sampson HA. Clinical reactivity to beef in children allergic to cow's milk. J Allergy Clin Immunol. 1997;99:293–300.

Wood RA, Sicherer SH, Vickery BP, Jones SM, Liu AH, Fleischer DM, et al. The natural history of milk allergy in an observational cohort. J Allergy Clin Immunol. 2013;131:805–12.

Worm M, Reese I, Ballmer-Weber B, et al. Guidelines on the management of IgE-mediated food allergies: S2k-Guidelines of the German Society for Allergology and Clinical Immunology (DGAKI) in collaboration with other German Medical Societies including the Association of the Scientific Medical Societies in Germany (AWMF). Allergo J Int. 2015;24:256–293.

Xepapadaki P, Fiocchi A, Grabenhenrich L, Roberts G, Grimshaw KE, Fiandor A, et al. Incidence and natural history of hen's egg allergy in the first 2 years of life-the EuroPrevall birth cohort study. Allergy. 2016;71:350–7.

Molecular and Extract-Based Diagnostics in Meat Allergy

16

C. Hilger, W. Hemmer, I. Swoboda, M. Morisset, J. Fischer, A. Tripathi, T. Platts-Mills, and T. Biedermann

16.1 Introduction to Molecular and Extract-Based Diagnostics in Meat Allergy

Meat allergy is increasingly recognized as cause of systemic type I reactions elicited by food. The origin of meat allergy may be manifold. As in other types of food allergy, it can be the result of cross-reactivity following sensitization to aeroallergens as in pork-cat or bird-egg syndrome leading to pork and poultry meat allergy,

C. Hilger, PhD (✉)
Allergology – Immunology – Inflammation Research Unit, Department of Infection and Immunity, Luxembourg Institute of Health, Esch-sur-Alzette, Luxembourg
e-mail: christiane.hilger@lih.lu; http://www.lih.lu/

W. Hemmer, MD, Assoc Prof.
FAZ – Floridsdorf Allergy Center, Vienna, Austria
e-mail: hemmer@faz.at

I. Swoboda, PhD, Prof.
Molecular Biotechnology Section, FH Campus Wien, University of Applied Sciences, Vienna, Austria

M. Morisset, MD
Immunology Allergology Unit, Centre Hospitalier de Luxembourg, Luxembourg, Luxembourg
e-mail: morisset.martine@chl.lu

J. Fischer, MD
Department of Dermatology, University Hospital Tübingen, Tübingen, Germany
e-mail: joerg.fischer@med.uni-tuebingen.de

A. Tripathi, MD • T. Platts-Mills, MD, Assoc Prof.
Division of Allergy, Asthma, & Immunology, Department of Medicine, University of Virginia Health System, Charlottesville, VA, USA
e-mail: AT3JX@hscmail.mcc.virginia.edu; tap2z@virginia.edu

T. Biedermann, MD, Prof.
Department of Dermatology and Allergology, Technical University of Munich, Munich, Germany
e-mail: tilo.biedermann@tum.de

J. Kleine-Tebbe, T. Jakob (eds.), *Molecular Allergy Diagnostics*,
DOI 10.1007/978-3-319-42499-6_16

respectively. Food allergy to milk or egg in children may be associated with simultaneous hypersensitivity to beef and chicken meat due to the concurrent presence of certain allergens in muscle tissue. Heat-stable meat proteins may also directly sensitize via the gastrointestinal tract and constitute genuine meat allergy. For peanut allergy, sensitization via the skin has been recognized as a major axis to establish food allergy. Interestingly, allergy to certain types of red meat and innards seems to be also acquired through the skin, because tick bites lead to IgE antibodies recognizing the carbohydrate side chain galactose-α-1,3-galactose.

This chapter introduces pork-cat syndrome and related syndromes based on cross-reactivity between pet dander and meat, type I reactions to galactose-α-1,3-galactose in red meat allergy with delayed and immediate onset of the symptoms, and the bird-egg syndrome as well as genuine poultry meat allergy. This chapter focuses on type I allergy to different meat types and does not cover: (i) allergic reactions due to other underlying mechanisms such as protein contact dermatitis or atopic dermatitis and (ii) allergic reactions to fish and seafood. Special emphasis is given to the allergens eliciting IgE-mediated reactions to meat and the diagnostic measures necessary to elucidate the underlying cause of this type I allergy. Extract-based skin and in vitro tests using meat of different sources can provide a first hint to establish a diagnosis. In the case of cross-reactivity with birds or pets, the respective extracts are used as circumstantial evidence to support the diagnosis. Molecular diagnostics will confirm or draw attention to the suspected diagnosis. Available tests are already well established in patient management, but tests utilizing additional single allergens are necessary for a complete workup of patients with suspected type I allergy to meat.

16.2 Pork-Cat Syndrome, a Link Between Pet Dander and Meat

16.2.1 Allergen Structure and Function

Serum albumins (SAs) are large, globular, non-glycosylated proteins with a molecular weight of 65–69 kDa. They are α-helical proteins composed of three flexible and structurally similar domains arranged into a heart-shaped form and stabilized by disulfide bridges. The crystal structures of bovine (Bos d 6) and horse (Equ c 3) SA have been resolved. The proteins are thermolabile – they unfold at temperatures above 50 °C and are easily denatured by cooking (Chruszcz et al. 2013).

Mammalian SAs have high sequence identities (72–82 %) relative to human SA. In comparison, avian serum albumins show only a moderate sequence identity (46–49 %) to human SA and to other mammalian SAs (42–48 %) (Chruszcz et al. 2013). Chicken SA, Gal d 5, formerly called α-livetin, is an allergen of egg yolk. Albumins are synthesized in the liver. They are abundant in plasma and contribute to the regulation of colloid osmotic pressure. They also transport a multitude of metabolites, nutrients, drugs, and other molecules. Currently, seven allergens are recognized by the IUIS Allergen Nomenclature Sub-committee: Bos d 6 (bovine), Can f 3 (dog), Cav p 4 (guinea pig), Equ c 3 (horse), Fel d 2 (cat), Gal d 5 (chicken), and Sus s 1 (pig). But SAs from a number of additional mammals were shown to bind IgE: sheep, goat, rabbit, hamster, and other mammals (Spitzauer et al. 1995).

16.2.2 Allergen Prevalence and Sensitization

Animal SAs are respiratory and food allergens as they are present in dander, milk, meat, and eggs. Mostly, contact with dander represents the primary event in the development of the IgE cross-reaction to SA. Up to 30 % of patients allergic to animal dander exhibited IgE antibodies reactive toward serum albumins (Spitzauer et al. 1995).

Serum albumins present in animal dander are considered allergens of low clinical relevance. However, there are some case reports of occupational asthma triggered by Bos d 6 [bovine serum albumin (BSA)] in laboratory workers (Choi et al. 2009; Voltolini et al. 2013). In contrast to its role as a respiratory allergen, Bos d 6 is known to elicit mild to severe symptoms as a food allergen. According to Werfel, beef allergy is present in 20 % of young children, especially those suffering from atopic dermatitis and cow's milk allergy (Werfel et al. 1997). In these children, the primary sensitizing source is mostly cow's milk, where Bos d 4 (alpha-lactalbumin), Bos d 5 (beta-lactoglobulin), and Bos d 8 (caseins) are the major allergens and Bos d 6 is a minor allergen. The symptoms with ingestion of beef are often mild and disappear naturally during the first 3 years of life, before resolution of cow's milk allergy (Martelli et al. 2002).

Bos d 6 is widely used in biochemical and immunological assays as well as in cell culture media. Several case reports have shown that, as an ingredient of the culture medium of spermatozoids, it has provoked severe anaphylactic reactions upon artificial insemination (Liccardi et al. 2011).

Cat SA (Fel d 2) and dog SA (Can f 3) are classified as intermediate allergens, with IgE antibodies present in up to 23 % of patients sensitized to cat (Hilger et al. 1997) and 35 % of those sensitized to dog dander (Spitzauer et al. 1994). Conversely, dogs may develop allergic manifestations involving IgE sensitization to human SA (Adamantos et al. 2009). The first clinical cases of cross-reactivity between mammalian meat SA and dander have been reported by Sabbah and Drouet in the 1990s in France with the "pork-cat syndrome" (Drouet and Sabbah 1996). The same authors subsequently published a fatal case after wild boar meat ingestion and stressed the role of cofactors, such as exercise or alcohol intake, which may contribute to the severity of the reaction (Drouet et al. 2001). The term pork-cat syndrome is somewhat misleading as the cat is the primary sensitization source. It would be preferable to redefine this syndrome as "cat-pork."

Hilger et al. analyzed two groups of cat-allergic patients: in a first group of patients with specific IgE to cat dander and a positive skin prick test to cat ($n=37$), 14 % had specific IgE to Fel d 2, and 2.7 % had IgE to porcine SA; in a second group of highly sensitized patients ($n=39$), 23 % were positive for Fel d 2, and 10.2 % had specific IgE to porcine SA. One out of three patients with specific IgE to porcine SA experienced clinical symptoms upon ingestion of pork meat (Hilger et al. 1997). Based on these data, it can be assumed that in highly sensitized cat-allergic patients, up to 3 % might experience clinical symptoms upon ingestion of raw pork such as ham and sausages. Inhibition experiments performed with cat SA and porcine SA demonstrated that sensitization to cat SA represents the primary event in the development of cross-reactive IgE. IgE antibodies directed against porcine SA could be completely inhibited by addition of cat SA. The pork-cat syndrome was nearly forgotten until eight new cases were reported in the United States by the team of Platts-Mills (Posthumus et al. 2013), and since awareness of delayed food anaphylaxis to red meat has increased.

The IgE cross-reactivity between Sus s 1 and Fel d 2 is the best-known association between animal dander and meat. However, due to the high sequence homology between mammalian SAs, clinically relevant cross-reactions occur also between other meat and dander SAs. Asero et al. have published the observation of a 16-year-old girl presenting with rhinoconjunctivitis to horse dander who later developed oropharyngeal pruritus after pork ingestion due to a cross-reactivity between the horse and porcine SAs (Asero et al. 1997). Another case of horse meat allergy was attributed to a cross-reactivity with hamster SA despite the fact that the RAST inhibitions have shown moderate inhibition below 30 %, using hamster epithelium or horse meat extract as inhibitor phase (Cisteró-Bahíma et al. 2003). Cross-reactivity between horse meat and horse epithelium has been documented in a case of horse meat anaphylaxis (Restani et al. 2009). Sequential allergy to pork and then to chicken has been reported in a patient employed in the pork processing industry (Hilger et al. 2010). Porcine and chicken SA as well as hemoglobin could be identified as cross-reactive allergens to which IgE are produced. An association between dog and beef has been shown in a dog-allergic cook experiencing cutaneous and respiratory symptoms when exposed to raw beef (San-Juan et al. 2005). He tolerated the ingestion of cooked beef.

We have recently reported anaphylaxis to horse meat in a female patient presenting with asthma in the presence of dogs (Morisset et al. 2016). Prick tests to aeroallergens were positive for pet dander and prick-to-prick tests were positive to all meats except poultry. The prick-to-prick test with cooked red meat resulted in a reduced wheal size. Specific IgE were strongly positive for dog dander and dog SA (Can f 3) and negative for α-Gal. IgE inhibition experiments confirmed a primary sensitization to Can f 3 and an IgE cross-reactivity to Equ c 3 (◉ Fig. 16.1). The patient was examined again 2 years after separating from her dog. Her asthma and rhinitis symptoms had resolved since she separated from her dog. She only reported symptoms during unanticipated exposure to dogs or cats. Specific IgE to mammalian SA were markedly decreased. She was still afraid to eat mammalian meat, but she tolerated fish and poultry without development of symptoms.

16.2.3 Diagnosis and Recommendations

Pork-cat syndrome has to be differentiated from the α-Gal syndrome. The most important clinical criterion is the onset of reaction: reactions to meat SAs are not delayed, but begin within 30–45 min after consumption. When meat allergy is suspected, specific IgE to pork, beef, porcine and beef SA as well as α-Gal should be quantified. Even low titers of specific IgE to porcine SA can lead to severe anaphylactic symptoms. A careful record of the clinical history will allow determination of potential primary sensitization to pets.

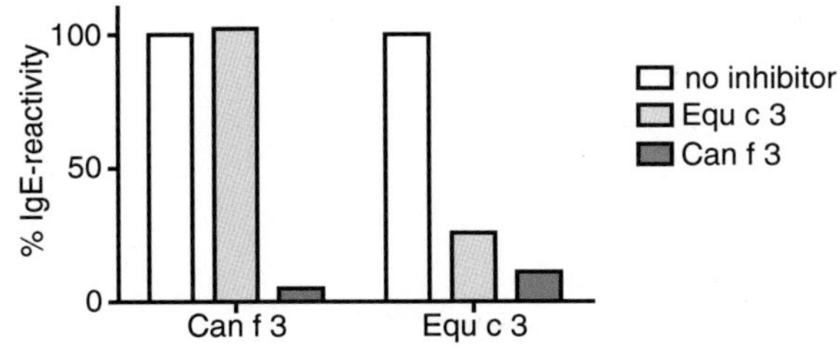

Fig. 16.1 ELISA inhibition assay. IgE reactivity to Can f 3 and Equ c 3 is monitored in the presence or absence of inhibitor. IgE reactivity to Can f 3 could not be inhibited by Equ c 3. In the reverse experiment, IgE reactivity to Equ c 3 could be largely inhibited by Can f 3

Pork-cat syndrome is certainly the most frequent cause of clinical cross-reactivity between mammalian meat and dander. Additional cases have been described for dog/hamster dander with horse meat and for horse dander with pork meat. As all mammalian SAs exhibit extensive amino acid homology, additional cases of clinically relevant cross-reactivity between different animal danders and meats are likely to be described in the future.

Sus s 1 and Fel d 2 have 79 % amino acid identity (◉ Fig. 16.2a) and Equ c 3 and Can f 3 have 76 % identity (◉ Fig. 16.2b). Amino acid sequence homology between SAs of cat and dog and SAs of pork, beef, and horse ranges between 74 % and 79 %. However, no clinical cross-reactivity between proteins of certain dander/meat combinations such as dog/pork, horse/beef, or cat/horse has yet been reported. Despite high overall sequence homology, there may be fewer identical conformational epitopes between, for example, Can f 3 and Sus s 1 than between Fel d 2 and Sus s 1.

Patients allergic to SAs react to raw or medium rare meat, but the majority tolerate boiled milk and well-cooked meat – as albumins are thermolabile proteins. In patients with pork-cat syndrome, reactivity to Bos d 6 is often variable (Hilger et al. 1997; Posthumus et al. 2013). Some patients are able to consume beef, whereas others cannot do so without developing symptoms. Avoidance of beef should not be recommended if patients report tolerating beef. Continued exposure to the sensitizing pet seems to be an important trigger for maintaining the sensitization to mammalian meat.

The use of Bos d 6 in culture medium used for in vitro fertilization may put women at risk that are highly sensitized to animal dander. Quantification of specific IgE to Bos d 6 or a skin test with medium is recommended.

16.3 Type I Hypersensitivity Reactions to Galactose-α-1,3-Galactose in Red Meat Allergy

16.3.1 Carbohydrate Side Chain Galactose-α-1,3-Galactose (α-Gal)

Carbohydrate side chains are often attached to proteins or lipids, and this attachment is referred to as glycosylation. Glycosylation increases the stability of proteins by protecting them from degradation processes, assures functioning by correct protein structure folding, and determines ligand binding to receptors (Schnaar 2015). The importance of certain glycans for the development of both Th2 immunity and IgE antibodies became apparent in research investigating immune defense against

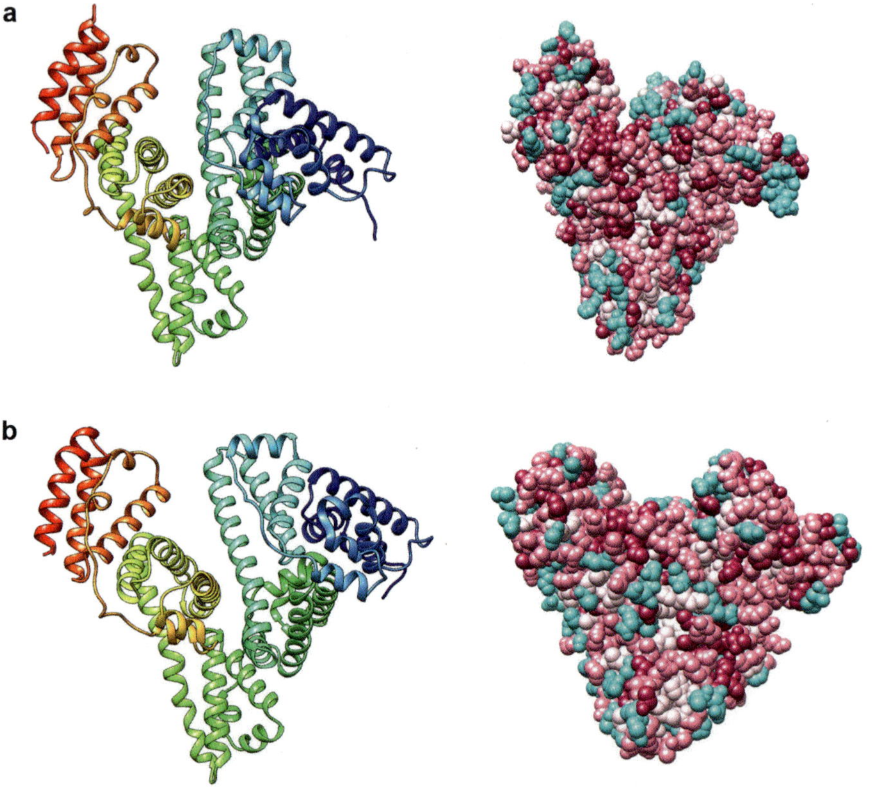

Fig. 16.2 Structures and surface comparisons between cross-reactive serum albumins. (**a**) Ribbon model of the three-dimensional structure of Fel d 2 and its surface representation, colored by sequence conservation with Sus s 1. (**b**) Ribbon model of the three-dimensional structure of Can f 3 and its surface representation, colored by sequence conservation with Equ c 3. In the surface representation, the highly variable sequences are colored as deep blue, the average is in *white*, and the conserved sequences are denoted in deep *red*

helminths. Helminths are known to be strong inducers of Th2- and IgE-dominated immune responses, and the relevance of IgE antibodies binding fucose- and xylose-containing carbohydrate side chains has been well documented (Okano et al. 2001; Faveeuw et al. 2003). In contrast, IgE binding to carbohydrate side chains in type I allergy was long classified as purely nonspecific and additionally as "cross-reactive," explicit in the term "cross-reactive carbohydrate determinants" (CCDs; see also Chap. 6 by U. Jappe). However, CCD-reactive IgE antibodies specifically bind to fucose-α-1,3, linked to N-glycans, and xylose (Wilson and Altmann 1998), both of which are epitopes identical to or very similar to the N-glycan structures that are relevant to recognition of helminths (Okano et al. 2001; Faveeuw et al. 2003). In contrast to CCD epitopes present on proteins from plants and insects, the glycan portion of glycoproteins in mammals was long classified as non-immunogenic. However, attempts to develop xenotransplantation for humans clearly showed that

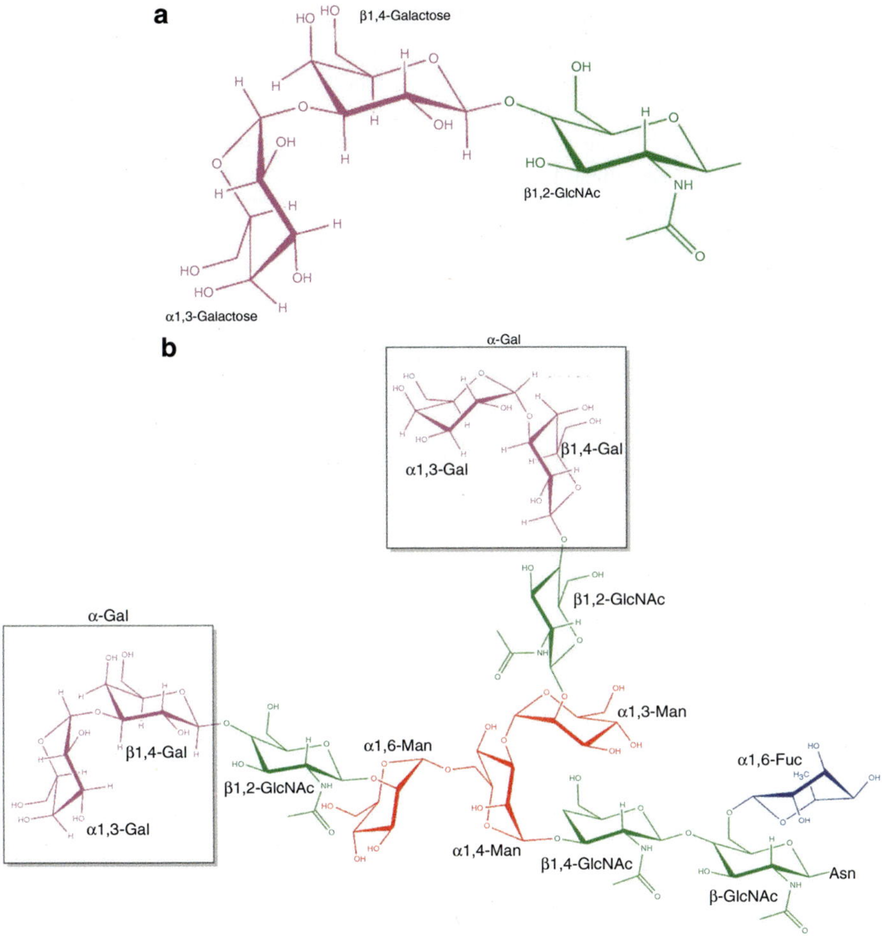

Fig. 16.3 Structure of galactose-α-1,3-galactose (α-Gal). The α-Gal epitope (**a**) is part of an N-glycan and (**b**) is present on mammalian proteins (non-primates, prosimians, and New World monkeys), but is not, however, present on human and Old World monkey proteins. As a result, α-Gal is immunogenic for humans and causes the production of specific IgG and sometimes also IgE antibodies. Although the α-Gal epitope is found on a variety of proteins, it is recognized by specific antibodies independent of the protein backbone. The gene that codes the enzyme necessary for the production of the α-Gal epitope, α-1,3-galactosyltransferase (β-galactosyl-α-1,3-galactosyltransferase), was inactivated in humans over the course of evolution by multiple mutations. *Asn* asparagine, *Fuc* fucose, *Gal* galactose, *GlcNac* N-acetylglucosamine, *Man* mannose (Figure reproduced with the kind permission from M. Schneider and Dr. S. Blank, Munich)

antibodies to carbohydrate side chains also occur in humans and other mammals. It was possible to show that preexisting antibodies that bind saccharide epitopes trigger acute immune responses to grafts in humans or Old World primates ("IgG-type xeno-reactive natural antibodies"). These IgG antibodies bind to galactose-α-1,3-galactose (α-Gal) (Galili et al. 1984) (◉ Fig. 16.3). Over the course of evolution, the terminal amino acid sequence of galactosyltransferase was lost in Old World monkeys due to mutation (Koike et al. 2002), and this glycan portion of mammalian glycoproteins became immunogenic for humans and Old World monkeys. These antibodies binding α-Gal are already present prior to exposure to the graft (Galili 2013). This means that the graft rejection mediated by these antibodies does not require a sensitization phase to the graft. Thus, it is assumed that IgG antibodies against α-Gal are induced early on in childhood, possibly as a result of contact with commensal microorganisms (Galili et al. 1988). α-Gal epitopes are also found on a variety of pathogens, such as viruses, bacteria, and protozoa (Almeida et al. 1991). Consequently, approximately 1 % of human B-lymphocytes produce IgM, IgG, and IgA antibodies that bind α-Gal epitopes with approximately 1 % of all immunoglobulins being directed against α-Gal (Galili et al. 1984; Galili et al. 1993).

16.3.2 Type I Allergy to α-Gal and the Role of Tick Bites

In contrast to IgG antibodies to α-Gal, IgE antibodies were discovered only recently. Primary anaphylaxis after initial administration of the anti-epidermal growth factor (EGF) receptor antibody cetuximab, a chimeric antibody first produced in mouse and then genetically humanized ("-imab"), was first observed in the Southeastern United States (Chung et al. 2008). The variable region specific for the EGF receptor is of murine origin and exhibits the α-Gal epitope (◉ Fig. 16.3). Patients with primary anaphylaxis to cetuximab had preformed IgE antibodies to these α-Gal-bearing glycoproteins. In 2009, the group of Platts-Mills described 24 patients with very particular histories: all patients exhibited urticaria, urticaria with angioedema, or anaphylaxis generally 3–6 h following ingestion of red meat. Of these patients, 10 described reactions following milk consumption. Further investigations detected specific IgE antibodies to α-Gal in all 24 patients (Commins et al. 2009). Although originally also described in the Southeastern United States, this clinical picture was then observed in many other countries around the world. Patients who developed immediate-type allergic symptoms to the regional specialty, "sauteed kidneys," had already attracted attention in Europe in the past (Biedermann and Röcken 2012; Morisset et al. 2012). Abnormalities had been observed in these patients even before the association with presence of IgE antibodies to α-Gal had been made: many of these patients reacted to ingestion of pork kidney, but tolerated ingestion of muscle meat (◉ Fig. 16.4). The patients that reacted to pork kidney exhibited skin test reactions in prick-to-prick testing, as well as in intradermal testing with extracts for beef or pork that were still available at that time; they also showed specific IgE antibodies to milk, cat, beef, and pork (Biedermann and Röcken 2012; Fischer et al. 2015). Investigations then revealed that these patients all had IgE antibodies to α-Gal. Twenty-five patients from Southern Germany were recently characterized in more detail: all of them reported a type I allergic reaction to pork innards. In total, 72 % of patients exhibited anaphylaxis, and 28 % exhibited urticaria with or without angioedema. Cofactors, such as exercise or ingestion of alcohol or ASA (acetylsalicylic acid), relevant to the onset of anaphylaxis were identified as having been

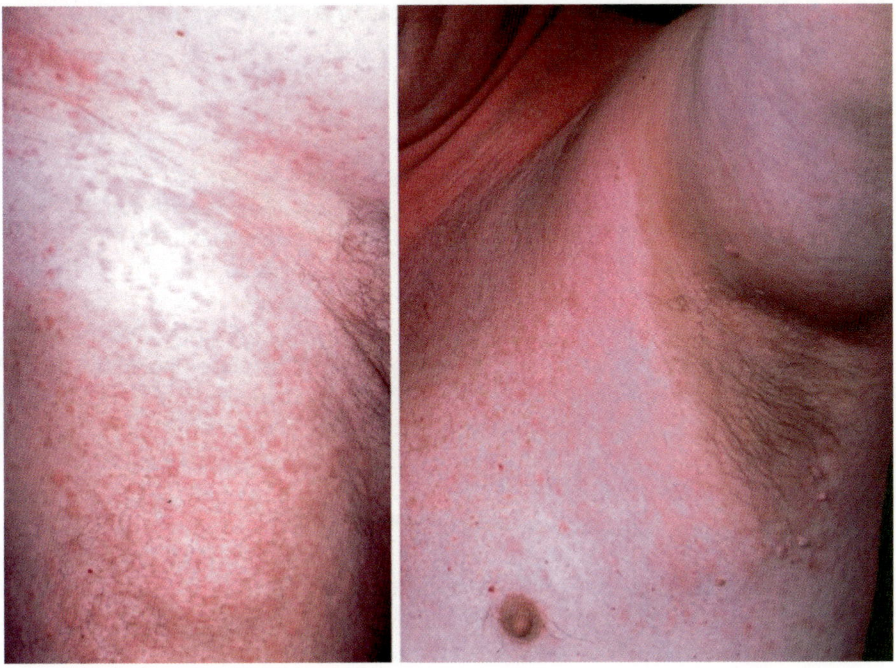

Fig. 16.4 Delayed skin symptoms of immediate-type allergy (From Biedermann and Röcken 2012)

present around the time of the reactions in over 80 % of the patients from their histories. Allergic reactions to other meat-containing foods, or even to gelatin-containing foods, were additionally described in over 50 % of the patients. Interestingly, besides the classic delayed type I hypersensitivity reactions, some of these patients also had immediate type I reactions (occurring within less than 3 hours after ingestion). Since the ingestion of pork kidneys primarily led to the short reaction times in these patients, it is assumed that pork kidney and other innards either contain or express more α-Gal epitopes (Fischer et al. 2014). Two cell membrane-bound peptidases were recently identified in pork kidney as α-Gal-carrying proteins (Hilger et al. 2016). Clinical relevance was confirmed by skin prick testing and basophil activation test. The clinical picture of type I allergy to red meat and innards, either of delayed or immediate onset, has since been diagnosed at numerous other centers worldwide (Tripathi et al. 2014). Precisely how and why this rare induction of IgE antibodies to α-Gal occurs is yet unclear. However, studies showed early on that tick bites could play a role (Commins et al. 2011). Indeed, primary anaphylaxis to the biologic agent cetuximab occurred primarily in individuals exposed to tick bites in the Southeastern United States. Furthermore, a Swedish working group successfully identified α-Gal-expressing proteins in ticks' intestine (Hamsten et al. 2013). Thus, it is assumed today that ticks are able to induce sensitization to the α-Gal epitope via the skin and, furthermore, provide the signals that can cause a switch to IgE production specific to α-Gal.

16.3.3 Diagnostic Measures in Delayed Type I Hypersensitivity Reactions to Red Meat and Innards

It was found that commercial skin prick test extracts have very low sensitivity in α-Gal-allergic patients. This applies to skin prick test extracts for pork, beef, lamb, and horse meat. On the other hand, prick-to-prick tests proved to be of diagnostic use. The use of pork or beef kidney in particular proved to be sensitive in the prick-to-prick test (◉ Fig. 16.5) and was more sensitive compared to muscle meat from a variety of other species. Although intradermal tests were significantly more sensitive, they are not available in many countries due to the tightening of regulations governing the marketing authorization of test extracts (Fischer et al. 2015). Cetuximab was long used as a test reagent and was also applied in intradermal testing. However, the required concentration of cetuximab was high, or the quantity of α-Gal needed to trigger degranulation in this medication was (too) low. It later became apparent that the gelatin-derived colloid, Gelafundin (a volume plasma expander), also caused anaphylaxis in patients with IgE antibodies to α-Gal (Mullins et al. 2012). Thus, this preparation was also deemed an alternative for intradermal testing. Sensitivity to Gelafundin in α-Gal-allergic patients is approximately 85 % (Fischer et al. 2014). The basophil activation test is also a suitable method to detect sensitization and α-Gal-rich proteins, as found in pork kidney extracts. The first commercially available test system for α-Gal-specific IgE antibodies uses purified bovine thyroglobulin, which naturally contains abundant α-Gal epitopes. Coupled to the ImmunoCAP solid phase system, this test has been available for routine diagnostic purposes since 2015 and helps to identify the cause of anaphylaxis in an increasing number of patients.

16.3.4 Clinical Relevance and Particular Features of Delayed Type I Hypersensitivity Reactions to Red Meat and Innards

Sensitization with IgE antibodies to α-Gal is more frequent in atopic compared with nonatopic individuals (Gonzalez-Quintela et al. 2014). From our own observations, it can be assumed that less than 10 % of patients sensitized to α-Gal (IgE) develop symptoms following the consumption of red meat or innards. With regard to the onset of symptoms and provocation testing, it should be pointed out that symptoms are more readily triggered by ingestion of pork kidney, possibly in conjunction with cofactors, compared with ingestion of muscle meat in the absence of cofactors (Fischer et al. 2014). The latter is also responsible for the considerable variation in the severity of reactions triggered by α-Gal-containing foods (Commins et al. 2014). Furthermore, the severity of reactions depends on the characteristics of the foodstuffs and their preparation. Raw meat is more hazardous compared with cured or cooked meat, indicating that at least some α-Gal-carrying proteins are degraded by "heat." In addition, innards such as pork kidney are more prone to elicit reactions compared with muscle meat. Of note, the severity of reactions varies considerably within individuals, and it is not possible to correlate the severity of the reaction with IgE antibody titers or with other predictive parameters. Some highly sensitized patients even react to gelatin-containing foods such as wine gums (Caponetto et al.

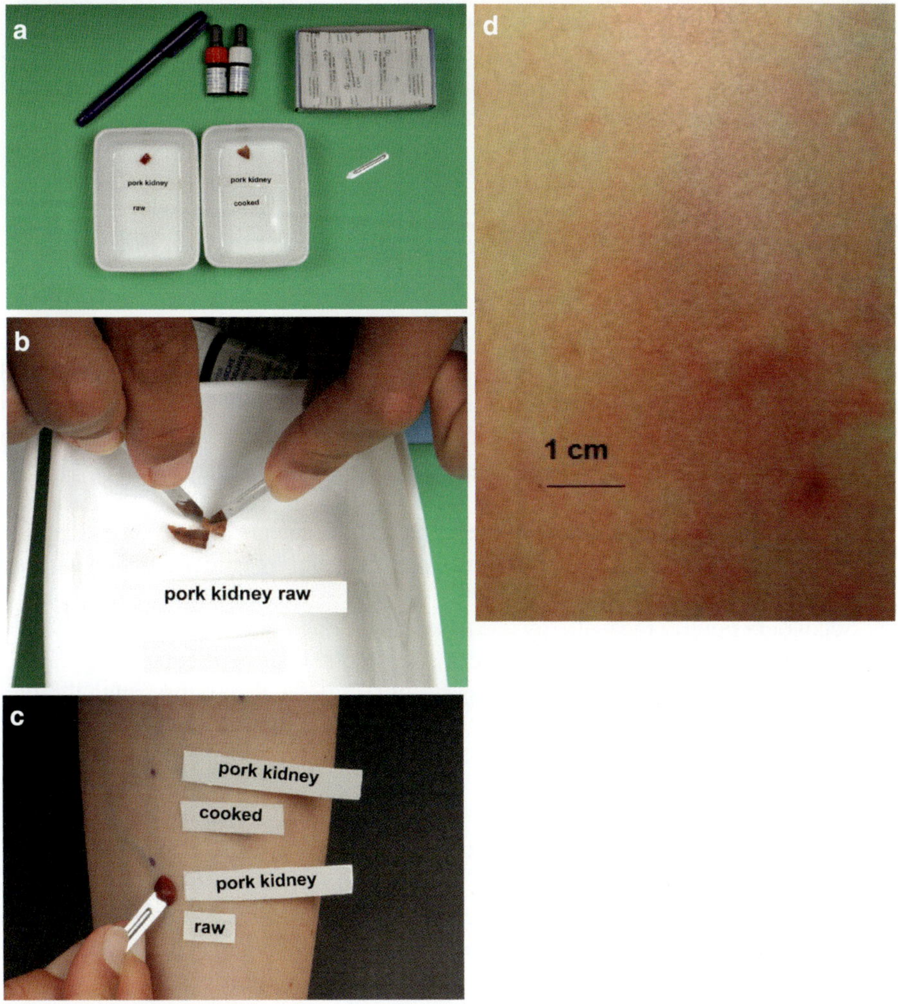

Fig. 16.5 (**a–d**) Prick-to-prick test with pork kidney. Skin prick tests for detection of type I sensitization to α-Gal is sensitive with prick-to-prick test using freshly prepared pork kidney (a, b). The use of raw pork kidney in particular is shown to be more sensitive than cooked pork kidney (c, d) and is more sensitive compared to muscle meat from a variety of other species

2013). As in other immediate-type allergies, α-Gal-sensitized patients with mastocytosis are also at higher risk of developing severe reactions following the consumption of foods containing only small amounts of α-Gal (Roenneberg et al. 2015).

Patients should also be informed that some medications could be hazardous to them. This of course applies most particularly to the anti-EGF receptor antibody, cetuximab. An alternative, panitumumab, also an anti-EGF receptor antibody, is now available – in contrast to "-imab" preparations," "-umab" preparations are fully human and have no α-Gal-containing glycoproteins (Caponetto et al. 2015). The gelatin-derived colloid, Gelafundin, can also cause severe anaphylactic reactions in α-Gal-allergic patients (Mullins et al. 2012). Thus, for the clarification of intraoperative anaphylaxis, testing of volume substitutes should always be included as well as testing for IgE antibodies to α-Gal. It is possible that other critical α-Gal-containing drugs or medical devices may be identified as relevant sources of α-Gal in the future – as anaphylaxis after implantation of biological heart valves in α-Gal IgE-positive patients was recently reported (Mozzicato et al. 2014).

16.4 Bird-Egg Syndrome and Genuine Poultry Meat Allergy

16.4.1 Types of Poultry Meat Allergy

Though in some cases there may be an immunologic link between poultry meat and red meat allergy, hypersensitivities to avian or mammalian meat are almost always distinct from each other. Poultry meat allergy can be further subdivided into two types, differing in sensitization routes and responsible allergens:

1. Primary (genuine) poultry meat allergy as a consequence of active sensitization to heat-resistant meat allergens most likely via the intestinal mucosa with no causal relationship to egg allergy.
2. Secondary poultry meat allergy due to sensitization to serum albumin and closely associated with simultaneous allergy to hen's egg, particularly egg yolk. Sensitization to serum albumins may occur (i) via the respiratory route through exposure to bird feathers (bird-egg syndrome) or alternatively (ii) through primary sensitization to egg yolk (egg-bird syndrome).

16.4.2 Allergen Structure and Function

Poultry meat allergens have not yet been studied in great detail. The responsible allergen in the bird-egg syndrome has been identified as serum albumin (Mandallaz et al. 1988; Szépfalusi et al. 1994; Quirce et al. 2001; Villas et al. 2009). Serum albumins are highly cross-reactive proteins conserved in amino acid sequence and protein structure with a molecular weight around 70 kDa. Chicken serum albumin (Gal d 5) can be found in all tissues, including muscle tissue, and is present in high amounts in egg yolk (α-livetin) as well. Sequence identity between avian and mammalian serum albumins is only moderate (42–49 %), and thus cross-reactivity between them is uncommon.

Allergens involved in genuine allergy to poultry meat are still poorly characterized. Studies identified major IgE-reactive proteins within the low molecular weight (LMW) range between 5 and 25 kDa (Liccardi et al. 1997; Cahen et al. 1998; Kelso et al. 1999). Studies using sera from sensitized patients also demonstrated strong cross-reactivity between LMW allergens from extracts from chicken and turkey meat (Cahen et al. 1998). Muscle α-parvalbumin was the first protein identified as a relevant allergen from chicken meat in a single patient (Kuehn et al. 2009). The patient's IgE also bound to α-parvalbumins from turkey, cow, horse, and frog suggesting cross-reactivity between the α-parvalbumins from all of these species. No reactivity was yet observed with β-parvalbumins, the major allergens in fish. A subsequent case study confirmed α-parvalbumin as a relevant allergen from chicken meat and, in addition, identified muscle myosin light chain (MLC)-1 as another candidate allergen (González-Mancebo et al. 2011).

MLCs were recently confirmed as major allergens from chicken meat in a large population of patients allergic to chicken meat (Klug et al. 2015; Hemmer et al. 2016). MLCs together with myosin heavy chains make up the subunits of the motor protein myosin (Crow et al. 1983), which, in concert with actin, triggers contraction of muscle fibers. MLCs are small proteins comprising several isoforms with a molecular weight of 16–24 kDa (Crow et al. 1983). By using IgE immunoblotting and subsequent identification of IgE-reactive proteins by peptide mass fingerprinting, MLC-1 (Gal d 7; ~23 kDa) and MLC-3 (~15 kDa), a truncated isoform of MLC-1 derived from the same gene by alternative transcription and splicing which deviates from MLC-1 by just a few amino acids, were identified as allergens from chicken meat recognized by the majority of patients (Klug et al. 2015; Hemmer et al. 2016). Following cDNA cloning of chicken MLC-1 and production as a recombinant protein, this allergen could be characterized more comprehensively: MLC-1 is a heat-stable allergen in chicken meat strongly cross-reactive with homologous proteins from turkey, goose, and duck (Klug et al. 2015).

Chicken serum albumin (Gal d 5) and chicken MLC-1 (Gal d 7) are the only avian meat allergens thus far recognized by the World Health Organization and International Union of Immunological Societies (WHO/IUIS) Allergen Nomenclature Sub-committee.

16.4.3 Allergen Prevalence and Sensitization in Bird-Egg Syndrome-Related Poultry Meat Allergy

Hypersensitivity to poultry meat in patients with bird-egg syndrome is due to the ubiquitous occurrence of serum albumin also in muscle tissue. In classical bird-egg syndrome, primary sensitization to serum albumins occurs via the respiratory route through exposure to pet birds (Mandallaz et al. 1988; Szépfalusi et al. 1994; Van Toorenbergen et al. 1994; de Blay et al. 1994). Classical bird-egg syndrome occurs mainly in adults and is uncommon in children (Añíbarro et al. 1993). Alternatively, the primary sensitizer may be serum albumin in egg yolk (α-livetin), particularly in atopic children with concomitant sensitization to egg white and egg yolk ("egg-bird syndrome") (Nevot Falcó et al. 2003; Cheikh Rouhou et al. 2012; Martínez Alonso et al. 2003). Co-sensitization to chicken meat may be encountered in up to 20 % of such children (Sampson 1983), and subsequent exposure to pet birds may cause respiratory symptoms (Cheikh Rouhou et al. 2012).

Patients with bird-egg syndrome may experience mild to moderately severe anaphylaxis after ingestion of raw or soft-boiled egg yolk, whereas hard-boiled egg yolk is well tolerated (Hoffman and Guenther 1988, Añibarro Bausela et al. 1991; Mandallaz et al. 1988; Szépfalusi et al. 1994; Quirce et al. 2001; Villas et al. 2009).

Clinical reactions to poultry meat are less common and mostly mild (e.g., oral allergy syndrome). Studies in children and adults with double sensitization to egg yolk and bird feathers revealed meat intolerance in 22 % and 12 % of subjects, respectively (Añibarro Bausela et al. 1991; Bausela et al. 1997). The main reason for the infrequence of clinical symptoms is the heat lability of serum albumins (Quirce et al. 2001). In case of ingestion of incompletely cooked meat, however, systemic reactions may occasionally occur (Añibarro Bausela et al. 1991; Cheikh Rouhou et al. 2012).

16.4.4 Allergen Prevalence and Sensitization in Primary Poultry Meat Allergy

Primary poultry meat allergy stands for a true type I food allergy against heat-stable meat allergens without a causal relationship to egg or bird feather allergy. There is a lack of studies investigating the prevalence of genuine poultry meat allergy, and most published work refers to case reports.

Primary poultry meat allergy has been described mainly in adolescents and young adults (◉ Table 16.1), but initial symptoms may have occurred already in the preschool and school age years (Liccardi et al. 1997; Cahen et al. 1998; Hemmer et al. 2016). In about 20 % of patients, the onset of meat intolerance occurred beyond the age of 20. Accordingly, primary allergy to poultry meat holds an intermediate position with regard to disease onset, starting later than typical early-childhood food allergies (such as milk, egg, and wheat), but earlier than pork-cat syndrome and α-Gal-associated allergy to red meat.

Symptoms associated with genuine poultry allergy include contact reactions, oral allergy syndrome (which may be severe and include breathing difficulties), and systemic reactions, which, however, are mostly moderate in severity and confined to the skin and gastrointestinal tract (urticaria, angioedema, nausea, emesis, diarrhea) (◉ Table 16.1). In contrast to α-Gal-mediated allergy to red meat, symptoms usually start within 30 min as is typical for immediate type I hypersensitivity reactions to food.

Chicken and turkey meat allergens are highly cross-reactive and account for most allergic reactions. Allergy testing nearly always reveals double-positive results to both birds. The meat from goose, duck, pheasant, and other birds is often tolerated or symptoms are mild (Kelso et al. 1999; Sokolova et al. 2009). Soups, sausages, and ham prepared from turkey meat are also relevant triggers of allergic reactions (Cahen et al. 1998; Kuehn et al. 2009; Ayuso et al. 1999). However, it should be noted that sausages of nonmammalian (poultry) meat are often encased in pork gut and can, therefore, cause allergic reactions unrelated to poultry, but due to the presence of α-Gal. Anaphylaxis from "hidden" poultry meat allergens, due to the replacement of pork ham by turkey ham, has been described (Cahen et al. 1998). In addition, cooking steams may cause allergic reactions in highly sensitive subjects (Polasani et al. 1997; Barnig et al. 2012).

Table 16.1 Published cases of genuine poultry meat allergy

Author	*n*	Age (years)	Onset (years)	Reported symptoms after ingestion of poultry meat	Other food allergies
Liccardi et al. (1997)	1	23	3?	U, AE, A	
Vila et al. (1998)	1	21	?	OAS	
Cahen et al. (1998)	2	10, 25	childhood	OAS, U, N, V	
Kelso et al. (1999)	3	18–19	?	OAS, A, U	
Zacharisen (2006)	1	41	?	GI, U, A	
Sokolova et al. (2009)	1	31	29	OAS, PR, E	
Kuehn et al. (2009)	1	54	?	OAS, V, HYPO	Fish
Theler et al. (2009)	1[a]	28	?	OAS, RC, AE, U, V	
Hilger et al. (2010)	1	42	?	RC, A	Pork
González-Mancebo et al. (2011)	1	20	?	OAS, U, AE, A	
González-de-Olano et al. (2012)	1	23	?	A	Fish
Barnig et al. (2012)	1	16	14	OAS, GI; A from cooking steams	
Can et al. (2014)	1	13	7	OAS, E, AE, RC	

A Asthma/dyspnea, *AE* Angioedema, *E* generalized erythema, *GI* gastrointestinal, *HYPO* hypotension, *N* nausea, *OAS* oral allergy syndrome, *PR* generalized pruritus, *RC* rhinoconjunctivitis, *U* urticaria, *V* vomitus
[a]Positive allergy test + positive DBPCFC

16.4.5 Immunologic Relationships Between Poultry Meat, Red Meat, and Other Foods

Simultaneous hypersensitivity to poultry and red meat is uncommon but does occur. Taking into account the prevalence of meat allergies, such double sensitivity is more likely due to cross-reactivity than true double sensitization.

Ayuso et al. studied 57 meat-allergic patients and observed double-positive test results to mammal and poultry meat in 35 % (Ayuso et al. 1999). However, the specificity of the blotting method used might have been limited, and no further characterization of potential cross-reactive allergens has been performed making the significance of these observations unclear. Hilger et al. described a patient with occupation-related pork allergy who later developed symptoms after ingestion of chicken meat (Hilger et al. 2010). The patient was found to be cross-sensitized to porcine and chicken hemoglobin α-chain (57 % sequence identity). In addition, he had IgE antibodies to pig serum albumin cross-reacting with chicken serum albumin. In general, however, cross-reactivity between mammalian and avian serum albumins appears to be uncommon (Restani et al. 1997).

In a study of 28 patients with primary allergy to chicken meat, 7 % (2/28) reported concurrent hypersensitivity to red meat (Hemmer et al. 2016). Both had double-positive test results to poultry and red meat, but neither was sensitized to serum albumins. Mammalian MLCs, showing up to 88 % sequence homology with chicken MLC-1, might represent potentially cross-reactive candidate allergens in red meat, but thus far this is not supported by experimental data. Another muscle protein shared by poultry and red meat is α-parvalbumin, which shows a high degree of homology (~80 %) between birds and mammals. In vitro cross-reactivity has been demonstrated in a single case between recombinant α-parvalbumins from chicken, turkey, cow, horse, and frog (Kuehn et al. 2009), but the clinical relevance of this cross-reactivity is not known.

Recent findings also indicate cross-reactivity of poultry meat allergens with fish and shellfish allergens. Thirty percent of chicken meat-allergic patients report concomitant fish allergy, and 50–60 % of sera show positive IgE binding to fish and shrimp extracts using ImmunoCAP (Hemmer et al. 2016). Concomitant fish allergy in patients allergic to poultry meat has already been observed in two earlier case reports where α-parvalbumin was identified as the responsible meat allergen (Kuehn et al. 2009; González-Mancebo et al. 2011), but only in one of these cases could cross-reactivity between poultry meat and fish extracts be proven. MLCs might represent another group of cross-reactive allergens in poultry meat, fish, and shellfish. MLCs have been already recognized as minor allergens in crustaceans (Ayuso et al. 2008), but minimally in fish. Cross-reactivity of chicken MLC might be expected particularly with fish MLCs, since they show a high degree of sequence identity (63–65 %). A polyclonal rabbit antiserum against chicken MLC-1 was found to bind to homologous proteins of similar molecular size in trout and carp extracts, and IgE-binding to these proteins could be inhibited by recombinant chicken MLC-1 (Hemmer et al. 2016), supporting a role of MLCs as cross-reactive allergens in poultry meat and fish.

16.4.6 Diagnosis and Recommendations

Diagnosis has to discriminate between bird-egg syndrome and primary poultry meat allergy. A history of egg/egg yolk allergy and exposure to pet birds gives important clues in regard to the origin of allergy to poultry meat. Patients with bird-egg syndrome show multiple positive tests for bird feathers, egg yolk, and chicken meat in vivo as well as in vitro (Szépfalusi et al. 1994). IgE levels are typically high for bird feathers and egg yolk and lower for chicken meat (Szépfalusi et al. 1994; Añíbarro et al. 1993). Chicken serum albumin (Gal d 5), a specific marker for bird-egg syndrome, is currently available for testing via ImmunoCAP ISAC, but is not available for testing by singleplex (◉ Table 16.2).

Making the diagnosis of "primary allergy" to poultry meat still relies on meat extracts. No recombinant or purified marker molecules are currently commercially available for in vitro testing. Although most patients with primary allergy to poultry meat lack a history of egg allergy, low-level IgE against egg white and/or egg yolk may be encountered in some of them (Hemmer et al. 2016). IgE levels to crude meat extracts are mostly low to moderate (class 1–2) and often borderline positive. Additional skin testing with extracts or native meat may be required to confirm the

Table 16.2 Helpful in vitro tests in the diagnosis of poultry meat allergy

		Singleplex assay with allergen extract	ImmunoCAP ISAC
Chicken meat	f83	x	
Turkey meat	f284	x	
Egg yolk	f75	x	
Gal d 5 (chicken serum albumin)			x
Budgerigar feathers	e78	x	
Parakeet feathers	e196	x	
Canary feathers	e201	x	
Hen's feathers	e85	x	

diagnosis. As simultaneous cross-sensitization to fish and shellfish might be widespread in poultry meat allergy, the diagnostic workup should also consider sensitization to fish, shrimp, and mollusks.

16.5 Advantage of Molecular Diagnostics

The quantification of specific IgE antibodies to α-Gal, Fel d 2, Can f 3, and Sus s 1 or Bos d 6 allows for discrimination of pork-cat syndrome from type I food allergy to red meat and innards. The use of whole extracts does not allow for discrimination between these differential diagnoses. In addition, meat extracts contain low quantities of α-Gal; therefore, specific IgE levels for whole-meat extracts remain low or can even be negative in affected patients. It became obvious that measuring IgE antibodies to α-Gal allows identification of red meat and innards as the eliciting foods in patients diagnosed with (i) idiopathic anaphylaxis and (ii) recurring episodes of acute urticaria or angioedema. With regard to poultry meat allergy, molecular diagnosis is currently limited to Gal d 5 (chicken serum albumin) which is a helpful marker in identifying patients with bird-egg syndrome. The availability of major allergens from muscle tissues, such as MLCs (Gal d 7) and α-parvalbumins, would greatly improve the proper diagnosis of primary poultry meat allergy, but these molecules are thus far not accessible for use in routine diagnosis.

16.6 Recommendations for Clinical Practice

Pork-cat syndrome is characterized by a primary respiratory sensitization to cat dander, followed by clinical symptoms upon ingestion of pork due to the presence of cross-reacting IgE antibodies directed against Fel d 2 and Sus s 1. Although the cross-reactivity between pork and cat SA is the most prevalent association, clinical cross-reactivity between different mammalian danders and meats has been reported as well. Clinical symptoms generally begin within 30–45 min after consumption.

In keeping with the fact that SAs are heat labile, most patients tolerate boiled or well-cooked versions of the inciting foods. Clinical diagnosis includes inquiry of respiratory symptoms with exposure to pets. Skin prick testing or measure of serum-specific IgE level using animal dander extract will confirm sensitization and presence of specific IgE to major allergens (Fel d 1, Can f 1, Can f 2, or Can f 5); sensitization to the respective SA should also be determined.

Type I allergy to the carbohydrate side chain α-Gal is coined "α-Gal syndrome"; characteristics include (i) type I allergic symptoms elicited by mammalian meat or innards with characteristic delayed onset or immediate onset of symptoms in response to ingestion of innards in some patients, (ii) possible dependence of these responses on presence of cofactors around the time of ingestion, and (iii) iatrogenic anaphylaxis due to α-Gal-containing drugs, such as chimeric antibodies or gelatin-derived plasma expanders. The diagnostic workup includes the detection of specific IgE to α-Gal, as well as skin testing and oral food challenge. Patients need to receive detailed information about the risks associated with certain foods and drugs.

Genuine (primary) allergy to poultry meat is regularly associated with anaphylaxis. Chicken and turkey meat proteins are highly cross-reactive, and their allergens remain intact in processed meat products. The meat from goose and duck is often tolerated, but some patients may suffer also from fish and/or seafood allergy. Secondary allergy to poultry meat, arising from sensitization to bird feathers, known as bird-egg syndrome, is rare and is mostly associated with mild reactions. Simultaneous testing for sensitization to egg yolk and bird feathers is essential to discriminate between primary and secondary allergy to poultry meat. Gal d 5 – the IgE level to which can be determined by means of ImmunoCAP ISAC testing – can be used as a marker for bird-egg syndrome. In patients with this syndrome, removal of pet birds from the patient's home may be a reasonable recommendation.

Conclusion

In summary, allergic reactions involving animal proteins and carbohydrates with differing methods and routes of sensitization have been increasingly recognized in the last 20 years. Various studies have now demonstrated that the use of molecular allergen diagnostics is necessary for accurate diagnosis of these allergy syndromes. Although methods to induce tolerance to the inciting causes in these syndromes are under investigation, accurate diagnosis using molecular assays has facilitated the development of successful recommendations for patients regarding allergen avoidance and dietary restriction.

References

Adamantos S, Chan DL, Goggs R, Humm K. Risk of immunologic reactions to human serum albumin solutions. J Small Anim Pract. 2009;50:206.

Almeida IC, Milani SR, Gorin PA, Travassos LR. Complement-mediated lysis of Trypanosoma cruzi trypomastigotes by human anti-a-galactosyl antibodies. J Immunol. 1991;146:2394–400.

Añíbarro B, García-Ara C, Ojeda JA. Bird-egg syndrome in childhood. J Allergy Clin Immunol. 1993;92:628–30.

Añibarro Bausela B, Martín Esteban M, Martínez Alzamora F, Pascual Marcos C, Ojeda Casas JA. Egg protein sensitization in patients with bird feather allergy. Allergy. 1991;46:614–8.
Asero R, Mistrello G, Falagiani P. Oral allergy syndrome from pork. Allergy. 1997;52:684–6.
Ayuso R, Grishina G, Bardina L, Carrillo T, Blanco C, Ibáñez MD, et al. Myosin light chain is a novel shrimp allergen, Lit v 3. J Allergy Clin Immunol. 2008;122:795–802.
Ayuso R, Lehrer SB, Tanaka L, Ibañez MD, Pascual C, Burks AW, et al. IgE antibody response to vertebrate meat proteins including tropomyosin. Ann Allergy Asthma Immunol. 1999;83:399–405.
Barnig C, Hilger C, Muti D, Blaumeiser M, Purohit A, Hentges F, et al. Anaphylaxis to vapors of roasting chicken controlled by omalizumab. J Investig Allergol Clin Immunol. 2012;22:439–40.
Bausela BA, Garcia-Ara MC, Martin Esteban M, Boyano Martinez TB, Diaz Pena JM, Ojeda Casas JA. Peculiarities of egg allergy in children with bird protein sensitization. Ann Allergy Asthma Immunol. 1997;78:213–6.
Biedermann T, Röcken M. Verzögert auftretende Symptome einer Soforttypallergie. Hautarzt. 2012;63 Suppl 1:76–9.
Cahen YD, Fritsch R, Wüthrich B. Food allergy with monovalent sensitivity to poultry meat. Clin Exp Allergy. 1998;28:1026–30.
Can C, Yazicioglu M, Ciplak G. Chicken meat anaphylaxis in a child with no allergies to eggs or feathers. Iran J Pediatr. 2014;24:786–7.
Caponetto P, Biedermann T, Yazdi A, Fischer J. Panitumumab: a safe option for oncologic patients sensitized to galactose-α-1,3-galactose. J Allergy Clin Immunol Pract. 2015;3:982–3.
Caponetto P, Fischer J, Biedermann T. Gelatin-containing sweets can elicit anaphylaxis in a patient with sensitization to galactose-α-1,3-galactose. J Allergy Clin Immunol Pract. 2013;1:302–3.
Cheikh Rouhou S, Bachouch I, Racil H, Chaouch N, Zarrouk M, Salmi L, et al. Anaphylaxis due to chicken meat. Rev Mal Respir. 2012;29:98–100.
Choi GS, Kim JH, Lee HN, Sung JM, Lee JW, Park HS. Occupational asthma caused by inhalation of bovine serum albumin powder. Allergy Asthma Immunol Res. 2009;1:45–7.
Chruszcz M, Mikolajczak K, Mank N, Majorek KA, Porebski PJ, Minor W. Serum albumins-unusual allergens. Biochim Biophys Acta. 2013;1830:5375–81.
Chung CH, Mirakhur B, Chan E, Le QT, Berlin J, Morse M, et al. Cetuximab-induced anaphylaxis and IgE specific for galactose-α-1,3-galactose. N Engl J Med. 2008;358:1109–17.
Cisteró-Bahíma A, Enrique E, San Miguel-Moncín MM, Alonso R, Bartra J, Fernández-Parra B, Lombardero M, Barber D. Meat allergy and cross-reactivity with hamster epithelium. Allergy. 2003;58:161–2.
Commins SP, James HR, Stevens W, Pochan SL, Land MH, King C, Mozzicato S, Platts-Mills TA. Delayed clinical and ex vivo response to mammalian meat in patients with IgE to galactose-alpha-1,3-galactose. J Allergy Clin Immunol. 2014;134:108–15.
Commins SP, James HR, Kelly LA, Pochan SL, Workman LJ, Perzanowski MS, Kocan KM, Fahy JV, Nganga LW, Ronmark E, Cooper PJ, Platts-Mills TA. The relevance of tick bites to the production of IgE antibodies to the mammalian oligosaccharide galactose-α-1,3-galactose. J Allergy Clin Immunol. 2011;127:1286–93.
Commins SP, Satinover SM, Hosen J, Mozena J, Borish L, Lewis BD, et al. Delayed anaphylaxis, angioedema, or urticaria after consumption of red meat in patients with IgE antibodies specific for galactose-α-1,3-galactose. J Allergy Clin Immunol. 2009;123:426–33.
Crow MT, Olson PS, Stockdale FE. Myosin light-chain expression during avian muscle development. J Cell Biol. 1983;96:736–44.
De Blay F, Hoyet C, Candolfi E, Thierry R, Pauli G. Identification of alpha livetin as a cross reacting allergen in a bird-egg syndrome. Allergy Proc. 1994;15:77–8.
Drouet M, Sabbah A. The pork/cat syndrome or crossed reactivity between cat epithelia and pork meat. Monogr Allergy. 1996;32:164–73.
Drouet M, Sabbah A, Le Sellin J, Bonneau JC, Gay G, Dubois-Gosnet C. Fatal anaphylaxis after eating wild boar meat in a patient with pork-cat syndrome. Allerg Immunol (Paris). 2001;33:163–5.
Faveeuw C, Mallevaey T, Paschinger K, Wilson IB, Fontaine J, Mollicone R, et al. Schistosome N-glycans containing core alpha 3-fucose and core beta 2-xylose epitopes are strong inducers of Th2 responses in mice. Eur J Immunol. 2003;33:1271–81.

Fischer J, Hebsaker J, Caponetto P, Platts-Mills TA, Biedermann T. Galactose-alpha-1,3-galactose sensitization is a prerequisite for pork-kidney allergy and cofactor-related mammalian meat anaphylaxis. J Allergy Clin Immunol. 2014;133:755–9.

Fischer J, Yazdi A, Biedermann T. Mammalian meat allergy: A diagnostic challenge. Allergo J Int. 2015;24:81–3.

Galili U. Anti-Gal: an abundant human natural antibody of multiple pathogeneses and clinical benefits. Immunology. 2013;140:1–11.

Galili U, Anaraki F, Thall A, Hill-Black C, Radic M. One percent of circulating B lymphocytes are capable of producing the natural anti-Gal antibody. Blood. 1993;82:2485–93.

Galili U, Mandrell RE, Hamadeh RM, Shohet SB, Griffiss JM. Interaction between human natural anti-alpha-galactosyl immunoglobulin G and bacteria of the human flora. Infect Immun. 1988;56:1730–7.

Galili U, Rachmilewitz EA, Peleg A, Flechner I. A unique natural human IgG antibody with anti-alpha-galactosyl specificity. J Exp Med. 1984;160:1519–31.

González-de-Olano D, Bartolomé B, Maroto AS, Vivanco F, Pastor-Vargas C. Asthma after chicken consumption due to cross-reactivity between fish and chicken parvalbumin. J Investig Allergol Clin Immunol. 2012;22:227–8.

González-Mancebo E, Pastor C, González-de-Olano D, et al. Identification of allergens in chicken meat allergy. J Investig Allergol Clin Immunol. 2011;21:326–7.

Gonzalez-Quintela A, Dam Laursen AS, Vidal C, Skaaby T, Gude F, Linneberg A. IgE antibodies to alpha-gal in the general adult population: relationship with tick bites, atopy, and cat ownership. Clin Exp Allergy. 2014;44:1061–8.

Hamsten C, Starkhammar M, Tran TA, Johansson M, Bengtsson U, Ahlen G, et al. Identification of galactose-alpha-1,3-galactose in the gastrointestinal tract of the tick Ixodes ricinus; possible relationship with red meat allergy. Allergy. 2013;68:549–52.

Hemmer W, Klug C, Swoboda I. Update on the bird-egg syndrome and genuine poultry meat allergy. Allergo J Int. 2016;25:68–75.

Hilger C, Kohnen M, Grigioni F, Lehners C, Hentges F. Allergic cross-reactions between cat and pig serum albumin. Study at the protein and DNA levels. Allergy. 1997;52:179–87.

Hilger C, Swiontek K, Hentges F, Donnay C, de Blay F, Pauli G. Occupational inhalant allergy to pork followed by food allergy to pork and chicken: sensitization to hemoglobin and serum albumin. Int Arch Allergy Immunol. 2010;151:173–8.

Hilger C, Fischer J, Swiontek K, Hentges F, Lehners C, Eberlein B, Morisset M, Biedermann T, Ollert M. Two galactose-α-1,3-galactose carrying peptidases from pork kidney mediate anaphylactogenic responses in delayed meat allergy. Allergy. 2016;71:711–9.

Hoffman DR, Guenther DM. Occupational allergy to avian proteins presenting as allergy to ingestion of egg yolk. J Allergy Clin Immunol. 1988;81:484–8.

Kelso JM, Cockrell GE, Helm RM, Burks AW. Common allergens in avian meats. J Allergy Clin Immunol. 1999;104:202–4.

Klug C, Hemmer W, Focke M, Wank H, Quirce S, Gaubitzer E, Swoboda I. Identification and characterisation of the muscle protein, myosin light chain 1, as a major chicken meat allergen. Allergy. 2015;70 Suppl 101:517.

Koike C, Fung JJ, Geller DA, et al. Molecular basis of evolutionary loss of the alpha 1,3-galactosyltransferase gene in higher primates. J Biol Chem. 2002;22:10114–20.

Kuehn A, Lehners C, Hilger C, Hentges F. Food allergy to chicken meat with IgE reactivity to muscle alpha-parvalbumin. Allergy. 2009;64:1557–8.

Liccardi G, Asero R, D'Amato M, D'Amato G. Role of sensitization to mammalian serum albumin in allergic disease. Curr Allergy Asthma Rep. 2011;11:421–6.

Liccardi G, Szepfalusi Z, Noschese P, Nentwich I, D'Amato M, D'Amato G. Allergy to chicken meat without sensitization to egg proteins: A case report. J Allergy Clin Immunol. 1997;100:577–9.

Mandallaz MM, de Weck AL, Dahinden CA. Bird-egg syndrome, Cross-reactivity between bird antigens and egg-yolk livetins in IgE-mediated hypersensitivity. Int Arch Allergy Appl Immunol. 1988;87:143–50.

Martelli A, De Chiara A, Corvo M, Restani P, Fiocchi A. Beef allergy in children with cow's milk allergy; cow's milk allergy in children with beef allergy. Ann Allergy Asthma Immunol. 2002;89:38–43.

Martínez Alonso JC, Domínguez Ortega FJ, Fuentes Gonzalo MJ. Angioedema due to sensitization to chicken meat. Allergol Immunopathol (Madr). 2003;31:50–2.
Morisset M, Arumugam K, Ollert M. Allergy to horse meat mediated by allergy to dog: report of an original case and review of the literature. Allergo J Int. 2016;25:76–81.
Morisset M, Richard C, Astier C, Jacquenet S, Croizier A, Beaudouin E, Cordebar V, Morel-Codreanu F, Petit N, Moneret-Vautrin DA, Kanny G. Anaphylaxis to pork kidney is related to IgE antibodies specific for galactose-alpha-1,3-galactose. Allergy. 2012;67:699–704.
Mozzicato SM, Tripathi A, Posthumus JB, Platts-Mills TA, Commins SP. Porcine or bovine valve replacement in 3 patients with IgE antibodies to the mammalian oligosaccharide galactose-alpha-1,3-galactose. J Allergy Clin Immunol Pract. 2014;2:637–8.
Mullins RJ, James H, Platts-Mills TA, Commins S. Relationship between red meat allergy and sensitization to gelatin and galactose-α-1,3-galactose. J Allergy Clin Immunol. 2012;129:1334–42.
Nevot Falcó S, Casas Ramisa R, Lleonart Bellfill R. Bird-egg syndrome in children. Allergol Immunopathol (Madr). 2003;31:161–5.
Okano M, Satoskar AR, Nishizaki K, Harn Jr DA. Lacto-Nfucopentaose III found on Schistosoma mansoni egg antigens functions as adjuvant for proteins by inducing Th2-type response. J Immunol. 2001;167:442–50.
Polasani R, Melgar L, Reisman RE, Ballow M. Hot dog vapor induced status asthmaticus. Ann Allergy Asthma Immunol. 1997;78:35–6.
Posthumus J, James HR, Lane CJ, Matos LA, Platts-Mills TAE, Commins SP. Initial description of pork-cat syndrome in the United States. J Allergy Clin Immunology. 2013;131:923–5.
Quirce S, Marañón F, Umpiérrez A, de las Heras M, Fernández-Caldas E, Sastre J. Chicken serum albumin (Gal d 5) is a partially heat-labile inhalant and food allergen implicated in the bird-egg syndrome. Allergy. 2001;56:754–62.
Restani P, Ballabio C, Tripodi S, Fiocchi A. Meat allergy. Curr Opin Allergy Clin Immunol. 2009;9:265–9.
Restani P, Fiocchi A, Beretta B, Velonà T, Giovannini M, Galli CL. Meat Allergy III Proteins involved and cross-reactivity between different animal species. J Am Coll Nutr. 1997;16:383–9.
Roenneberg et al. JACI in practice in press. 2015.
Sampson HA. Role of immediate food hypersensitivity in the pathogenesis of atopic dermatitis. J Allergy Clin Immunol. 1983;71:473–80.
San-Juan S, Lezaun A, Caballero ML, Moneo I. Occupational allergy to raw beef due to cross-reactivity with dog epithelium. Allergy. 2005;60:839–40.
Schnaar RL. Glycans and glycan-binding proteins in immune regulation: A concise introduction to glycobiology for the allergist. J Allergy Clin Immunol. 2015;135:609–15.
Sokolova A, Costa AC, Santos MC, Bartolomé B, Barbosa MP. Severe allergy to poultry meat without sensitisation to egg proteins with concomitant Leguminosae allergy. Case report. Allergol Immunopathol. 2009;37:165–72.
Spitzauer S, Pandjaitan B, Soregi G, Muhl S, Ebner C, Kraft D, Valenta R, Rumpold H. IgE cross-reactivities against albumins in patients allergic to animals. J Allergy Clin Immunol. 1995;96:951–9.
Spitzauer S, Schweiger C, Sperr WR, Pandjaitan B, Valent P, Muhl S, Ebner C, Scheiner O, Kraft D, Rumpold H, Valenta R. Molecular characterization of dog albumin as a cross-reactive allergen. J Allergy Clin Immunol. 1994;93:614–27.
Szépfalusi Z, Ebner C, Pandjaitan R, Orlicek F, Scheiner O, Boltz-Nitulescu G, et al. Egg yolk alpha-livetin (chicken serum albumin) is a cross-reactive allergen in the bird-egg syndrome. J Allergy Clin Immunol. 1994;93:932–42.
Theler B, Brockow K, Ballmer-Weber BK. Clinical presentation and diagnosis of meat allergy in Switzerland and Southern Germany. Swiss Med Wkly. 2009;139:264–70.
Tripathi A, Commins SP, Heymann PW, Platts-Mills TA. Delayed anaphylaxis to red meat masquerading as idiopathic anaphylaxis. J Allergy Clin Immunol Pract. 2014;2:259–65.
Van Toorenbergen AW, Huijskesheins MIE, Van Wijk RG. Different pattern of IgE binding to chicken egg yolk between patients with inhalant allergy to birds and food-allergic children. Int Arch Allergy Immunol. 1994;104:199–203.
Vila L, Barbarin E, Sanz ML. Chicken meat induces oral allergy syndrome: a case report. Ann Allergy Asthma Immunol. 1998;80:195–6.

Villas F, Compes E, Fernández-Nieto M, Muñoz MP, Bartolome B, de las Heras M. Bird-egg syndrome caused by Agapornis species (lovebird). J Investig Allergol Clin Immunol. 2009; 19:71–2.

Voltolini S, Spigno F, Cioè A, Casnati P, Bignardi D, Minale P. Bovine Serum Albumin: a double allergy risk. Eur Ann Allergy Clin Immunol. 2013;45:144–7.

Werfel SJ, Cooke SK, Sampson HA. Clinical reactivity to beef in children allergic to cow's milk. J Allergy Clin Immunol. 1997;99:293–300.

Wilson IB, Altmann F. Structural analysis of N-glycans from allergenic grass, ragweed and tree pollens: core 1,3-linked fucose and xylose present in all pollens examined. Glycoconj J. 1998;15:1055–70.

Zacharisen MC. Severe allergy to chicken meat. WMJ. 2006;105:50–2.

Molecular Diagnostics in Food-Dependent Exercise-Induced Anaphylaxis

17

S.C. Hofmann and T. Jakob

17.1 Introduction

Food-dependent exercise-induced anaphylaxis (FDEIA) belongs to the group of "summation" anaphylaxis, an entity which requires both an allergen exposure and the presence of a second factor (e.g., physical exercise, drug, infection). It differs from the classic form of food anaphylaxis, as patients generally tolerate the causative food through normal ingestion and only experience an anaphylactic reaction when the food is consumed in combination with an augmentation factor. FDEIA usually manifests clinically in the form of generalized urticaria with or without angioedema (grade 1 anaphylaxis according to Ring and Messmer); however, gastrointestinal, bronchopulmonary, or cardiovascular symptoms, including cardiovascular arrest, are seen in more severe cases.

FDEIA was first described in 1979 by Maulitz et al. in reference to a patient who experienced an anaphylactic reaction to seafood when consumed in a temporal relationship to physical activity (Maulitz et al. 1979). Over the years, wheat-dependent

---

The present chapter is based on, and modified from, an article by the same authors that appeared in 2013 in *Allergo Journal* (Hofmann SC, Jakob T: Molecular diagnostics in food-dependent exercise-induced anaphylaxis. Allergo J 2013; 22: 308–311).
The authors gratefully thank Prof. Sarbjit S. Saini, Division of Allergy and Clinical Immunology, Department of Medicine, Johns Hopkins Asthma & Allergy Center, Baltimore, MD, USA, for reviewing the manuscript, editorial assistance, and helpful suggestions regarding this chapter.

S.C. Hofmann, MD (✉)
Center for Dermatology, Allergy and Dermatosurgery, HELIOS University Hospital Wuppertal, University Witten/Herdecke, Wuppertal, Germany
e-mail: silke.hofmann@helios-kliniken.de

T. Jakob, MD, Prof.
Department of Dermatology and Allergology, University Medical Center Giessen (UKGM), Justus-Liebig-University, Giessen, Germany
e-mail: thilo.jakob@derma.med.uni-giessen.de

J. Kleine-Tebbe, T. Jakob (eds.), *Molecular Allergy Diagnostics*,
DOI 10.1007/978-3-319-42499-6_17

exercise-induced anaphylaxis (WDEIA) became the best characterized form of FDEIA (Wong and Krishna 2013). WDEIA causes immediate-type allergic reactions following the consumption of wheat, e.g., bread, pizza, or pasta in combination with a cofactor. In addition to seafood and wheat, a number of other foods (e.g., fruit, celery, tomato, peanut, hazelnut, soy, cow's milk, or red meat) can trigger FDEIA (Romano et al. 2012).

IgE-mediated and non-IgE-mediated mechanisms act synergistically in the pathophysiology of FDEIA. The essential presence of an amplification factor in addition to type I sensitization to a food explains why the FDEIA attacks in an individual generally occur sporadically and with a time delay following food intake. The augmentation factors themselves can be as variable as the eliciting food: physical exertion within 1–6 h of food intake, alcohol consumption, and the use of a nonsteroidal anti-inflammatory agent (NSAID) are the most commonly described cofactors. More rarely, infections, stress, and hormonal factors (menstrual cycle) in combination with particular foods elicit FDEIA. Mast cell activation due to c-KIT mutation has also been described in one case as augmentation factor.

Augmentation Factors in FDEIA

- Physical activity (variable intensity)
- Medications (in particular aspirin and other NSAID)
- Alcohol
- Infections
- Fatigue and stress
- Hormonal factors (in particular menstruation)

In some patients, anaphylaxis only occurs when two different cofactors (e.g., exercise and an infection) are present simultaneously alongside the relevant food. The intensity of augmentation factors can also vary widely, as evidenced by the fact that a light stroll following food consumption can trigger FDEIA in some patients, while intense physical activity, e.g., playing football or competitive sports, is required in others.

Until a few years ago, the diagnosis of FDEIA was challenging due to the multitude of possible allergens, its clinical variability, and the low sensitivity of prick tests or conventional serological tests. Due to the availability of molecular allergy diagnostics, numerous FDEIA patients previously classified as idiopathic anaphylaxis for many years can now be given a clear diagnosis by means of serological testing that identifies the triggering allergen. The present chapter provides an overview of the most important FDEIA allergens and their structural and functional characteristics. Current serological diagnostics using recombinant allergens for the purposes of diagnostic confirmation will then be discussed. The various FDEIA allergens are discussed in each section successively. In terms of treatment, avoidance of the eliciting food, at least in conjunction with the relevant cofactor, always takes precedence, in addition to the prescription of an adrenaline autoinjector as emergency medication.

17.2 Allergen Identification

Like all cereals, wheat belongs to the grass family (Poaceae). Allergic reactions to wheat (*Triticum aestivum*) are caused by one of several protein families.

Wheat proteins can be subdivided as follows:

1. Water-soluble albumins (including the α-amylase inhibitor)
2. Salt-soluble globulins
3. Water- and salt-insoluble glutens (⊙ Fig. 17.1).

The gluten group comprises:

(a) Monomeric gliadins (α/β-, γ-, and ω1–ω5-gliadins)

(b) Polymeric gliadins [high molecular weight (HMW) and low molecular weight (LMW) glutenins]

Monomeric gliadins are classified according to their electrophoretic mobility. Although more than 20 wheat proteins are known to trigger allergies, the group of WDEIA allergens identified to date is restricted to storage proteins from the gluten family (⊙ Table 17.1). A number of European and Japanese working groups (Matsuo et al. 2004; Palosuo et al. 2003) identified and confirmed ω-5-gliadin (Tri a 19) as a major allergen; with a molecular weight of 65 kDa, it is a fast-moving ω-gliadin. Other allergens capable of eliciting WDEIA include HMW glutenin (Tri a 26), α/β-gliadin (Tri a 21), and γ-gliadin.

A number of cases of FDEIA due to sensitization to nonspecific lipid transfer proteins (nsLTP) in vegetables, fruit, pulses (in particular peanut), or tree nuts have

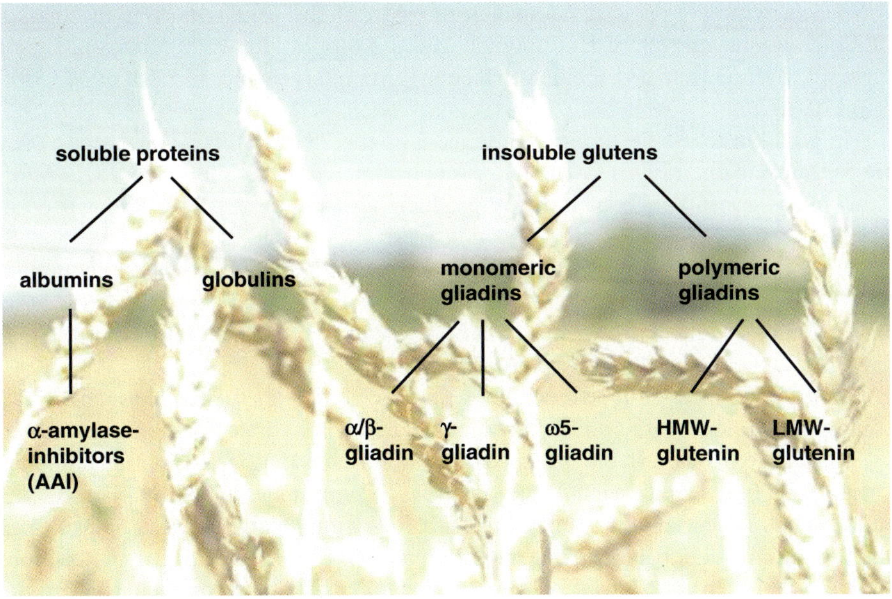

Fig. 17.1 Classification of the wheat proteins

Table 17.1 WDEIA-associated allergens

Wheat allergen	Protein	MW (kDa)	Sensitivity/specificity in WDEIA	Reference
Tri a 14	nsLTP	9	Low (more commonly triggers baker's asthma and cofactor-independent anaphylaxis)	Palacin et al. (2010)
Tri a 19	ω-5-gliadin	65	78 %/96 %[a] (also a marker allergen for severe wheat allergy in children)	Matsuo et al. (2005a)
Tri a 21	α/β-gliadin	31–45	53 %/100 %[a]	Hofmann et al. (2012)
Tri a 26	HMW glutenin	90[b]	17 %/93 %[a]	Takahashi et al. (2012)
Tri a 36	LMW glutenin GluB3-23	40	(80 % of all wheat-allergic individuals/ low specificity for WDEIA)	Baar et al. (2012)
Tri a γ-Gliadin	γ-gliadin	36	76 %/100 %[a]	Hofmann et al. (2012)

WDEIA wheat-dependent exercise-induced anaphylaxis, *nsLTP* nonspecific lipid transfer protein, *MW* molecular weight, *HMW* high molecular weight, *LMW* low molecular weight
[a]Specificity relates to control subjects with no wheat allergy
[b]Recombinant HMW glutenin

been described in the Mediterranean region, most notably in Spain (Romano et al. 2012). nsLTP are widespread plant panallergens with a molecular weight of 9 kDa and high allergenic potency (Petersen and Scheurer 2011). Peach (*Prunus persica*) is the most frequent sensitizer in the Mediterranean region. Thus, Pru p 3, the nsLTP of peach, which is primarily found in the skin of the fruit, serves as the marker allergen. Other relevant nsLTP include Mal d 3 (apple), Pru av 3 (cherry), Vit v 1 (grape), Lyc e 3 (tomato), Cor a 8 (hazelnut), Ara h 9 (peanut), and Zea m 14 (corn) (⦿ Fig. 17.2).

In addition to nsLTP, storage proteins, e.g., the 7S-globulin β-conglycinin (Gly m 5), can also elicit FDEIA. The latter is considered a major allergen in FDEIA following the consumption of tofu/soy products (Adachi et al. 2009; Radauer et al. 2012).

In Asia, the consumption of seafood (prawns, mussels, squid, etc.) in combination with sport or other cofactors is known to have triggered anaphylaxis (Maulitz et al. 1979). The muscle protein tropomyosin (Pen m 1), with a molecular weight of 36 kDa, is the major allergen in crustaceans.

A further immediate-type food allergy in which cofactors such as physical activity may play a role is based on sensitization to the carbohydrate allergen galactose-α-1,3-galactose (α-Gal). In the presence of relevant sensitization, α-Gal in mammalian meat triggers delayed anaphylactic reactions (Commins et al. 2009). These often manifest as urticaria with a delay of 4–6 h following enteral allergen uptake (e.g., after consuming lamb, pork, game meat, or innards) (Commins et al. 2014). Reactions of this kind were previously considered as idiopathic due to this latency. From a pathophysiological perspective, the late onset of anaphylaxis may be explained by

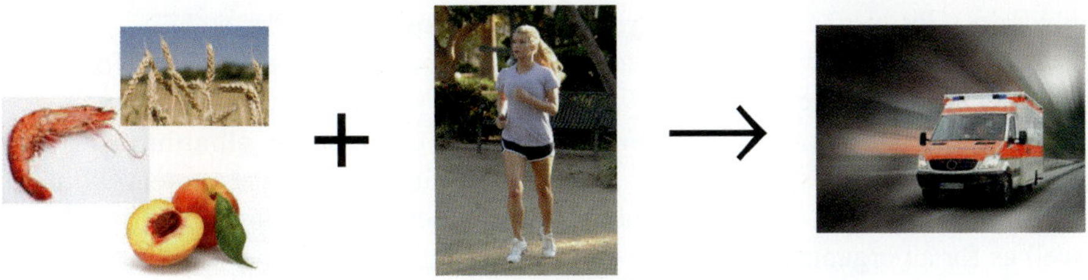

Allergen	Protein	Allergen Source
Tri a 19	ω_5 -gliadin	wheat
Pen m 1	tropomyosin	shrimps, shellfish
Gly m 5	β-conglycinin	soy
Pru p 3	nsLTP	peach
Mal d 3	nsLTP	apple
Vit v 1	nsLTP	grape
Lyc e 3	nsLTP	tomato
Cor a 8	nsLTP	hazelnut
Ara h 9	nsLTP	peanut
Zea m 14	nsLTP	maise
α-Gal	galactose- α-1,3-galactose	meat, giblets (pluck)

Fig. 17.2 Relevant allergens in food-dependent exercise-induced anaphylaxis (*nsLTP* nonspecific lipid transfer proteins)

the fact that the allergen first reaches the bloodstream (where it causes basophil activation) from the gastrointestinal tract 3–5 h following meat consumption.

17.3 Structure, Function, and Importance of the Allergens

Wheat glutens (gliadins and glutenins) are thermo- and digestion-stable storage proteins with a high glutamine, proline, glycine, and phenylalanine content (Baar et al. 2012). They are found in wheat seeds, roots, and tubers and account for 80 % of the total protein in wheat. Together with water, glutens form a continuous network responsible for dough elasticity, pore formation, and the firmness of crumbs in baked goods. Due to their proline- and glutamine-rich amino acid sequence, gliadins (e.g., ω5-gliadin) and glutamines are only partially split by gastric and pancreatic enzymes and resorbed to a limited extent. Therefore, large volumes of proteins and/or cofactors are required to trigger an allergic reaction. Physical activity (similarly to ethanol and acetylsalicylic acid) causes a drop in gastric pH, thereby resulting in greater gluten solubility and increased absorption (Matsuo et al. 2005 b). IgE antibodies in WDEIA are directed against linear, sequential epitopes, most notably of ω5-gliadin.

nsLTP are heat- and digestion-stable panallergens, which, as stress proteins, bind lipids and contribute to cell membrane development. They are found in numerous types of fruit, vegetable, grain, and nuts (Palacin et al. 2010). nsLTP are not a pollen-associated allergen, since sensitization occurs in the gastrointestinal tract (Petersen and Scheurer 2011). Storage proteins such as β-conglycinin (Gly m 5) and glycinin (Gly m 6) from soy (*Glycine maxima*) exhibit similar stability (Radauer et al. 2012). The reader is referred to ▶ Chaps. 4 and 5 for more detailed information on nsLTP and storage proteins.

The muscle protein *tropomyosin* (Pen m 1) is expressed in all arthropods (seafood as well as house dust mite). As an actin-binding filament protein with two α-helical coiled-coil domains, tropomyosin is essential for cytoskeletal function as well as for an organism's capacity for muscle contraction.

Galactose-α-1,3-galactose (α-Gal) is a sugar structure (galactose in α-1,3 coupled to another galactose; Galα1-3Galβ1-4GlcNAc-R) that is ubiquitous on mammalian glycolipids and glycoproteins—with the exception of primates (Commins and Platts-Mills 2013). α-Gal is produced enzymatically by α-1,3-galactosyltransferase activity. IgG to α-Gal account for approximately 1 % of all circulating human immunoglobulins and mediates the hyperacute rejection of porcine xenografts (Commins et al. 2009). IgE to α-Gal were first identified in 2008 in patients with hypersensitivity reactions to the chimeric monoclonal antibody cetuximab. This is explained by the fact that the α-Gal epitope also occurs on asparagine at position 88 in the murine heavy chain portion of cetuximab. α-Gal was identified as an allergen in delayed meat allergy shortly after this finding was made. It was recently shown that circulating IgE antibodies (anti-α-Gal-IgE) in Japanese patients with delayed allergy to beef bind to 240-kDa and 140-kDa proteins from beef extract. These proteins were identified as beef laminin γ-1 and collagen α-1 (VI) using two-dimensional gel electrophoresis (Takahashi et al. 2014). Bound α-Gal was detected on the surface of both proteins. In a different study, two major IgE-binding proteins were identified in pork kidney: porcine angiotensin-I-converting enzyme (ACE I) and aminopeptidase N (AP-N), both being able to activate patient basophils and elicit positive responses in skin prick tests (Hilger et al. 2016).

The carbohydrate epitope α-Gal is also found in infusion solutions containing gelatin (e.g., Gelafundin) and can cause anaphylaxis when administered parenterally. Primary sensitization to α-Gal likely occurs through tick bites, in particular ticks belonging to the *Amblyomma americanum* species, which transfer α-Gal-containing proteins via saliva (Commins et al. 2009). In Europe, sensitization probably occurs via ticks belonging to the *Ixodes ricinus* species, as recently demonstrated in a study by Hamsten et al. (2013): mono- and polyclonal antibodies against α-Gal, as well as anti-α-Gal-IgE from patients with meat allergy, stained the gastrointestinal tract of *I. ricinus* using cryostat cut sections.

17.4 Sensitization Prevalences/Distribution

Whereas wheat allergies are relatively common in children (with a prevalence of up to 9 %), only around 0.4 % of adults develop a food allergy to wheat.

However, WDEIA represents one of the most important and potentially severe forms of wheat allergy in adults.

ω5-Gliadin was identified as an allergen in WDEIA in 1999 (Palosuo et al. 2003). As shown by numerous studies in recent years, sensitization to ω-5-gliadin is detected in the majority of WDEIA patients; as a result, ω-5-gliadin is now considered a major allergen in classic WDEIA. Hydrolyzed wheat proteins (HWP) in soap were recently identified in Japan as triggers of a WDEIA variant (HWP-WDEIA). In these cases, sensitization occurs percutaneously via the nasal mucosa or conjunctiva (Fukutomi et al. 2011). The triggering of an immediate-type allergy may then cause contact urticaria (e.g., eyelid edema) upon renewed contact with the skin as well as anaphylaxis upon consumption of wheat products in combination with physical activity. ω-5-gliadin plays a minor role as an allergen in these special forms of WDEIA. In reality, other gliadins (in particular γ-gliadin) or glutenins are considered more relevant allergens (Yokooji et al. 2013).

IgE antibodies to nsLTP were detected in 80 % of Italian FDEIA patients, highlighting the relevance of the Pru p 3 allergen and other nsLTP in FDEIA (Romano et al. 2012). Immediate-type allergies in the setting of nsLTP sensitization often follow a severe course; therefore, identifying the triggering allergen is of great importance for patients.

Delayed anaphylaxis following the consumption of red meat in the setting of sensitization to α-Gal has been described in the USA, Europe, and Japan. This phenomenon is likely to be more widespread than currently assumed, since tests for IgE to α-Gal only recently became commercially available. The prevalence of anti-α-Gal-IgE is estimated at <2.5 % in the European population, whereby most patients report a history of tick bites and/or atopy or keep a cat as a pet (Gonzalez-Quintela et al. 2014).

17.5 Cross-Reactive Versus Marker Allergens

In all, 80 % of WDEIA patients exhibit specific IgE antibodies to ω-5-gliadin, which is considered a major allergen for WDEIA. The detection of IgE to ω-5-gliadin in adult patients has an extremely high specificity of approximately 96 %. In contrast, IgE to ω-5-gliadin in children primarily suggests a classic IgE-mediated immediate-type allergy to wheat, which often follows a severe course. Cross-reactivity between ω-5-gliadin IgE and rye protein (γ-70 secalin and γ-35 secalin) or with barley (γ-3 hordein) has been described (Morita et al. 2003; Varjonen et al. 2000). Therefore, WDEIA patients should adhere to a gluten-free diet. IgE antibodies in grass pollen allergy sufferers often also bind to wheat allergens (in particular albumins and globulins); however, this is usually of no clinical relevance (Sander et al. 1997). On the other hand, no cross-reactivity appears to exist between wheat nsLTP (Tri a 14), LMW glutenin (Tri a 36), ω5-gliadin (Tri a 19), and grass pollen allergens.

Cross-reactivity within the nsLTP family depends on the degree of structural similarity of individual proteins. Peach and apple nsLTP most frequently show cross-reactivity, while wheat LTP, for instance, only rarely causes cross-reactivity (Petersen and Scheurer 2011). Pen m 1 is a muscle protein, a tropomyosin, expressed in all arthropods. This gives rise to possible cross-reactivity between prawn, crab, langouste, and lobster.

Tropomyosin from crustaceans also exhibits cross-reactivity with the tropomyosin and minor allergen from house dust mites Der p 10 and Der f 10.

The soy storage proteins Gly m 5 and Gly m 6 exhibit in vitro cross-reactivity with peanut proteins (Ara h 1 and Ara h 3), which is likely to be clinically irrelevant. The Bet v 1-homologous soy protein Gly m 4 primarily plays a role as an allergen in birch pollen-related allergy to soy in the sense of oral allergy syndrome. However, cases of FDEIA due to Gly m 4 sensitization have also been described.

α-Gal-sensitized patients with meat allergy sometimes experience anaphylactic reactions following the ingestion of cow's milk. This may be explained by the finding that cow's milk proteins also carry the α-Gal epitope (Commins et al. 2009). Cross-reactivity with cat dander and the increased incidence of α-Gal-sensitization among cat owners is explained by the presence of the α-Gal epitope on the cat allergen, Fel d 5 (cat IgA) (Gronlund et al. 2009). Anaphylaxis in an α-Gal-sensitized patient following the consumption of gelatin-containing wine gums was recently described (Caponetto et al. 2013).

Due to the possibility of cross-reactivity, gelatin-containing foods and drugs (colloidal infusions) should be strictly avoided by patients with delayed meat allergy. A note to this effect should be made in the allergy passports in this patient group.

17.6 Diagnostic Workup

Prick tests using commercial wheat extracts are of limited reliability in the diagnosis of WDEIA as positive reactions are seen in only 30 % of WDEIA patients. Prick tests using native flour (e.g., type 405 wheat flour) have a diagnostic sensitivity of around 80 % (Hofmann et al. 2012), albeit with only low specificity. Patients with "classic" (exercise-independent) wheat allergy also show positive reactions.

Due to their low sensitivity and specificity, IgE tests with (aqueous) wheat whole-allergen extract (f4) are poorly suited to the diagnosis of WDEIA. This is likely explained by ω-5-gliadin's poor water solubility, rendering it underrepresented in the wheat extract.

IgE detection against recombinant ω5-gliadin (Tri a 19) has become established in routine diagnosis. This method provides a reliable diagnosis in around 80 % of WDEIA patients paired with high specificity.

The test is also useful in patients with intermittent urticaria of unknown origin, which may be explained by WDEIA (see ⊙ Fig. 17.3 for a diagnostic algorithm). However, ω5-gliadin-specific IgE tests reveal a diagnostic gap of 20 % in the molecular diagnosis of WDEIA. Combining various wheat allergens seems to offer a solution: HMW glutenin (Tri a 26) has also been described by Japanese working groups as an important WDEIA allergen (Matsuo et al. 2005a). In total, 97 % of Japanese WDEIA patients could be diagnosed using combined ω5-gliadin and HMW glutenin testing (Takahashi et al. 2012). Although many WDEIA patients showed IgE antibodies to HMW glutenin in an own study, this was not necessarily the case in the minority of ω5-gliadin-negative patients (Hofmann et al. 2012). Our results suggest that IgE antibodies to α/β-gliadin (Tri a 21; IgE detectable in around 53 % of WDEIA patients) or to γ-gliadin (IgE detectable in around 76 %) are of greater relevance than HMW glutenin (Tri a 26) in European patients. To date, γ-gliadin in

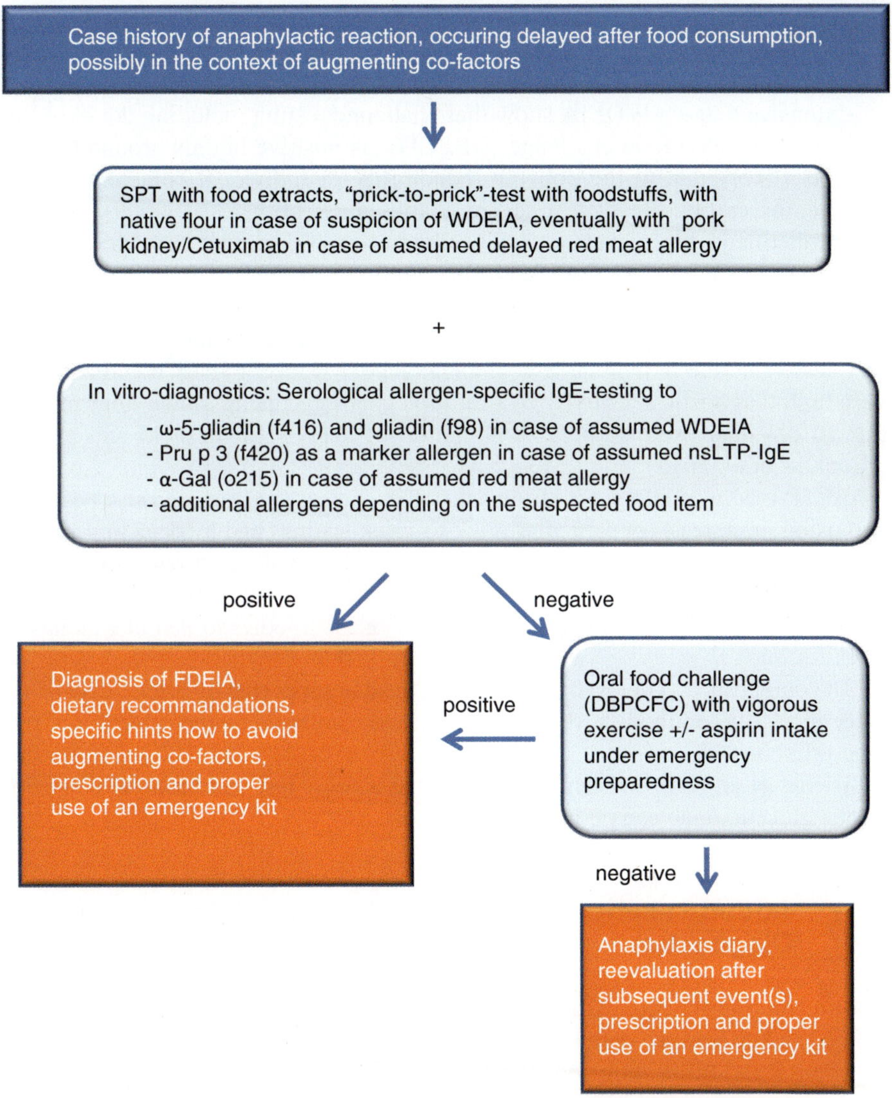

Fig. 17.3 Diagnostic algorithm in suspected food-dependent exercise-induced anaphylaxis based on patient history. Skin testing and in vitro detection of IgE should be performed in parallel. Double-blind, placebo-controlled food challenge (DBPCFC), combined with physical exertion and/or aspirin administration, is the only method capable of assessing individual cofactors and a patient's individual risk of anaphylaxis

particular has been detected as the sole triggering allergen in three Japanese and one German WDEIA patient (Hofmann et al. 2012; Morita et al. 2001). An ImmunoCAP test recently became available for the detection of specific IgE antibodies to gliadin (f98), which could help to close this diagnostic gap.

Oral challenge tests with the suspected foodstuff followed by exertion on an ergometer or aspirin and alcohol administration represent the gold standard for the conclusive diagnosis of FDEIA.

Extensive data on WDEIA show that challenge testing including double-blind placebo-controlled food challenge (DBPCFC) is positive in only around 60 % of patients (likely due to the poor reproducibility of individual cofactors) and in some cases carries the risk of severe anaphylaxis (Loibl et al. 2009). In cases where distinctly high levels of IgE antibodies to ω-5-gliadin are detected, it is often possible, due to the test's high specificity, to abstain from challenge testing as a means of confirming the diagnosis. However, challenge testing serves not only to confirm the diagnosis but also as a means to analyze individual cofactors and determine the individual risk of anaphylaxis. A recent study demonstrated a very high diagnostic sensitivity by oral food challenge using gluten flour in addition to physical exercise or a combination of acetylsalicylic acid and alcohol (Brockow et al. 2015).

nsLTP-mediated allergies to fruit, vegetables, pulses, and nuts can also be identified using prick tests (in particular prick-to-prick testing) and by detecting specific IgE antibodies to Pru p 3 (the prototype of an nsLTP and often sufficient on its own), Mal d 3, Cor a 8, or Ara h 9, for example. The diagnostic workup of FDEIA caused by seafood also includes the determination of IgE antibodies to Pen m 1 alongside prick testing.

The diagnosis of a delayed allergy to red meat is supported by prick tests and the detection of IgE antibodies to pork and beef and confirmed by the detection of specific IgE to α-Gal.

Michel et al. (2014) recently reported that a prick test and basophil activation tests with cetuximab can point to the diagnosis.

17.7 Added Benefits Conferred by Molecular Allergy Diagnostics

Prior to the introduction of molecular allergy diagnostics, WDEIA was a poorly defined and difficult-to-diagnose clinical entity, in particular due to the low sensitivity of prick and IgE testing with aqueous wheat extracts. Many patients were incorrectly diagnosed with "idiopathic anaphylaxis" (Heaps et al. 2014). The recombinant expression of the major allergen ω-5-gliadin (Tri a 19) and its use in routine diagnostics has since made it possible to confirm the diagnosis of WDEIA with high specificity in the majority of patients (Hofmann and Jakob 2013). Sensitizations to HMW glutenin (particularly in Japan) or to other gliadins (α/β-gliadin, γ-gliadin) can generally be detected in patients lacking IgE antibodies to ω-5-gliadin (Hofmann et al. 2012; Morita et al. 2001). The determination of IgE to gliadin can be helpful as an adjunctive test.

In FDEIA caused by food (e.g., peach or soy), precise identification of the triggering single allergen, e.g., Pru p 3 in peach allergy, can permit conclusions to be drawn about the severity and further course to be expected.

Patients sensitized to Pru p 3, Gly m 5, or Gly m 6, for example, need to be instructed to avoid all consumption of peach or soy, since nsLTP similar to storage proteins are heat-stable, not denatured by gastric acids, and can cause anaphylaxis even in minute amounts.

Detailed knowledge about relevant allergens enables patients to deal safely with their allergy and improve their quality of life.

The added benefit conferred by molecular allergy diagnostics in delayed anaphylaxis due to red meat is also obvious: prick tests with extracts from beef, pork, and lamb generally produce only a small wheal (<4 mm); it was only with the recent introduction of commercially available tests to detect specific IgE to α-Gal that a contribution was made to the characterization of this relatively new clinical entity and to distinctly improved diagnostics.

17.8 Therapy and Recommendations

In the case of WDEIA, wheat-containing foods should be avoided for up to 6 h prior to physical activity and/or alcohol consumption or NSAID use. Some patients also develop FDEIA over time after switching to spelt-containing foods, which can be explained by the described cross-reactivity with other gluten-containing cereal types (barley, rye, spelt). A gluten-free diet is advised in such cases. Complete resolution of WDEIA can be achieved in the rarer form of HWP-WDEIA (described to date only in Japan) by avoiding HWP-containing soaps (Hiragun et al. 2013).

Among safe foods for individuals with nsLTP allergy are carrots, potatoes, bananas, and melon. It is possible that the fruit's sensitization potential can be reduced by scrubbing the peach surface fluff, which harbors large quantities of nsLTP. As a basic principle, patients with α-Gal allergy should avoid red meat, whereas chicken, turkey, and fish are tolerated. Cetuximab and gelatin-containing products should also be avoided.

All FDEIA patients should carry emergency medication with them, including an adrenalin autoinjector, for self-medication purposes.

No specific immunotherapy is as yet available. Individual cases of the successful prophylactic use of ketotifen, cromoglicic acid, antihistamines, montelukast, or gastric acid blockers such as misoprostol have been reported.

17.9 Perspectives

The detection of IgE antibodies to ω-5-gliadin, in conjunction with a patient's history and possibly oral challenge testing, currently serves to confirm the diagnosis of WDEIA. Future studies will reveal whether the detection of specific IgE antibodies to additional wheat proteins (HMW glutenin, α/β-gliadin, and γ-gliadin) will further improve the diagnostic sensitivity and specificity of serum diagnostics and which of these recently identified epitopes are clinically relevant. It is possible that the daily life of WDEIA patients can be improved in the future by means of genetically transformed wheat plants: wheat in which expression of the ω-5-gliadin-encoding gene is silenced has been produced in the USA. Thus, it should be possible to minimize the immunogenic potential of wheat in the future (Altenbach and Allen 2011). Similar research is under way to silence the expression of nsLTP in fruits. This has already been achieved in the tomato: Lyc e 3-deficient transgenic tomato fruits exhibit significantly reduced allergenicity (Le et al. 2010).

Diagnostics need to be optimized in particular in FDEIA caused by allergens other than wheat proteins or α-Gal. Not all these cases can be explained by sensitization to LTP, storage proteins, or tropomyosin from crustaceans. For example, a number of cases of FDEIA due to peach in the absence of evidence of IgE to Pru p 3 have been published. Further epitopes of plant allergens will undoubtedly be identified in the future and new serological test options made commercially available. Highly specific allergen chips containing all FDEIA-associated single allergens may allow for targeted FDEIA diagnostics in the future. The development of a biomarker to identify patients predisposed to cofactor-associated anaphylaxis is also desirable.

Conclusions

Well-characterized WDEIA can be seen as a model disease for FDEIA in general. Allergists should always ask patients specifically about foods and cofactors such as physical exertion in cases of anaphylaxis of unclear etiology that are not directly temporally related to food intake. If patients' history points to FDEIA, specific IgE antibodies against the following allergens should be determined:

- Recombinantly produced ω-5-gliadin in suspected WDEIA
- α-Gal in suspected delayed meat allergy
- Pru p 3 as a marker allergen in suspected LTP sensitization
- If the patient's history unequivocally points to a particular food: IgE against the relevant storage protein or nsLTP

These novel diagnostic options have significantly contributed to the diagnosis of previously unclear anaphylaxis, and the ongoing characterization of epitopes has expanded our understanding of immediate-type allergies.

References

Adachi A, Horikawa T, Shimizu H, et al. Soybean beta-conglycinin as the main allergen in a patient with food-dependent exercise-induced anaphylaxis by tofu: food processing alters pepsin resistance. Clin Exp Allergy. 2009;39:167–73.

Altenbach SB, Allen PV. Transformation of the US bread wheat 'Butte 86' and silencing of omega-5 gliadin genes. GM Crops. 2011;2:66–73.

Baar A, Pahr S, Constantin C, et al. Molecular and immunological characterization of Tri a 36, a low molecular weight glutenin, as a novel major wheat food allergen. J Immunol. 2012;189:3018–25.
Brockow K, Kneissl D, Valentini L, et al. Using a gluten oral food challenge protocol to improve diagnosis of wheat-dependent exercise-induced anaphylaxis. J Allergy Clin Immunol. 2015;135:977–84.
Caponetto P, Fischer J, Biedermann T. Gelatin-containing sweets can elicit anaphylaxis in a patient with sensitization to galactose-alpha-1,3-galactose. J Allergy Clin Immunol Pract. 2013;1:302–3.
Commins SP, James HR, Stevens W, et al. Delayed clinical and ex vivo response to mammalian meat in patients with IgE to galactose-alpha-1,3-galactose. J Allergy Clin Immunol. 2014;134:108–15.
Commins SP, Platts-Mills TA. Tick bites and red meat allergy. Curr Opin Allergy Clin Immunol. 2013;13:354–9.
Commins SP, Satinover SM, Hosen J, et al. Delayed anaphylaxis, angioedema, or urticaria after consumption of red meat in patients with IgE antibodies specific for galactose-alpha-1,3-galactose. J Allergy Clin Immunol. 2009;123:426–33.
Fukutomi Y, Itagaki Y, Taniguchi M, et al. Rhinoconjunctival sensitization to hydrolyzed wheat protein in facial soap can induce wheat-dependent exercise-induced anaphylaxis. J Allergy Clin Immunol. 2011;127:532–3.
Gonzalez-Quintela A, Dam Laursen AS, et al. IgE antibodies to alpha-gal in the general adult population. Relationship with tick bites, atopy, and cat ownership. Clin Exp Allergy. 2014;44:1061–8.
Gronlund H, Adedoyin J, Commins SP, et al. The carbohydrate galactose-alpha-1,3-galactose is a major IgE-binding epitope on cat IgA. J Allergy Clin Immunol. 2009;123:1189–91.
Hamsten C, Starkhammar M, Tran TA, et al. Identification of galactose-alpha-1,3-galactose in the gastrointestinal tract of the tick Ixodes ricinus; possible relationship with red meat allergy. Allergy. 2013;68:549–52.
Heaps A, Carter S, Selwood C, et al. The utility of the ISAC Allergen Array in the investigation of Idiopathic Anaphylaxis. Clin Exp Immunol. 2014;177:483–90.
Hilger C, Fischer J, Swiontek K, et al. Two galactose-alpha-1,3-galactose carrying peptidases from pork kidney mediate anaphylactogenic responses in delayed meat allergy. Allergy. 2016;71:711–9.
Hiragun M, Ishii K, Hiragun T, et al. The sensitivity and clinical course of patients with wheat-dependent exercise-induced anaphylaxis sensitized to hydrolyzed wheat protein in facial soap – secondary publication. Allergol Int. 2013;62:351–8.
Hofmann SC, Jakob T. Molekulare Diagnostik bei nahrungsmittelabhängiger anstrengungsinduzierter Anaphylaxie. Allergo J. 2013;22:308–11.
Hofmann SC, Fischer J, Eriksson C, et al. IgE detection to alpha/beta/gamma-gliadin and its clinical relevance in wheat-dependent exercise-induced anaphylaxis. Allergy. 2012;67:1457–60.
Le LQ, Mahler V, Scheurer S, et al. Yeast profilin complements profilin deficiency in transgenic tomato fruits and allows development of hypoallergenic tomato fruits. FASEB J. 2010;24:4939–47.
Loibl M, Schwarz S, Ring J, et al. Definition of an exercise intensity threshold in a challenge test to diagnose food-dependent exercise-induced anaphylaxis. Allergy. 2009;64:1560–1.
Matsuo H, Morita E, Tatham AS, et al. Identification of the IgE-binding epitope in omega-5 gliadin, a major allergen in wheat-dependent exercise-induced anaphylaxis. J Biol Chem. 2004;279:12135–40.
Matsuo H, Kohno K, Niihara H, et al. Specific IgE determination to epitope peptides of omega-5 gliadin and high molecular weight glutenin subunit is a useful tool for diagnosis of wheat-dependent exercise-induced anaphylaxis. J Immunol. 2005a;175:8116–22.
Matsuo H, Morimoto K, Akaki T, et al. Exercise and aspirin increase levels of circulating gliadin peptides in patients with wheat-dependent exercise-induced anaphylaxis. Clin Exp Allergy. 2005b;35:461–6.

Maulitz RM, Pratt DS, Schocket AL. Exercise-induced anaphylactic reaction to shellfish. J Allergy Clin Immunol. 1979;63:433–4.
Michel S, Scherer K, Heijnen IA, et al. Skin prick test and basophil reactivity to cetuximab in patients with IgE to alpha-gal and allergy to red meat. Allergy. 2014;69:403–5.
Morita E, Kameyoshi Y, Mihara S, et al. gamma-Gliadin: a presumptive allergen causing wheat-dependent exercise-induced anaphylaxis. Br J Dermatol. 2001;145:182–4.
Morita E, Matsuo H, Mihara S, et al. Fast omega-gliadin is a major allergen in wheat-dependent exercise-induced anaphylaxis. J Dermatol Sci. 2003;33:99–104.
Palacin A, Bartra J, Munoz R, et al. Anaphylaxis to wheat flour-derived foodstuffs and the lipid transfer protein syndrome: a potential role of wheat lipid transfer protein Tri a 14. Int Arch Allergy Immunol. 2010;152:178–83.
Palosuo K, Varjonen E, Nurkkala J, et al. Transglutaminase-mediated cross-linking of a peptic fraction of omega-5 gliadin enhances IgE reactivity in wheat-dependent, exercise-induced anaphylaxis. J Allergy Clin Immunol. 2003;111:1386–92.
Petersen A, Scheurer S. Stabile pflanzliche Nahrungsmittelallergene: Lipid-Transfer-Proteine. Allergo J. 2011;20:384–6.
Radauer C, Kleine-Tebbe J, Beyer K. Stabile pflanzliche Nahrungsmittelallergene: Speicherproteine. Allergo J. 2012;21:8888–92.
Romano A, Scala E, Rumi G, et al. Lipid transfer proteins: the most frequent sensitizer in Italian subjects with food-dependent exercise-induced anaphylaxis. Clin Exp Allergy. 2012;42: 1643–53.
Sander I, Raulf-Heimsoth M, Duser M, et al. Differentiation between cosensitization and cross-reactivity in wheat flour and grass pollen-sensitized subjects. Int Arch Allergy Immunol. 1997;112:378–85.
Takahashi H, Matsuo H, Chinuki Y, et al. Recombinant high molecular weight-glutenin subunit-specific IgE detection is useful in identifying wheat-dependent exercise-induced anaphylaxis complementary to recombinant omega-5 gliadin-specific IgE test. Clin Exp Allergy. 2012;42:1293–8.
Takahashi H, Chinuki Y, Tanaka A, et al. Laminin gamma-1 and collagen alpha-1 (VI) chain are galactose-alpha-1, 3-galactose-bound allergens in beef. Allergy. 2014;69:199–207.
Varjonen E, Vainio E, Kalimo K. Antigliadin IgE—indicator of wheat allergy in atopic dermatitis. Allergy. 2000;55:386–91.
Wong GK, Krishna MT. Food-dependent exercise-induced anaphylaxis: is wheat unique? Curr Allergy Asthma Rep. 2013;13:639–44.
Yokooji T, Kurihara S, Murakami T, et al. Characterization of causative allergens for wheat-dependent exercise-induced anaphylaxis sensitized with hydrolyzed wheat proteins in facial soap. Allergol Int. 2013;62:435–45.

Benefits and Limitations of Recombinant Allergens in Diagnostics of Insect Venom Allergy

18

T. Jakob, S. Blank, and E. Spillner

18.1 Introduction

Insect venom allergies belong to the classical immunoglobulin-E-(IgE)-mediated allergies and are often manifest as severe anaphylactic reactions that can even be lethal. According to the recommendations of current guidelines for diagnosis and therapy of insect venom allergies, a diagnostic work-up is recommended for patients with systemic insect sting reactions to demonstrate an IgE-mediated sensitization to the venom of the stinging insect (Przybilla et al. 2011).

For patients with systemic sting reactions, venom immunotherapy (VIT) offers a high degree of protection against anaphylactic reactions to subsequent stings. A prerequisite for initiating VIT is the unequivocal demonstration of an IgE-mediated

This chapter is based on a publication by the authors that was published in *Allergo Journal* 2012 (Spillner E, Blank S, Jakob T: Potentials, pitfalls and current state of molecular diagnostics in insect venom allergy. Allergo J 2012;21:249–56) and has now been extended and updated as book chapter.
The authors gratefully thank Dr. David B. K. Golden, Allergy Division of Internal Medicine at MedStar Franklin Square Medical Center and Johns Hopkins University School of Medicine, Baltimore, MD, USA, for reviewing the manuscript, editorial assistance, and many helpful suggestions regarding this chapter.

T. Jakob, MD, Prof. (✉)
Department of Dermatology and Allergology, University Medical Center Giessen (UKGM), Justus-Liebig-University, Giessen, Germany
e-mail: thilo.jakob@derma.med.uni-giessen.de

S. Blank, PhD
Center of Allergy and Environment (ZAUM), Technical University of Munich and Helmholtz Center Munich, Munich, Germany
e-mail: simon.blank@tum.de

E. Spillner, PhD, Prof.
Immunological Engineering, Department of Engineering, Aarhus University, Aarhus, Denmark
e-mail: e.spillner@eng.au.dk

J. Kleine-Tebbe, T. Jakob (eds.), *Molecular Allergy Diagnostics*,
DOI 10.1007/978-3-319-42499-6_18

sensitization against the venom of the culprit insect, which in Central and Northern Europe is predominantly honeybee or yellow jacket (Przybilla et al. 2011) (◉ Fig. 18.1).

The diagnosis of insect venom allergy is based on a positive history of a systemic sting reaction and the demonstration of an IgE-mediated sensitization to the insect venom (◉ Fig. 18.2), which is obtained either by skin testing or by measuring specific IgE antibodies against honeybee or yellow jacket venom using unfractionated venom preparations.

In daily practice, however, test results are often difficult to interpret, particularly when specific IgE tests show positive results for both honeybee and yellow jacket venom. In this case it cannot be distinguished whether double-positive test results are due to cross-reactivity or genuine double sensitization. Unfortunately this is not a rare event. In our own cohort, 47 % of patients with Hymenoptera venom allergy displayed double-positive results when tested for sIgE to honeybee and yellow jacket venom (◉ Fig. 18.3).

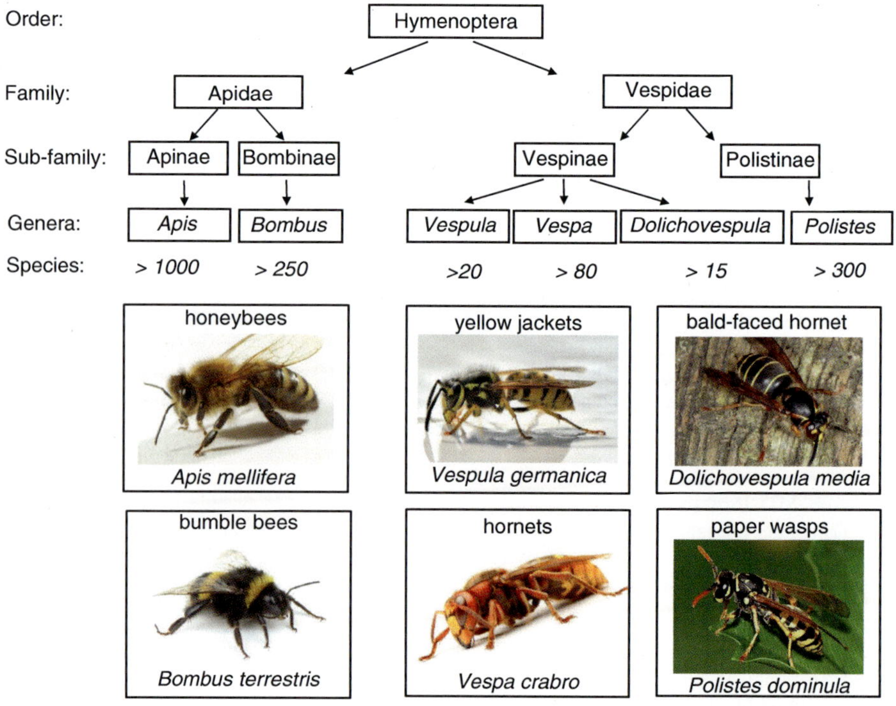

Fig. 18.1 Major elicitors of insect venom allergy (Source and copyright: *Apis mellifera* © Tomo Jesenicnik/fotolia.com; *Vespula germanica* © Sabine Schmidt/fotolia.com; *Bombus terrestris* © Roman Ivaschenko/fotolia.com; *Dolichovespula media* © Fritz Geller-Grimm/wikipedia.de; *Polistes dominula* © Fritz Geller-Grimm/wikipedia.de; *Vespa crabro* © Szasz-Fabian Erika/fotolia.com)

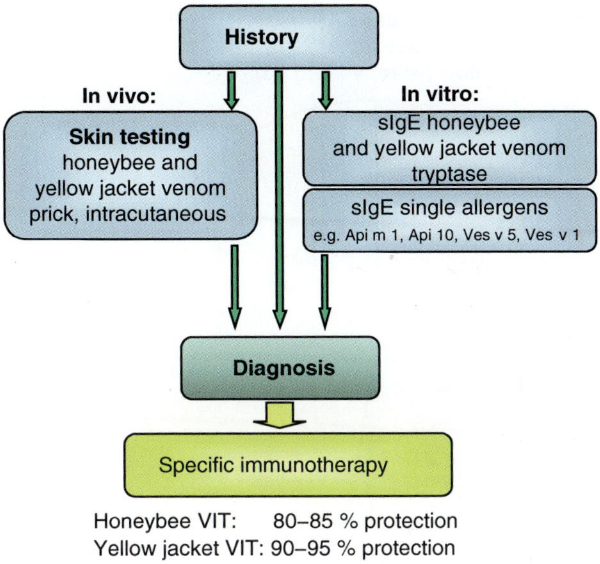

Fig. 18.2 Diagnosis of insect venom allergy is based on a positive history of a systemic insect sting reaction and the detection of IgE-mediated insect venom sensitization, either by skin test or by in vitro detection of sIgE against yellow jacket and honeybee venom extracts and/or recombinant single allergens

IgE reactivity against both honeybee and yellow jacket venom can either reflect a genuine double sensitization or be caused by cross-reactive structures present in both venoms. IgE cross-reactivity may be based on common protein epitopes, e.g., of homologous allergens, that are present in both venoms and have a high degree of sequence identity as described for hyaluronidases, dipeptidylpeptidases, and vitellogenins. Alternatively cross-reactivities can be attributed to so-called cross-reactive carbohydrate determinants (CCD). CCD reactivity of IgE antibodies is thought to be primarily due to sensitization to CCD-positive plant-derived allergens.

Recombinantly produced CCD-free insect venom allergens now allow for a better differentiation of genuine double sensitization and cross-reactivity and represent an important advancement in the diagnostics of insect venom allergy (Jakob et al. 2014; Jakob and Ollert 2011; Müller and Helbling 2013; Spillner et al. 2012, 2014) (◉ Fig. 18.4).

Patients with a convincing history of an anaphylactic sting reaction, but negative venom sIgE, represent another difficult to interpret clinical constellation. At least in yellow jacket venom allergy, the introduction of recombinantly produced insect venom allergens resulted in a significant improvement of diagnostic sensitivity that allowed the detection of IgE-mediated sensitization in the majority of yellow jacket venom extract-negative patients.

Here we present the currently known Hymenoptera venom allergens and discuss the benefit and limitations for improved diagnostics in Hymenoptera venom allergy.

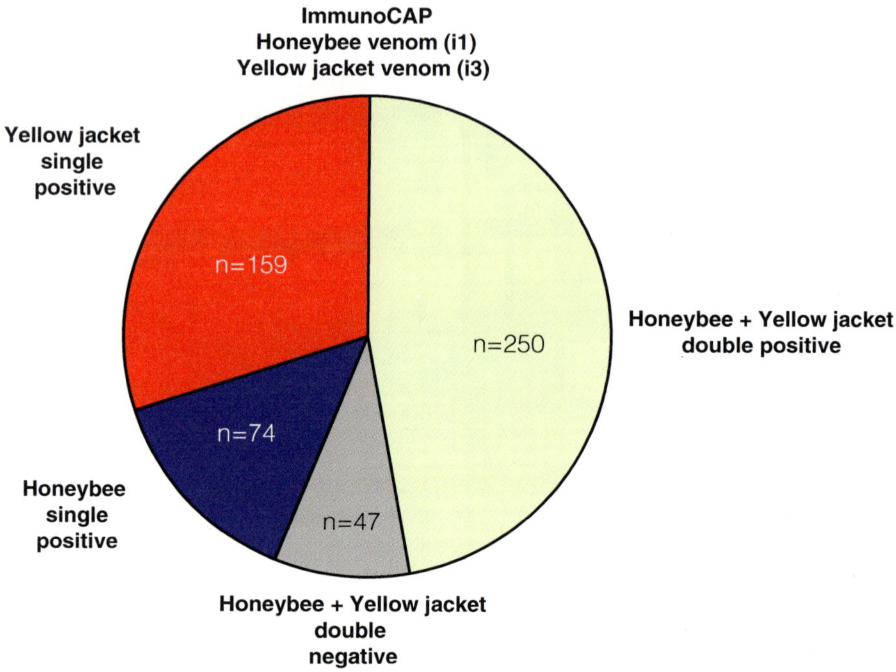

Fig. 18.3 Distribution of insect venom sensitizations in conventional, extract-based diagnostics ($n=530$ patients with anaphylactic sting reaction: 112 honeybee, 231 yellow jacket, 187 sting by unknown insect). Double-positive results are obtained in 47 % of the patients for which it remains unclear if the double-positive test results reflect genuine double sensitization or are due to cross-reactivity

Individual aspects were published by the authors before in different review articles (Jakob et al. 2014; Jakob and Ollert 2011; Spillner et al. 2012, 2014) and are summarized here in an updated form.

18.2 Structure, Function, and Relevance of Hymenoptera Venom Allergens

The advancement in the field of molecular characterization of the composition of Hymenoptera venoms is best exemplified by the venom allergen components of the honeybee (*Apis mellifera*) and the common yellow jacket (*Vespula vulgaris*). A list of the allergens that are currently known and available in databases is given in ◉ Table 18.1.

The most prominent honeybee venom (HBV) allergens include phospholipase A2 (Api m 1), hyaluronidase (Api m 2), and the basic 26 amino acid peptide melittin (Api m 4) (Arbesman et al. 1976), which together constitute the majority of venom proteins with estimated amounts of 12 %, 2 %, and 50 % of the venom dry weight, respectively (Müller 1988). Classical yellow jacket venom (YJV) allergens are

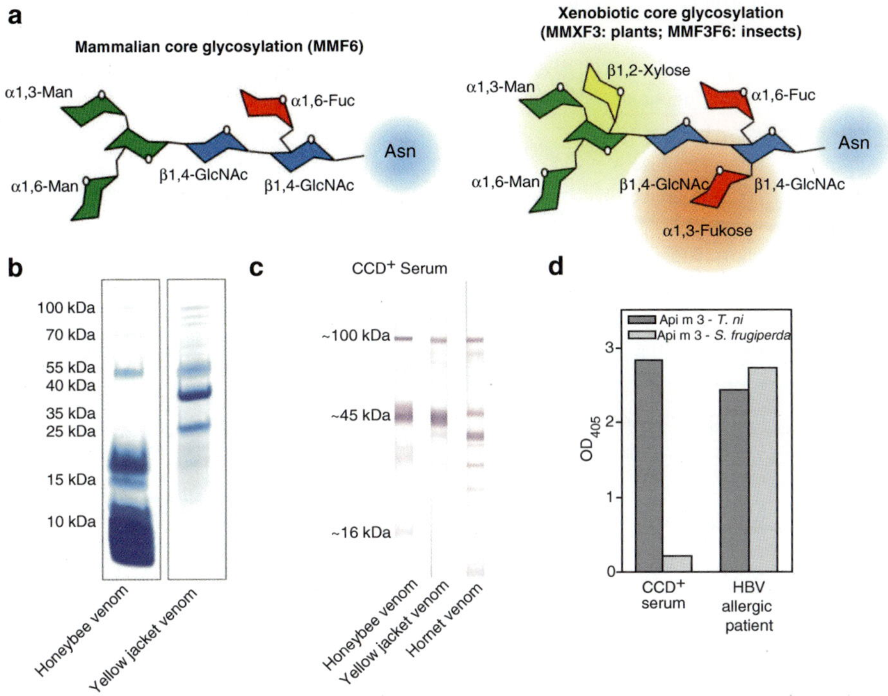

Fig. 18.4 Cross-reactive carbohydrate determinants (CCDs) in honeybee and yellow jacket venom and their relevance on sIgE reactivities: (**a**) Simplified, exemplary representation of the core glycosylation of mammals such as humans as compared to the xenobiotic glycosylation of insects and plants. The latter ones carry an additional α-1,3-linked fucose residue and in plants a β-1,2-linked xylose residue (*GlcNAc* N-acetylglucosamine, *Man* mannose, *Fuc* Fucose). (**b**) Highly variant distribution of high and low abundance components of honeybee and yellow jacket venom in a gelelectrophoretic analysis. (**c**) Exemplary sIgE reactivity of a CCD-positive serum with honeybee, yellow jacket, and hornet venom in immunoblotting. (**d**) sIgE reactivity of a CCD-positive serum and the serum of a honeybee venom-allergic patient with recombinant Api m 3 from *S. frugiperda* and *T. ni* insect cells in ELISA. In contrast to the pronounced CCD reactivity of Api m 3 produced in *T. ni* insect cells, the CCD reactivity of Api m 3 from Sf9 cells is immunologically not detectable

phospholipase A1 (Ves v 1), hyaluronidase (Ves v 2), and antigen 5 (Ves v 5) (King et al. 1983), the function of which remains unknown, which represent 6–14 %, 1–3 %, and 5–10 % of the venom dry weight. In recent years, however, significant progress has been made in identification of novel molecules of lower abundance. For some the allergic potential had already been described, such as the acid phosphatase of HBV (Api m 3); however, the gene was identified and recombinantly expressed only recently (Arbesman et al. 1976; Grunwald et al. 2006). Moreover, with the identification of the 100 kDa allergen C of HBV and its YJV homolog as dipeptidylpeptidases IV, a novel class of Hymenoptera venom enzymes could be described (Blank et al. 2010; Hoffman et al. 1977). In YJV in addition to the classical hyaluronidase (Ves v 2.0101), an inactive isoform (Ves v 2.0201) was identified, which seems to be the dominating isoform in the venom (Kolarich et al. 2005).

Table 18.1 Overview of the known allergens of the families Apidae and Vespidae

Allergen	Name/function	MW [kDa]	% DW	Potential N-glycosylation sites	Bacterial expression	Eukaryotic expression
Honeybees (e.g., *Apis mellifera*)						
Api m 1	Phospholipase A_2	17	12	1	+	+
Api m 2[a]	Hyaluronidase	45	2	3	+	+
Api m 3	Saure phosphatase	49	1–2	2		+
Api m 4	Melittin	3	50	–		–
Api m 5[b]	Allergen C/DPP IV	100	<1	6		+
Api m 6	Protease inhibitor	8	1–2	–		+
Api m 7[e]	Protease	39	?	3		+
Api m 8	Carboxylesterase	70	?	4		+
Api m 9	Carboxypeptidase	60	?	4		+
Api m 10	CRP/icarapin	55	<1	2	+	+
Api m 11.0101	MRJP 8	65	?	6		+
Api m 11.0201	MRJP 9	60	?	3		+
Api m 12[c]	Vitellogenin	200	?	1		+
Bumble bees (e.g., *Bombus terrestris*)						
Bom t 1	Phospholipase A_2	16		1		
Bom t 4	Protease	27		1		
Yellow jackets (e.g., *Vespula vulgaris*)						
Ves v 1	Phospholipase A_1	35	6–14	–		+
Ves v 2.0101[a]	Hyaluronidase	45	1–3	4	+	+
Ves v 2.0201[a]	Hyaluronidase[f]	45	?	2		+
Ves v 3[b]	DPP IV	100	?	6		+
Ves v 5[d]	Antigen 5	25	5–10	–	+	+
Ves v 6[c]	Vitellogenin	200	?	4		+
Hornets (e.g., *Vespa crabro*)						
Vesp c 1	Phospholipase A_1	34		–		
Vesp c 5[d]	Antigen 5	23		–		+
Bald-faced hornet (e.g., *Dolichovespula maculata*)						
Dol m 1	Phospholipase A_1	34		2		
Dol m 2	Hyaluronidase	42		2		
Dol m 5[d]	Antigen 5	23		–		+
European paper wasps (e.g., *Polistes dominula*)						
Pol d 1	Phospholipase A_1	34		1		+

Table 18.1 (continued)

Allergen	Name/function	MW [kDa]	% DW	Potential N-glycosylation sites	Bacterial expression	Eukaryotic expression
Pol d 4	Protease	33		6		+
Pol d 5[d]	Antigen 5	23		–		+
American paper wasps (e.g, *Polistes annularis*)						
Pol a 1	Phospholipase A_1	34		3		+
Pol a 2	Hyaluronidase	38		–		
Pol a 4	Protease	?		2		+
Pol a 5[d]	Antigen 5	23		–		+

CRP carbohydrate-rich protein, *DPP IV* dipeptidylpeptidase IV, *MRJP* major royal jelly protein, *DW* dry weight
[a, b, c]Corresponding cross-reactive allergens in honeybee and yellow jacket venom
[d]Corresponding and potentially cross-reactive allergens in venoms of yellow jacket, hornet, bald-faced hornet, and paper wasps
[e]A homologous protease was identified in yellow jacket venom, but not described as allergen
[f]Inactive isoform

Furthermore, it was demonstrated that Api m 10 represents a novel major allergen of HBV with potentially high impact for diagnostic and therapeutic applications (Blank et al. 2011a; Köhler et al. 2014). Other IgE-reactive proteins of HBV include a putative protease inhibitor (Kettner et al. 2001), a protease (Winningham et al. 2004), an esterase, and a peptidase whose relevance is currently investigated. The newest allergens are the two major royal jelly proteins (MRJP) 8 and 9 (2 isoforms of Api m 11) from HBV (Blank et al. 2012) as well as novel pan-allergens, the vitellogenins Api m 12 and Ves v 6 (Blank et al. 2013a).

It should also be mentioned here that nearly all and, in particular, the new allergens are glycoproteins, a finding of significant relevance.

In addition to these components with documented allergenic nature, some other components such as a C1q-like protein (de Graaf et al. 2010), a PDGF/VEGF (platelet-derived growth factor/vascular endothelial growth factor)-like protein (Peiren et al. 2005), and hexamerin (Schmidt et al. 2005) were recently identified. The allergenic nature of these components still has to be evaluated.

With an increasing application of proteomic and genomic approaches, it is evident that the number of relevant identified allergens will rise significantly in the future. How many and, most importantly, which ones of the allergens will become essential and important for molecular diagnostics and in which form they will be used in routine diagnostic procedures remain impossible to predict at this point in time.

Transcriptomics very recently suggested the presence of an antigen 5-like protein in the venom of winter bees (Van Vaerenbergh et al. 2013). Even the season (and most likely the climate and geographic region) seems to have a profound impact on the venom. Proteomics revealed the presence of the antimicrobial peptide apidaecin (Van Vaerenbergh et al. 2013) further demonstrating that the complexity of the venom is not restricted to larger proteins. The lower molecular weight fraction of the venom contains a variety of peptidic components with unique biophysical and clinical characteristics. Their contributions to the sting reaction beyond IgE reactivity however still need to be addressed.

By increasing application of advanced proteomic, peptidomic, and genomic approaches, the venom and thereby the number of allergens certainly will significantly increase in the future. The most recent proteomic analysis of honey bee venom revealed >100 different components (Van Vaerenbergh et al. 2014). Furthermore, another level of complexity is achieved by the generation of additional isoforms and posttranslational modification. All available data however suggest that the apparent plasticity of the venom makes its final definition a never ending story. As HBV and YJV can be considered prototypic for other Hymenoptera venoms, their composition is reflected in other species including the bumble bee (Bombus terrestris and the American *Bombus pennsylvanicus*), the venom composition of which closely resembles that of the honeybee. Bumble bees gained particular importance for pollination industry workers. By analogy, venom allergens of diverse other *Vespidae* species such as the white-faced hornet (*Dolichovespula maculata*) or the European hornet (*Vespa crabro*) are fairly similar to those of the yellow jacket.

Allergy to venom of the phylogenetically more-distant paper wasps (Polistinae) is common in North America as well as in Europe, especially in Mediterranean areas. Important *Polistes* species in Europe are *P. dominula* and *P. gallicus*, whereas in Northern America other species such as *P. annularis*, *P. apachus*, *P. exclamans*, *P. fuscatus*, and *P. metricus* are dominant. In the last decades, *P. dominula* has increasingly spread across the North American continent and central and northern parts of Europe. The IgE cross-reactivity between European and American *Polistes* species is described as rather low because they belong to different subgenera. In contrast, cross-reactivity between Polistinae and Vespinae (*Vespula*, *Dolichovespula*, and *Vespa*) venoms and purified venom proteins (Monsalve et al. 2012) is frequently observed, especially for *Vespula* and both American and European *Polistes* venom (Caruso et al. 2007).

For all these species, only a limited set of allergens has been identified so far although it is quite likely that all venoms will contain conserved allergens such as hyaluronidases, dipeptidylpeptidases, and vitellogenins that in part contribute to molecular cross-reactivity. Other protein families such as proteases (Api m 7, Pol d 4, Ves v 4) show clear molecular differences, and it remains open if these proteases will be found in all Hymenoptera venoms.

Moreover, it is widely accepted that IgE cross-reactivity between different insect venoms can be attributed to cross-reactive carbohydrate determinants (CCD) that are present on a large number of venom allergens.

The only exceptions are apparently venoms of *Polistes* species that seem to lack the alpha 1,3-linked fucose residue that is responsible for IgE reactivity to CCDs (Blank et al. 2013b).

18.3 Methodological Aspects for the Production of Recombinant Hymenoptera Venom Allergens

Until recently only a very limited number of venom allergens such as Api m 1, Api m 4, and Ves v 5 was available either as native or recombinant proteins (King and Spangfort 2000; Müller 2003). Their use and the possibility to perform analyses on a molecular level resulted in a clear improvement of diagnostic precision.

Inherent problems and general considerations however apply for the isolation and production of venom allergens. Purification of native proteins from venom is a suitable approach for high abundance allergens only (such as Api m 1, Api m 4, Ves v 1, Ves v 5), but even then you run the risk of having contaminating residual components in the preparation that may distort the picture at a molecular level. For example, the removal of Api m 4 as predominant component in honeybee venom is highly difficult.

When using recombinant technologies, this particular problem does not exist, but difficulties rather lie in the establishment of an adequate and efficient production system.

For the first recombinant expressions of insect venom allergens, the bacterial system was employed which definitely is suited to easily and quickly obtain large amounts of protein. Apart from efficient production, however, authentic conformational structure and immunoreactivity of the allergens have to be guaranteed. Their toxic nature and enzymatic activities may also have an impact on efficacy of production and the characteristics of the resulting recombinant proteins. Selected insect venom allergens nevertheless could be produced in a functional form in bacteria, primarily for structural analyses (◉ Table 18.1) (Dudler et al. 1992; Gmachl and Kreil 1993; Henriksen et al. 2001; Kuchler et al. 1989; Skov et al. 2006; Soldatova et al. 1998). The efficiency of the prokaryotic approach is often compromised by the need for extensive folding steps limiting its use to structurally relatively simple and small molecules.

In summary it is evident from the available data that purification is only suitable occasionally and a bacterial expression is suitable only for few, non-glycosylated allergens of primarily lower molecular weight.

18.3.1 Recombinant Allergens from Eukaryotic Cells

Eukaryotic cells grow more slowly and provide reduced yields of recombinant proteins, but result in proteins with invariant alterations in the form of posttranslational modifications.

In contrast to *Escherichia coli*, eukaryotic cells such as yeasts as well as insect cells and mammalian cells add oligosaccharides that have a similar core structure mimicking the glycan of the native glycosylated allergen and influence both folding and immunoreactivity (Soldatova et al. 1998).

The majority of IgE epitopes appear to be conformational and demand an intact surface. Hence the eukaryotic approach for expression of allergens is superior for diagnostic purposes, and posttranslational modifications are essential for the formation of correct three-dimensional structures of many eukaryotic proteins.

Although recognized early (Soldatova et al. 1998), in the last few years, expression in insect cells was established as an appropriate system for insect venom allergens. The functionality of proteins, the epitope authenticity, and the correct folding of resulting proteins could be demonstrated for a large number of allergens (◉ Table 18.1) (Blank et al. 2010; Soldatova et al. 1998; Seismann et al. 2010a). As an indicator for the latter, the enzymatic activity – if existing – can be considered, as shown for insect cell-derived phospholipase A_1 (Ves v 1) (Seismann et al. 2010b), hyaluronidases (Api m 2, Ves v 2) (Soldatova et al. 1998; Seismann et al. 2010a), and dipeptidylpeptidases IV (Api m 5, Ves v 3) (Blank et al. 2010).

Api m 1 serves as an additional example for the potential of recombinant approaches. It has a single glycosylation site that can be occupied with a oligomannosidic N-glycan. In addition Api m 1 carries an alpha 1,3-linked fucose on the N-glycan core structure and thus is reactive with IgE directed against CCDs. Hence Api m 1 exists in nature in different glycoforms. Expression of Api m 1 in E. coli results in a homogenous protein without glycan. Expression in eukaryotic systems yields a heterogenous set of glycoforms also present in the natural form that also could be produced on demand (Blank et al. 2011b). A mutation of the glycosylation site again results in a homogenous protein. Different variants of recombinant forms of Api m 1 are or will become commercially available.

18.4 Benefits of Molecular Diagnostics

The utility of molecular diagnostics is evident in particular in situations when conventional extract-based diagnostics is limited. These limitations primarily include false-positive and false-negative test results as well as questions for individual reactivity of selected allergens. In the following some of these issues are described.

18.4.1 Molecular Diagnostics for Differentiation of Double Sensitizations

Apart from a genuine double sensitization to honeybee and yellow jacket venom, cross-reactivities in extract-based diagnostic tests can result in false-positive results. This phenomenon may be based on common protein epitopes of homologous allergens of both venoms as described for hyaluronidases (Api m 2, Ves v 2) and dipeptidylpeptidases (Api m 5, Ves v 3) and for and the new 200 kDa vitellogenin allergens (Api m 12, Ves v 6) which are present in both venoms (◉ Fig. 18.5).

Alternatively a majority of cross-reactivities can be attributed to IgE antibodies directed against cross-reactive glyco-epitopes of the allergens (cross-reactive carbohydrate determinants, CCD) (Hemmer et al. 2004; Jappe et al. 2006; Aalberse et al. 2001). This is of particular importance, since most honeybee and yellow jacket venom allergens are glycoproteins with one or more of such carbohydrate structures (◉ Table 18.1).

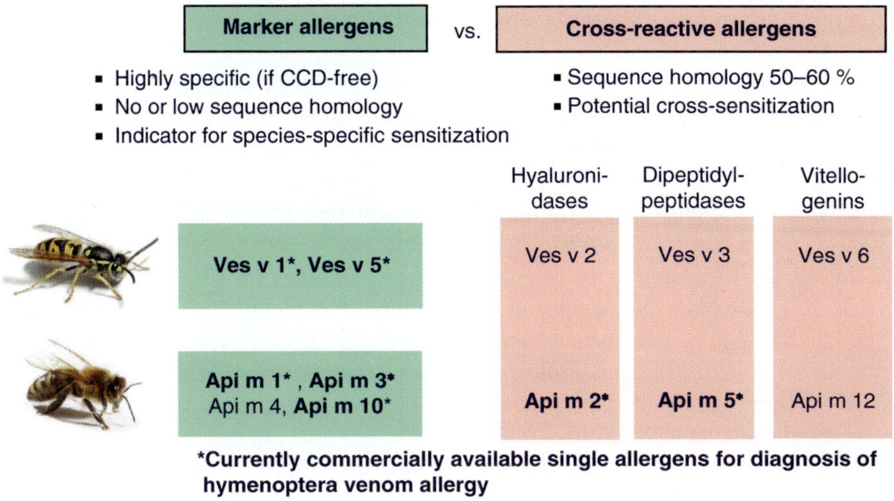

Fig. 18.5 Recombinant insect venom allergens that can be used for differentiation of genuine sensitization and cross-reactivity. Marker allergens (e.g., Ves v 1, Ves 5, and Api m 1, Api m 3, Api m 10) allow for identification of genuine sensitization (e.g., to yellow jacket and honeybee venom). In contrast, cross-reactive allergens such as hyaluronidases (Ves v 2, Api m 2), dipeptidylpeptidases (Ves v 3, Api m 5), or vitellogenins (Ves v 6, Api m 12) are homologous proteins in different venoms and therefore do not provide reliable information about genuine sensitization or cross-reactivity

Causative for the phenomenon of cross-reactivity are IgE antibodies that are directed against an alpha 1,3-linked fucose residue of the N-glycan core established by insects and plants (◉ Fig. 18.4a). A beta 1,2-xylose residue at the core glycan to which IgE also can be directed is found in plants, but not in insects. Such xenobiotic modifications represent highly immunogenic epitopes which can induce specific immunoglobulin-G (IgG) as well as IgE antibodies (Jin et al. 2008). CCD-specific IgE antibodies against the fucose-based epitope have been reported to be responsible for the majority of double sensitizations to honeybee and yellow jacket venom (Jappe et al. 2006), complicating the choice of the appropriate therapeutic intervention. The clinical relevance of CCD reactive IgE antibodies is controversial, but in the case of insect venom allergy appears to be low or non-existing.

Nevertheless, anti-CCD IgE represents an undoubted pitfall of in vitro allergy diagnostics, since they cause multiple reactivities with any glycosylated plant (food, pollen) or insect venom allergen and thereby interfere with the detection of clinically relevant sensitization to protein epitopes (◉ Fig. 18.4b, c).

For determination of CCD-specific antibodies, different reagents are now available (bromelain, MUXF; horseradish peroxidase, HRP; ascorbatoxidase). As natural proteins they have to be considered a phenomenological indicator rather than exact glycan structure and do not allow for conclusions on relevance of other sensitizations.

The use of glycosylated, species-specific allergens such as Api m 1 (◉ Table 18.1) is only an inferior option, and the deletion of glycosylation sites – as realized in a commercial product – de facto is not feasible for proteins with multiple glycans, e.g., Api m 3 and Api m 5.

The use of Sf9 insect cells from *Spodoptera frugiperda* as the expression system results in allergens with functional glycosylation, proper folding, and complete epitope spectrum but not showing any immunologically detectable CCD reactivity (◉ Fig. 18.4d). This phenomenon is obviously based on the specific absence of alpha 1,3-core fucosylation (Seismann et al. 2010a). Other insect cells however such as those from *Trichoplusia ni* are able to establish the authentic phenotype including the CCD reactivity.

So far, molecular diagnostics applying non-glycosylated species-specific allergens such as Api m 1 and Ves v 5 led to a significant benefit in the dissection of true double sensitization versus cross-reactivity (Hofmann et al. 2011a; Müller et al. 2009). The potential of this approach can be realized in the future by additional species-specific as well as cross-reactive, but CCD-free allergens.

Furthermore, CCD-free-engineered and correctly folded allergens allow for the first time the assessment of their relevance regardless of their natural glycosylation bypassing complex inhibition analyses. Using CCD-free, correctly folded Ves v 2.0101 and Ves v 2.0201, we were able to clearly demonstrate that hyaluronidases – contrary to previous assumptions – do not play a significant role as major allergens of yellow jacket venom (Seismann et al. 2010a), a fact that was corroborated by findings of others (Jin et al. 2010; Seppala et al. 2009). In contrast, even for highly glycosylated proteins such as Api m 5, Api m 10, and Api m 11, a pronounced IgE reactivity beyond CCDs with clinical relevance was demonstrated (Blank et al. 2011b, 2012).

These approaches recently allowed a first systematic analysis of IgE reactivities to six individual allergens from honeybee venom (Köhler et al. 2014).

It was shown that much more of the venom proteins represent major allergens than anticipated. Moreover patients exhibited highly individual and complex reactivity profiles that often include sIgE antibodies to components that are only occasionally present in extracts (Blank et al. 2011a).

In summary the use of such defined recombinant molecules that do not reflect the natural, but the diagnostically and clinically important IgE reactivity will shed light on the relevance of individual allergens and may allow the charcterization of comprehensive sensitization profiles.

18.4.2 Use of Recombinant Insect Venom Allergens in Clinical Routine Diagnostics

Until recently only few individual major allergens have been available as recombinantly expressed products for routine diagnostics in insect venom allergy. These include phospholipase A_2 (Api m 1) and icarapin (Api m 10) from honeybee venom, the antigen 5 from yellow jacket (Ves v 5), the phospholipase A_1 (Ves v 1) from yellow jacket, and the antigen 5 from paper wasps (Pol d 5).

The main field of application of recombinant insect venom allergens is the differentiation of true double sensitization and cross-reactivity in patients who exhibit IgE reactivity against both honeybee venom and yellow jacket venom (◉ Fig. 18.5).

This is particularly true when the culprit insect could not reliably be identified by the patient. The current guidelines recommend immunotherapy with both venoms in cases in which the culprit insect was not identified and the skin testing and/or sIgE testing demonstrate a double sensitization to both venoms. Since the anaphylactic reaction usually was mediated by the sting of one insect species only, this double immunotherapy usually represents an overtreatment and could be avoided, provided that reliable laboratory parameters would be available that allow a clear-cut differentiation of cross-reactivity and genuine sensitization.

Prerequisite for a reliable differentiation using recombinant insect venom allergens is a sufficient prevalence of sensitization to the tested allergens and a sufficient sensitivity of the test used. Since the introduction of test reagents for routine diagnostic work-up, a plethora of studies were published which could be summarized as follows.

The recombinant marker allergens available for diagnosis of yellow jacket allergy, i.e., Ves v 5 and Ves v 1, detect 94–97 % of yellow jacket-allergic patients (Jakob and Ollert 2011; Hofmann et al. 2011a; Ebo et al. 2013; Müller et al. 2012; Vos et al. 2013).

Here a diagnostic gap of 3–6 % is remaining, which would be nice to close, e.g., by additional recombinant yellow jacket allergens. Unfortunately the other established yellow jacket allergens Ves v 2, Ves v 3, and Ves v 6 are only partially suited for this, since all of them have homologous allergens in honeybee venom. It remains open if additional marker allergens in yellow jacket venom can be identified that close the remaining diagnostic gap.

The situation is completely different for the molecular diagnosis of honeybee venom allergy. Initially there was only Api m 1 available as a recombinant marker allergen for honeybee venom allergy. Specific IgE to Api m 1 was found for 97 % of bee venom-allergic patients in the first study (Müller et al. 2009). Here a bacterially produced Api m 1 was used for analysis in a fluid phase test system (Advia) that is not available for routine diagnosis anymore. The included honeybee venom-allergic patients were strictly selected for a history of an anaphylactic sting reaction within the last 12 months and positive skin test. Follow-up studies using Api m 1 now available for routine diagnostics on a solid-phase assay system, the ImmunoCAP platform, showed lower sensitization rates. Based on these data, the prevalence of Api m 1 sensitization in patients with honeybee venom allergy is now reported as approximately 70 % only (57–82 %) (Köhler et al. 2014; Müller et al. 2012; Hofmann et al. 2011b; Jakob et al. 2012; Korosec et al. 2011).

The significant differences in sensitization rates to Api m 1 in the different studies were explained by some authors as regional variations of analyzed study populations (Sturm et al. 2012). According to our interpretation, the differences more likely rely on the varying definition of patient populations. Here very stringent criteria were applied, e.g., anaphylaxis after bee sting within the last 12 months, positive skin test, positive serology, and identification of the culprit insect by the patient, whereas other studies employed less stringent inclusion criteria.

Another approach to explain the low prevalence for recombinant Api m 1 is the estimation that the expression system used here is not optimal. A head-to-head comparison of natural and recombinant Api m 1 reported significant differences (Korosec et al. 2011). Follow-up studies however documented that increased sensitization rates for natural Api m 1 are primarily caused by elevated CCD reactivities and that patients without CCD reactivity showed similar sensitization rates for natural and recombinant Api m 1 (Jakob et al. 2012).

Apart from speculations about why large differences in prevalence of Api m 1 sensitization are observed, it is clear that a substantial part of honeybee venom-allergic patients (30 %; a range of 18–43 %) cannot be detected by using recombinant Api m 1 only.

This significant diagnostic gap means in clinical routine that a honeybee venom allergy cannot be ruled out reliably by an Api m 1-negative test result. Here an extension of the diagnostic spectrum by additional marker allergens is urgently needed.

In this context we recently established detailed sensitization profiles in a large cohort of honeybee venom-allergic patients by using ImmunoCAP research prototypes of Api m 2, Api m 3, Api m 4, Api m 5, and Api m 10 (Köhler et al. 2014). From this study of more than 140 patients with honeybee venom allergy, it became evident that – in addition to Api m 1 – Api m 3, Api m 5, and Api m 10, with sensitization rates of more than 50 %, have to be considered as major allergens in honeybee venom. The rate of sensitization to Api m 1 was found at 72 % in the study group. By combination of all analyzed allergens, 95 % of the honeybee venom-allergic patients could be identified. Against this background Api m 2, Api m 3, Api m 5, and Api m 10 are currently being developed for routine diagnostics. The use of Api m 10 and Api m 3 as additional marker allergens in a routine setting allowed the detection of a significant sensitization in 50 % of the Api m 1-negative honey bee venom-allergic patients (Frick et al. 2015). Api m 10 has been introduced into the market in June 2015, and the release of additional honeybee allergens such as Api m 2, Api m 3, and Api m 5 is expected by the end of 2016.

18.4.3 Improvement of Test Sensitivity by Recombinant Allergens

Another diagnostic difficulty arises in patients with a well-documented history of an anaphylactic sting reaction, but negative venom sIgE test results. A possible reason might be that venom extracts represent heterogeneous mixtures in which components are present in widely varying concentrations and that particular allergens can be lost or degraded during processing (Blank et al. 2011a).

Already in the very first study on the benefits of using sIgE to Api m 1 and Ves v 5 in the diagnostics of Hymenoptera venom allergy, it was reported that for patients with a convincing history of an anaphylactic yellow jacket sting reaction but negative serology to yellow jacket venom (ImmunoCAP I3), positive specific IgE level against the marker allergen Ves v 5 was determined in five out of eight cases (Hofmann et al. 2011b). These results were verified in a larger follow-up study of 308 patients with yellow jacket venom allergy (Vos et al. 2013). In this population 83.4 % of patients displayed a sensitization as determined by sIgE (≥0,35 kU/l) to yellow jacket venom extract (i3). In contrast, 96 % of this population displayed an IgE sensitization when tested for sIgE to single allergens Ves v 1 and Ves v 5. Among patients with a history of yellow jacket sting anaphylaxis but negative IgE test results to yellow jacket venom extract, 84.4 % could be diagnosed by using recombinant Ves v 5. Comparative analyses of IgE reactivity against yellow jacket venom and Ves v 5 revealed a significantly higher IgE reactivity to the single component as compared to the extract. These observations suggested that IgE reactivity to Ves v 5 was underrepresented in the whole venom extract.

Causative for such a phenomenon could be different mechanisms, such as:

- A lack of the allergen Ves v 5 in whole yellow jacket venom extract
- An insufficient coupling of Ves v 5 of the natural yellow jacket venom extract to the solid support of the test system
- A steric blockade of relevant IgE epitopes of Ves v 5

In the meantime the obviously lacking IgE immunoreactivity in the conventional ImmunoCAP i3 has been compensated by addition of recombinant Ves v 5 to yellow jacket venom (Vos et al. 2013). Comparison of the conventional yellow jacket venom ImmunoCAP with the Ves v 5-spiked ImmunoCAP showed significantly increased IgE reactivity for Ves v 5-positive patients. Ves v 5-negative patients had comparable results on both CAP variants.

Addition ("spiking") of rVes v 5 increased test sensitivity of the yellow jacket ImmunoCAP from 83.4 to 96.8 %. The observed increase of sensitivity was not associated with decreased specificity of the test system. Based on these data, the Ves v 5-spiked yellow jacket venom has been introduced in the market in 2012. After a transition phase, the conventional (not Ves v 5-spiked) yellow jacket venom ImmunoCAP i3 was discontinued. Unfortunately the manufacturer failed to communicate this change appropriately and failed to label the different variants in a way that would allow an easy identification which variant was used. This was particularly relevant for therapeutic monitoring during specific immunotherapy since the new spiked ImmunoCAP (i3) in most cases gave higher readings. In general it can be assumed that determinations of specific IgE to yellow jacket venom (i3) performed prior to 2012 were done on the "old," i.e., non-spiked ImmunoCAP (i3). All determinations performed after 2012 were analyzed with the new, rVes v 5-spiked ImmunoCAP (i3).

The significant increase of sensitivity by addition of recombinant Ves v 5 led to the assumption that other single allergens such as Ves v 1, Ves v 2, and Ves v 3 could be used for improvement of the test performance. Analysis of sera from patients with a clear history of yellow jacket sting anaphylaxis, but without specific IgE against Ves v 5-spiked yellow jacket venom, however, showed that this is not the case (Rafei-Shamsabadi et al. 2014). The same also seems to be true for additional allergens in honeybee venom allergy. For patients with clear history of honeybee venom allergy but without positive specific IgE against honeybee venom extract, the use of additional allergens (Api m 1, Api m 2, Api m 3, Api m 4, Api m 5, and Api m 10) did not result in an improved test sensitivity (Köhler et al. 2014; Rafei-Shamsabadi et al. 2014).

For patients with a convincing history of sting anaphylaxis and negative results in serology and skin tests, cellular test systems have gained significant importance. Today the flow cytometric basophil activation test is the most frequently used and best standardized cellular test for the detection of an IgE-mediated sensitization to insect venom. The basophil activation test was able to detect an IgE-mediated sensitization in approx. 60 % of patients with a convincing history of insect sting anaphylaxis but negative sIgE to the corresponding venom (Eberlein-Koenig and Ring 2004; Korosec et al. 2009, 2013). Although the basophil activation test has obviously a higher sensitivity compared to serology, it is also limited by the same problems of cross-reactive carbohydrate determinants and cross-reacting insect venom allergens when performed with whole venom preparations. Using well-standardized, CCD-free, recombinant marker allergens would allow to circumvent these problems of cross-reactivity and simultaneously enable us to use the increased sensitivity of the basophil activation test.

18.4.4 Potential Relevance for Specific Immunotherapy

Specific immunotherapy with insect venom offers a high grade of protection against future anaphylactic sting reactions (80–84 % for honeybee venom allergy and 90–95 % for the yellow jacket venom allergy) (Biló and Bonifazi 2009). A current study reported a protection rate of 84 % for honeybee venom immunotherapy and 96 % for yellow jacket venom immunotherapy (Rueff et al. 2014). This difference between therapy with honeybee venom and yellow jacket venom has been known for decades and has been explained by variations in quality and quantity of the venoms. Very recent advances in the molecular characterization of venoms revealed that honeybee venom proteins of limited concentration such as Api m 3, Api m 5, and Api m 10 play an important and so far underestimated role as allergens (Grunwald et al. 2006; Blank et al. 2010, 2011a). Although these proteins are present in low amounts only, they have to be considered as major allergens (Köhler et al. 2014). Notably two of these allergens, Api m 3 and Api m 10, were reported to be lacking or to be underrepresented in therapeutic venom preparations (Blank et al. 2011a).

In honeybee venom-allergic patients, IgE against Api m 3 and/or Api m 10 was detectable in 68 % of sera, and in 5 % of patients IgE was directed exclusively against Api m 3 and/or Api m 10 (Köhler et al. 2014). Another indirect hint for the lack or underrepresentation of Api m 3 and Api m 10 in therapeutic venom preparations was the fact that absent or very low induction of Api m 3- and Api m 10-specific IgG_4 antibodies could be observed upon immunotherapy, in contrast to the pronounced induction of IgG_4 antibodies against Api m 1, Api m 2, and Api m 4 (Kohler et al. 2014). Based on these findings, it was tempting to speculate that the relative lack of allergens in therapeutic venom preparation may account for the reduced efficacy of VIT in bee venom-allergic patients, a hypothesis that has been addressed in a very recent study (Frick et al. 2016). The retrospective analysis of component-resolved sensitization profiles in HBV-allergic patients that had undergone controlled HB sting challenge after at least 6 months of HBV immunotherapy demonstrated that predominant Api m 10 sensitization (>50 % of sIgE to HBV) was the best discriminator for treatment failure with an odds ratio of 8.444 (2.127–33.53; $p=0.0013$). Interestingly, some but not all therapeutic HBV preparations displayed a lack of Api m 10, while Api m 1 and Api m 3 immunoreactivity was comparable to that of crude HBV (Frick et al. 2016). In line with this, significant Api m 10 IgG_4 induction was only observed in patients treated with HBV in which Api m 10 was detectable. In conclusion, this retrospective study suggested that HBV-allergic patients with dominant sensitization to Api m 10 are at increased risk for treatment failure in HBV immunotherapy and should benefit from treatment with Api m 10 containing preparations.

18.5 Open Questions and Future Perspectives

The current availability of recombinant allergens for routine diagnostics is still limited. In yellow jacket allergy, the two major allergens Ves v 1 and Ves v 5 allow the detection of up to 97 % of the patients. In contrast, in honeybee venom allergy, the two currently available allergens Api m 1 and Api m 10 only detect approx. 80 % of the patients. This is a substantial diagnostic gap which needs to be closed as soon as possible. Based on study data, additional honeybee venom allergens are being standardized and hopefully will become available for routine diagnostics in the near future.

Advances in proteome analysis suggest that the list of insect venom allergens known so far is still incomplete. Novel candidates have been identified and are currently under investigation. Hence it is expected that the number of relevant insect venom allergens will continue to increase. Another level of complexity is achieved by the generation of additional isoforms, as described for the yellow jacket venom hyaluronidase (Ves v 2) or icarapin (Api m 10) from honeybee venom (Van Vaerenbergh et al. 2015). The ongoing development of molecular diagnostics using recombinant insect venom allergens should enable us in the future to increase the precision in diagnosing genuine double sensitization in patients with IgE reactivities to different insect species.

While differentiation of honeybee and yellow jacket venom allergy is of central relevance in Central Europe, differentiation between members of the yellow jackets (Vespinae) and the paper wasps (Polistinae) is highly relevant in the Mediterranean countries. The so far available recombinant allergens of the antigen 5 group (Ves v 5 and Pol d 5) exhibit a high degree of cross-reactivity and are not sufficiently suited for a differential diagnosis. An urgent quest is ongoing for allergens that are expressed differentially in only one but not the other venom and therefore allow for a differentiation of sensitization with improved precision. The more recombinant, CCD-free allergens become available, the better we can characterize the sensitization profiles of our patients. Currently we mostly use these profiles for diagnostic purposes. Subsequent studies need to address, whether these profiles can be used as predictive markers for therapeutic success or failure of specific immunotherapy.

18.6 Conclusion for Daily Practice

The molecular diagnostics available right now for honeybee and yellow jacket venom allergy offer elegant strategies for the differentiation of genuine double sensitization from cross-reactivity. In the molecular diagnostics of yellow jacket venom allergy, we obtain a satisfactory sensitivity using the available allergens Ves v 1 and Ves v 5. For the molecular diagnostics of honeybee venom allergy, the currently available allergens Api m 1 and Api m 10 are not sufficient. There is a clear need for additional allergens that are currently under development. Even more difficult is the situation for differentiation of members of yellow jackets (Vespinae) and paper wasps (Polistinae). So far no allergens exist that allow for a reliable differentiation.

In practical use, a combination of extract-based and molecular tools is recommended, at best in a stepwise approach. The baseline diagnostics are best performed using sIgE to whole venom preparations. In case of double-positive test results or discrepancies between history, skin test, and serology, molecular diagnostics using sIgE to available single-venom allergens (e.g., Ves v 5, Ves v 1, Api m 1, Api m 10, et al.) will provide important additional information and facilitate therapeutic decision for a specific immunotherapy (◉ Fig. 18.6).

By using an extending panel of CCD-free, specific marker allergens, and homologous recombinant allergens, molecular diagnostics will increasingly allow for establishment of individual sensitization profiles of patients. This approach can be

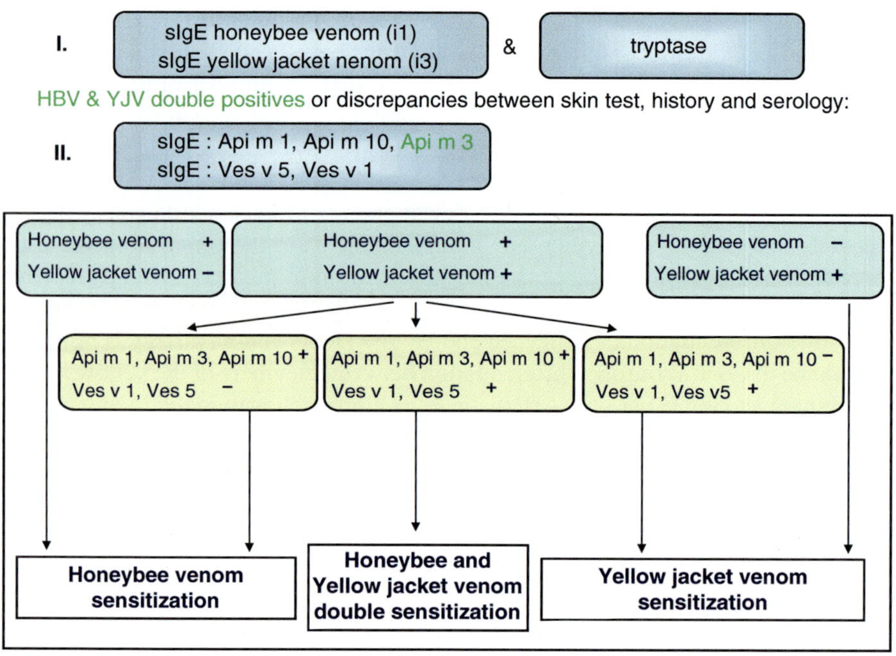

Fig. 18.6 Algorithm for the in vitro diagnostics of insect venom allergy

used to monitor therapeutic intervention, to recognize intervention-induced neo-sensitizations, and potentially to develop prognostic markers for treatment success in venom immunotherapy.

References

Aalberse RC, Akkerdaas J, van Ree R. Cross-reactivity of IgE antibodies to allergens. Allergy. 2001;56:478–90.

Arbesman CE, Reisman RE, Wypych JI. Allergenic potency of bee antigens measured by RAST inhibition. Clin Allergy. 1976;6:587–95.

Bilo MB, Bonifazi F. The natural history and epidemiology of insect venom allergy: clinical implications. Clin Exp Allergy. 2009;39:1467–76.

Blank S, Seismann H, Bockisch B, Braren I, Cifuentes L, McIntyre M, Ruhl D, Ring J, Bredehorst R, Ollert MW, Grunwald T, Spillner E. Identification, recombinant expression, and characterization of the 100 kDa high molecular weight Hymenoptera venom allergens Api m 5 and Ves v 3. J Immunol. 2010;184:5403–13.

Blank S, Seismann H, Michel Y, McIntyre M, Cifuentes L, Braren I, Grunwald T, Darsow U, Ring J, Bredehorst R, Ollert M, Spillner E. Api m 10, a genuine A. mellifera venom allergen, is clinically relevant but underrepresented in therapeutic extracts. Allergy. 2011a;66:1322–9.

Blank S, Michel Y, Seismann H, Plum M, Greunke K, Grunwald T, Bredehorst R, Ollert M, Braren I, Spillner E. Evaluation of different glycoforms of honeybee venom major allergen phospholipase A2 (Api m 1) produced in insect cells. Protein Pept Lett. 2011b;18:415–22.

Blank S, Bantleon FI, McIntyre M, Ollert M, Spillner E. The major royal jelly proteins 8 and 9 (Api m 11) are glycosylated components of Apis mellifera venom with allergenic potential beyond carbohydrate-based reactivity. Clin Exp Allergy. 2012;42:976–85.

Blank S, Neu C, Hasche D, Bantleon FI, Jakob T, Spillner E. Polistes species venom is devoid of carbohydrate-based cross-reactivity and allows interference-free diagnostics. J Allergy Clin Immunol. 2013b;131:1239–42.

Caruso B, Bonadonna P, Severino MG, Manfredi M, Dama A, Schiappoli M, Rizzotti P, Senna G, Passalacqua G. Evaluation of the IgE cross-reactions among vespid venoms. A possible approach for the choice of immunotherapy. Allergy. 2007;62:561–4.

de Graaf DC, Brunain M, Scharlaken B, Peiren N, Devreese B, Ebo DG, Stevens WJ, Desjardins CA, Werren JH, Jacobs FJ. Two novel proteins expressed by the venom glands of Apis mellifera and Nasonia vitripennis share an ancient C1q-like domain. Insect Mol Biol. 2010;19 Suppl 1:1–10.

Dudler T, Chen WQ, Wang S, Schneider T, Annand RR, Dempcy RO, Crameri R, Gmachl M, Suter M, Gelb MH. High-level expression in Escherichia coli and rapid purification of enzymatically active honey bee venom phospholipase A2. Biochim Biophys Acta. 1992;1165:201–10.

Eberlein-Koenig B, Ring J. Diagnosis of IgE-mediated hymenoptera venom anaphylaxis in patients with negative skin tests and negative RAST using cellular in vitro tests. J Allergy Clin Immunol. 2004;113:1223; author reply 1223–1224.

Ebo DG, Faber M, Sabato V, Leysen J, Bridts CH, De Clerck LS. Component-resolved diagnosis of wasp (yellow jacket) venom allergy. Clin Exp Allergy. 2013;43:255–61.

Frick M, Müller S, Bantleon F, Huss-Marp J, Lidholm J, Spillner E, Jakob T. rApi m 3 and rApi m 10 improve detection of honey bee sensitization in Hymenoptera venom-allergic patients with double sensitization to honey bee and yellow jacket venom. Allergy. 2015;70:1665–8.

Frick M, Fischer J, Helbling A, Rueff F, Wieczorek D, Ollert M, Pfützner W, Müller S, Huss-Marp J Dorn B, Biedermann T, Lidholm J, Ruecker G, Bantleon F, Mühe M, Spillner E, Jakob T. Predominant Api m 10 sensitization as risk factor for treatment failure in honey bee venom immunotherapy. J Allergy Clin Immunol. 2016;138:1663–71.

Gmachl M, Kreil G. Bee venom hyaluronidase is homologous to a membrane protein of mammalian sperm. Proc Natl Acad Sci U S A. 1993;90:3569–73.

Grunwald T, Bockisch B, Spillner E, Ring J, Bredehorst R, Ollert MW. Molecular cloning and expression in insect cells of honeybee venom allergen acid phosphatase (Api m 3). J Allergy Clin Immunol. 2006;117:848–54.

Hemmer W, Focke M, Kolarich D, Dalik I, Gotz M, Jarisch R. Identification by immunoblot of venom glycoproteins displaying immunoglobulin E-binding N-glycans as cross-reactive allergens in honeybee and yellow jacket venom. Clin Exp Allergy. 2004;34:460–9.

Henriksen A, King TP, Mirza O, Monsalve RI, Meno K, Ipsen H, Larsen JN, Gajhede M, Spangfort MD. Major venom allergen of yellow jackets, Ves v 5: structural characterization of a pathogenesis-related protein superfamily. Proteins. 2001;45:438–48.

Hoffman DR, Shipman WH, Babin D. Allergens in bee venom II. Two new high molecular weight allergenic specificities. J Allergy Clin Immunol. 1977;59:147–53.

Hofmann S, Pfender N, Weckesser S, Blank S, Johannes HM, Spillner E, Jakob T. Use of a panel of species-specific major allergens improves diagnosis of hymenoptera venom allergy. J Invest Dermatol. 2011a;131:S41.

Hofmann SC, Pfender N, Weckesser S, Huss-Marp J, Jakob T. Added value of IgE detection to rApi m 1 and rVes v 5 in patients with Hymenoptera venom allergy. J Allergy Clin Immunol. 2011b;127:265–7.

Jakob T, Ollert M. Rekombinante Insektengiftallergene – Nutzen in der Abgrenzung von Kreuzsensibilisierungen und echten Doppelsensibilisierungen. Allergo J. 2011;20:22–3.

Jakob T, Köhler J, Blank S, Magnusson U, Huss-Marp J, Spillner E, Lidholm J. Comparable IgE reactivity to natural and recombinant Api m 1 in cross-reactive carbohydrate determinant-negative patients with bee venom allergy. J Allergy Clin Immunol. 2012;130:276–8. author reply 278–279.

Jakob T, Müller S, Rafei-Shamsabadi D, Bantleon F, Spillner E. State of the art and new developments in diagnostics of insect venom allergy using recombinant allergens. Allergologie. 2014;37:362–7.

Jappe U, Raulf-Heimsoth M, Hoffmann M, Burow G, Hubsch-Muller C, Enk A. In vitro hymenoptera venom allergy diagnosis: improved by screening for cross-reactive carbohydrate determinants and reciprocal inhibition. Allergy. 2006;61:1220–9.

Jin C, Hantusch B, Hemmer W, Stadlmann J, Altmann F. Affinity of IgE and IgG against cross-reactive carbohydrate determinants on plant and insect glycoproteins. J Allergy Clin Immunol. 2008;121:185–90.

Jin C, Focke M, Leonard R, Jarisch R, Altmann F, Hemmer W. Reassessing the role of hyaluronidase in yellow jacket venom allergy. J Allergy Clin Immunol. 2010;125(184–190):e181.

Kettner A, Hughes GJ, Frutiger S, Astori M, Roggero M, Spertini F, Corradin G. Api m 6: a new bee venom allergen. J Allergy Clin Immunol. 2001;107:914–20.

King TP, Spangfort MD. Structure and biology of stinging insect venom allergens. Int Arch Allergy Immunol. 2000;123:99–106.

King TP, Alagon AC, Kuan J, Sobotka AK, Lichtenstein LM. Immunochemical studies of yellow-jacket venom proteins. Mol Immunol. 1983;20:297–308.

Köhler J, Blank S, Müller S, Bantleon F, Frick M, Huss-Marp J, Lidholm J, Spillner E, Jakob T. Component resolution reveals additional major allergens in patients with honeybee venom allergy. J Allergy Clin Immunol. 2014;133:1383–9.

Kolarich D, Leonard R, Hemmer W, Altmann F. The N-glycans of yellow jacket venom hyaluronidases and the protein sequence of its major isoform in Vespula vulgaris. FEBS J. 2005;272:5182–90.

Korosec P, Erzen R, Silar M, Bajrovic N, Kopac P, Kosnik M. Basophil responsiveness in patients with insect sting allergies and negative venom-specific immunoglobulin E and skin prick test results. Clin Exp Allergy. 2009;39:1730–7.

Korosec P, Mavsar N, Bajrovic N, Silar M, Mrhar A, Kosnik M. Basophil responsiveness and clinical picture of acetylsalicylic acid intolerance. Int Arch Allergy Immunol. 2011;155:257–62.

Korosec P, Silar M, Erzen R, Celesnik N, Bajrovic N, Zidarn M, Kosnik M. Clinical routine utility of basophil activation testing for diagnosis of hymenoptera-allergic patients with emphasis on individuals with negative venom-specific IgE antibodies. Int Arch Allergy Immunol. 2013;161:363–8.

Kuchler K, Gmachl M, Sippl MJ, Kreil G. Analysis of the cDNA for phospholipase A2 from honeybee venom glands. The deduced amino acid sequence reveals homology to the corresponding vertebrate enzymes. Eur J Biochem. 1989;184:249–54.

Monsalve RI, Vega A, Marques L, Miranda A, Fernandez J, Soriano V, Cruz S, Dominguez-Noche C, Sanchez-Morillas L, Armisen-Gil M, Guspi R, Barber D. Component-resolved diagnosis of vespid venom-allergic individuals: phospholipases and antigen 5s are necessary to identify Vespula or Polistes sensitization. Allergy. 2012;67:528–36.

Müller UR. Insektenstichallergie: Klinik, Diagnostik und Therapie. Stuttgart/New York: Fischer; 1988.

Müller UR. Recent developments and future strategies for immunotherapy of insect venom allergy. Curr Opin Allergy Clin Immunol. 2003;3:299–303.

Müller UR, Helbling A. Update on Hymenoptera venom allergy with focus on diagnostics and therapy. Allergo J. 2013;22:265–73.

Müller UR, Johansen N, Petersen AB, Fromberg-Nielsen J, Haeberli G. Hymenoptera venom allergy: analysis of double positivity to honey bee and Vespula venom by estimation of IgE antibodies to species-specific major allergens Api m1 and Ves v5. Allergy. 2009;64:543–8.

Müller U, Schmid-Grendelmeier P, Hausmann O, Helbling A. IgE to recombinant allergens Api m 1, Ves v 1, and Ves v 5 distinguish double sensitization from crossreaction in venom allergy. Allergy. 2012;67:1069–73.

Ollert M, Wolf S, Bantleon FI, Spillner E. Vitellogenins are new high molecular weight components and allergens (Api m 12 and Ves v 6) of Apis mellifera and Vespula vulgaris venom. PLoS One. 2013a;8:e62009.

Peiren N, Vanrobaeys F, de Graaf DC, Devreese B, Van Beeumen J, Jacobs FJ. The protein composition of honeybee venom reconsidered by a proteomic approach. Biochim Biophys Acta. 2005;1752:1–5.

Przybilla B, Ruëff F, Walker A, Helen-Caroline Räwer HC, Aberer W, Bauer CP, Berdel D, Biedermann T, Brockow K, Forster J, Fuchs T, Hamelmann E, Jakob T, Jarisch R, Merk HF, Müller U, Ott H, Sitter W, Urbanek R, Wedi B. S2 Guideline (AWMF 061-020) Diagnosis and therapy of bee and wasp venom allergy. Allergo J. 2011;20:318–39.

Rafei-Shamsabadi D, Müller S, Pfützner W, Spillner E, Rueff F, Jakob T. Recombinant allergens rarely allow identification of Hymenoptera venom-allergic patients with negative specific IgE to whole venom preparations. J Allergy Clin Immunol. 2014;134:493–4.

Rueff F, Vos B, Oude Elberink J, Bender A, Chatelain R, Dugas-Breit S, Horny HP, Kuchenhoff H, Linhardt A, Mastnik S, Sotlar K, Stretz E, Vollrath R, Przybilla B, Flaig M. Predictors of clinical effectiveness of Hymenoptera venom immunotherapy. Clin Exp Allergy. 2014;44:736–46.

Schmidt M, Weimer ET, Sakell RH, Hoffman DR. Proteins in the high molecular weight fraction of honeybee venom. J Allergy Clin Immunol. 2005;115:S107.

Seismann H, Blank S, Braren I, Greunke K, Cifuentes L, Grunwald T, Bredehorst R, Ollert M, Spillner E. Dissecting cross-reactivity in hymenoptera venom allergy by circumvention of alpha-1,3-core fucosylation. Mol Immunol. 2010a;47:799–808.

Seismann H, Blank S, Cifuentes L, Braren I, Bredehorst R, Grunwald T, Ollert M, Spillner E. Recombinant phospholipase A1 (Ves v 1) from yellow jacket venom for improved diagnosis of hymenoptera venom hypersensitivity. Clin Mol Allergy. 2010b;8:7.

Seppala U, Selby D, Monsalve R, King TP, Ebner C, Roepstorff P, Bohle B. Structural and immunological characterization of the N-glycans from the major yellow jacket allergen Ves v 2: the N-glycan structures are needed for the human antibody recognition. Mol Immunol. 2009;46:2014–21.

Skov LK, Seppala U, Coen JJ, Crickmore N, King TP, Monsalve R, Kastrup JS, Spangfort MD, Gajhede M. Structure of recombinant Ves v 2 at 2.0 Angstrom resolution: structural analysis of an allergenic hyaluronidase from wasp venom. Acta Crystallogr D Biol Crystallogr. 2006;62:595–604.

Soldatova LN, Crameri R, Gmachl M, Kemeny DM, Schmidt M, Weber M, Mueller UR. Superior biologic activity of the recombinant bee venom allergen hyaluronidase expressed in baculovirus-infected insect cells as compared with Escherichia coli. J Allergy Clin Immunol. 1998;101:691–8.

Spillner E, Blank S, Jakob T. Potentials, pitfalls and current state of molecular diagnostics in insect venom allergy. Allergo J. 2012;21:249–56.

Spillner E, Blank S, Jakob T. Hymenoptera allergens: from venom to "venome". Front Immunol. 2014;5:77.

Sturm GJ, Bilo MB, Bonadonna P, Hemmer W, Caruso B, Bokanovic D, Aberer W. Ves v 5 can establish the diagnosis in patients without detectable specific IgE to wasp venom and a possible north–south difference in Api m 1 sensitization in Europe. J Allergy Clin Immunol. 2012;130:817. author reply 818–819.

Van Vaerenbergh M, Cardoen D, Formesyn EM, Brunain M, Van Driessche G, Blank S, Spillner E, Verleyen P, Wenseleers T, Schoofs L, Devreese B, de Graaf DC. Extending the honey bee venome with the antimicrobial peptide apidaecin and a protein resembling wasp antigen 5. Insect Mol Biol. 2013;22:199–210.

Van Vaerenbergh M, Debyser G, Devreese B, de Graaf DC. Exploring the hidden honeybee (Apis mellifera) venom proteome by integrating a combinatorial peptide ligand library approach with FTMS. J Proteomics. 2014;99:169–78.

Van Vaerenbergh M, De Smet L, Rafei-Shamsabadi D, Blank S, Spillner E, Ebo DG, Devreese B, Jakob T, de Graaf DC. IgE recognition of chimeric isoforms of the honeybee (Apis mellifera) venom allergen Api m 10 evaluated by protein array technology. Mol Immunol. 2015;63:449–55.

Vos B, Köhler J, Muller S, Stretz E, Rueff F, Jakob T. Spiking venom with rVes v 5 improves sensitivity of IgE detection in patients with allergy to Vespula venom. J Allergy Clin Immunol. 2013;131:1225–1227:e1221.

Winningham KM, Fitch CD, Schmidt M, Hoffman DR. Hymenoptera venom protease allergens. J Allergy Clin Immunol. 2004;114:928–33.

Molecular Diagnostics in Allergy to Mammals

19

C. Hilger, J. Kleine-Tebbe, and M. van Hage

19.1 Introduction

Mammals being rich sources of allergens are interesting from an allergological point of view. Their proteins frequently result in allergic symptoms in both domestic and work environments. In Europe and the USA, pets are very popular: depending on the region, 30–60 % of all households have one or more. The most common pet animals are dogs and cats, followed by fish, small mammals (such as rabbits, guinea pigs, and hamsters), and birds. Many of the allergens present in animal fur and epithelium are now well characterized. In addition to the two main families, the lipocalins and the serum albumins, there are individual allergens belonging to other protein families such as secretoglobins, cystatins, kallikreins, and latherins. Other members of these protein families will most likely be identified as allergens in the future.

This contribution is based on a publication by the authors that appeared in the *Allergo Journal* in 2011 (Hilger C, Kleine-Tebbe J. Inhalative Säugetierallergene: Lipokaline und Serumalbumine. Allergo J 2011;20:142–4) and which has now been updated, expanded, and translated into English as a chapter for this book.

C. Hilger, PhD (✉)
Allergology – Immunology – Inflammation Research Unit, Department of Infection and Immunity, Luxembourg Institute of Health, Esch-sur-Alzette, Luxembourg
e-mail: christiane.hilger@lih.lu

J. Kleine-Tebbe, MD, Prof.
Allergy and Asthma Center Westend, Outpatient Clinic Hanf, Ackermann & Kleine-Tebbe, Berlin, Germany
e-mail: kleine-tebbe@allergie-experten.de

M. van Hage, MD, Prof.
Immunology and Allergy Unit, Department of Medicine Solna, Karolinska Institutet and Karolinska University Hospital, Stockholm, Sweden
e-mail: marianne.van.hage@ki.se

J. Kleine-Tebbe, T. Jakob (eds.), *Molecular Allergy Diagnostics*,
DOI 10.1007/978-3-319-42499-6_19

The disadvantage of animal hair and epithelial extracts used in skin tests and in vitro IgE diagnosis is that they are hard to standardize and contain cross-reactive molecules. They are mainly serum albumins, although recently several cross-reactive lipocalins have also been identified. Diagnosis using single allergens has the potential to specifically determine the animal species triggering the allergy, meaning that patients can be advised better and provided with suitable immunotherapy.

19.2 Protein Structure and Function

Most allergenic molecules of animal origin belong to one of two protein families: the lipocalins or the serum albumins.

Allergens of the lipocalin family have been identified in all mammals investigated. Lipocalins form a group of proteins found universally in nature, even in bacteria and the plant kingdom (Grzyb et al. 2006). There are numerous types, performing different functions. Some are involved in transport and storage of substances with poor solubility; others are immunomodulators, have defense roles, or are important for the sense of smell.

Lipocalins are characterized by a shared tertiary structure consisting of an eight-stranded β-sheet that forms an internal binding pocket (Flower et al. 2000). This is closed at one end by the N-terminal 3_{10} helix (◉ Fig. 19.1). Lipocalins are small molecules with a molecular weight (mw) of 16–22 kDa; and despite their similar three-dimensional structure, they have very different amino acid sequences. The sequence identity is often as low as 20 %. According to recent findings, there is, however, a subgroup of lipocalins that have a relatively high amino acid identity of 47–67 % and can also induce IgE cross-reactions (Hilger et al. 2012b).

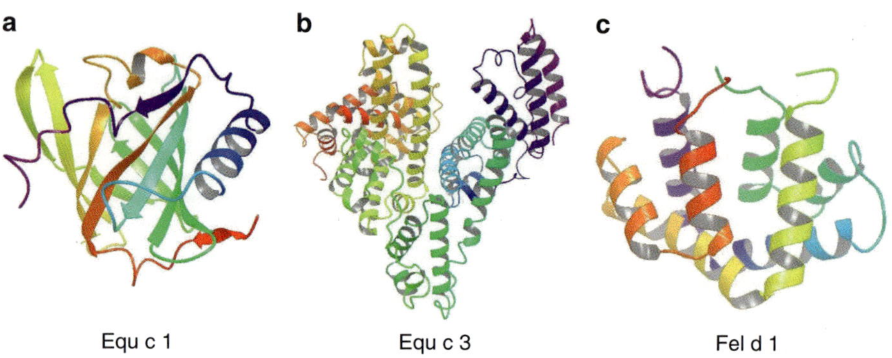

Fig. 19.1 Ribbon models illustrating the three-dimensional structure of Equ c 1, Equ c 3, and Fel d 1. Equ c 1 (**a**) is based on the crystal molecule 1EW3; Equ c 3 (**b**) is based on 4F5U. The N-terminal end is shown in *red*, the C-terminal end in *violet*. Fel d 1 (**c**) is based on the crystal molecule 1PU0. Chain A is depicted in *red* to *yellow-green*, chain B in *green* to *violet*. The N-terminal end is marked *red*, the C-terminal end *violet* (By kind permission of Karthik Arumugam, LIH, Luxemburg)

Some of the allergenic mammalian lipocalins transport small hydrophobic molecules (e.g., lipids, pheromones, steroids) in their binding pocket. Different lipocalins excreted in the urine have had a social-behavioral function ascribed to them, as they transport pheromones and fragrances. The precise roles of the allergenic members of this family are, however, still largely unknown.

Serum albumins are large, globular proteins with α-helical structures that are stabilized by several disulfide bridges (◉ Fig. 19.1b). They have a molecular weight of 66 kDa and are not glycosylated. The amino acid identity between albumins of different mammals is high (75–80 % on average) (Chruszcz et al. 2013). Identity between serum albumins in mammals and birds is, however, only around 45 %. Serum albumin is synthesized in the liver and as the main protein constituent of plasma, regulates the colloid-osmotic pressure. Additionally, due to its high protein-binding capacity, it transports fatty acids, hormones, bilirubin, and other substances. Serum albumins are thermolabile and easily denatured.

19.3 Current Status of Identified Allergenic Molecules from Different Mammalian Allergen Sources

19.3.1 Cat Allergenic Molecules

Fel d 1 (*Felis domesticus* 1) is a uteroglobin synthesized in the salivary glands and in the skin (Morgenstern et al. 1991) (◉ Fig. 19.1c). Uteroglobins belong to the family of secretoglobins; they are small, dimeric molecules linked by disulfide bridges and only occur in mammals. Their physiological role is still largely not understood. Over 90 % of all persons allergic to cat have specific IgE to Fel d 1, the major cat allergen, which consists of two molecules linked by disulfide bridges that form heterodimers, and two heterodimers together form a tetramer.

Fel d 2, serum albumin, is regarded as a minor allergen. Depending on the individual patient group, rates of sensitization fluctuate between 14 and 23 %. Fel d 2 is responsible for cross-reactions with raw or medium cooked pork or beef, such as ham and salami (Hilger et al. 1997) (◉ Fig. 19.2).

Fel d 3, a cystatin, has been isolated from the skin (Ichikawa et al. 2001). It is a small molecule with a molecular weight of 11 kDa and is recognized by only around 10 % of individuals with cat allergy.

Fel d 4 was the first cat lipocalin to be isolated from cat, specifically from the salivary gland (Smith et al. 2004). It is the second most important major allergen, with 63 % of persons allergic to cat having specific IgE to Fel d 4.

The two immunoglobulins A (IgA) and M (IgM) are named **Fel d 5** and **Fel d 6** (Adedoyin et al. 2007). Both carry a carbohydrate side chain designated as α-gal (galactose-α-1,3-galactose) (Commins et al. 2011; Gronlund et al. 2009) (◉ Fig. 19.2). Red meat allergic patients may be sensitized to cat due to IgE reactivity to α-gal on cat IgA or cat IgM (Commins et al. 2011; Hamsten et al. 2013).

Another lipocalin, **Fel d 7**, has been isolated from the tongue. It is found in cat saliva and hair (Smith et al. 2011). Fel d 7 has high amino acid identity with Can f

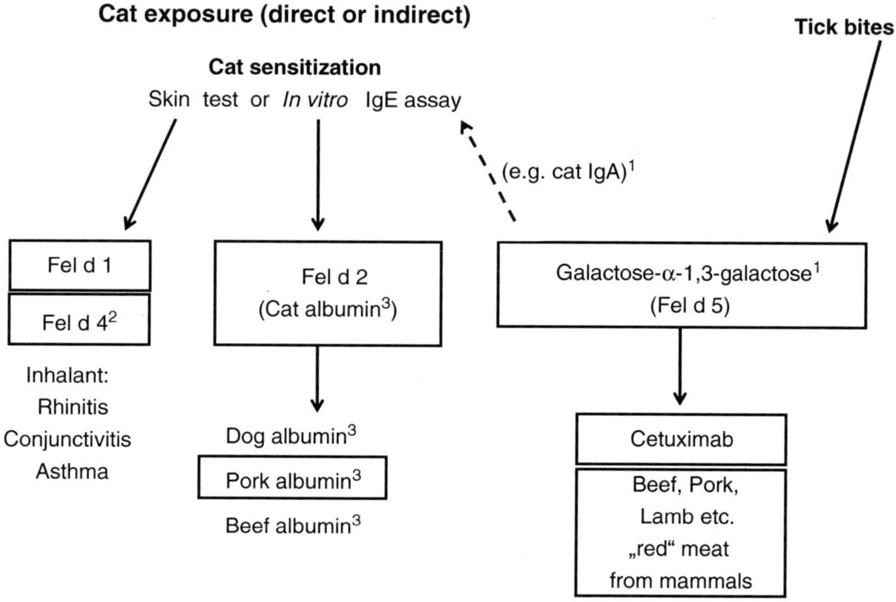

Fig. 19.2 Cat allergens and corresponding clinical symptoms. IgE sensitization to various cat allergen molecules can be triggered by different exposures and associated with inhalant symptoms or two different forms of a food allergy. [1]Levels of cat IgA and other cat proteins with α-gal side chains are lower in extracts from cat dander than those from cat epithilia. [2]Fel d 4 is a lipocalin with cross-reactivity to Can f 6 and Equ c 1. [3]Albumins are generally cross-reactive, although cross-reactivity between cat albumins and certain albumins from other mammals (e.g. dog, pig) appears more pronounced than those between cat and beef albumin (Adapted by kind permission from Konradsen et al. 2015)

1 (62 %). Cross-reactivity between Fel d 7 and Can f 1 has been described (Apostolovic et al. 2016).

Fel d 8 has been identified in the submandibular gland. It belongs to the family of latherins that are proteins with surface-active, tenside-like properties (Smith et al. 2011). An allergen from the same protein family, Equ c 4, is present in the horse. Amino acid identity to Fel d 8 is, however, only 46 %. Cross-reactions have not yet been reported.

Of those allergic to cat hair, 38 % and 19 % have IgE antibodies to Fel d 7 and Fel d 8, respectively (Smith et al. 2011).

19.3.2 Dog Allergenic Molecules

Lipocalins are the most important group of allergens in dogs.

Can f 1 (*Canis familiaris* 1) and **Can f 2**, both lipocalins, have been isolated from the salivary glands (Konieczny et al. 1997). Can f 1 is a major allergen and is recognized by the IgE repertoire in 50–75 % of all individuals allergic to dog. For Can f 2, the proportion is only 22–30 %.

Can f 3, dog serum albumin, has been proved to be a strongly cross-reactive allergen, and in an early study, up to 35 % of all patients had specific IgE to Can f 3 (Spitzauer et al. 1994).

Can f 4, the third lipocalin, has been isolated from dog epithelium. About 35 % of persons with dog allergy have specific IgE to this allergen (Mattson et al. 2010).

Can f 5, a prostate kallikrein, has been isolated from the urine of male dogs. It exhibits a high degree of homology to human prostate antigen and appears to be responsible for IgE-mediated reactions to sperm (Mattson et al. 2009). Around 70 % of all patients allergic to dog have specific IgE to Can f 5.

Can f 6 is the most recently isolated lipocalin. It has what is, for lipocalins, an atypically high identity to other lipocalins such as Equ c 1 (horse) and Fel d 4 (Hilger et al. 2012a, b; Nilsson et al. 2012). Not only have strong IgE cross-reactions been detected in vitro, but also clinically relevant cross-reactions between horse and dog have been detected (Jakob et al. 2013). Sensitization to Can f 6 has, depending on the study, been detected in 38–61 % of patients (Hilger et al. 2012a, b; Nilsson et al. 2012).

19.3.3 Horse Allergenic Molecules

Equ c 1 (*Equus caballus* 1) is the major horse allergen. It is a lipocalin that occurs in high concentrations in the saliva of horses, in their coats, and, in small amounts, in their urine (Dandeu et al. 1993; Gregoire et al. 1996). Equ c 1 has surface-active properties (Goubran Boutos et al. 2001). Equ c 1 has been shown to cross-react with the dog lipocalin Can f 6 (Nilsson et al. 2012).

Equ c 2, another lipocalin, has been characterized only in part but is recognized by around 50 % of individuals with horse allergy (Bulone et al. 1998).

Horse serum albumin is designated **Equ c 3** and is strongly cross-reactive with other albumins. About 20 % of the horse-allergic patients had detectable IgE against Equ c 3 (Cabanas et al. 2000).

Equ c 4 belongs to the latherin family. It has tenside-like properties and appears to be involved in sweat distribution and evaporation. 77 % of the horse-allergic patients, have specific IgE to Equ c 4 (Goubran Boutos et al. 2001). The previously described Equ c 5 is identical to Equ c 4 and has been removed from the official list of allergens (IUIS/WHO nomenclature).

19.3.4 Cattle Allergenic Molecules

The main allergen sources are the hair and epithelia of cattle, but also urine has been described as a relevant source. Of the various allergens, **Bos d 2** (*Bos domesticus* 2), a lipocalin, appears to be the major allergen (Ylönen et al. 1992). Cattle allergens play an important role in the induction of occupational asthma in farmers. In a German study, about 9 % of occupational respiratory diseases were caused by cattle (Heutelbeck et al. 2007).

Another inhalant cattle allergen is the thus-far rather poorly characterized **Bos d 3**. This is a small protein that was found in the skin and exhibits a high degree of homology (63 % identity) to human psoriasin. Of 16 test subjects, seven had specific IgE to Bos d 3 (Rautiainen et al. 1995).

Cattle allergens have been detected in large quantities in deposited dust in cattle housing and can also spread to adjacent human living space (Zahradnik et al. 2011). The other known cattle allergens are food allergens in meat and milk.

19.3.5 Rabbit Allergenic Molecules

To date, there have been few studies on rabbit allergens. Older publications report that most of the allergens are found in saliva, although many can also be found in urine and fur (Price and Longbottom 1988). Two allergens, **Ory c 1** (*Oryctolagus cuniculus* 1) and **Ory c 2**, have been incompletely characterized and assigned, based on available information about sequences, to the lipocalins (Baker et al. 2001).

A new allergen, **Ory c 3**, has recently been identified. It belongs to the secretoglobin family and exhibits close structural similarity to Fel d 1 (both allergens consist of two chains forming heterodimers which join to form tetramers) (Hilger et al. 2014a). At the amino acid level, however, there is little similarity. No cross-reactions with Fel d 1 have been found. Of all rabbit-allergic individuals, 77 % had specific IgE to Ory c 3 (Hilger et al. 2014b). This allergen has been detected in dust from rabbit owners' homes. Commercial tests are not yet available.

Another allergen, **Ory c 4**, has been identified. This is a lipocalin that is highly similar to Fel d 4 and Can f 6 and is probably IgE cross-reactive (Hilger et al. 2014b). Of 35 patients tested, 46 % had specific IgE to Ory c 4.

19.3.6 Mouse and Rat Allergenic Molecules

High levels of rat and mouse allergens are detected in these animals' urine. Saliva, fur extracts, and dust samples also contain many IgE-reactive proteins (Gordon et al. 2001). Both **Rat n 1** (*Rattus norvegicus* 1) and **Mus m 1** (*Mus musculus* 1) are lipocalins belonging to the group of urinary proteins (Cavaggioni and Mucignat-Caretta 2000). Both are regarded as marker allergens for sensitization and for allergen detection. They are synthesized in the liver and excreted in the urine of adult mice and rats, with males excreting much higher quantities than females. The mouse has some 35 different genes that code for urinary proteins, although not all of them are expressed in each mouse line.

Rat n 1 and Mus m 1 exhibit a high sequence identity of amino acids, 64 %; thus, IgE cross-reactions are highly probable. Cross-reactivity has been demonstrated indirectly in a study on the sensitization of laboratory workers (Jeal et al. 2009): 62 % of the individuals sensitized to rat also had specific IgE to mouse allergens. In the reverse case, 91 % of persons sensitized to mouse had IgE to rat. Marked cross-reactivity has been detected between the allergens in rat and mouse urine.

Although mice and rats are not very commonly kept as pets, one environment in which they are frequently found is research laboratories, where up to one-third of staff may be affected. Nevertheless, the crucial factor in sensitization appears to be the type and extent of exposure (Jeal and Jones 2010).

19.3.7 Guinea Pig Allergenic Molecules

In the guinea pig, too, the major allergens are found mainly in urine, saliva, and epithelium.

Cav p 1 (*Cavia porcellus* 1) has been incompletely characterized; it is, however, widely considered to be a lipocalin (Fahlbusch et al. 2002).

Cav p 2 and **Cav p 3** are also lipocalins detected in hair extracts, subsequently being isolated from accessory (i.e., Harder's) lacrimal glands and the submandibular glands (Hilger et al. 2011). Both are major allergens; of 26 guinea pig-allergic patients tested, 65 % exhibited specific IgE to Cav p 2, and 54 % specific IgE to Cav p 3. Neither of these two lipocalins showed cross-reactions with dog and cat allergens, making them good potential markers for guinea pig allergy.

As with dog, cat, and horse, the serum albumin, **Cav p 4**, is regarded as a minor allergen.

19.3.8 Hamster Allergenic Molecules

Although hamsters are not among the more common pets, several case reports exist on anaphylactic reactions following hamster bites and on asthmatic symptoms following exposure to these animals. Hamsters are not a uniform animal group, but are subdivided into different species. The most common pets are the golden hamster (*Mesocricetus auratus*), and two of the Phodopus hamsters, the Roborovski hamster (*Phodopus roborovskii*) and the Djungarian hamster (*Phodopus sungorus*).

The major allergen of the Djungarian hamster has recently been identified as a lipocalin (Torres et al. 2014). This allergen has a high sequence identity to the allergen of the Roborovski hamster. Both are strongly IgE cross-reactive .

By contrast, the recently reported major allergen **Mes a 1** of the golden hamster is different from those of the two Phodopus hamsters (Hilger et al. 2015; Torres et al. 2014). This is particularly relevant, as conventional skin test solutions are all derived from golden hamster or field hamster. Accordingly, various case reports show that skin tests for suspected allergy to the Djungarian hamster are generally negative.

19.4 Prevalence of Sensitization/Distribution

In Germany, around 38 % of households have a pet; in families with children, however, the proportion rises to 58 %. About 19 % of all homes have a cat, 14 % a dog, and 6 % a small mammal (German Industrial Association of Pet Care Producers

(IVH); ▶ www.ivh-online.de). There are also occupationally exposed groups such as farmers, riding-stable employees, and veterinarians, as well as workers in pet shops, zoos, and research laboratories. Studies have shown that sensitization and exposure to furry animals is a risk factor for the development of allergic diseases, such as asthma and rhinitis (Desjardins et al. 1993; Konradsen et al. 2015; Perzanowski et al. 2002).

Rates of sensitization to animal allergens vary greatly from region to region. In a multicenter European study, some 3,000 patients were tested who presented at an allergy center with respiratory symptoms (Heinzerling et al. 2009). Sensitization rates averaged around 27 % to dog and/or cat, making rates of sensitization to animal epithelia very similar to rates for house dust mites (31 %). The rate of sensitization to dog reached 56 % in Denmark, but was only 16 % in Austria. A current German investigation on the prevalence of sensitization to inhalant and food allergens, based on a sample of around 7,000 adults, yielded a sensitization rate of 10 % to animal epithelia (Haftenberger et al. 2013). Frequency within the 18–29-year age group was around 15 %. Additionally, a cross-sectional study between 2003 and 2006 found that children in Germany showed increasing animal sensitization to cat, dog, and horse as a function of age: 5.7 % (3–6 years), 11.5 % (7–10 years), 15 % (11–13 years), and 17.2 % (14–17 years). From Sweden, the population-based birth-cohort BAMSE has recently reported that there is an increase in sensitization to cat (from 6.4 to 19.0 %), dog (from 4.8 to 22.6 %), and horse (from 3.1 to 10.6 %) in children followed from 4 to 16 years (Wickman et al. 2014).

As a proportion of the entire sample (almost 13, 000 subjects), specific IgE to cat was detected in 8.1 % of children and adolescents (3–17 years). The figures for dog and horse were 9.7 % and 4.4 %, respectively (Schmitz et al. 2013).

There are numerous international studies addressing the measurement of exposure to animal hair allergens in indoor spaces (Zahradnik and Raulf 2014). Animal allergens are, evidently, ubiquitous. They enter the environment via shed hair and danders, as well as secretion of bodily fluids such as saliva and urine. They bind to small dust particles and can thus be spread to rooms that the animals do not usually visit. Levels are found to be high in homes of animal owners and via clothing; they are also introduced into schools and other public buildings.

19.5 Cross-Reactive Versus Marker Allergens in Mammals

Due to the high sequential and structural identity of the albumins, IgE antibodies that are formed against albumins, e.g. cat serum albumin, also bind serum albumins of other mammals (such as dog, rabbit, guinea pig, horse, and pig).

Serum albumin from chicken (Gal d 5) has a lower sequence identity to mammalian serum albumins (46 %) but may, in rare cases, also lead to cross-sensitization (Hilger et al. 2010).

Although lipocalins have a similar structure, they have low sequence identity. Cross-reactions were previously considered to be unlikely. The only such responses reported are various weak cross-reactions of as-yet-unknown clinical relevance

(Saarelainen et al. 2008). With the identification of the dog allergen Can f 6, however, a subgroup of lipocalins that exhibit very high mutual sequence identities of 47–67 % seems to be emerging (Hentges et al. 2014). Marked IgE cross-reactions between Equ c 1, Fel d 4, and Can f 6 have been detected. It would seem that some of these are clinically relevant, as was demonstrated in the case of a horse- and dog-allergic person. This individual had specific IgE to Equ c 1 and Can f 6, but did not have IgE to any of the other dog allergens (Jakob et al. 2013).

Fel d 1, regarded as a marker allergen in the cat, is recognized by more than 90 % of all individuals with cat allergy. IgE testing with just Fel d 1 has lately been reported to be as good as IgE testing to cat allergen extract (Asarnoj et al. 2016). With respect to Fel d 7, this allergen has recently shown to be of importance in a Swedish cat-sensitized population. More than 40 % of the patients had IgE antibodies to Fel d 7. As Fel d 7 cross-reacts with the major dog allergen Can f 1, it may contribute to symptoms not only in cat allergic but also in dog-allergic patients (Apostolovic et al. 2016).

Equivalents in the dog are Can f 1 and Can f 2. IgE to the major dog allergen Can f 1 has shown in a birth cohort study to be the most important prognostic marker of dog allergy and superior to IgE assessed with dog allergen extract (Asarnoj et al. 2016). Many patients are also sensitized to the new allergen Can f 5. The diagnostic sensitivity of the various dog allergens is, however, relatively low owing to limited sensitization rates; thus, several components need to be tested if a satisfactory level of sensitivity is to be achieved.

Equ c 1 was widely considered a marker allergen for horse hair allergy. This must, however, now be seen in relative terms due to the demonstrated cross-reactions with Fel d 4 and Can f 6.

The rodent allergens Mus m 1 and Rat n 1 are cross-reactive and hence not suitable for species-specific diagnosis. In the other small mammals, Cav p 2 and Ory c 3 appear to be good marker allergens, although they are not yet available for IgE diagnostics.

Finally, further studies with well-characterized pateint populations are required in order to clarify which animal allergens can be definitively regarded as species-specific marker allergens and which are cross-reactive (◉ Fig. 19.3).

19.6 Problems in Diagnosing Sensitization to Animals

Animal hair extracts in diagnostics do not allow unambiguous identification of the allergen source. This is based on the fact that one-third of patients with animal allergies is sensitized to, for example, serum albumin, and may therefore react to various animal hair extracts.

The recent identification of some cross-reactive lipocalins has increased the number of known cross-reactive allergens in animal hair extract. This impedes also the clear determination of the sensitization source within the context of conventional diagnostics with animal hair extracts.

Nevertheless, the use of isolated single allergens for in vitro diagnostics could enable the causative animal species to be more precisely identified as the allergen

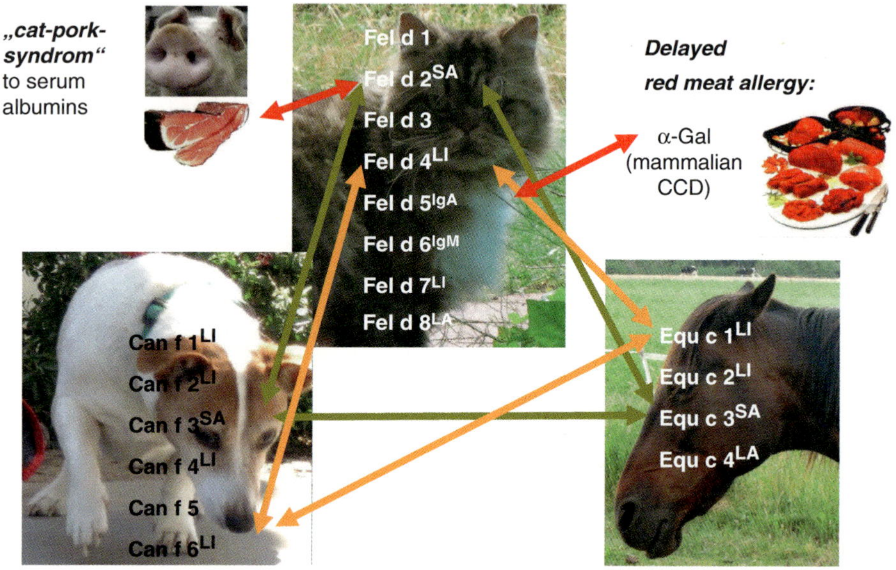

Fig. 19.3 Identified animal allergens and their structural relatedness (potential cross-reactivity) (*arrows*) (*IgA* immunoglobulin A, *IgM* immunoglobulin M, *LA* latherin, *LI* lipocalin, *SA* serum albumin)

source. Owing to the complexity of the situation, as well as the relatedness of some allergens and the heterogenous sensitization patterns, the principles and arguments for molecular allergy diagnostics in cases of suspected animal sensitization cannot be directly adopted:

- An individual, dominant marker allergen has, to date, been established only for the cat (Fel d 1).
- Sensitization to other animal species can probably be specifically (i.e., unambiguously) detected only by using several single allergens.
- Certain animal allergens may potentially enhance test sensitivity (limit of quantification, LoQ), especially if they are under-represented in animal extracts.
- In order to make use of an LoQ which is much less effective, all single allergens that are under-represented in the extract would ideally have to be diagnostically available. This is not yet the case.
- Most likely not all significant animal allergens have yet been identified, and hence their potential marker function as well as cross-reactivity have not yet been assessed.

The discovery and characterization of new animal hair allergens is currently progressing well, continuously providing new findings about the protein families involved and their family relationships between the various animal species. Unfortunately, it takes a fairly long time for a given molecule to be introduced into diagnostics, and as such the scope for systematic evaluation and use of molecular IgE testing currently remains limited.

19.7 Current Additional Benefits from Molecular Diagnostics

The combined use of marker allergens and cross-reactive allergens (e.g., serum albumin) for IgE testing already renders a more reliable identification of the correct allergen source possible.

While Fel d 1 is regarded as the marker allergen of the cat, Can f 1 and Can f 2 are marker allergens in the dog.

Explanation: when a patient has specific IgE to Fel d 1 (and possibly Fel d 2), but not to Can f 1 or Can f 2, then cat is the major allergen source (primary sensitization to cat). If diagnosis was carried out using total extract, both cat and dog may result positive and a distinction between primary sensitization and co-sensitization would be impossible primary sensitization from cross-sensitization.

When observing a primary sensitization to horse, it is very likely that the total extracts from cat and dog are also positive, as Equ c 1 cross-reacts with both Fel d 4 and Can f 6. The marker allergens Fel d 1, Can f 1, and Can f 2 would, however, be negative. There are, of course, also persons that show co-sensitization to two or more allergen sources.

Sensitization to serum albumins from pets may, due to cross-reactivity, lead to beef/pork allergy.

The clinical relevance of serum albumins must be clarified on an individual basis. Reactions mainly occur to meat which has been poorly or not cooked and are not always reproducible. Detection of IgE to serum albumin of one animal species allows for potential cross-sensitization to be predicted. There is very limited data on sensitization to serum albumins and symptoms. High levels of IgE to Fel d 2 have been associated with atopic dermatitis in children with cat allergy (Wisniewski et al. 2013).

Recently, an increasing number of cases have been reported involving a delayed reaction to red meat or innards, these evidently being due to sensitization toward the mammalian oligosaccharide galactose-alpha-1,3-galactose (α-gal) (◉ Fig. 19.2). This carbohydrate chain is present on proteins from mammals other than primates. It also occurs on Fel d 5 and Fel d 6, and, therefore, specific IgE to cat extract can be detected in these individuals.

19.8 Therapy and Recommendations

The eliciting allergen should, in the future, be established as precisely as possible by means of patient interviews and molecular diagnostics (if available), thus enabling specific recommendations to be given. Once the diagnosis of a clinically relevant allergy is confirmed, the animal should, if possible, be removed from the home environment.

If a patient is not sensitized to any serum albumin, (i.e., Equ c 1, Fel d 4, Can f 6), current knowledge enables the clinician to recommend an alternative pet as a cross-sensitization to another furry animal is unlikely. However, the development of a new allergy to a different animal cannot be ruled out in the case of increased susceptibility to allergy.

In occupational animal allergy, the relevant notifiable health-and-safety authorities must be informed as soon as possible that an occupational condition is suspected. With their support, the first step should be to take technical or individual preventive measures and to see where reduced exposure to the allergen can prevent the continuation of symptoms, worsening of the condition, and, ultimately, the patient having to give up the occupation altogether.

19.9 Outlook

Thus far, few single allergens are commercially available to diagnose animal allergy (◉ Table 19.1). Many other single allergens have, however, already been identified, and it is to be hoped that these will soon be introduced into routine diagnostic practice.

Fel d 1 is the best-characterized animal allergen. Due to its high clinical relevance, research on immunotherapy primarily focuses on this allergen. Fel d 1 is developed recombinantly or as a "cocktail" of relevant peptides of Fel d 1 for immunotherapy (van Hage and Pauli, 2014). An early clinical study with a peptide mix containing dominant T cell epitopes revealed an improvement in rhinoconjunctivitis symptoms after only four injections (Patel et al. 2013). Recombinant "designer molecules" represent another advance. One of these is a Fel d 1 protein fused with the hepatitis B virus PreS antigen, which consists of two non-allergenic peptides. Using an animal model, undesirable side effects mediated by IgE and T cells were prevented and it proved possible to boost production of blocking IgG antibodies (Niespodziana et al. 2011). In another clinical investigation, Fel d 1 was specifically modulated in order to optimize antigen presentation and achieve effective antigen-specific T cell tolerance. Injection directly into a lymph node also allows the use of lower doses of antigen (Senti et al. 2012). Here, too, the findings are promising, with enhanced tolerance generated after only three injections.

19.10 Conclusion: Potential for Routine Clinical Practice

With the use of cat and dog allergen components, genuine sensitization can be distinguished from cross-reactivity. For certain other mammals such as rabbit, guinea pig, hamster, and rat, no individual components are yet available. The current marker allergen for horse, Equ c 1, is cross-reactive with allergens from cat and dog. However, the list of available single allergens for routine diagnostics is still incomplete. In diagnostics using crude extract, it must be kept in mind that extracts contain different cross-reactive components such as serum albumins and various lipocalins. Here, the specific, additional use of marker allergens can provide clarification regarding primary sensitization. Thus, sensitization to, e.g., cat extract can be associated with two distinct forms of food allergy, pork-cat syndrome (IgE to serum

Table 19.1 Inhalant mammalian allergens

Animal species	Allergen	Protein family	UniProtKB accession no.	Apparent mol. wt. in kDa
Bos domesticus (domestic cattle)	Bos d 2	Lipocalin	Q28133	20
	Bos d 3	S100 Ca-binding protein	Q28050	11
Canis familiaris (dog)	**Can f 1**	Lipocalin	O18873	23–25
	Can f 2	Lipocalin	O18874	19
	Can f 3	Serum albumin	P49822	69
	Can f 4	Lipocalin	D7PBH4	18
	Can f 5	Kallikrein	P09582	28
	Can f 6	Lipocalin	H2B3G5	27–29
Cavia porcellus (guinea pig)	Cav p 1	Lipocalin	P83507	20
	Cav p 2	Lipocalin	F0UZ11	17
	Cav p 3	Lipocalin	F0UZ12	18
	Cav p 4	Serum albumin	Q6WDN9	66
	Cav p 6	Lipocalin	S0BDX9	18
Equus caballus (horse)	**Equ c 1**	Lipocalin	Q95182	25
	Equ c 2	Lipocalin	P81216, P81217	17
	Equ c 3	Serum albumin	P35747	67
	Equ c 4	Latherin	P82615	17; 20.5
Felis domesticus (cat)	**Fel d 1**	Secretoglobin	P30438; P30440	18
	Fel d 2	Serum albumin	P49064	69
	Fel d 3	Cystatin	Q8WNR9	11
	Fel d 4	Lipocalin	Q5VFH6	22
	Fel d 5	IgA	–	400
	Fel d 6	IgM	–	800–1000
	Fel d 7	Lipocalin	E5D2Z5	17.5
	Fel d 8	Latherin	F6K0R4	24
Mesocricetus auratus (golden hamster)	Mes a 1	Lipocalin	Q9QXU1	20.5; 24
Mus musculus (mouse)	**Mus m 1**	Lipocalin	P02762, P11589	17
Oryctolagus cuniculus (rabbit)	Ory c 1	Lipocalin	–	17–18
	Ory c 2[a]	Lipocalin	–	21
	Ory c 3	Secretoglobin	Q9GK63; Q9GK67	19–21
	Ory c 4	Lipocalin	U6C8D6	24
Phodopus sungorus (Djungarian hamster)	Pho s 21 kDa[a]	Lipocalin	S5ZYD3	18; 21; 23
Rattus norvegicus (rat)	Rat n 1	Lipocalin	P02761	17

Bold type: allergen available for specific IgE detection
[a]Name not registered with the WHO/IUIS Allergen Nomenclature Sub-Committee

albumin) and red meat allergy (due to IgE reactivity to α gal on cat IgA or cat IgM), as well as with inhalant allergy (Konradsen et al. 2015).

References

Adedoyin J, Gronlund H, Oman H, Johansson SGO, van Hage M. Cat IgA, representative of new carbohydrate cross-reactive allergens. J Allergy Clin Immunol. 2007;119:640–5.

Apostolovic D, Sánchez-Vidaurre S, Waden K, Curin M, Grundström J, Gafvelin G, Cirkovic Velickovic T, Grönlund H, Thomas WR, Valenta R, Hamsten C, van Hage M. The cat lipocalin Fel d 7 and its cross-reactivity with the dog lipocalin Can f 1. Allergy. 2016;71:1490–5.

Asarnoj A, Hamsten C, Wadén K, Lupinek C, Andersson N, Kull I, Curin M, Anto J, Bousquet J, Valenta R, Wickman M, van Hage M. Sensitization to cat and dog allergen molecules in childhood and prediction of symptoms of cat and dog allergy in adolescence: a BAMSE/MeDALL study. J Allergy Clin Immunol. 2016;137:813–21.

Baker J, Berry A, Boscato LM, Gordon S, Walsh BJ, Stuart MC. Identification of some rabbit allergens as lipocalins. Clin Exp Allergy. 2001;31:303–12.

Bulone V, Krogstad-Johnsen T, Smestad-Paulsen B. Separation of horse dander allergen proteins by two-dimensional electrophoresis–molecular characterisation and identification of Equ c 2.0101 and Equ c 2.0102 as lipocalin proteins. Eur J Biochem. 1998;253:202–11.

Cabañas R, López-Serrano MC, Carreira J, Ventas P, Polo F, Caballero MT, Contreras J, Barranco P, Moreno-Ancillo A. Importance of albumin in cross-reactivity among cat, dog and horse allergens. J Investig Allergol Clin Immunol. 2000;10:71–7.

Cavaggioni A, Mucignat-Caretta C. Major urinary proteins, [alpha]2U-globulins and aphrodisin. Biochim Biophys Acta. 2000;1482:218–28.

Chruszcz M, Mikolajczak K, Mank N, Majorek KA, Porebski PJ, Minor W. Serum albumins-unusual allergens. Biochim Biophys Acta. 2013;1830:5375–81.

Commins SP, James HR, Kelly LA, Pochan SL, Workman LJ, Perzanowski MS, Kocan KM, Fahy JV, Nganga LW, Ronmark E, Cooper PJ, Platts-Mills TAE. The relevance of tick bites to the production of IgE antibodies to the mammalian oligosaccharide galactose-α-1,3-galactose. J Allergy Clin Immunol. 2011;127:1286–93.

Dandeu JP, Rabillon J, Divanovic A, Carmi-Leroy A, David B. Hydrophobic interaction chromatography for isolation and purification of Equ.cl, the horse major allergen. J Chromatogr. 1993;621:23–31.

Desjardins A, Benoit C, Ghezzo H, L'Archeveque J, Leblanc C, Paquette L, et al. Exposure to domestic animals and risk of immunologic sensitization in subjects with asthma. J Allergy Clin Immunol. 1993;91:979–86.

Fahlbusch B, Rudeschko O, Szilagyi U, Schlott B, Henzgen M, Schlenvoigt G, Schubert H. Purification and partial characterization of the major allergen, Cav p 1, from guinea pig Cavia porcellus. Allergy. 2002;57:417–22.

Flower DR, North ACT, Sansom CE. The lipocalin protein family: structural and sequence overview. Biochim Biophys Acta. 2000;1482:9–24.

Gordon S, Tee RD, Stuart MC, Newman Taylor AJ. Analysis of allergens in rat fur and saliva. Allergy. 2001;56:563–7.

Goubran Botros H, Poncet P, Rabillon J, Fontaine T, Laval JM, David B. Biochemical characterization and surfactant properties of horse allergens. Eur J Biochem. 2001;268:3126–36.

Gregoire C, Rosinski-Chupin I, Rabillon J, Alzari PM, David B, Dandeu JP. cDNA cloning and sequencing reveal the major horse allergen Equ c1 to be a glycoprotein member of the lipocalin superfamily. J Biol Chem. 1996;271:32951–9.

Gronlund H, Adedoyin J, Commins SP, Platts-Mills TA, van Hage M. The carbohydrate galactose-alpha-1,3-galactose is a major IgE-binding epitope on cat IgA. J Allergy Clin Immunol. 2009;123:1189–91.

Grzyb J, Latowski D, Strzalka K. Lipocalins – a family portrait. J Plant Physiol. 2006;163:895–915.

Haftenberger M, Laußmann D, Ellert U, Kalcklösch M, Langen U, Schlaud M, Schmitz R, Thamm M. Prävalenz von Sensibilisierungen gegen Inhalations- und Nahrungsmittelallergene (DEGS1). Bundesgesundheitsblatt Gesundheitsforschung Gesundheitsschutz. 2013;56:687–97.

Hamsten C, Tran TA, Starkhammar M, Brauner A, Commins SP, Platts-Mills TA, van Hage M. Red meat allergy in Sweden: association with tick sensitization and B-negative blood groups. J Allergy Clin Immunol. 2013;132:1431–4.

Heinzerling LM, Burbach GJ, Edenharter G, Bachert C, Bindslev-Jensen C, Bonini S, Bousquet J, Bousquet-Rouanet L, Bousquet PJ, Bresciani M, Bruno A, Burney P, Canonica GW, Darsow U, Demoly P, Durham S, Fokkens WJ, Giavi S, Gjomarkaj M, Gramiccioni C, Haahtela T, Kowalski ML, Magyar P, Muraközi G, Orosz M, Papadopoulos NG, Röhnelt C, Stingl G, Todo-Bom A, von Mutius E, Wiesner A, Wöhrl S, Zuberbier T. GA 2 LEN skin test study I: GA^{2}LEN harmonization of skin prick testing: novel sensitization patterns for inhalant allergens in Europe. Allergy. 2009;64:1498–506.

Hentges F, Léonard C, Arumugam K, Hilger C. Immune responses to inhalant Mammalian allergens. Front Immunol. 2014;5:234.

Heutelbeck AR, Janicke N, Hilgers R, Kütting B, Drexler H, Hallier E, Bickeböller H. German cattle allergy study (CAS): public health relevance of cattle-allergic farmers. Int Arch Occup Environ Health. 2007;81:201–8.

Hilger C, Kohnen M, Grigioni F, Lehners C, Hentges F. Allergic cross-reactions between cat and pig serum albumin. Study at the protein and DNA levels. Allergy. 1997;52:179–87.

Hilger C, Swiontek K, Hentges F, Donnay C, de Blay F, Pauli G. Occupational inhalant allergy to pork followed by food allergy to pork and chicken: sensitization to hemoglobin and serum albumin. Int Arch Allergy Immunol. 2010;151:173–8.

Hilger C, Swiontek K, Kler S, Diederich C, Lehners C, Vogel L, Vieths S, Hentges F. Evaluation of two new recombinant guinea-pig lipocalins, Cav p 2 and Cav p 3, in the diagnosis of guinea-pig allergy. Clin Exp Allergy. 2011;41:899–908.

Hilger C, Swiontek K, Arumugam K, Lehners C, Hentges F. Identification of a new major dog allergen highly cross-reactive with Fel d 4 in a population of cat- and dog-sensitized patients. J Allergy Clin Immunol. 2012;129:1149–51.

Hilger C, Kuehn A, Hentges F. Animal lipocalin allergens. Curr Allergy Asthma Rep. 2012;12:438–47.

Hilger C, Kler S, Arumugam K, Revets D, Muller CP, Charpentier C, Lehners C, Morisset M, Hentges F. Identification and isolation of a Fel d 1-like molecule as a major rabbit allergen. J Allergy Clin Immunol. 2014;133:759–66.

Hilger C, Kler S, Hentges F. Reply. J Allergy Clin Immunol. 2014;133:284–5.

Hilger C, Dubey VP, Lentz D, Davril C, Revets D, Muller CP, Diederic C, De La Barrière H, Codreanu-More F, Morisset M, Lehners C, De PK, Hentges F. Male-specific submaxillary gland protein, a lipocalin allergen of Golden hamster, differs from lipocalin allergens of Siberian and Roborovski dwarf hamsters. Int Arch Allergy Immunol. 2015;166:30–40.

Ichikawa K, Vailes LD, Pomes A, Chapman MD. Molecular cloning, expression and modelling of cat allergen, cystatin (Fel d 3), a cysteine protease inhibitor. Clin Exp Allergy. 2001;31:1279–86.

Jakob T, Hilger C, Hentges F. Clinical relevance of sensitization to cross-reactive lipocalin Can f 6. Allergy. 2013;68:690–1.

Jeal H, Harris J, Draper A, Taylor AN, Cullinan P, Jones M. Dual sensitization to rat and mouse urinary allergens reflects cross-reactive molecules rather than atopy. Allergy. 2009;64: 855–61.

Jeal H, Jones M. Allergy to rodents: an update. Clin Exp Allergy. 2010;40:1593–601.

Konieczny A, Morgenstern JP, Bizinkauskas CB, Lilley CH, Brauer AW, Bond JF, Aalberse RC, Wallner BP, Kasaian MT. The major dog allergens, Can f 1 and Can f 2, are salivary lipocalin proteins: cloning and immunological characterization of the recombinant forms. Immunology. 1997;92:577–86.

Konradsen JR, Fujisawa T, van Hage M, Hedlin G, Hilger C, Kleine-Tebbe J, Matsui EC, Roberts G, Rönmark E, Platts-Mills T. Allergy to furry animals: new insights, diagnostic approaches, and challenges. J Allergy Clin Immunol. 2015;135:616–25.

Mattsson L, Lundgren T, Everberg H, Larsson H, Lidholm J. Prostatic kallikrein: a new major dog allergen. J Allergy Clin Immunol. 2009;123:362–8.

Mattsson L, Lundgren T, Olsson P, Sundberg M, Lidholm J. Molecular and immunological characterization of Can f 4: a dog dander allergen cross-reactive with a 23 kDa odorant-binding protein in cow dander. Clin Exp Allergy. 2010;40:1276–87.

Morgenstern JP, Griffith IJ, Brauer AW, Rogers BL, Bond JF, Chapman MD, Kuo MC. Amino acid sequence of Fel dI, the major allergen of the domestic cat: protein sequence analysis and cDNA cloning. Proc Natl Acad Sci U S A. 1991;88:9690–4.

Niespodziana K, Focke-Tejkl M, Linhart B, Civaj V, Blatt K, Valent P, van Hage M, Grönlund H, Valenta R. A hypoallergenic cat vaccine based on Fel d 1-derived peptides fused to hepatitis B PreS. J Allergy Clin Immunol. 2011;127:1562–70.

Nilsson OB, Binnmyr J, Zoltowska A, Saarne T, van Hage M, Grönlund H. Characterization of the dog lipocalin allergen Can f 6: the role in cross-reactivity with cat and horse. Allergy. 2012;67:751–7.

Patel D, Couroux P, Hickey P, Salapatek AM, Laidler P, Larché M, Hafner RP. Fel d 1-derived peptide antigen desensitization shows a persistent treatment effect 1 year after the start of dosing: a randomized, placebo-controlled study. J Allergy Clin Immunol. 2013;131: 103–9.

Perzanowski MS, Ronmark E, Platts-Mills TA, Lundback B. Effect of cat and dog ownership on sensitization and development of asthma among preteenage children. Am J Respir Crit Care Med. 2002;166:696–702.

Price JA, Longbottom JL. Allergy to rabbits. II. Identification and characterization of a major rabbit allergen. Allergy. 1988;43:39–48.

Rautiainen J, Rytkönen M, Parkkinen S, Pentikäinen J, Linnala-Kankkunen A, Virtanen T, Pelkonen J, Mäntyjärvi R. cDNA cloning and protein analysis of a bovine dermal allergen with homology to psoriasin. J Invest Dermatol. 1995;105:660–3.

Schmitz R, Ellert U, Kalcklösch M, Dahm S, Thamm M. Patterns of sensitization to inhalant and food allergens – findings from the german health interview and examination survey for children and adolescents. Int Arch Allergy Immunol. 2013;162:263–70.

Saarelainen S, Rytkonen-Nissinen M, Rouvinen J, Taivainen A, Auriola S, Kauppinen A, Kinnunen T, Virtanen T. Animal-derived lipocalin allergens exhibit immunoglobulin E cross-reactivity. Clin Exp Allergy. 2008;38:374–81.

Senti G, Crameri R, Kuster D, Johansen P, Martinez-Gomez JM, Graf N, Steiner M, Hothorn LA, Grönlund H, Tivig C, Zaleska A, Soyer O, van Hage M, Akdis CA, Akdis M, Rose H, Kündig TM. Intralymphatic immunotherapy for cat allergy induces tolerance after only 3 injections. J Allergy Clin Immunol. 2012;129:1290–6.

Smith W, Butler AJ, Hazell LA, Chapman MD, Pomés A, Nickels DG, Thomas WR. Fel d 4, a cat lipocalin allergen. Clin Exp Allergy. 2004;34:1732–8.

Smith W, O'Neil SE, Hales BJ, Chai TLY, Hazell LA, Tanyaratsrisakul S, Piboonpocanum S, Thomas WR. Two newly identified Cat allergens: the von ebner gland protein Fel d 7 and the latherin-like protein Fel d 8. Int Arch Allergy Immunol. 2011;156:159–70.

Spitzauer S, Schweiger C, Sperr WR, Pandjaitan B, Valent P, Mühl S, Ebner C, Scheiner O, Kraft D, Rumpold H. Molecular characterization of dog albumin as a cross-reactive allergen. J Allergy Clin Immunol. 1994;93:614–27.

Torres JA, de Las Heras M, Maroto AS, Vivanco F, Sastre J, Pastor-Vargas C. Molecular and immunological characterization of the first allergenic lipocalin in hamster: the major allergen from Siberian hamster (Phodopus sungorus). J Biol Chem. 2014;289:23382–8.

van Hage M, Pauli G. New vaccines for Mammalian allergy using molecular approaches. Front Immunol. 2014;5:81.

Wickman M, Asarnoj A, Tillander H, Andersson N, Bergström A, Kull I, Melén E, Pershagen G, Ahlstedt S, Lilja G. van Hage M; MeDALL consortium. Childhood-to-adolescence evolution

of IgE antibodies to pollens and plant foods in the BAMSE cohort. J Allergy Clin Immunol. 2014;133:580–2.
Wisniewski JA, Agrawal R, Minnicozzi S, Xin W, Patrie J, Heymann PW, Workman L, Platts-Mills TA, Song TW, Moloney M, Woodfolk JA. Sensitization to food and inhalant allergens in relation to age and wheeze among children with atopic dermatitis. Allergy. 2013;43:1160–70.
Ylonen J, Mantyjarvi R, Taivainen A, Virtanen T. IgG and IgE antibody responses to cow dander and urine in farmers with cow-induced asthma. Clin Exp Allergy. 1992;22:83–90.
Zahradnik E, Sander I, Bruckmaier L, Flagge A, Fleischer C, Schierl R, Nowak D, Sültz J, Spickenheuer A, Noss I, Brüning T, Raulf-Heimsoth M. Development of a sandwich ELISA to measure exposure to occupational cow hair allergens. Int Arch Allergy Immunol. 2011;155:225–33.
Zahradnik E, Raulf M. Animal allergens and their presence in the environment. Front Immunol. 2014;5:76.

Extract-Based and Molecular Diagnostics in Fish Allergy

20

A. Kuehn, C. Radauer, A.L. Lopata, J. Kleine-Tebbe, and I. Swoboda

20.1 Introduction

The increasing trend toward healthy nutrition has seen a substantial increase in the global demand for fish and fish products due to the valuable source of ω-3 fatty acids, essential amino acids, and fat-soluble vitamins (www.fischinfo.de). Among

This contribution is based on a publication by the authors that appeared in the *Allergo Journal* in 2012 (Kuehn A, Radauer C, Swoboda I, Kleine-Tebbe J: Fischallergie – Parvalbumine und andere Allergene. Allergo J. 2012;21:16–18) and which has now been updated, expanded, and translated into English as a chapter for this book.

A. Kuehn, PhD (✉)
Allergology – Immunology – Inflammation Research Unit, Department of Infection and Immunity, Luxembourg Institute of Health, Esch-sur-Alzette, Luxembourg
e-mail: annette.kuehn@lih.lu

C. Radauer, PhD, Prof.
Department of Pathophysiology and Allergy Research, Center for Pathophysiology, Infectiology and Immunology, Medical University of Vienna, Vienna, Austria
e-mail: christian.radauer@meduniwien.ac.at

A.L. Lopata, PhD, Prof.
Molecular Allergy Research Laboratory, Centre for Biodiscovery and Molecular Development of Therapeutics, Australian Institute of Tropical Health and Medicine, James Cook University, Townsville, QLD, Australia
e-mail: andreas.lopata@jcu.edu.au

J. Kleine-Tebbe, MD, Prof.
Allergy and Asthma Center Westend, Outpatient Clinic Hanf, Ackermann and Kleine-Tebbe, Berlin, Germany
e-mail: kleine-tebbe@allergie-experten.de

I. Swoboda, PhD, Prof.
Molecular Biotechnology Section, FH Campus Wien, University of Applied Sciences, Vienna, Austria
e-mail: ines.swoboda@fh-campuswien.ac.at

J. Kleine-Tebbe, T. Jakob (eds.), *Molecular Allergy Diagnostics*,
DOI 10.1007/978-3-319-42499-6_20

the most popular species of marine fish consumed in Germany are Alaska pollock, herring, salmon, tuna, and cod.

Fish is considered to be one of the eight food groups with the highest allergenic potential, besides cow's milk, hen's eggs, peanuts, true nuts, wheat, soy, and crustaceans. Allergic sensitization is elicited through consumption, skin contact, or inhalation of allergens during fish processing (Jeebhay and Lopata 2012; Sharp and Lopata 2013). Fish can cause allergic reactions even in small quantities. Symptoms usually manifest within minutes, but in some cases can take up to 48 hours to appear. Often, the skin (e.g. urticaria, Quincke's edema), the digestive tract (e.g. diarrhea, vomiting), or the respiratory tract (e.g. bronchioconstriction) is affected. These symptoms can occur alone or in combination and might in extreme cases cause anaphylactic shock reactions.

20.2 Allergens: Nomenclature

Allergic reactions to fish are mainly induced by one specific protein family: parvalbumins (Sharp and Lopata 2013). Atlantic cod parvalbumin was the first food allergen to be identified in the early 1970s (Elsayed and Aas 1971). Since then, this allergen has been reported in a number of widely consumed fish species, including carp, Atlantic salmon, mackerel, Alaska pollock, tuna, herring, sardine, and swordfish (Beale et al. 2009; Kuehn et al. 2014c). The last few years have seen an increasing number of reports on other fish allergens. Among these recently described allergens are the β-enolases and the aldolases derived from Atlantic cod, salmon, and tuna, as well as tropomyosin from Mozambique tilapia (Kuehn et al. 2013; Liu et al. 2013). Vitellogenin, an egg yolk protein, has been identified in the eggs of various fish as an allergen (Perez-Gordo et al. 2008). Collagen (gelatin), mainly found in the skin of fish, has been previously described in case reports and small case series but recently identified in a large patient cohort (Sakaguchi et al. 2000; Kuehn et al. 2009; Kobayashi et al. 2016).

Other fish allergens, such as aldehyde phosphate dehydrogenase (Atlantic cod: Gad c APDH) (Das Dores et al. 2002), are not dealt with in this chapter. Their allergenic potency has not yet been clarified. It is possible that they either only rarely lead to sensitization or are relevant only for individual fish species.

20.3 Allergens: Structure

Parvalbumins

are acidic proteins with a low molecular weight of approximately 12 kDa. They are typical members of the protein family of calcium-binding EF-hand proteins, which includes important allergens of animal and plant origin (Radauer et al. 2008). EF-hand proteins are characterized by specific segments of the protein structure: a helix, a loop, and a second helix (◉ Fig. 20.1), with the two helices arranged like the spread thumb and index finger on a human hand. The designation "EF hand" is

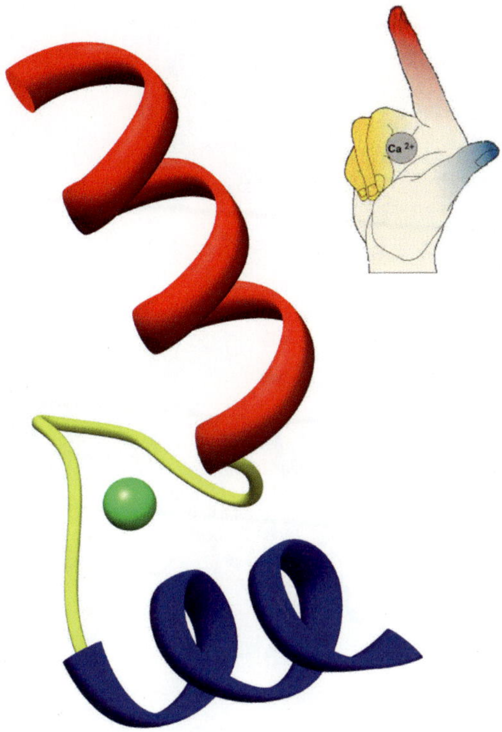

Fig. 20.1 Calcium-binding EF-hand domain, "helix–loop–helix" (*red*, E helix; *blue*, F helix; *green*, bound calcium ion). Owing to the two flanking helices (thumb and index finger), the structure resembles an outstretched hand (Adapted from www.chemgapedia.de)

derived from the nomenclature of helices in the structure of parvalbumins, which are numbered from A to F. The C, D, E, and F helices form the prototypical EF-hand structures. These EF-hand motifs are binding sites for both calcium and magnesium ions (◉ Fig. 20.2a, see below). Ionic bonding is important for the stabilization of the protein structure (Griesmeier et al. 2010). For four parvalbumins, including allergens of carp and hake (Kumar et al. 1990; Richardson et al. 2000), three-dimensional structures have already been elucidated by means of X-ray structure analysis. Two parvalbumin isoform linages are found in fish, the α- and β- linages, whereas the latter one is the main allergenic parvalbumin, present in all bony fish (Sharp and Lopata 2013). In contrast, the α-lineage parvalbumin is mainly found in cartilaginous fish, sharks, and rays, which seem to be nonallergenic.

Enolases
are homodimeric proteins whose subunits have a molecular weight of approximately 50 kDa. These subunits consist of two domains: a small N-terminal domain and a larger C-terminal domain, forming the so-called TIM barrel structure – a barrel-like fold consisting of one α-helix and one β-sheet. TIM barrels are found in a number of non-related enzymes, such as the eponymous triosephosphate

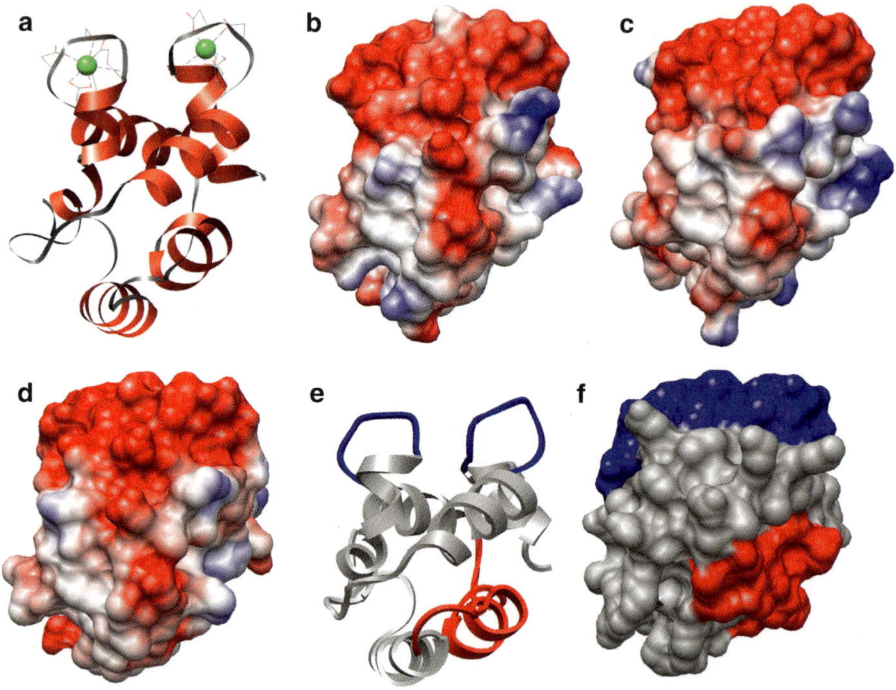

Fig. 20.2 Structure of parvalbumins: their great structural similarity is the cause of the high level of cross-reactivity, which can also be observed between parvalbumins of distantly related species. (**a**) Ribbon diagram of the parvalbumin structure in carp. The bound calcium ions (*green*) contribute toward the unusually high molecular stability. (**b–d**) Surface charge (*red*, positive; *blue*, negative) of parvalbumins in various fish species: (**b**) carp, (**c**) hake, (**d**) pike. However, some patients react only to specific types of fish, which can be explained by species-specific IgE-binding sites. (**e**, **f**) Salmon parvalbumin (*red*, specific epitope; *blue*, calcium-binding site)

isomerase (TIM). For their enzyme activity, enolases require two magnesium ions that are bound in their active center. Three isoforms (α, β, and γ) are found in vertebrates, the β-isoform being the one expressed in muscle.

Aldolases
(more precisely: fructose 1,6-biophosphate aldolases) are tetrameric proteins with subunits of around 40 kDa. They are divided into two distantly related classes: those occurring in plants and animals are exclusively class I enzymes. Aldolases also exhibit TIM barrel folding. In vertebrate animals, three tissue-specific isoforms (A, B, and C) are found, of which aldolase A is the one expressed in muscle.

Collagen
is a rod-shaped molecule of about 330 kDa which is characterized by a triple-helix structure consisting of three supercoiled polypeptide chains, called α-chains (Boran and Regenstein 2010). The primary structure of the α-chains is composed of multiple

repetitions of "Glycine-X-Y" motifs: "X" is often proline and "Y" the rare amino acid hydroxyproline. During the production of fish gelatin, collagen is hydrolyzed into three main fractions (α-, β-, and γ-chain) and degradation products thereof.

Tropomyosins
are proteins of approximately 32 kDa, belonging to a family of highly conserved proteins occurring in different isoforms (Nevzorov and Levitsky 2011). Tropomyosin is a rod-shaped molecule consisting of two helical molecules coiled into a double-helix shape. Protein structures of allergenic fish tropomyosin have yet to be reported but are assumed to correspond with those of known tropomyosins in other organisms.

Vitellogenins
are macromolecular glycolipoproteins (>150 kDa) belonging to the group of lipid transport proteins. They are composed of different subunits: a light and a heavy chain (Finn 2007). Vitellogenins are egg yolk precursor proteins, examples being lipovitellin and phosvitin. Data on the structure of allergenic vitellogenin are not available but have been obtained for lipovitellin–phosvitin complexes in other organisms (Raag et al. 1988).

20.4 Allergens: Function

Parvalbumins
are found in the muscle tissue of all vertebrates in which these calcium buffer proteins are involved in muscle relaxation (Arif 2009). Rapidly contracting muscles contain large amounts of parvalbumin. The highest concentration has been detected in the extremely fast-contracting white muscle fibers of fish, with up to 0.5 % of the total protein content. Fish also have red, slow-contracting muscle tissue with lower levels of parvalbumins. The distribution of white and dark muscle fibers – and thus the parvalbumin content – may vary greatly between different fish species (Kobayashi et al. 2006). In frequently consumed species such as herring, parvalbumin levels are about twice as high as in Atlantic cod or salmon and ten times as high as in mackerel (Kuehn et al. 2010). The parvalbumin content in tuna, which has predominantly red muscle tissue, is so low that canned tuna is often used as a placebo in oral challenges (Kelso et al. 2003). However, the low contents of parvalbumin in canned tuna might also be due to the type of food processing, which is particularly forceful during the canning process.

Enolases and Aldolases
are elementary enzymes involved in the general metabolism of glucose. During cellular energy production, the aldolases catalyze the fourth step of glycolysis (cleavage of fructose 1,6-bisphosphate into dihydroxyacetone phosphate and glyceraldehyde 3-phosphate), while the enolases are responsible for the penultimate step (dehydration of 2-phospho-D-glycerate to form phosphoenolpyruvate)

(Garfinkel and Garfinkel 1985). As they are the key enzymes of carbohydrate metabolism, significant amounts are present in muscle tissue; the content of allergenic enzymes is thus similar to that of parvalbumin.

Collagen
is an important structure protein and, thus, a main constituent of fish skin, bone, and connective tissue. Different collagen types (type I, II, etc.) of mostly tissue-specific distribution are known, while type I collagen is the main protein. Fish collagen is mostly isolated from fish skin. Fish gelatin which is not a naturally occurring protein is produced from collagen by partial hydrolysis. Fish gelatin is used in many industrial applications such as foods, pharmaceuticals, and cosmetics as stabilizer and structure protein.

Tropomyosin
is an important structural protein in the muscle cell, which is also found in other cells. It regulates muscle contraction together with troponin. A complex consisting of troponin and tropomyosin interacts with binding sites of myosin, the muscle fiber protein, thus allowing muscle contraction (Perry 2001). Tropomyosin constitutes approximately 3 % of total myofibrillar protein.

Vitellogenins
are egg yolk precursor proteins that supply the embryo with lipid (lipovitin) and phosphate (phosvitin) reserves (Ding et al. 1989). These proteins account for almost the total content of egg yolk proteins.

20.5 Allergens: Relevance

Parvalbumins
show a strong sensitization potential. The reasons for this are twofold: the remarkable stability of proteins to heat and denaturing agents (Elsayed and Aas 1971; Griesmeier et al. 2010; Saptarshi et al. 2014) and the high degree of cross-reactivity between parvalbumins of different species (◉ Fig. 20.2b–d) (van Do et al. 2005). Parvalbumins can be modified by industrial food processing, inducing, for example, the formation of oligomers or peptide fragments with altered epitopes; these are recognized differently by patients' individual IgE repertoires, resulting in increased or decreased IgE-binding activity (Sletten et al. 2010).

Fish Enolases and Aldolases
have only recently been discovered as new allergens in Atlantic cod, salmon, and tuna (Kuehn et al. 2013). IgE antibodies to these proteins can be produced by patients both with and without sensitization to parvalbumin. The clinical relevance of this cosensitization is not yet fully understood. Enolases and aldolases seem to be much less stable to (physical and chemical) food preparation-related influences than parvalbumins. It has not yet been shown how this instability influences their potential as food allergens.

Fish Collagen
as well as fish gelatin has been identified as inducers of allergic sensitization (Sakaguchi et al. 2000; Kuehn et al. 2009). Fish-allergic patients may be cosensitized to parvalbumin in parallel to fish collagen. A recent study pointed out that the allergenicity of fish collagen and gelatin might be not equal as important epitopes could be destroyed by hydrolysis during the production of fish gelatin (Kobayashi et al. 2016). Still, the final proof of the clinical relevance of collagen or gelatin as fish allergens is still missing, and food challenges would be required to proof the in vivo reactivity of collagen and gelatin.

Fish Tropomyosins
have been described as allergens in only one type of fish to date: tilapia (Liu et al. 2013). Among the patients in this study, who were sensitized to tropomyosin, sensitization to parvalbumin played only a tangential role. Since other allergenic tropomyosins, such as those derived from shrimp (Shanti et al. 1993), have been reported as being extremely stable proteins, it can be expected that homologous fish tropomyosin also demonstrates thermal stability.

Vitellogenins
are important allergens derived from fish eggs, which have thus far been identified in salmon, trout, and sturgeon. Investigations on protein stability showed that these allergens exhibit a high level of resistance to enzymatic digestion (Fujita et al. 2012). This stability, and the high concentration of proteins in fish eggs, explains their allergenic potential. Vitellogenins derived from fish eggs are probably thermostable proteins that possess properties similar to Gal d 6, a homologous allergen from egg yolk (Amo et al. 2010).

20.6 Sensitization Prevalence

Fish is not only one of the most common triggers of IgE-mediated food allergies but also the leading cause of occupational allergy (Douglas et al. 1995; Jeebhay et al. 2008; Jeebhay and Lopata 2012). Allergic reactions to fish are, therefore, frequently found in areas with high fish consumption where the fish-processing industry is one of the most important economic sectors. One individual in 1,000 can be expected to be affected by fish allergy in such regions (Aas 1987).

Most fish-allergic patients are sensitized to parvalbumins. The general prevalence (frequency of sensitization among those with fish allergy) varies, depending on the type of fish and the sensitized population group, between 70 and 95 %. β-enolase and aldolase have recently been successfully purified from muscle tissue of Atlantic cod, salmon, and tuna (Kuehn et al. 2013). These proteins now represent two additional fish allergens, which could in the future be used for more accurate diagnostics. Initial investigations have found that the prevalence of IgE reactivity to enolase and aldolase may be approximately 63 % and 50 %, respectively. Sensitization to these allergens appears to be especially relevant in patients who show no reaction to parvalbumins (Kuehn et al. 2013).

Sensitization to fish collagen was first assessed in single studies with low numbers of patients, but a recent study showed that collagen sensitization might be more prevalent as previously indicated. A study among Japanese patients with fish allergy even demonstrated higher sensitivity to collagen (50 %) than to parvalbumin (Kobayashi et al. 2016). It still needs to be clarified whether this prevalence is a population-specific phenomenon.

So far, the data available on tropomyosins as fish allergens are insufficient to draw conclusions about the relative impact and prevalence of IgE sensitization.

As fish eggs are merely considered as a culinary delicacy, this sensitization does not occur frequently. It has, however, been proven that vitellogenin and its related proteins are the major allergens of caviar (Fujita et al. 2012; Perez-Gordo et al. 2008).

20.7 Cross-Reactive Versus Marker Allergens

IgE antibodies to the parvalbumin of a given fish species often also recognize parvalbumins of other fish species (van Do et al. 2005) (◉ Figs. 20.2b–d and ◉ 20.3). The basis of this cross-reactivity is the high level of sequence identity (>70 %) and structural similarity between fish parvalbumins (Swoboda et al. 2002b). The more closely fish species are related, the more similar are their parvalbumins. Highest levels of sequence similarity are found in the calcium-binding domains; these domains can form conformational epitopes and bind IgE antibodies (Bugajska-Schretter et al. 2000). As the IgE reactivity of parvalbumins is reduced in the absence of calcium, binding of calcium ions probably influences the conformation of IgE epitopes.

Although the majority of patients have allergic reactions to several fish species, some patients show monosensitization or oligosensitization to individual fish species (Kuehn et al. 2011; Raith et al. 2014; Swoboda et al. 2013) as well as different IgE reactivity to different allergen isoforms (Sharp et al. 2014). Differences in parvalbumin content and species-specific IgE-binding epitopes provide possible explanations why patients, all with their own IgE repertoires, react differently to various fish species (◉ Fig. 20.2e–f).

The cross-reactivity of the β-enolases and the aldolases purified from Atlantic cod, salmon, and tuna was also investigated (first study by Kuehn et al. 2013). Cross-reactivity between the aldolases varied strongly between individuals. One interesting finding was that, of all the enolases investigated, Atlantic cod enolase was the one able to inhibit IgE binding to other enolases most successfully (Kuehn et al. 2013). The cause of the high inhibition potential of Atlantic cod enolase may be the patients' primary sensitization to this fish. Should these results be confirmed in a larger patient population, quantitative assessment of specific IgE antibodies toward a number of enolases could help to identify primary sensitizing enolases and corresponding fish species (Kuehn et al. 2013, 2014a).

Data on the in vivo and in vitro cross-reactivity of fish collagens are scarce. The first study to demonstrate that collagen is a potential fish allergen in a large patient

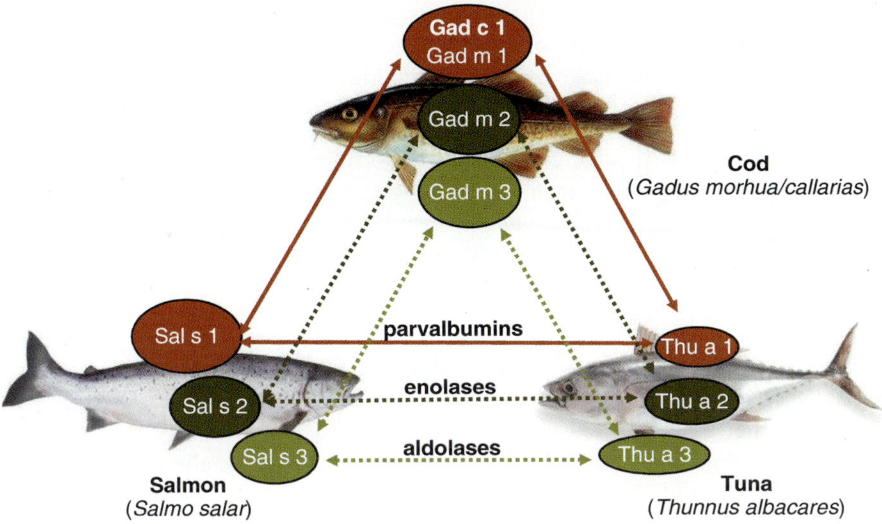

Fig. 20.3 Identified allergens of three frequently consumed fish species: the allergen content of parvalbumin is higher in salmon and Atlantic cod than in tuna. Cross-reactivity between parvalbumins is pronounced, whereas that between minor allergens (enolases, aldolases) is variable. (**Bold type**: available for in vitro diagnostics)

cohort was conducted in on mackerel. It was shown that there was a high cross-reactivity between mackerel collagen and collagens from 22 other fish species (87–98 %) (Kobayashi et al. 2016). Further studies will be required to define the cross-reactivity of fish collagens.

For tropomyosin from the fish tilapia, it was shown that the isolated protein cross-reacts with tropomyosin, the major allergen of shrimp (Lopata et al. 2010; Liu et al. 2011). However, the amino acid homology between tilapia and shrimp tropomyosin is very low with only 57 %, which would not predict significant immunological cross-reactivity. The clinical relevance of this serological IgE reactivity, a potential cross-reaction between fish and seafood, requires further clarification.

To date, it has been shown for vitellogenin, the allergen derived from fish eggs, that IgE antibodies are able to bind to homologous members of different fish species (Shimizu et al. 2009). Clinical reactivity seems to be variable but is apparently often directed specifically against individual types of caviar. No cross-reactivity could be found to similar proteins derived from hen's eggs (Perez-Gordo et al. 2008).

20.8 Diagnostics

Routine diagnostic procedures are performed using fish extracts or fish products in vivo by means of skin tests and in vitro by detecting fish-specific IgE antibodies. To date, around 30 extracts of various fish species – but no extracts of fish eggs – and two recombinant parvalbumins are available for testing specific IgE antibodies (◉ Table 20.1). Minor allergens are not yet available as isolated components for in vitro diagnostics (see also Matricardi et al. 2016).

> Clinical reactivity can be verified by performing oral challenges, especially if the aim is to determine whether patients can tolerate particular fish species. However, the risks and the cost, time, and effort involved in such provocation tests justify this examination only in exceptional cases.

20.9 Additional Benefit from Molecular Diagnostics

Just like other extracts used in allergy diagnostics, commercially produced fish extracts are subject to considerable variability as far as their allergen and protein content is concerned. Thus, the reliability of the diagnostic findings obtained using these extracts is often unsatisfactory (Kuehn et al. 2010).

Molecular biological and biotechnological procedures now enable recombinant production of fish allergens and extraction of allergens in their pure form from fish muscle tissue (Kuehn et al. 2013; Swoboda et al. 2002a; Sharp et al. 2014). The use of recombinant and pure natural allergens allows more precise diagnosis of fish allergy and makes it possible to accurately analyze patients' individual sensitization profiles (Matricardi et al. 2016). By using purified natural parvalbumins, β-enolases, and aldolases from Atlantic cod, salmon, and tuna in IgE ELISA experiments, it is not only possible to determine which fish species the patients are primarily sensitized toward but also to identify the underlying molecular components (component diagnostics) (Kuehn et al. 2013, 2014a).

Additional potential advantages of using individual fish allergens for the evaluation of IgE sensitization are as follows (▶ Chap. 7):

- Increased test sensitivity (decreased limit of quantification, LoQ)
- Improved analytical specificity (selectivity) for certain fish allergens with already known clinical characteristics (i.e., sensitization associated with severe reactions)
- Used as potential markers for cross-reactions
- Used as potential markers for species-specific sensitization

Polysensitization to numerous fish allergens (parvalbumins, enolases, aldolases, collagen) together with high IgE levels seems to be more associated with severe clinical reactions (Kuehn et al. 2013, 2014b) – presumably indicating a wider IgE repertoire which could have developed concurrently with increased IgE

Table 20.1 Identified fish allergens

Order	Species	Parvalbumin	Other allergens
Anguilliformes	Eel	"Ang a 1"	–
Perciformes	Atlantic horse mackerel	"Tra j 1"	Gelatin
	Mackerel[a]	"Sco s 1"	–
	Chub mackerel	"Sco j 1"	–
	Snapper	–	–
	Swordfish	Xip g 1	–
	Smallmouth bass	–	–
	Tuna[a]	Thu a 1	Collagen (gelatin) Thu a 2 (enolase) Thu a 3 (aldolase)
	Tilapia	"Ore ni 1"	Ore m 4 (tropomyosin)
	Asian sea bass	Lat c 1	–
Gadiformes	Baltic Sea cod	**Gad c 1**	–
	Atlantic cod[a]	Gad m 1	Aldehyde phosphate dehydrogenase Gad m 2 (enolase) Gad m 3 (aldolase) Gelatin
	Saithe	"Pol vi 1"	–
	Hake	"Mer mr 1"	–
	Alaska pollock	"The ch 1"	–
Scorpaeniformes	Japanese stingfish	"Seb in 1"	–
	Ocean perch	Seb m 1	–
Clupeiformes	Atlantic herring[a]	Clu h 1	–
	South American pilchard	Sar sa 1	–
	European pilchard	"Sar p 1"	–
Cypriniformes	Common carp [a]	**Cyp c 1**	–
	Anchovy	"Eng e 1"	–
Salmoniformes	Rainbow trout	Onc m 1	Collagen Aldolase Serum albumin, triosephosphate isomerase Vitellogenin
	Chum salmon	–	Onc k 5 (vitellogenin)
	Char	"Sal f 1"	–
	Atlantic salmon [a]	Sal s 1	Gelatin Sal s 2 (enolase) Sal s 3 (aldolase)

(continued)

Table 20.1 (continued)

Order	Species	Parvalbumin	Other allergens
Pleuronectiformes	Megrim	Lep w 1	–
	Atlantic halibut	"Hip h 1"	–
	Common sole	"Sol so 1"	Triosephosphate isomerase
Acipenseriformes	Beluga sturgeon	–	Vitellogenin
Siluriformes	Brown bullhead	"Ict pu 1"	–

Fish classified by order (in alphabetical order) and species (second column): species, of which extracts are available for in vitro diagnostics, are listed. For most fish species, parvalbumin has been described as an allergen. Third column: Official IUIS allergen nomenclature (www.allergen.org); unofficial allergen names in quotation marks. Further allergens are known for some fish species (fourth column)

Bold type: recombinant parvalbumins, available for in vitro diagnostics (ImmunoCAP, ISAC; Phadia-Thermofisher, Upsala, Sweden)

[a]Potentially useful for in vitro diagnostics as representative of a fish family

to fish allergens. However, to date, it is not possible to use specific IgE toward certain fish allergens to predict clinical reactivity; no threshold values are available.

A different study was able to demonstrate the advantage of in vitro diagnostics with recombinant parvalbumin over diagnostics involving fish extracts. In this research, a child with confirmed fish allergy showed increased levels of IgE antibodies to recombinant parvalbumin (in this case, rCyp c 1), but to none of the tested fish extracts (Agabriel et al. 2010). This indicates that IgE tests with recombinant fish allergens can be highly useful due to the potentially enhanced sensitivity (as measured by LoQ) of such testing, especially when IgE detection with fish extracts yields negative results despite clinical suspicion.

The additional benefit of using individual components to diagnose fish allergy has recently been investigated (Kuehn et al. 2014c). Fifty-eight percent of those study participants who had cross-reacting IgE antibodies to parvalbumin were all positively diagnosed using Atlantic cod parvalbumin. However, ImmunoCAP testing with Atlantic cod extract also generated a positive outcome in all these subjects. In 42 % of cases, improved test sensitivity (i.e., decreased LoQ) was established by means of component diagnostics. Most of these patients (81 %) were positively tested using salmon parvalbumin or the recently identified single allergens (enolases, aldolases, fish gelatin). It was also observed that component diagnostics, using newly discovered allergens, appears to be especially useful for parvalbumin-negative patients, as the majority (71 %) of these individuals had specific IgE to these allergens.

In summary, fish extracts can be stated to have (thus far) been regarded as sufficiently sensitive for use in sensitization testing to identify fish allergens. This is because the most important group of major allergens, the parvalbumins, is not only well represented in extracts (native, heated) because of their high levels and stability but is also available in IgE-reactive form. However, more recent studies have indicated the additional benefit from diagnostic procedures using individual components (parvalbumins, enolases, aldolases, fish gelatin). Parvalbumins should be regarded only as markers for pronounced cross-reactivity between numerous fish species and not generally as markers of species-specific fish sensitization.

Clinically speaking, it is sufficient, in highly sensitized fish-allergic individuals, to identify IgE antibodies to a single parvalbumin instead of toward all members of the parvalbumin family. However, in patients with species-specific allergies, it is entirely appropriate to test for IgE antibodies to a wider range of different parvalbumins (and, in the future, to other fish allergens).

In this way, these allergic patients can be provided with a differential diagnosis to enable them to distinguish between fish species they must avoid and those they may tolerate.

20.10 Therapy and Recommendation

No specific immunotherapy is currently available to treat fish allergy, as the risk of anaphylactic side effects induced by this therapy is high. Patients are therefore advised to strictly avoid all types of fish (although a number of species would probably be tolerated by some individuals). Food manufacturers in EU member states are obliged to label fish as an ingredient in packaged goods (Allergen Labelling Directive; Commission Directive 2007/68/EC).

Caution is, nevertheless, warranted with respect to a range of highly processed food products which may contain fish including surimi, paella, and Worcester sauce or may contain fish gelatin such as some kosher products.

20.11 Outlook

1. The use of molecular biological methods in allergology has led to new strategies aimed at developing molecules for effective immunotherapy with few adverse reactions (Valenta et al. 2010). As far as the major fish allergen – parvalbumin – is concerned, calcium depletion experiments have shown that its IgE reactivity is decreased if calcium is absent (Bugajska-Schretter et al. 2000; Swoboda et al. 2002a). Through targeted insertion of mutations in calcium-binding EF-hand motifs of carp parvalbumin, Swoboda et al. (2007) succeeded in the production of a hypoallergenic variant with significantly reduced IgE reactivity and biological activity which should lead to comparatively few side effects during medical treatment. This protein is currently being evaluated in clinical studies and could serve as an important future tool in immunotherapy.
2. Studies on the clinical relevance of minor fish allergens could potentially improve future in vitro diagnostics of fish allergy. One conceivable option would be to test for IgE to representative minor allergens in individual cases where sensitiza-

tion to fish parvalbumin is not present (this being the case in up to 30 % of patients). Thus, the use of enolases, aldolases, and fish gelatin would probably increase the test sensitivity of component diagnostics in fish allergy as this would allow parvalbumin-negative patients to be identified as sensitized. The sensitivity of testing can be assumed to be higher (i.e., with LoQ lower) compared to only using fish extracts. IgE detection would increase in sensitivity – a great advantage for sensitization at low thresholds or for exclusion diagnostics with a view to invalidating IgE sensitization by means of negative results. Additionally, the analysis of specific IgE antibodies to minor allergens may allow conclusions regarding which fish species the patient is primarily sensitized toward and with which fish species cross-reactions occur. In cases of rare isolated sensitization to minor allergens, the clinical risk potential would have to be investigated, especially as to the extent to which cooking or other forms of processing may mitigate the allergenicity of these fish allergens. This would be important for individualized consultations with fish-allergic patients.

20.12 Conclusions: Potential for Everyday Clinical Practice

Fish extracts and recombinant allergens currently available allow reliable serological diagnostics of fish allergy. As highly sensitized fish-allergic patients tend to react to parvalbumin, it is in most cases (about 70–80 %) possible to achieve confirmation of sensitization toward fish by means of one of the recombinant parvalbumins obtainable for routine diagnostic purposes (Gad c 1 derived from Atlantic cod or Cyp c 1 from carp) (◉ Fig. 20.3). As some patients are sensitized to minor allergens in fish and some demonstrate species-specific fish allergy, the recombinant parvalbumins cannot as yet completely replace fish extracts. In order to avoid having to test all fish extracts, representative extracts of individual fish families should be selected (◉ Table 20.1), as cross-reactions often occur between closely related fish species. As soon as minor allergens and a larger number of different parvalbumin proteins can be used in routine diagnostics – either purified natural or in recombinant form – it will be possible to replace extract-based diagnostics with diagnostics focused on individual components.

At present, the only recommended action for fish-allergic individuals is strict avoidance of the food item triggering the allergy. However, the use of molecular biological and biotechnological methods has already led to the development of the first hypoallergenic molecules, which may allow effective therapy of fish allergies with few side effects.

References

Aas K. Fish allergy and the cod allergen model. In: Brostoff J, Challacombe ST, editors. Food allergy and intolerance. London: Balliere Tindall; 1987. p. 356.

Agabriel C, Robert P, Bongrand P, Sarles J, Vitte J. Fish allergy: in Cyp c1 we trust. Allergy. 2010;65:1483–4.

Amo A, Rodríguez-Pérez R, Blanco J, Villota J, Juste S, Moneo I, Caballero ML. Gal d 6 is the second allergen characterized from egg yolk. J Agric Food Chem. 2010;58:7453–7.
Arif SH. A Ca(2+)-binding protein with numerous roles and uses: parvalbumin in molecular biology and physiology. Bioessays. 2009;31:410–21.
Beale JE, Jeebhay MF, Lopata AL. Characterisation of purified parvalbumin from five fish species and nucleotide sequencing of this major allergen from Pacific pilchard, Sardinops sagax. Mol Immunol. 2009;46:2958–93.
Boran G, Regenstein JM. Fish gelatin. Adv Food Nutr Res. 2010;60:119–43.
Bugajska-Schretter A, Grote M, Vangelista L, Valent P, Sperr WR, Rumpold H, Pastore A, Reichelt R, Valenta R, Spitzauer S. Purification, biochemical, and immunological characterisation of a major food allergen: different immunoglobulin E recognition of the apo- and calcium-bound forms of carp parvalbumin. Gut. 2000;46:661–9.
Das Dores S, Chopin C, Romano A, Galland-Irmouli AV, Quaratino D, Pascual C, Fleurence J, Gueant JL. IgE-binding and cross-reactivity of a new 41 kDa allergen of codfish. Allergy. 2002;57:84–7.
Ding JL, Hee PL, Lam TJ. Two forms of vitellogenin in the plasma and gonads of male Oreochromis aureus. Comp Biochem Phys Part B. 1989;93:363–70.
Douglas JD, McSharry C, Blaikie L, Morrow T, Miles S, Franklin D. Occupational asthma caused by automated salmon processing. Lancet. 1995;346:737–40.
Elsayed S, Aas K. Characterization of a major allergen (cod). Observations on effect of denaturation on the allergenic activity. J Allergy. 1971;47:283–91.
Finn RN. Vertebrate yolk complexes and the functional implications of phosvitins and other subdomains in vitellogenins. Biol Reprod. 2007;76:926–35.
Fujita S, Shimizu Y, Kishimura H, Watanabe K, Hara A, Saeki H. In vitro digestion of major allergen in salmon roe and its peptide portion with proteolytic resistance. Food Chem. 2012;130:644–50.
Griesmeier U, Bublin M, Radauer C, Vázquez-Cortés S, Ma Y, Fernández-Rivas M, Breiteneder H. Physicochemical properties and thermal stability of Lep w 1, the major allergen of whiff. Mol Nutr Food Res. 2010;54:861–9.
Garfinkel L, Garfinkel D. Magnesium regulation of the glycolytic pathway and the enzymes involved. Magnesium. 1985;4:60–72.
Jeebhay MF, Robins TG, Malo J-L, Miller M, Bateman E, Smuts M, Baatjies R, Lopata AL. Occupational allergy and asthma among salt water bony-fish processing workers. Am J Ind Med. 2008;51:899–910.
Jeebhay MF, Lopata AL. Occupational allergies in seafood processing workers. Adv Food Nutr Res. 2012;66:47–73.
Kelso JM, Bardina L, Beyer K. Allergy to canned tuna. J Allergy Clin Immunol. 2003;111:901.
Kobayashi A, Tanaka H, Hamada Y, Ishizaki S, Nagashima Y, Shiomi K. Comparison of allergenicity and allergens between fish white and dark muscles. Allergy. 2006;61:357–63.
Kobayashi Y, Akiyama H, Huge J, Kubota H, Chikazawa S, Satoh T, Miyake T, Uhara H, Okuyama R, Nakagawara R, Aihara M, Hamada-Sato N. Fish collagen is an important panallergen in the Japanese population. Allergy. 2016;71:720–3.
Kuehn A, Hilger C, Hentges F. Anaphylaxis provoked by ingestion of marshmallows containing fish gelatin. J Allergy Clin Immunol. 2009;123:708–9.
Kuehn A, Scheuermann T, Hilger C, Hentges F. Important variations in parvalbumin content in common fish species: a factor possibly contributing to variable allergenicity. Int Arch Allergy Immunol. 2010;153:359–66.
Kuehn A, Hutt-Kempf E, Hilger C, Hentges F. Clinical monosensitivity to salmonid fish linked to specific IgE-epitopes on salmon and trout beta-parvalbumins. Allergy. 2011;66:299–301.
Kuehn A, Hilger C, Lehners-Weber C, Codreanu-Morel F, Morisset M, Metz-Favre C, Pauli G, de Blay F, Revets D, Muller CP, Vogel L, Vieths S, Hentges F. Identification of enolases and aldolases as important fish allergens in cod, salmon and tuna: component resolved diagnosis using parvalbumin and the new allergens. Clin Exp Allergy. 2013;43:811–22.

Kuehn A, Fischer J, Hilger C, Sparla C, Biedermann T, Hentges F. Correlation of clinical monosensitivity to cod with specific IgE to enolase and aldolase. Ann Allergy Asthma Immunol. 2014a;113:670–1.

Kuehn A, Metz-Favre C, Pauli G, Lehners-Weber C, Codreanu-Morel F, Hentges F, Auriol P, Bienvenu F, Braun C, Crepin C, Foessel A, Guenard L, Krieger P, Renaudin JM, Tuyeras JF, de Blay F, Morisset M, Hilger C. A study comparing the clinical phenotypes of fish-allergic patients with their specific IgE profiles to fish parvalbumin, enolase, aldolase and gelatin. Rev Fr d'Allergol. 2014b;54:51–60.

Kuehn A, Swoboda I, Arumugam K, Hilger C, Hentges F. Fish allergens at a glance: variable allergenicity of parvalbumins, the major fish allergens. Front Immunol. 2014c;5:179. doi:10.3389/fimmu.2014.00179.

Kumar VD, Lee L, Edwards BF. Refined crystal structure of calcium-liganded carp parvalbumin 4.25 at 1.5-A resolution. Biochemistry. 1990;29:1404–12.

Liu R, Krishnan HB, Xue W, Liu C. Characterization of allergens isolated from the freshwater fish blunt snout bream (Megalobrama amblycephala). J Agric Food Chem. 2011;59:458–63.

Liu R, Holck AL, Yang E, Liu C, Xue W. Tropomyosin from tilapia (Oreochromis mossambicus) as an allergen. Clin Exp Allergy. 2013;43:365–77.

Lopata AL, O'Hehir R, Lehrer SL. Shellfish allergy – clinical and diagnostic approaches. Clin Exp Allergy Rev. 2010;40:850–8.

Nevzorov IA, Levitsky DI. Tropomyosin: double helix from the protein world. Biochemistry. 2011;76:1507–27.

Perez-Gordo M, Sanchez-Garcia S, Cases B, Pastor C, Vivanco F, Cuesta-Herranz J. Identification of vitellogenin as an allergen in Beluga caviar allergy. Allergy. 2008;63:479–80.

Perry SV. Vertebrate tropomyosin: distribution, properties and function. J Muscle Res Cell Motil. 2001;22:5–49.

Raag R, Appelt K, Xuong NH, Banaszak L. Structure of the lamprey yolk lipid-protein complex lipovitellin-phosvitin at 2.8 A resolution. J Mol Biol. 1988;200:553–69.

Radauer C, Bublin M, Wagner S, Mari A, Breiteneder H. Allergens are distributed into few protein families and possess a restricted number of biochemical functions. J Allergy Clin Immunol. 2008;121:847–52.

Raith M, Klug C, Sesztak-Greinecker G, Balic N, Focke M, Linhart B, Hemmer W, Swoboda I. Unusual sensitization to parvalbumins from only certain fish species. Ann Allergy Asthma Immunol. 2014;113:571–2.

Richardson RC, King NM, Harrington DJ, Sun H, Royer WE, Nelson DJ. X-Ray crystal structure and molecular dynamics simulations of silver hake parvalbumin (Isoform B). Protein Sci. 2000;9:73–82.

Sakaguchi M, Toda M, Ebihara T, Irie S, Hori H, Imai A, Yanagida M, Miyazawa H, Ohsuna H, Ikezawa Z, Inouye S. IgE antibody to fish gelatin (type I collagen) in patients with fish allergy. J Allergy Clin Immunol. 2000;106:579–84.

Saptarshi SR, Sharp MF, Kamath SD, Lopata AL. Effect of heat processing on antibody reactivity to allergen variants and fragments of black tiger prawn: a comprehensive allergenomic approach. Food Chem. 2014;58:1144–55.

Shanti KN, Martin BM, Nagpal S, Metcalfe DD, Rao PV. Identification of tropomyosin as the major shrimp allergen and characterization of its IgE-binding epitopes. J Immunol. 1993;151:5354–63.

Sharp MF, Lopata AL. Fish allergy: in review. Clin Rev Allergy Immunol. 2013;46:258–71.

Sharp MF, Kamath SD, Koeberl M, Jerry DR, O'Hehir RE, Campbell DE, Lopata AL. Differential IgE binding to isoallergens from Asian seabass (Lates calcarifer) in children and adults. Mol Immunol. 2014;62:77–85.

Shimizu Y, Nakamura A, Kishimura H, Hara A, Watanabe K, Saeki H. Major allergen and its IgE cross-reactivity among salmonid fish roe allergy. J Agric Food Chem. 2009;57:2314–9.

Sletten G, Van Do T, Lindvik H, Egaas E, Florvaag E. Effects of industrial processing on the immunogenicity of commonly ingested fish species. Int Arch Allergy Immunol. 2010;151:223–36.

Swoboda I, Bugajska-Schretter A, Verdino P, Keller W, Sperr WR, Valent P, Valenta R, Spitzauer S. Recombinant carp parvalbumin, the major cross-reactive fish allergen: a tool for diagnosis and therapy of fish allergy. J Immunol. 2002a;168:4576–84.
Swoboda I, Bugajska-Schretter A, Valenta R, Spitzauer S. Recombinant fish parvalbumins: candidates for diagnosis and treatment of fish allergy. Allergy. 2002b;57 Suppl 72:94–6.
Swoboda I, Bugajska-Schretter A, Linhart B, Verdino P, Keller W, Schulmeister U, Sperr WR, Valent P, Peltre G, Quirce S, Douladiris N, Papadopoulos NG, Valenta R, Spitzauer S. A recombinant hypoallergenic parvalbumin mutant for immunotherapy of IgE-mediated fish allergy. J Immunol. 2007;178:290–6.
Swoboda I, Balic N, Klug C, Focke M, Weber M, Spitzauer S, Neubauer A, Quirce S, Douladiris N, Papadopoulos NG, Valenta R. A general strategy for the generation of hypoallergenic molecules for the immunotherapy of fish allergy. J Allergy Clin Immunol. 2013;132:979–81.
Valenta R, Ferreira F, Focke-Tejkl M, Linhart B, Niederberger V, Swoboda I, Vrtala S. From allergen genes to allergy vaccines. Annu Rev Immunol. 2010;28:211–41.
van Do T, Elsayed S, Florvaag E, Hordvik I, Endresen C. Allergy to fish parvalbumins: studies on the cross-reactivity of allergens from 9 commonly consumed fish. J Allergy Clin Immunol. 2005;116:1314–20.

Allergens and Molecular Diagnostics of Shellfish Allergy

21

A.L. Lopata, J. Kleine-Tebbe, and S.D. Kamath

21.1 Background

In recent years, there has been a steady growth in the production and consumption of seafood and partial shellfish. This increased consumption has led to an increase in adverse health problems among consumers including allergic reactions.

The pattern of allergic symptoms after ingestion of crustaceans appears similar to the symptoms experienced due to other foods. Reactions are immediate and reported mostly within 2 hours; however, late-phase reactions have been reported up to 8 hours after ingestion, particularly to snow crab, cuttlefish, limpet, and abalone (Lopata et al. 1997; Villacis et al. 2006). Patients may have a single symptom but often there is a multi-organ involvement. Importantly, respiratory reactions are often

This contribution is based on a publication by the authors that appeared in the *Allergo Journal Int* in 2016 (Lopata AL, Kleine-Tebbe J, Kamath SD. Allergens and molecular diagnostics of shellfish allergy. Allergo J Int. 2016;25:210–8. DOI: 10.1007/s40629-016-0124-2) and which has been updated and expanded as a chapter for this book.

A.L. Lopata, PhD, Prof. (✉) • S.D. Kamath, PhD
Molecular Allergy Research Laboratory, Centre for Biodiscovery and Molecular Development of Therapeutics, Australian Institute of Tropical Health and Medicine, James Cook University, Townsville, QLD, Australia
e-mail: andreas.lopata@jcu.edu.au; sandip.kamath@jcu.edu.au

J. Kleine-Tebbe, MD, Prof.
Allergy and Asthma Center Westend, Outpatient Clinic Hanf, Ackermann and Kleine-Tebbe, Berlin, Germany
e-mail: kleine-tebbe@allergie-experten.de

J. Kleine-Tebbe, T. Jakob (eds.), *Molecular Allergy Diagnostics*,
DOI 10.1007/978-3-319-42499-6_21

seen after ingestion of allergenic seafood and frequently anaphylactic reactions (Matricardi et al. 2016). Particularly, the oral allergy syndrome (OAS) seems to be very often experienced by crustacean allergic subjects. Shrimp has also been implicated in food-dependent exercise-induced anaphylaxis (Zhang et al. 2006).

Currently, 2 % of the general world population is affected by shellfish allergy, with much higher rates in countries with high seafood consumption. Unlike many other food allergies, most shellfish allergy persists for life in the affected individual.

21.2 Classification of Shellfish Groups

Patients with allergy to shellfish may fail to identify the offending seafood species, often as a result of confusion regarding the different common names used to describe diverse seafood. The two invertebrate phyla of arthropods and mollusks are generally referred to as "shellfish" (see ◉ Fig. 21.1).

Crustaceans are, perhaps surprisingly, classified as arthropods together with spiders and insects. This might provide an explanation for the observed molecular and clinical cross-reactivity discussed in detail below. Over 30,000 living crustacean

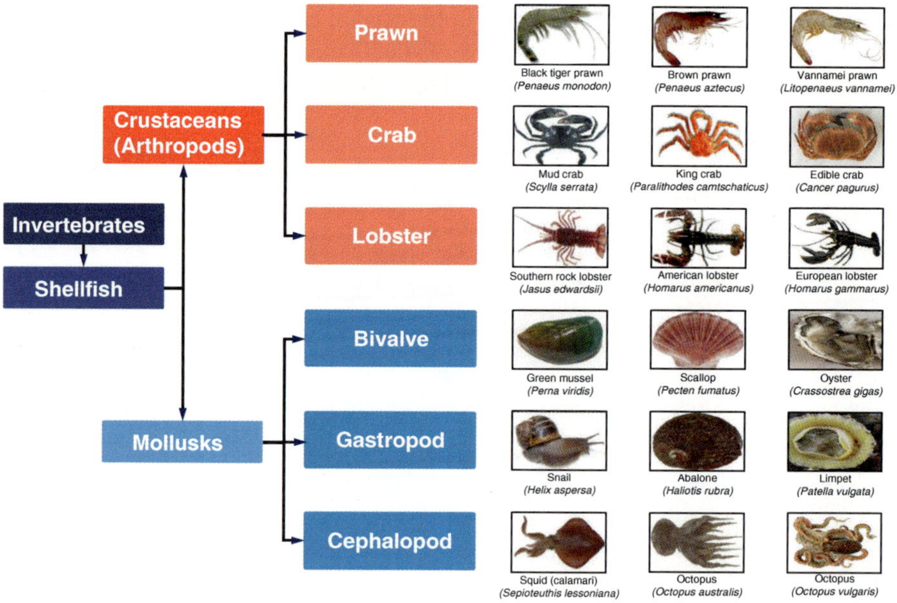

Fig. 21.1 Schematic classification of most commonly consumed shellfish species

species are found worldwide, and large varieties are consumed raw or cooked worldwide.

The group of mollusks is a large and diverse group, subdivided into the classes' bivalve, gastropod and cephalopod. This group comprises over 100,000 different species, including several important seafood groups including mussels, oysters, abalone, snails, and squid (calamari).

21.3 Prevalence of Shellfish Allergy

The prevalence of allergic reactions to seafood is usually higher when the consumption plays a greater part in the diet of the observed community (see ◉ Table 21.1) (Lopata et al. 2016). It is generally considered that crustacean and mollusk are among the foods that most commonly provoke severe anaphylaxis (Tham et al. 2008). A recent study established surprisingly that seafood allergies are a significant health concern affecting approximately 6.5 million people in the USA – more than twice as common as peanut allergy. The telephone survey among 14,948 individuals reported 5.9 % with shellfish allergy, and seafood allergy was almost five times more common among adults compared to children. Of all the subjects with allergies to crustacean and mollusk, only 38 % and 49 %, respectively, reported reactions to multiple species, and only 14 % reacted to both shellfish groups (Sicherer et al. 2004).

In France, a study by Andre and co-worker among 580 patients with adverse reactions to food, 34 % were identified having specific IgE to crab (Andre et al. 1994). A study by Crespo et al. in Spain established that 6.8 % of patients reacted to crustaceans (Crespo et al. 1995). A study from South Africa including 105 individuals with perceived adverse reactions to seafood confirmed sensitization to shrimps and rock lobster in almost 50 % (Lopata et al. 1997; Zinn et al. 1997).

While seafood allergy is common in Western countries such as Europe, the USA, and Australia, it seems that in Asian countries, allergic reactions to shellfish are of greater importance among adults and children (Goh et al. 1999; Shek et al. 2010; Thalayasingam et al. 2015). This clearly supports the view that the likelihood of becoming sensitized to shellfish seems to correlate with geographical eating habits and is most likely underreported in many Asian populations.

Not only ingestion of shellfish can cause sensitization but also exposure during processing in factories and domestic environment. There seems to be a strong correlation between high concentration of airborne allergens and increased allergic sensitization (Baatjies et al. 2015; Kamath et al. 2014a). Crustaceans seem to produce the strongest allergic response during processing of seafood and reach prevalence rates of up to 30 % (Bonlokke et al. 2012; Gautrin et al. 2010).

Table 21.1 List of identified and characterized shellfish allergens according to the International Union of Immunological Societies (IUIS) allergen nomenclature

	Biochemical name	Molecular weight	Heat stability and IgE binding	Route of exposure	IgE sensitization (%) (*n* = subjects tested)	Physiological function
1	Tropomyosin	34–38 kDa	Highly heat stable and IgE reactive	Ingestion Inhalation	Pen a 1, 51 % (*n* = 45) Gámez et al. (2011) Lit v 1, 61 % (*n* = 19) Ayuso et al. (2010) Pen m 1, 62 % (*n* = 16) Kamath et al. (2014b)	Coiled-coil protein that binds to actin and regulates interaction of troponin and myosin
2	Arginine kinase	40–45 kDa	Labile but can elicit IgE binding	Ingestion Inhalation	Pen m 2, 50 % (*n* = 16) Kamath et al. (2014b) Lit v 2, 21 % (*n* = 19) Ayuso et al. (2010)	A kinase that catalyzes reversible transfer of phosphoryl group from ATP to arginine
3	Myosin light chain	17–20 kDa	Stable	Ingestion	Pen m 3, 31 % (*n* = 16) Kamath et al. (2014b) Lit v 3, 31 % (*n* = 19) Ayuso et al. (2010)	Regulatory function in smooth muscle contraction when phosphorylated by MLC kinase
4	Sarcoplasmic calcium-binding protein	20–25 kDa	Stable	Ingestion	Pen m 4, 19 % (*n* = 16) Kamath et al. (2014b) Lit v 4, 21 % (*n* = 19) Ayuso et al. (2010)	Binds to cytosolic calcium (Ca^{2+}) and acts as a calcium buffer regulating calcium-based signaling
5	Troponin C	20–21 kDa	Unknown	Ingestion	Cra c 6, 29 % (*n* = 31) Bauermeister et al. (2011)	Regulates interaction of actin and myosin during muscle contraction on binding to calcium
6	Triose-phosphate isomerase	28 kDa	Labile	Ingestion Inhalation	Pen m 8, 19 % (*n* = 16) Kamath et al. (2014b) Cra c 8, 23 % (*n* = 31) Bauermeister et al. (2011)	Key enzyme in glycolysis; catalyzes conversion of dihydroxyacetone phosphate to glyceraldehyde 3-phosphate

21.4 Structure and Biological Functions of Shellfish Allergens

Over the past 20 years, several shellfish allergens, particularly in crustaceans, have been identified and sequenced (◉ Table 21.2). Currently, 34 allergens have been identified and characterized in detail from various crustacean and mollusk species and registered with the International Union of Immunological Societies (IUIS) Allergen Database (Radauer et al. 2008). Most of these allergens belong to six different protein families. The biochemical characteristics of shellfish allergenic proteins are typically low molecular weight, high water solubility, high heat stability, and an acidic isoelectric point. Almost all of the known characterized allergens are found in the edible portions of various shellfish species. For example, the major shellfish allergen tropomyosin is found in the abdominal part of prawns, pincer and tail of crabs and lobsters, as well as body or arm/tentacles of octopus and squid. However, some protease-based allergens, which cause clinical reactions through the protease-activated receptor (PAR) pathway (non-IgE mediated), are present in the gastrointestinal regions of the different shellfish species (Sun and Lopata 2010). The allergen family-specific properties of shellfish allergens are described below (see ◉ Table 21.1):

1. *Tropomyosin (TM) Pen m 1*
   Tropomyosin is the major allergenic protein across all edible crustacean and mollusk species. It is also the most abundant allergen in shellfish, constituting up to 20 % of the total protein. More than 60 % of shellfish-allergic patients are sensitized and react to TM, often leading to severe systemic reactions. Tropomyosin-specific IgE is frequently used to predict clinical outcomes of shrimp allergy with a positive predictive value of 0.72 (Gámez et al. 2011; Pascal et al. 2015).

   Tropomyosin forms a large family of proteins, which are associated to actin filaments and play a critical role in the regulation of actin filaments in muscle and non-muscle cells (Oguchi et al. 2011). This allergen is an alpha-helical coiled-coil dimeric protein that binds along the length of actin and regulates the cooperation of troponin and myosin, thus controlling the contraction of muscle fibers (Oguchi et al. 2011). Due to TM's primary role in muscle contraction regulation, the primary structure is highly conserved across various invertebrate species. This seems the main reason for high IgE-mediated allergenic cross-reactivity across various shellfish species as described below in detail. Depending on alternate splicing mechanisms, different isoforms of tropomyosin are generated, with structural and functional differences (Reese et al. 1999). In crustacean species, the fast twitch and the slow twitch isoforms were identified in the tail and pincer muscles, respectively (Motoyama et al. 2007). Interestingly, even though crustacean and mollusk tropomyosins are allergenic, they share only very low amino acid sequence identities of 55–70 %.

   Allergenic TMs have generally molecular weights of between 33 kDa and 38 kDa and are highly stable to heat treatment, capable of retaining allergenicity

Table 21.2 Characterized allergens in crustacean and mollusk species

	Shellfish species	Common names	Tropomyosin	Arginine kinase	Myosin light chain 1 and 2	Sarcoplasmic calcium-binding protein	Troponin C, troponin I	Triose-phosphate isomerase
Prawn	*Penaeus monodon*	Black tiger prawn, giant tiger prawn, Asian tiger shrimp	Pen m 1[b]	Pen m 2[b]	Pen m 3	Pen m 4[b]	Pen m 6	Cra c 8
	Penaeus aztecus	Brown shrimp	Pen a 1[a]	–	–	–	–	–
	Crangon crangon	North Sea shrimp, common shrimp	Cra c 1	Cra c 2	Cra c 5	Cra c 4	Cra c 6	–
	Litopenaeus vannamei	Pacific white shrimp, vannamei shrimp	Lit v 1	Lit v 2	Lit v 3	Lit v 4	–	–
	Melicertus latisulcatus	King prawns, Western king prawns	Mel l 1	–	–	–	–	–
	Pandalus borealis	Northern shrimp, pink shrimp	Pan b 1	–	–	–	–	–
	Penaeus indicus	Indian white prawn	Pen i 1	–	–	–	–	–
	Metapenaeus ensis	Greasyback shrimp, sand shrimp	Met e 1	–	–	–	–	–
	Archaeopotamobius sibiriensis	ND	–	–	–	–	–	Arc s 8
Crab	*Charybdis feriatus*	Crucifix crab	Cha f 1	–	–	–	–	–
	Portunus pelagicus	Blue swimmer crab	Por p 1	–	–	–	–	–
Lobster	*Homarus americanus*	American lobster	Hom a 1		Hom a 3		Hom a 6	
	Panulirus stimpsoni	Spiny lobster	Pan s 1	–	–	–	–	–
	Pontastacus leptodactylus	Narrow-clawed crayfish	Pon i 1	–	–	–	–	–
Bivalve	*ND*		–	–	–	–	–	–
Gastropod	*Helix aspersa*	Garden snail	Hel as 1	–	–	–	–	–
	Haliotis midae	South African abalone	Hal m 1	–	–	–	–	–
Cephalopod	*Todarodes pacificus*	Pacific squid	Tod p 1	–	–	–	–	–

Allergens stated are registered with the IUIS allergen nomenclature
"–"and "ND" indicates not determined
[a]Allergens included in ImmunoCAP
[b]Allergens included in ISAC

even after cooking and high-pressure processing. However, some studies have demonstrated modulation of IgE recognition to tropomyosin due to heat-induced Maillard reaction, which may occur in some shellfish species (Nakamura et al. 2005, 2006.

According to the AllFam database, the TM family is the largest "food" allergen family in animal sources, consisting of currently 47 identified TMs, mostly from crustacean species (Radauer et al. 2008). Examples of well-characterized TM are Pen m 1, Pen a 1, Lit v 1, and Hom a 1.

2. *Arginine kinase (AK) Pen m 2*

   Arginine kinase was first characterized as an allergen in Indian meal moth (Binder et al. 2001). Since then, AK has been identified in over six crustacean and one mollusk species. Arginine kinase belongs to a class of kinases that catalyze the reversible transfer of the high-energy phosphoryl group from ATP to arginine, thus yielding ADP and *N*-phosphoarginine (Yu et al. 2003). These phosphagens then serve as high energy source from which ATP can be replenished in many invertebrate species (Pereira et al. 2000). Creatinine kinase serves this purpose in higher vertebrates.

   IgE sensitization to AK has been demonstrated in 21–50 % of adults and 67 % of children (Kamath et al. 2014b; Yang et al. 2010). However, the frequency of clinical reactivity to AK has not been investigated in detail. Invertebrate AK has a molecular weight of 40–42 kDa and is not stable to acid or alkali treatment. Unlike tropomyosin, AK is also not stable to heat treatment. However, IgE binding has been demonstrated to AK in heat-treated shrimps, which may be due to remaining intact IgE epitopes on aggregated AK (Kamath et al. 2014b; Shen et al. 2012). Interestingly, crustacean AK along with TM has also been implicated in inhalational exposure and sensitization among crab-processing workers (Abdel Rahman et al. 2011). Crustacean AK has been demonstrated to cross-react to ingested insect AK as well as being implicated in seafood-mite cross-reactivity (Srinroch et al. 2015; Gamez et al. 2014).

3. *Myosin light chain (MLC) Pen m 3*

   The EF-hand domain superfamily is the second largest group of all allergens, after profilins, which encompasses both food and inhalant allergens from animal and plant sources. Three classes of shellfish allergens are EF-hand domain proteins, which include MLC, sarcoplasmic calcium-binding proteins, and troponin. Interestingly, the major allergen in fish is parvalbumin, which is also an EF-hand domain allergen.

   MLC is mainly found in smooth muscles in complex with myosin heavy chain motor domains. During muscle contraction, the calcium-calmodulin complex, MLC kinase is activated, which in turn phosphorylates myosin light chain, regulating the smooth muscle movement (Kamm and Stull 1985). Two isoforms are currently known, the essential MLC and regulatory MLC. As an EF-hand domain protein, the regulatory MLC binds metal ions, mostly with magnesium (Trybus 1994). Myosin light chains have a molecular weight between 17 and 20 kDa, are well characterized in four crustacean species, and seem to be heat stable. Currently, there is a lack of data on immunological cross-reactivity of

MLC among crustaceans, mollusks, or other invertebrate species. An amino acid sequence alignment for MLC based on sequences available on GenBank estimates an identity ranging between 86 and100 %; although this is highly dependent on the isoforms sequenced.

4. *Sarcoplasmic calcium-binding protein (SCBP) Pen m 4*
   Sarcoplasmic calcium-binding proteins are also members of the EF-hand calcium-binding protein family incorporating the helix-loop-helix motif in the primary amino acid sequence. It is believed to function as the invertebrate counterpart of vertebrate parvalbumin. Its main activity is the regulation of the cytosolic calcium (Ca2+) concentration, thus assisting in calcium-dependent cell signaling. SCBP is ubiquitously expressed throughout the organism, but more abundant in the abdominal muscle (Gao et al. 2006). In mollusks, it is located in a tissue-specific manner (Hermann and Cox 1995). It has a molecular weight of approximately 20 kDa and an isoelectric point of 5 and can elicit IgE binding even after heat treatment (Kamath et al. 2014b). Due to its similar molecular weight with that of MLC, it is difficult to establish the IgE recognition pattern using traditional immunochemical methods such as immunoblotting. Recent studies have highlighted the relevance of SCBP as a shellfish allergen. Ayuso et al. demonstrated IgE recognition in 85 % of shrimp-allergic children, which is much higher compared to tropomyosin (Ayuso et al. 2009). More importantly, it has been shown that specific IgE to SCBP, in addition to that of TM, is associated with clinical reactivity to shrimps (Pascal et al. 2015).
5. *Troponin C (TnC) Cra c 6*
   Troponin C has been characterized in shrimps, but also as important cockroach allergen (Bla g 6 and Per a 6). Similar to SCBP and MLC, TnC is an EF-hand calcium-binding protein. Troponin C forms a complex with troponin I and TM. Based on conformational changes to the complex, due to calcium influx, it regulates the interaction of actin and myosin during muscle contraction (Hindley et al. 2006). Troponin C is approximately 20 kDa in size and its possible heat stability is not fully understood. Interestingly, it was demonstrated that IgE binding to Bla g 6 (cockroach) increased after addition of calcium in previously depleted serum, indicating the possible presence of calcium-dependent conformational IgE epitopes on TnC. The IgE-binding frequency to TnC is with 15 % lower as reactivity to TM, AK, or SCBP.
6. *Triose-phosphate isomerase (TIM) Cra c 8*
   Triose-phosphate isomerase plays an important role in the glycolysis involved in energy production. TIM catalyzes the conversion of dihydroxyacetone phosphate to glyceraldehyde 3-phosphate, the final product of this metabolic pathway being pyruvate. This allergen has been characterized in shrimps (Cra c 8), crayfish (Arc s 8), and cockroach (Bla g TPI). It has an approximate molecular weight of 28 kDa and is probably heat sensitive (Bauermeister et al. 2011). The clinical and immunological cross-reactivity of TIM among various invertebrate species are not well understood and amino acid sequences have not been performed.

21.5 Clinical and Immunological Cross-Reactivity

True sensitization to shellfish-specific allergens can be hampered due the highly cross-reactive nature of some allergenic proteins. The best-known panallergen is tropomyosin, being the major cause for reported clinical cross-reactivity among and between crustacean and mollusk, but also other invertebrates, including mites, cockroaches, and parasites (see ◉ Fig. 21.2). Some conserved regions of IgE-binding epitope of tropomyosin seem to be shared between crustaceans and mollusks. It is known that tropomyosin has mainly linear IgE epitopes and is of great importance in determining the degree of cross-reactivity between different shellfish species. A direct amino acid sequence alignment and comparison of amino acid sequences of IgE-binding epitopes may be able to predict the level of IgE cross-reactivity. However, tropomyosin is highly conserved among various crustacean species such as prawns, crabs, and lobsters with amino acid identities reaching 95–100%. Therefore, IgE cross-reactivity is very frequent among crustacean species (Zhang et al. 2006; Abramovitch et al. 2013; Nakano et al. 2008; Motoyama et al. 2007; Ayuso et al. 2002).

Within the mollusk group, hypersensitivity cross-reaction is often seen in allergic individuals, as determined for ten different species of cephalopods (Motoyama et al. 2006). Similar results were shown for four species of gastropods (disk abalone, turban shell, whelk, and *Middendorf s buccinum*) and seven species of bivalves

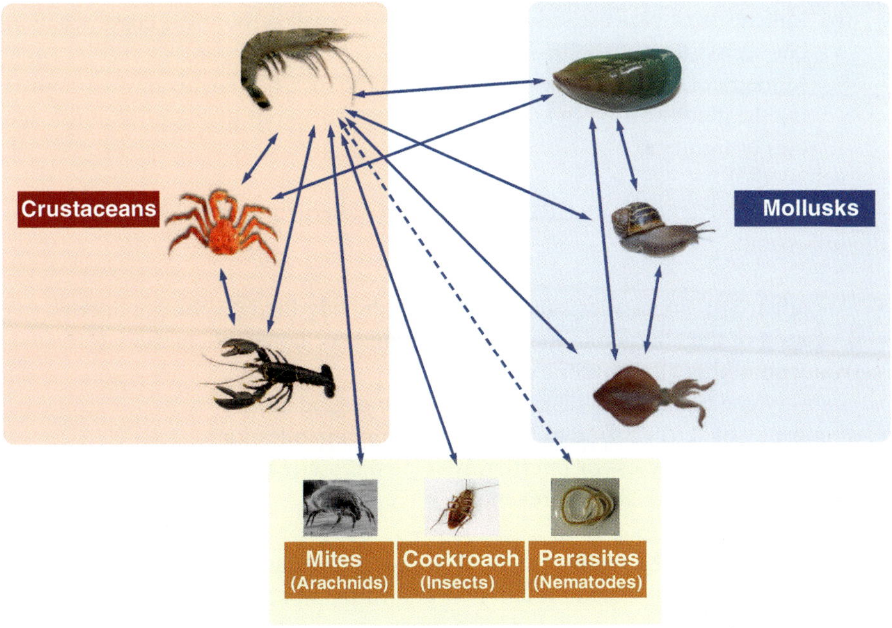

Fig. 21.2 Graphical representation of immunological cross-reactivity among crustacean and mollusk species as well as to mites, insects, and nematodes

(bloody cockle, Japanese oyster, Japanese cockle, surf clam, horse clam, razor clam, and short neck clam) (Emoto et al. 2009).

Increasingly important seems to be IgE cross-sensitization between tropomyosin from shellfish and other important allergenic invertebrates, including dust mites and cockroaches (◉ Fig. 21.2). It was demonstrated that IgE against mite tropomyosin (Der p 10) reacted very strongly to shrimp tropomyosin, although tropomyosin is present in very low concentrations in house dust mites (Arlian et al. 2009). More interestingly, reactivity to shrimp has been demonstrated in subjects with house dust mite allergy, who have never been exposed to shrimps due to religious eating habits (Fernandes et al. 2003).

21.5.1 Potential Advantages of Component-Resolved Diagnosis (CRD) in Shellfish Allergy

Applying single allergenic molecules (Matricardi et al. 2016) from shellfish for allergen-specific IgE detection could potentially modify the following:

1. Test sensitivity (improving the limit of quantitation to shellfish allergens of rare abundance or low stability)
2. Analytical specificity, particularly if specific IgE is detectable to:
   (a) Risk-associated molecules (being more likely responsible for severe reactions and/or more specific for children or adults)
   (b) Indicators of cross-reactivity (involved in broad serological cross-reactions between different shellfish species)
   (c) Markers of primary species- and/or family-specific sensitizations (facilitating the identification of unique allergic sensitizations to certain shellfish species or families)

The listed advantages of CRD require some allergen-related knowledge about the following:

- Abundance of single allergens in the shellfish body (and resulting extracts)
- Location of the allergen in the organism (edible or nonedible parts)
- Water solubility (for proper extraction)
- Stability and behavior to thermal and gastric degradation
- Frequency of sensitization to the single allergen in question
- Degree of interspecies- or interfamily-related cross-reactivity
- Risk to elicit severe allergic reactions

Specific IgE to TM, thanks to its high abundance and stability, is picked up reasonably easy using heated protein extracts from probably most shellfish species. Thus, there is no particular need to further increase test sensitivity. However, increased analytical specificity of TM in molecular-based serological tests will help to identify patients at risk for severe allergic reactions and, in addition, indicate broad cross-reactivity to TM from other shellfish species and perhaps insects and mites. Testing IgE to more than one TM is probably providing more information about cross-reactivity between crustaceans and mollusks.

Similar assumptions are related to the other described shellfish allergens (see above), i.e., AK, MLC, SCBP, TnC, and TIM: Being part of the edible part of shellfish, with basic functions in muscle fibers or general energy metabolism, they are presumably also highly conserved, showing variable degrees of cross-reactivity, which has not been studied yet. Increasing test sensitivity through the use of single molecules might be useful in less-stable allergens (i.e., AK, TIM), but not necessarily for more robust proteins (i.e., MLC, SCBP). Increased analytical specificity can assist uncovering associated risks, i.e., in case of IgE to SCBP (Pascal et al. 2015). However, none of these candidates might serve as a single marker for species-specific sensitization due to variable degrees of IgE-related cross-reactivity, which still needs to be addressed. Recent advances in PCR-based allergen-specific IgE quantification have further improved the sensitivity and specificity of tests to single allergens, using serum from a fingerprick, which is of particular advantage for infant allergy testing (Johnston et al. 2014).

In conclusion, no species-specific allergens have been identified so far, making it difficult to precisely diagnose allergy to a specific crustacean or mollusk species with the use of allergen molecules (Matricardi et al. 2016; Aalberse 2015)). If more of the already identified and additional allergens are available for diagnostics, it might be helpful to test one per protein family, ensuring maximum test sensitivity and enhanced molecular specificity, particularly if TM is not the major allergen. This does, however, not solve the question of potential clinical cross-reactions to closely related shellfish species: Only anamnestic data or oral challenges can indicate or rule out clinically relevant allergic reactions to certain shellfish species.

21.6 Diagnostics Separating IgE-Mediated Allergy from Other Reactions

Serum-based IgE quantification tests are available for a wide variety of crustacean and mollusk species as well as for cross-reactive invertebrate species such as dust mites and cockroaches. IgE quantification tests for single-component allergens are currently only available for shrimp tropomyosin (rPen a 1). However, some additional shellfish allergens are available in multiplex (microarray) format for prawn tropomyosin (nPen m 1), arginine kinase (nPen m 2), and sarcoplasmic calcium-binding protein (rPen m 4).

Approximately 60 % of patients with clinical allergy to crustacean demonstrate specific IgE binding to tropomyosin. It has been suggested that IgE reactivity to tropomyosin is a better predictor of shrimp allergy as compared to SPT or IgE to whole shrimp extract (Gámez et al. 2011; Yang et al. 2010). However, also sarcoplasmic calcium-binding protein (Pen m 4) reactivity has been associated with clinical reactivity to shrimp. The combination of reactivity to both allergens might increase the sensitivity to detect clinically allergic patients, but has still to be confirmed.

The consumption of seafood is very different from most other food allergen sources. It can trigger clinical adverse symptoms, although nonallergic in origin, being similar in clinical presentation to true IgE-mediated allergic reactions. These substances are found in seafood much more frequently as compared to any other food source. An atypical clinical history or an inconsistent history always suggests a nonatopic etiology, such as contamination with marine biotoxins, parasites, bacteria, and viruses (Lopata et al. 2010; Lopata and Kamath 2012). Because of the similarity in clinical reactions of affected individuals, it is essential to differentiate adverse reactions from true shellfish allergy and understand the molecular nature of the offending allergens for improved component-resolved diagnosis.

Food challenge or double-blind placebo-controlled food challenge (DBPCFC) can be performed to confirm clinical reactivity to crustacean and mollusk species. However, such provocation tests are not performed routinely because of increased risk and costs and are only performed for investigating individual cases.

21.7 Outlook for Future Diagnostic Options

Most of the clinical studies on cross-reactivity have been conducted using tropomyosin as the major pan-allergen. However, other shellfish allergens may play a role in immunological cross-sensitization. A recent study has shown that allergens other than tropomyosin, such as arginine kinase, might also be responsible for cross-reactivity between shellfish and inhalant invertebrate allergen sources (Gamez et al. 2014; Marinho et al. 2006). In addition, hemocyanin has been demonstrated to be cross-reactive and also is a known cockroach allergen (Giuffrida et al. 2014; Khurana et al. 2014).

However, an in-depth investigation into the conservation or relevance of specific IgE epitopes between pan-allergens from crustaceans and mollusks and clinical cross-reactivity to mites and cockroaches have not been conducted or confirmed using a larger number of shellfish-allergic patients.

21.8 Suggestions for Present Clinical Practice

Diagnosis of shellfish allergy is based on:

- Clinical history
- Sensitization tests (allergen-specific IgE tests; skin tests)
- Oral challenge test, if needed

In case of severe allergic reaction, allergen-specific IgE should precede any in vivo tests, i.e., skin prick test (SPT), to avoid any risks for the shellfish-allergic patient.

IgE diagnostics should include:

- Total IgE (for improved interpretation of the quantitative allergen-specific IgE values)

- Allergen-specific IgE preferably to the reaction-eliciting (or biologically closely related) shellfish species
- Allergen-specific IgE to Pen a 1, at the present only available TM for singleplex testing from brown shrimp (*Penaeus aztecus*):
  A. If extract- and TM-specific IgE results are positive with quantitative IgE levels being higher to TM than to the whole extract, immunodominant sensitization to shellfish TM is likely, and broad (serological) cross-reactivity to other shellfish species is to be expected. During interpretation of the test, concordance between recorded symptoms and the identified shellfish species should be checked. Only in case of corresponding symptoms and a positive sensitization test, clinically relevant allergy has successfully been demonstrated.
  B. If only the extract-specific IgE, but not the TM-specific IgE is positive, sensitization to TM is unlikely, but other shellfish allergens might be involved.
  C. If both IgE tests (shellfish extract- and TM-specific IgE) turn out to be negative, it is mandatory to perform a skin test, i.e., SPT with a commercial shellfish extract and/or a (titrated) SPT with native material (i.e., prick-prick test with fresh shellfish species, if possible raw and cooked).
  D. In case of a clearly positive SPT result, an immediate-type sensitization is likely, particularly if healthy control individuals do not react to the applied skin test material.
  E. In case of clearly negative skin test results, IgE-mediated sensitization to the tested shellfish species becomes very unlikely, and differential diagnoses other than IgE-mediated allergic reactions to shellfish should be considered.
  F. Additional testing with other shellfish species has limited value for subsequent consulting of the patient: In case of positive skin or IgE test results, serological cross-reactivity has been demonstrated, which does not always translate into clinical cross-reactivity. However, in case of a clearly negative skin and/or IgE response to related or biologically more distant shellfish specifies (serological), cross-reactivity and subsequent clinical cross-reactivity becomes unlikely.
  G. In case of doubt or mismatch between case history and diagnostic results, carefully titrated oral challenge tests with the suspected shellfish species might solve the discrepancies. However, due to the risk for the patient in case of previous severe allergic reactions and limited specialized centers, they are not frequently performed. A negative provocation test, if previous sensitizations tests turned out negative, is usually safe and an appropriate way to rule out a present food allergy to shellfish.

In general, patients with proven shellfish allergy should avoid a broad range of related shellfish species (crustacean or mollusk), unless they have already tolerated other (presumably biologically more distant) shellfish species. This rather cautious approach takes into account that allergic subjects are not necessarily familiar with huge variety of present shellfish species, their biological relationship, and the composition in mixed seafood dishes, particularly from nonself-prepared meals.

Due to the often long-lasting nature of IgE-mediated allergies to shellfish species, patients with proven allergic reactions should avoid shellfish permanently, unless subsequent controlled challenges have ruled out a still-present clinical reactivity.

References

Aalberse RC. Shrimp serology: We need tests with more and less cross-reactivity. J Allergy Clin Immunol Pract. 2015;3:530–1.

Abdel Rahman AM, Kamath SD, Lopata AL, Robinson JJ, Helleur RJ. Biomolecular characterization of allergenic proteins in snow crab (*Chionoecetes opilio*) and de novo sequencing of the second allergen arginine kinase using tandem mass spectrometry. J Proteomics. 2011;74:231–41.

Abramovitch JB, Kamath S, Varese N, Zubrinich C, Lopata AL, O'Hehir RE, et al. IgE reactivity of blue swimmer crab *portunus pelagicus* tropomyosin, Por p 1, and other allergens; cross-reactivity with black tiger prawn and effects of heating. PLoS One. 2013;8:e67487.

Andre F, Andre C, Colin L, Cacaraci F, Cavagna S. Role of new allergens and of allergens consumption in the increased incidence of food sensitizations in France. Toxicology. 1994;93:77–83.

Arlian L, Morgan M, Vyszenski-Moher D, Sharra D. Cross-reactivity between storage and dust mites and between mites and shrimp. Exp Appl Acarol. 2009;47:159–72.

Ayuso R, Reese G, Leong-Kee S, Plante M, Lehrer SB. Molecular basis of arthropod cross-reactivity: IgE-binding cross-reactive epitopes of shrimp, house dust mite and cockroach tropomyosins. Int Arch Allergy Immunol. 2002;129:38–48.

Ayuso R, Grishina G, Ibanez MD, Blanco C, Carrillo T, Bencharitiwong R, et al. Sarcoplasmic calcium-binding protein is an EF-hand-type protein identified as a new shrimp allergen. J Allergy Clin Immunol. 2009;124:114–20.

Ayuso R, Sanchez-Garcia S, Lin J, Fu ZY, Ibanez MD, Carrillo T, et al. Greater epitope recognition of shrimp allergens by children than by adults suggests that shrimp sensitization decreases with age. J Allergy Clin Immunol. 2010;125:1286–93.

Baatjies R, Meijster T, Heederik D, Jeebhay MF. Exposure-response relationships for inhalant wheat allergen exposure and asthma. Occup Environ Med. 2015;72:200–7.

Bauermeister K, Wangorsch A, Garoffo LP, Reuter A, Conti A, Taylor SL, et al. Generation of a comprehensive panel of crustacean allergens from the North Sea Shrimp Crangon crangon. Mol Immunol. 2011;48:1983–92.

Binder M, Mahler V, Hayek B, Sperr WR, Scholler M, Prozell S, et al. Molecular and immunological characterization of arginine kinase from the Indianmeal moth, Plodia interpunctella, a novel cross-reactive invertebrate pan-allergen. J Immunol. 2001;167:5470–7.

Bonlokke JH, Gautrin D, Sigsgaard T, Lehrer SB, Maghni K, Cartier A. Snow crab allergy and asthma among Greenlandic workers–a pilot study. Int J Circumpolar Health. 2012;71:19126.

Crespo JF, Pascual C, Burks AW, Helm RM, Esteban MM. Frequency of food allergy in a pediatric population from Spain. Pediatr Allergy Immunol. 1995;6:39–43.

Emoto A, Ishizaki S, Shiomi K. Tropomyosins in gastropods and bivalves: identification as major allergens and amino acid sequence features. Food Chem. 2009;114:634–41.

Fernandes J, Reshef A, Patton L, Ayuso R, Reese G, Lehrer SB. Immunoglobulin E antibody reactivity to the major shrimp allergen, tropomyosin, in unexposed Orthodox Jews. Clin Exp Allergy. 2003;33:956–61.

Gámez C, Sánchez-García S, Ibáñez MD, López R, Aguado E, López E, et al. Tropomyosin IgE-positive results are a good predictor of shrimp allergy. Allergy. 2011;66:1375–83.

Gamez C, Zafra MP, Boquete M, Sanz V, Mazzeo C, Ibanez MD et al. New shrimp IgE-binding proteins involved in mite-seafood cross-reactivity. Mol Nutr Food Res. 2014;58:1915–25.

Gao Y, Gillen CM, Wheatly MG. Molecular characterization of the sarcoplasmic calcium-binding protein (SCP) from crayfish Procambarus clarkii. Comp Biochem Physiol B Biochem Mol Biol. 2006;144:478–87.

Gautrin D, Cartier A, Howse D, Horth-Susin L, Jong M, Swanson M, et al. Occupational asthma and allergy in snow crab processing in Newfoundland and Labrador. Occup Environ Med. 2010;67:17–23.

Giuffrida MG, Villalta D, Mistrello G, Amato S, Asero R. Shrimp allergy beyond Tropomyosin in Italy: clinical relevance of Arginine Kinase, Sarcoplasmic calcium binding protein and Hemocyanin. Eur Ann Allergy Clin Immunol. 2014;46:172–7.

Goh DL, Lau YN, Chew FT, Shek LP, Lee BW. Pattern of food-induced anaphylaxis in children of an Asian community. Allergy. 1999;54:84–6.

Hermann A, Cox JA. Sarcoplasmic calcium-binding protein. Comp Biochem Physiol B Biochem Mol Biol. 1995;111:337–45.

Hindley J, Wunschmann S, Satinover SM, Woodfolk JA, Chew FT, Chapman MD, et al. Bla g 6: a troponin C allergen from Blattella germanica with IgE binding calcium dependence. J Allergy Clin Immunol. 2006;117:1389–95.

Johnston EB, Kamath SD, Lopata AL, Schaeffer PM. Tus-Ter-lock immuno-PCR assays for the sensitive detection of tropomyosin-specific IgE antibodies. Bioanalysis. 2014;6:465–76.

Kamath SD, Thomassen MR, Saptarshi SR, Nguyen HM, Aasmoe L, Bang BE, et al. Molecular and immunological approaches in quantifying the air-borne food allergen tropomyosin in crab processing facilities. Int J Hyg Environ Health. 2014a;217:740–50.

Kamath SD, Rahman AM, Voskamp A, Komoda T, Rolland JM, O'Hehir RE, et al. Effect of heat processing on antibody reactivity to allergen variants and fragments of black tiger prawn: a comprehensive allergenomic approach. Mol Nutr Food Res. 2014b;58:1144–55.

Kamm KE, Stull JT. The function of myosin and myosin light chain kinase phosphorylation in smooth muscle. Annu Rev Pharmacol Toxicol. 1985;25:593–620.

Khurana T, Collison M, Chew FT, Slater JE. Bla g 3: a novel allergen of German cockroach identified using cockroach-specific avian single-chain variable fragment antibody. Ann Allergy Asthma Immunol. 2014;112:140–5.e1.

Lopata AL, Kamath S. Shellfish allergy diagnosis–gaps and needs. Curr Allergy Clin Immunol. 2012;25:60–6.

Lopata AL, Zinn C, Potter PC. Characteristics of hypersensitivity reactions and identification of a unique 49 kd IgE-binding protein (Hal-m-1) in abalone (Haliotis midae). J Allergy Clin Immunol. 1997;100:642–8.

Lopata AL, O'Hehir RE, Lehrer SB. Shellfish allergy. Clin Exp Allergy. 2010;40:850–8.

Lopata AL, SD K. Allergy to crustacean and mollusks (shellfish). In: Matricardi PM K-TJ, Hoffmann HJ, Valenta R, Ollert M, editor. EAACI molecular allergology user's guide: published by the European Academy of Allergy and Clinical Immunology. 2016. p. 173–83.

Marinho S, Morais-Almeida M, Gaspar A, Santa-Marta C, Pires G, Postigo I, et al. Barnacle allergy: allergen characterization and cross-reactivity with mites. J Investig Allergol Clin Immunol. 2006;16:117–22.

Matricardi PM, Kleine-Tebbe J, Hoffmann HJ, Valenta R, Hilger C, Hofmaier S, et al. EAACI molecular allergology user's guide. Pediatr Allergy Immunol. 2016;27 Suppl 23:1–250.

Motoyama K, Ishizaki S, Nagashima Y, Shiomi K. Cephalopod tropomyosins: identification as major allergens and molecular cloning. Food Chem Toxicol. 2006;44:1997–2002.

Motoyama K, Suma Y, Ishizaki S, Nagashima Y, Shiomi K. Molecular cloning of tropomyosins identified as allergens in six species of crustaceans. J Agric Food Chem. 2007;55:985–91.

Nakamura A, Watanabe K, Ojima T, Ahn DH, Saeki H. Effect of Maillard reaction on allergenicity of scallop tropomyosin. J Agric Food Chem. 2005;53:7559–64.

Nakamura A, Sasaki F, Watanabe K, Ojima T, Ahn DH, Saeki H. Changes in allergenicity and digestibility of squid tropomyosin during the maillard reaction with ribose. J Agric Food Chem. 2006;54:9529–34.

Nakano S, Yoshinuma T, Yamada T. Reactivity of shrimp allergy-related IgE antibodies to krill tropomyosin. Int Arch Allergy Immunol. 2008;145:175–81.

Oguchi Y, Ishizuka J, Hitchcock-DeGregori SE, Ishiwata S, Kawai M. The role of tropomyosin domains in cooperative activation of the actin-myosin interaction. J Mol Biol. 2011;414:667–80.

Pascal M, Grishina G, Yang AC, Sanchez-Garcia S, Lin J, Towle D, et al. Molecular diagnosis of shrimp allergy: efficiency of several allergens to predict clinical reactivity. J Allergy Clin Immunol Pract. 2015;3:521–9.e10.

Pereira CA, Alonso GD, Paveto MC, Iribarren A, Cabanas ML, Torres HN, et al. Trypanosoma cruzi arginine kinase characterization and cloning. A novel energetic pathway in protozoan parasites. J Biol Chem. 2000;275:1495–501.

Radauer C, Bublin M, Wagner S, Mari A, Breiteneder H. Allergens are distributed into few protein families and possess a restricted number of biochemical functions. J Allergy Clin Immunol. 2008;121:847–52.e7.

Reese G, Ayuso R, Lehrer SB. Tropomyosin: an invertebrate pan–allergen. Int Arch Allergy Immunol. 1999;119:247–58.

Shek LPC, Cabrera-Morales EA, Soh SE, Gerez I, Ng PZ, Yi FC, et al. A population-based questionnaire survey on the prevalence of peanut, tree nut, and shellfish allergy in 2 Asian populations. J Allergy Clin Immunol. 2010;126:324–U50.

Shen HW, Cao MJ, Cai QF, Ruan MM, Mao HY, Su WJ, et al. Purification, cloning, and immunological characterization of arginine kinase, a novel allergen of *octopus fangsiao*. J Agric Food Chem. 2012;60:2190–9.

Sicherer SH, Munoz-Furlong A, Sampson HA. Prevalence of seafood allergy in the United States determined by a random telephone survey. J Allergy Clin Immunol. 2004;114:159–65.

Srinroch C, Srisomsap C, Chokchaichamnankit D, Punyarit P, Phiriyangkul P. Identification of novel allergen in edible insect, Gryllus bimaculatus and its cross-reactivity with Macrobrachium spp. allergens. Food Chem. 2015;184:160–6.

Sun S, Lopata A. The role of shellfish proteases in allergic diseases and inflammation. Current Allergy Clin Immunol. 2010;23:174–9.

Thalayasingam M, Gerez IF, Yap GC, Llanora GV, Chia IP, Chua L, et al. Clinical and immunochemical profiles of food challenge proven or anaphylactic shrimp allergy in tropical Singapore. Clin Exp Allergy. 2015;45:687–97.

Tham EH, Tay SY, Lim DLC, Shek LPC, Goh AEN, Giam YC, et al. Epinephrine auto-injector prescriptions as a reflection of the pattern of anaphylaxis in an Asian population. Allergy Asthma Proc. 2008;29:211–5.

Trybus K. Role of myosin light chains. J Muscle Res Cell Motil. 1994;15:587–94.

Villacis J, Rice TR, Bucci LR, El-Dahr JM, Wild L, Demerell D, et al. Do shrimp-allergic individuals tolerate shrimp-derived glucosamine? Clin Exp Allergy. 2006;36:1457–61.

Yang AC, Arruda LK, Santos ABR, Barbosa MCR, Chapman MD, Galvao CES, et al. Measurement of IgE antibodies to shrimp tropomyosin is superior to skin prick testing with commercial extract and measurement of IgE to shrimp for predicting clinically relevant allergic reactions after shrimp ingestion. J Allergy Clin Immunol. 2010;125:872–8.

Yu CJ, Lin YF, Chiang BL, Chow LP. Proteomics and immunological analysis of a novel shrimp allergen, Pen m 2. J Immunol. 2003;170:445–53.

Zhang Y, Matsuo H, Morita E. Cross-reactivity among shrimp, crab and scallops in a patient with a seafood allergy. J Dermatol. 2006;33:174–7.

Zinn C, Lopata A, Visser M, Potter PC. The spectrum of allergy to South African bony fish (Teleosti). Evaluation by double-blind, placebo-controlled challenge. S Afr Med J. 1997;87:146–52.

Allergens, Diagnostics, and Therapeutic Aspects in House Dust Mite Allergy

22

S. Vrtala, S. Kull, and J. Kleine-Tebbe

22.1 Introduction

House dust is the most important elicitor of allergic reactions worldwide, and already in the 1960s mites were identified as the most important allergen source in house dust (Voorhorst et al. 1964). Up to 20 % of the population is sensitized to mites constituting about 50 % of all atopic persons (Boulet et al. 1997). During childhood, mite allergy is the major risk factor for the development of asthma, and more than 80 % of all asthmatics are allergic to house dust mites (Platts-Mills et al. 2000). House dust mites of the genus *Dermatophagoides* were identified as the most important elicitors of allergic reactions indoors.

This contribution is based on a publication by the authors that appeared in the *Allergo Journal* in 2013 (Vrtala S, Kleine-Tebbe J: Hausstaubmilbenallergene und ihre Bedeutung. Allergo J 2013; 22(8):546–9) and which has now been updated, expanded, and translated into English as a chapter for this book.
The authors gratefully thank Prof. Wayne Thomas, PhD, Telethon Kids Institute, West Perth, Western Australia, Australia, for reviewing the manuscript, editorial assistance, and many helpful suggestions regarding this chapter.

S. Vrtala, PhD, Prof. (✉)
Department of Pathophysiology and Allergy Research, Center for Pathophysiology, Infectiology and Immunology, Medical University of Vienna, Vienna, Austria
e-mail: susanne.vrtala@meduniwien.ac.at

S. Kull, PhD
Clinical and Molecular Allergology, Research Center Borstel, Leibniz-Center for Medicine and Biosciences, Borstel, Germany
e-mail: skull@fz-borstel.de

J. Kleine-Tebbe, MD, Prof.
Allergy & Asthma Center Westend, Outpatient Clinic Hanf, Ackermann & Kleine-Tebbe, Berlin, Germany
e-mail: kleine-tebbe@allergie-experten.de

J. Kleine-Tebbe, T. Jakob (eds.), *Molecular Allergy Diagnostics*,
DOI 10.1007/978-3-319-42499-6_22

Allergy to storage mites was once only regarded as health problem for certain occupations (e.g., farmers, bakers) (Van Hage-Hamsten et al. 1985), but other studies show that storage mites are also present in house dust and can induce allergic reactions (Wraith et al. 1979).

Diagnosis and immunotherapy of house dust mite allergy are performed with allergen extracts that contain a mixture of allergenic and nonallergenic components. These extracts are difficult to standardize, and the allergen content varies considerably depending on the culture conditions of the mites and the extraction procedures. Therefore, important allergens can be absent from the extracts or present in insufficient amounts, or the extracts can be contaminated with allergens from other allergen sources or medium components (Brunetto et al. 2010; Casset et al. 2012). Consequently, some house dust mite-allergic patients cannot be diagnosed with certain allergen extracts, and immunotherapy with house dust mite extracts is less efficient than immunotherapy with pollen extracts (Mellerup et al. 2000).

The introduction of molecular biological methods in allergy research has allowed producing the most important allergens as recombinant proteins. Today, more than 30 allergens of house dust mites have been identified, and most of them were produced as recombinant proteins (Thomas et al. 2002; Weghofer et al. 2013). The use of recombinant allergens would allow component-resolved diagnosis (for review (Matricardi et al. 2016)) and, following the lead of successful trials for pollen allergens (Niederberger et al. 2004; Pauli et al. 2008), potential improvements in immunotherapy by the application of recombinant allergens and genetically engineered hypoallergenic derivatives.

22.2 Designation of Allergens

In Europe, house dust mites of the genus *Dermatophagoides* are the major elicitors of mite allergy. More than 30 allergens of house dust mites have been identified and are named according to the mite species (e.g., *Dermatophagoides pteronyssinus* and *Dermatophagoides farinae*) as Der p or Der f 1–33 (◉ Table 22.1).

22.3 Structure and Function of Allergens

House dust mite allergens have different functions and structures that might influence the allergenic activity of these substances. Some allergens have an enzymatic activity, whereas others are lipid-binding or chitinase-binding proteins or are associated with calcium. The function of certain house dust mite allergens is so far unknown or not sufficiently studied. ◉ Table 22.1 shows the function of the known *Dermatophagoides* allergens, and in ◉ Fig. 22.1, structures of *Dermatophagoides* allergens are shown.

The *group 1, 3, 6, and 9* allergens are proteases with the group 1 being a cysteine protease and the serine proteases 3, 6, and 9, respectively, being trypsin, a collagenolytic protease, and chymotrypsin (Chua et al. 1988; King et al. 1996; Stewart et al. 1992; Yasueda et al. 1993).

Table 22.1 List of the allergens from *D. pteronyssinus* and *D. farinae*

Der p	Der f	Biochemical function	MW SDS-PAGE [kDa]	IgE reactivity [%]
1	1	Cysteine protease	25	64–100
2	2	Lipid-binding protein	15	63–100
3	3	Trypsin	31	9–97
4		α-Amylase	57	28–74
5		Unknown	15	6–74
6	6	Chymotrypsin	25	41–65
7	7	Unknown	26, 29, 31	13–57
8		Glutathione S-transferase	26	9–96
9		Serine protease	30	92
10	10	Tropomyosin	37	6–55
11	11	Paramyosin	96	50, 75
	13	Fatty-acid-binding protein	15	?
14	14	Lipid transfer protein	177	?
15	15	Chitinase	98, 105	70
	16	Gelsolin-like protein	53	47
	17	Calcium-binding protein	53	35
18	18	Chitinase-like protein	60	63
20		Arginine kinase	40	15–44
21		Unknown	15	26
	22	Unknown	?	?
23		Chitin-binding protein	8	61, 85
	24	Ubiquinol-cytochrome C reductase-binding protein (homolog)	13	100
	25	Triosephosphate isomerase	34	75
	26	Myosin	18	?
	27	Serpin	48	?
	28	Heat shock protein 70	70	11
	29	Peptidyl-prolyl cis-trans isomerase	16	85
	30	Ferritin	16	63
	31	Cofilin	15	?
	32	Pyrophosphatase	35	?
	33	Tubulin	52	?

Like most proteases, the mite proteases are synthesized as inactive precursor molecules, and the activation of the precursor molecule for catalytic function has been reported to occur with the help of the mite allergen Der p 1 (Herman et al. 2014).

Active Der p 1 can destroy the barrier function of the bronchial epithelium, by disrupting the transmembrane molecules occludin and claudin (Wan et al. 1999), so this and similar hydrolysis by other proteases could contribute to an increased permeability of the bronchial epithelium, allowing these allergens as well as the non-proteolytic allergens to obtain access to dendritic cells.

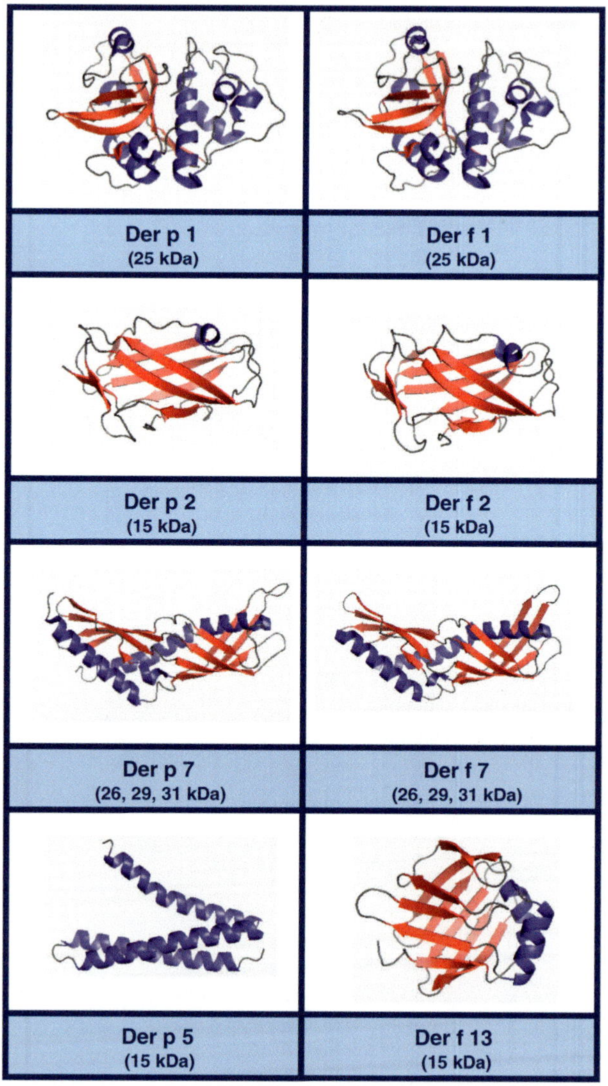

Fig. 22.1 Structures of some Dermatophagoides allergens: Der p 1 (pdb: 2AS8), Der f 1 (pdb: 3D6S), Der p 2 (pdb: 1KTJ), Der f 2 (pdb: 1WRF), Der p 5 (pdb: 3MQ1), Der p 7 (pdb: 3H47), Der f 7 (pdb: 3UV1), and Der f 13 (pdb: 2A0A)

Additionally, Der p 1, Der p 3, and Der p 9 can induce the formation of proinflammatory substances by activation of the protease-activated receptor 2 (PAR-2) (Asokananthan et al. 2002; Sun et al. 2001). In contrast to other proteases of house dust mites, group 3 (Der f 3) can produce anaphylatoxins (e.g., C3a and C5a) through proteolytic processing of complement proteins (Maruo et al. 1997).

Besides allergens with protease activity, several allergens with lipid-binding functions can be found in house dust mites. More than 50 % of the classified major allergens represent lipid-binding proteins (Thomas et al. 2005). It is speculated that allergens with lipid-binding functions have an intrinsic adjuvant effect which is responsible for the allergenicity of these molecules (Trompette et al. 2009). However, allergens with lipophilic functions are often underrepresented or are even lacking from aqueous extracts used for diagnosis and are thus difficult to characterize as natural proteins (Casset et al. 2012). Complete characterization of these allergens and their natural lipid ligands needs suitable purification strategies with lipophilic extraction procedures to complement the studies done with recombinant proteins.

The *group 2, 5, 7, 13, and 14* allergens from house dust mites were shown to have similarity to lipid-binding proteins.

The *group 2* allergens have an immunoglobulin-like tertiary region around a hydrophobic cavity (Derewenda et al. 2002). The structure of group 2 allergens contains an MD-2-related lipid-recognition domain (Inohara and Nunez 2002), which can bind lipopolysaccharides (LPS). Because of this, these allergens can activate the toll-like receptor 4 (TLR4) and induce an innate immune response (Trompette et al. 2009).

Group 5 house dust mite allergens are mainly monomers with a helical structure. However, also multimers were found, such as the Der p 5 dimer, which contains a hydrophobic binding site (Mueller et al. 2010a). Although the structure of group 5 allergens has been resolved, the function of group 5 allergens is so far unknown. *Group 7* allergens have a structural similarity to LPS-binding proteins, but as reported to date, the recombinant allergens could not bind to LPS rather showing weak affinity to the bacterial lipopeptide polymyxin B (Mueller et al. 2010b).

Group 13 allergens are fatty-acid-binding proteins. So far, only Der f 13 was described as allergen with a molecular weight of ~15 kDa (Chan et al. 2006). *Group 14* house dust mite allergens represent lipid transfer proteins with an apolipophorin-like structure in the N-terminal region. Der p 14 has the highest molecular weight (~177 kDa) of all known house dust mite allergens (Epton et al. 1999).

The muscle proteins of the house dust mite (*groups 10 and 11*) can also elicit allergic reactions. Group 10 allergens are tropomyosins, whereas group 11 allergens are paramyosins (Aki et al. 1995; Tsai et al. 1998). The sequences of tropomyosins are highly conserved (amino acid identity between Der p 10 and Der f 10 is ~98 %) (Asturias et al. 1998). Similarly an amino acid sequence identity with crustaceans of about 80 % results in a high cross-reactivity responsible for the relationship between house dust mite allergy and food allergy.

The sequences of *group 15, 18, and 23* allergens have homology to chitin-binding proteins (O'Neil et al. 2006; An et al. 2013a). Der p 15 contains an O-glycosylation site in a region which is rich in amino acids proline (P), glutamate (E), serine (S), and threonine (T) (PEST region). This is one of three domains which are typical for chitin-binding proteins. The other two domains are an N-terminal glycosyl hydrolase catalytic region and a C-terminal chitin-binding region with 4–6 cysteine residues, which form disulfide bonds (O'Neil et al. 2006). In contrast to the group 15 allergens, the group 18 allergens with a molecular weight of ~60 kDa lack the PEST region. Additionally, the N-terminal glycosyl hydrolase catalytic region is truncated and lacks the glutamate needed for catalytic activity. However, Der p 18 possesses the C-terminal chitin-binding peritrophin A domain and thus probably belongs to the non-catalytic chitinases (O'neil et al. 2006). The recently identified Der p 23 is a peritrophin-like protein with a molecular weight of ~8 kDa. In contrast to Der p 15 and Der p 18, Der p 23 lacks the glycosyl hydrolase catalytic region but possesses a PEST region as well as a peritrophin A domain (Weghofer et al. 2013).

Further allergens with known functions are the *group 4* (α-amylase), *group 8* (glutathione S-transferase), *group 16* (gelsolin-like protein), *group 17* (calcium-binding protein), *group 20* (arginine kinase), *group 25* (triosephosphate isomerase), *group 26* (myosin), *group 27* (serpin), *group 28* (heat shock protein 70), *group 29* (peptidyl-prolyl cis-trans isomerase), *group 30* (ferritin), *group 31* (cofilin), *group 32* (pyrophosphatase), and *group 33* allergens (tubulin) (An et al. 2013a). The function of *group 21* (~15 kDa) and *group 22* allergens is so far unknown. However, it has been shown that Der p 21 has structural similarity to Der p 5 (Weghofer et al. 2008a).

The *group 24* allergens are ubiquinol-cytochrome C reductase-binding proteins with a molecular weight of ~13 kDa as denominated by the IUIS (International Union of Immunological Societies Allergen Database) (Chan et al. 2015) although an α-actinin protein with a molecular weight of 90 kDa was erroneously called Der f 24 (An et al. 2013b).

22.4 Importance of the Allergens

Der p 1 and Der p 2 (◉ Fig. 22.1) are the major allergens of the house dust mite *D. pteronyssinus*, and about 80–90 % of all mite-allergic patients are sensitized to one or both of these two allergens (Batard et al. 2016). Both allergens elicit strong allergic symptoms and are found in huge amounts in house dust (Custovic et al. 1996; Wahn et al. 1997). Recently, Der p 23 was identified as third major allergen, to which about 70 % of the patients are sensitized and which is of high clinical importance (Weghofer et al. 2013).

Der p 5, Der p 7, and Der p 21 are recognized by approximately 30 % of house dust mite-allergic patients, and the IgE reactivity to these allergens is often as strong as to the major allergens (Thomas 2015). The serine proteases Der p 3, Der p 6, and Der p 9 only show weak IgE reactivity, and also most of the other known mite allergens seem to be of low importance for house dust mite allergy (Weghofer et al. 2008b).

Der p 10, mite tropomyosin, is recognized by only 10 % of house dust mite-allergic patients in Europe. However, it represents an important cross-reactive allergen, due to its high sequence identity to tropomyosins from other invertebrates (Reese et al. 1999). Several allergens (mainly those allergens with high molecular weight, e.g., Der p 11, Der p 14, Der p 15, and Der p 18) are not sufficiently characterized regarding their clinical importance (◉ Table 22.1). Recently, a new allergen (Der f 24) was identified, which bound IgE from all tested mite-allergic patients (Chan et al. 2015). However, further investigations are needed to determine the importance of this allergen. For the recently identified HDM allergens Der f 25–Der f 33, quantitative or comparative IgE binding has not been determined (An et al. 2013a). The most important allergens of the tropical mite *B. tropicalis* are Blo t 5 and the related allergen Blo t 21 (the group 5 and 21 allergens) (Chua et al. 2007). In contrast, little is known about the importance of the group 1 and 2 allergens from *B. tropicalis*.

22.5 Frequency of Sensitization/Distribution

More than 20 % of children and adolescents between 3 and 17 years in Germany were shown to be sensitized to house dust mites, accounting for 50 % of all atopic persons (Schmitz et al. 2013). House dust mite allergy is a major risk factor for the development of asthma (Platts-Mills et al. 2000) and is responsible for clinical symptoms in approximately 18 % of asthmatic patients in Europe (Sunyer et al. 2004). Exposure to house dust mites in early childhood can lead to sensitization (Casas et al. 2015), and it has been shown that more than 2 μg allergen/g dust increases the risk of sensitization (Huss et al. 2001).

House dust mites are found almost worldwide and house dust mite allergy is a major health problem in all continents. In arid and cold regions, only few mites can be found, e.g., Alps, Rocky Mountains, and Arctic regions (Arlian et al. 2002). Mites are mainly found in mattresses, carpets, and upholstered furniture and can also be present in large amounts in public buildings.

Mite allergy is mainly caused by mite feces, which also contain the most important allergens (Tovey et al. 1981). The most important mite species are *D. pteronyssinus*, the European house dust mite, and *D. farinae*, the American house dust mite, but in most regions both mite species are present in house dust. *D. farinae* predominates in arid regions, whereas *D. pteronyssinus* is more often found in coastal regions. In tropical areas, the tropical mite *Blomia tropicalis* is predominant. Additionally, also storage mites (e.g., *Lepidoglyphus destructor*, *Tyrophagus putrescentiae*, *Glycyphagus domesticus*) can be found in house dust and can elicit allergic reactions.

22.6 Cross-Reactive Allergens/Marker Allergens

Most allergens of the house dust mite *D. pteronyssinus* show high sequence identity of 80–85 % to the respective allergens of *D. farinae*. Therefore, IgE antibodies raised to allergens of one mite species often also recognize homologous allergens of the other mite species. Allergens with sequence homology to house dust mite allergens are also found in tropical mites (*B. tropicalis*) and in different species of storage mites (e.g., *Lepidoglyphus destructor*, *Tyrophagus putrescentiae*). However, the sequence identity between most allergens of house dust mites and storage mites is rather low (not more than 50 %); thus no relevant cross-reactivity can be found between allergens of house dust mites and storage mites (Van Hage-Hamsten et al. 1987).

Tropomyosin (Der p 10) represents an important panallergen among invertebrates and plays a major role in seafood allergy. Whereas in most European countries, only about 10 % of house dust mite-allergic patients are sensitized to Der p 10, tropomyosin represents a major allergen in seafood allergy, and more than 80 % of shrimp-allergic patients are sensitized to tropomyosin (Reese et al. 1999). Der p 10 shows a sequence identity of 80 % to tropomyosin from cockroach, and a high cross-reactivity was found between these two allergens (Satinover et al. 2005). The sequence identity between Der p 10 and tropomyosin from vertebrates is 50–60 %, and no cross-reactivity can be found.

22.7 Diagnosis

Diagnosis of house dust mite allergy is performed routinely with allergen extracts. Evidence of sensitization is given in vivo by prick tests and/or in vitro by the presence of mite-specific IgE antibodies. In most cases it is sufficient to test one species of house dust mites (*D. pteronyssinus* or *D. farinae*), because of the high cross-reactivity between these two species. If a diagnosis is unclear, conjunctival or nasal provocation with allergen extracts (*D. pteronyssinus* or *D. farinae*) can be performed to determine the clinical relevance of the house dust mite allergy.

House dust mite extracts are difficult to standardize being composed of a mixture of allergenic and nonallergenic components. The allergen content of these extracts varies depending on the culture conditions of the mites and the extraction methods; thus the major allergens of house dust mites Der p 1 (group 1) and Der p 2 (group 2) are present in variable amounts in extracts from different manufacturers. Other important allergens, e.g., Der p 23, are only present in small amounts in many commercial house dust mite extracts and often not detectable (Casset et al. 2012). Accordingly some house dust mite-allergic patients cannot be diagnosed with allergen extracts, in particular patients without sensitization to group 1 or group 2 allergens. A component-specific diagnosis with all important house dust mite allergens would allow the diagnosis to include these patients.

Today, it is possible to determine specific IgE to nDer p 1 (d202, ImmunoCAP, Thermo Fisher, Uppsala, Sweden), rDer p 2 (d203), and to the panallergen tropomyosin from house dust mites, rDer p 10 (d205). So far, no advantage has been shown compared to diagnosis with allergen extracts, probably because group 1 and group 2 house dust mite allergens are present in sufficient amounts in most of the available house dust mite extracts. However, it would be advisable to test sensitization to group 1 and group 2 house dust mite allergens before specific immunotherapy, since most house dust mite extracts are mainly standardized for these two major allergens.

The current IgE microarray (ImmunoCAP ISAC, Thermo Fisher) contains 112 allergens from 51 allergen sources. It allows the determination of specific IgE to nDer p 1, nDer f 1, rDer p 2, rDer f 2, and rDer p 10 (mite tropomyosin) as well as to tropomyosin from different seafood species and cockroach. Additionally, the IgE microarray contains the major allergen of the storage mite *Lepidoglyphus destructor* (rLep d 2) and the major allergen of the tropical mite *Blomia tropicalis* (Blo t 5). Whereas the ISAC test showed good correlation to extract-based tests for most allergen sources, a considerably lower correlation was found for *Dermatophagoides pteronyssinus*, indicating that certain relevant house dust mite allergens (e.g., Der p 5, Der p 7, Der p 21, and Der p 23) need to be added to the ISAC chip (Huss-Marp et al. 2015).

22.8 Added Value of Molecular Diagnosis

House dust mite extracts are difficult to standardize and contain a mixture of allergens in variable amounts. The concentration of the allergens in extracts depends on the amount of these proteins in the mites and thus cannot be influenced. Consequently, certain allergens are only present in tiny amounts in extracts, and house dust mite-allergic patients, which are exclusively sensitized to such allergens, cannot be diagnosed with these extracts (Casset et al. 2012). Moreover, diagnosis with house dust mite extracts only determines if a patient is sensitized to house dust mites and cannot determine the allergens responsible for the allergy.

A component-specific diagnosis with purified natural or recombinant allergens (Matricardi et al. 2016) would allow the determination of the exact sensitization profile of a patient, thus precisely elucidating the house dust mite allergens responsible for the sensitization (◉ Fig. 22.2).

In particular, a component-specific diagnosis would be important to determine whether a patient is genuinely sensitized to house dust mites (e.g., IgE reactivity to Der p 1 or Der p 2) or if the reaction to house dust mites is caused by cross-reactivity (e.g., exclusive sensitization to the cross-reactive panallergen Der p 10 in shrimp-allergic patients (Reese et al. 1999) or low anti-Der p 1 and 2 IgE titers in combination with high anti-Der p 4 and 20 IgE titers in scabies-infected subjects (Walton et al. 2016)).

Additionally, a component-specific diagnosis with purified natural or recombinant house dust mite allergens would allow an improved selection of patients for specific immunotherapy.

Since house dust mite extracts used for immunotherapy are only standardized for the major allergens (Der p 1 and Der p 2) and other allergens are often only present in insufficient amounts in the extracts, a component-specific diagnosis would help to select those patients which are suitable and might benefit from specific immunotherapy with house dust mite extracts.

22.9 Therapy and Recommendations

Specific immunotherapy (SIT) is performed by applying high doses of house dust mite extracts sublingually or subcutaneously to the house dust mite-allergic patient. The extracts can be chemically modified (allergoids) and administered with an adjuvant (e.g., aluminum hydroxide) for injection therapy. SIT with house dust mite

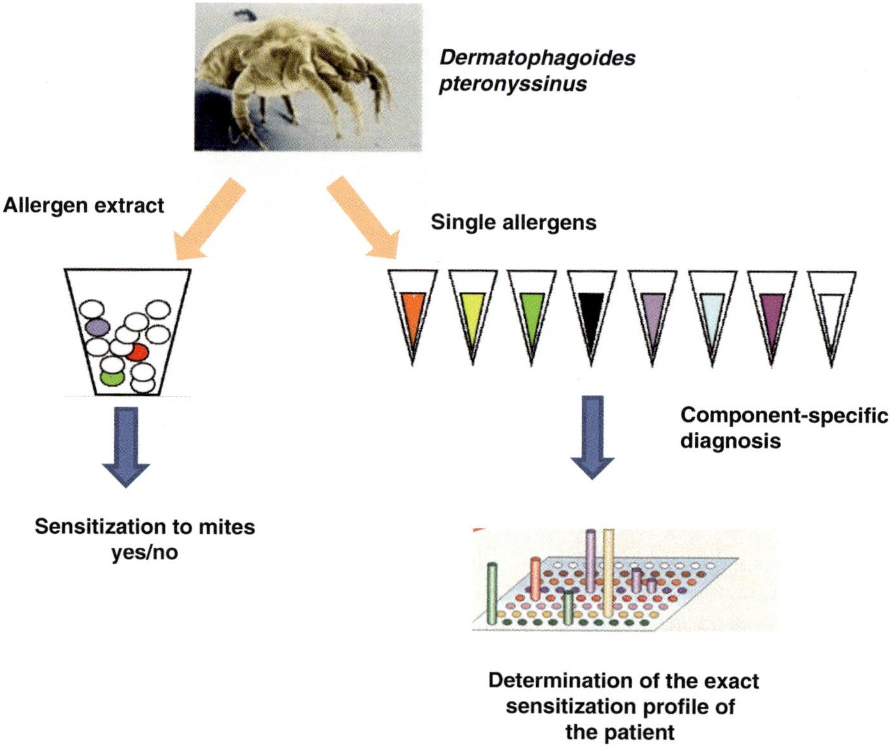

Fig. 22.2 Diagnosis of house dust mite allergy

extracts is less efficient than therapy with pollen extracts (Bousquet and Michel 1994). The reason for this might be the variable and often bad quality of the house dust mite extracts used for SIT, which probably do not contain all important house dust mite allergens in sufficient amounts (Casset et al. 2012).

A possible solution to improve house dust mite SIT would be to add those allergens that are missing or only present in tiny amounts in house dust mite extracts as purified single allergens to the existing house dust mite extracts. A second possibility would be to perform immunotherapy with purified natural or recombinant house dust mite allergens.

In case of pollen allergy, it has already been shown that patients can be treated successfully with recombinant allergens or hypoallergenic derivatives of these allergens (Niederberger et al. 2004; Pauli et al. 2008).

Because of these promising results, hypoallergenic derivatives with reduced allergenic activity were produced from the most important house dust mite allergens (i.e., Der p 1, Der p 2, and Der p 23). Mutants of group 2 allergens from *D. pteronyssinus* (Der p 2) and *D. farinae* (Der f 2) were produced by in vitro mutagenesis with the aim to destroy one of the three disulfide bonds and thus the three-dimensional structure and conformational epitopes of these allergens (Smith and Chapman 1996; Takai et al. 1997). However, controversial results were obtained regarding the best mutant, and another variant of group 2 allergens, produced by in vitro mutagenesis of IgE epitopes, only showed weak reduction of the allergenic activity (Takai et al. 2001).

Additionally, N- and C-terminal deletion variants were produced from group 2 allergens as well as fragments and hybrids, where the fragments were reassembled in inverse order (Takai et al. 1999; Chen et al. 2008a). All these variants showed reduced IgE-binding capacity and reduced allergenic activity.

Hybrid molecules, consisting of hypoallergenic variants of Der p 1 and Der p 2, showed reduced IgE-binding capacity and induced blocking antibodies in animal models (Asturias et al. 2009; Chen et al. 2008b). With the aim to reduce IgE- and T-cell mediated side effects, peptides from Der p 2 were synthesized. When coupled to the carrier protein KLH, the Der p 2 peptides induced allergen-specific antibodies in animal models, which inhibited binding of patients' IgE to the wild-type Der p 2 (Chen et al. 2008b). In the case of Der p 23, peptides were synthesized with reduced IgE-binding capacity and allergenic activity. The hypoallergenic Der p 23 peptides were expressed together with the hepatitis B surface antigen PreS in the form of fusion proteins and induced specific antibodies in animal models, which inhibited mite-allergic patients' IgE binding to Der p 23 (Banerjee et al. 2014).

22.10 Perspectives

Today, only nDer p 1, rDer p 2, and rDer p 10 are available as single allergens for diagnosis of house dust mite allergy. The availability of further important house dust mite allergens (e.g., Der p 5, Der p 7, Der p 21, and Der p 23) as single allergens could improve considerably diagnosis of house dust mite allergy. Hypoallergenic variants have already been produced of the most important house dust mite allergens by genetic engineering. The hypoallergenic variants of house dust mite allergens induce allergen-specific antibodies in animal models, which inhibit binding of patients' IgE to the wild-type allergens (Chen et al. 2008a, b). If shown to be successful in clinical tests, these hypoallergenic variants could lead to improved immunotherapy of house dust mite-allergic patients in the future.

Today it is supposed that the house dust mite allergens Der p 1, Der p 2 (the major group 1 and group 2 allergens), Der p 5, Der p 7, Der p 21, and Der p 23 are sufficient for immunotherapy with single components.

Conclusion

House dust mite extracts are difficult to standardize and do not contain all important allergens in sufficient amounts. Consequently, not all house dust mite-allergic patients can be diagnosed and treated successfully with these extracts. Purified, natural, or recombinant single allergens could improve diagnosis and immunotherapy of house dust mite allergy; however, today only Der p 1, Der p 2, and Der p 10 are available for routine diagnosis.

References

Aki T, Kodama T, Fujikawa A, et al. Immunochemical characterization of recombinant and native tropomyosins as a new allergen from the house dust mite, Dermatophagoides farinae. J Allergy Clin Immunol. 1995;96:74–83.

An S, Chen L, Long C, et al. Dermatophagoides farinae allergens diversity identification by proteomics. Mol Cell Proteomics. 2013a;12:1818–28.

An S, Shen C, Liu X, et al. Alpha-actinin is a new type of house dust mite allergen. PLoS One. 2013b;8:e81377.

Arlian LG, Morgan MS, Neal JS. Dust mite allergens: ecology and distribution. Curr Allergy Asthma Rep. 2002;2:401–11.

Asokananthan N, Graham PT, Stewart DJ, et al. House dust mite allergens induce proinflammatory cytokines from respiratory epithelial cells: the cysteine protease allergen, Der p 1, activates protease-activated receptor (PAR)-2 and inactivates PAR-1. J Immunol. 2002;169:4572–8.

Asturias JA, Arilla MC, Gomez-Bayon N, et al. Sequencing and high level expression in Escherichia coli of the tropomyosin allergen (Der p 10) from Dermatophagoides pteronyssinus. Biochim Biophys Acta. 1998;1397:27–30.

Asturias JA, Ibarrola I, Arilla MC, et al. Engineering of major house dust mite allergens Der p 1 and Der p 2 for allergen-specific immunotherapy. Clin Exp Allergy. 2009;39:1088–98.

Banerjee S, Weber M, Blatt K, et al. Conversion of Der p 23, a new major house dust mite allergen, into a hypoallergenic vaccine. J Immunol. 2014;192:4867–75.

Batard T, Baron-Bodo V, Martelet A, et al. Patterns of IgE sensitization in house dust mite-allergic patients: implications for allergen immunotherapy. Allergy. 2016;71:220–9.

Boulet LP, Turcotte H, Laprise C, et al. Comparative degree and type of sensitization to common indoor and outdoor allergens in subjects with allergic rhinitis and/or asthma. Clin Exp Allergy. 1997;27:52–9.

Bousquet J, Michel FB. Specific immunotherapy in asthma. Allergy Proc. 1994;15:329–33.

Brunetto B, Tinghino R, Braschi MC, et al. Characterization and comparison of commercially available mite extracts for in vivo diagnosis. Allergy. 2010;65:184–90.

Casas L, Sunyer J, Tischer C, et al. Early-life house dust mite allergens, childhood mite sensitization, and respiratory outcomes. Allergy. 2015;70:820–7.

Casset A, Mari A, Purohit A, et al. Varying allergen composition and content affects the in vivo allergenic activity of commercial Dermatophagoides pteronyssinus extracts. Int Arch Allergy Immunol. 2012;159:253–62.

Chan SL, Ong ST, Ong SY, et al. Nuclear magnetic resonance structure-based epitope mapping and modulation of dust mite group 13 allergen as a hypoallergen. J Immunol. 2006;176: 4852–60.

Chan TF, Ji KM, Yim AK, et al. The draft genome, transcriptome, and microbiome of Dermatophagoides farinae reveal a broad spectrum of dust mite allergens. J Allergy Clin Immunol. 2015;135:539–48.

Chen KW, Fuchs G, Sonneck K, et al. Reduction of the in vivo allergenicity of Der p 2, the major house-dust mite allergen, by genetic engineering. Mol Immunol. 2008;45:2486–98.

Chua KY, Stewart GA, Thomas WR, et al. Sequence analysis of cDNA coding for a major house dust mite allergen, Der p 1. Homology with cysteine proteases. J Exp Med. 1988;167:175–82.

Chua KY, Cheong N, Kuo IC, et al. The Blomia tropicalis allergens. Protein Pept Lett. 2007;14:325–33.

Custovic A, Taggart SC, Francis HC, et al. Exposure to house dust mite allergens and the clinical activity of asthma. J Allergy Clin Immunol. 1996;98:64–72.

Derewenda U, Li J, Derewenda Z, et al. The crystal structure of a major dust mite allergen Der p 2, and its biological implications. J Mol Biol. 2002;318:189–97.

Epton MJ, Dilworth RJ, Smith W, et al. High-molecular-weight allergens of the house dust mite: an apolipophorin-like cDNA has sequence identity with the major M-177 allergen and the IgE-binding peptide fragments Mag1 and Mag3. Int Arch Allergy Immunol. 1999;120:185–91.

Herman J, Thelen N, Smargiasso N, et al. Der p 1 is the primary activator of Der p 3, Der p 6 and Der p 9 the proteolytic allergens produced by the house dust mite Dermatophagoides pteronyssinus. Biochim Biophys Acta. 2014;1840:1117–24.
Huss K, Adkinson Jr NF, Eggleston PA, et al. House dust mite and cockroach exposure are strong risk factors for positive allergy skin test responses in the Childhood Asthma Management Program. J Allergy Clin Immunol. 2001;107:48–54.
Huss-Marp J, Gutermuth J, Schaffner I, et al. Comparison of molecular and extract-based allergy diagnostics with multiplex and singleplex analysis. Allergo J Int. 2015;24:46–53.
Inohara N, Nunez G. ML -- a conserved domain involved in innate immunity and lipid metabolism. Trends Biochem Sci. 2002;27:219–21.
King C, Simpson RJ, Moritz RL, et al. The isolation and characterization of a novel collagenolytic serine protease allergen (Der p 9) from the dust mite Dermatophagoides pteronyssinus. J Allergy Clin Immunol. 1996;98:739–47.
Maruo K, Akaike T, Ono T, et al. Generation of anaphylatoxins through proteolytic processing of C3 and C5 by house dust mite protease. J Allergy Clin Immunol. 1997;100:253–60.
Matricardi PM, Kleine-Tebbe J, Hoffmann HJ, et al. EAACI molecular allergology user's guide. Pediatr Allergy Immunol. 2016;27(suppl23):1–250.
Mellerup MT, Hahn GW, Poulsen LK, et al. Safety of allergen-specific immunotherapy. Relation between dosage regimen, allergen extract, disease and systemic side-effects during induction treatment. Clin Exp Allergy. 2000;30:1423–9.
Mueller GA, Gosavi RA, Krahn JM, et al. Der p 5 crystal structure provides insight into the group 5 dust mite allergens. J Biol Chem. 2010a;285:25394–401.
Mueller GA, Edwards LL, Aloor JJ, et al. The structure of the dust mite allergen Der p 7 reveals similarities to innate immune proteins. J Allergy Clin Immunol. 2010b;125:909–17.
Niederberger V, Horak F, Vrtala S, et al. Vaccination with genetically engineered allergens prevents progression of allergic disease. Proc Natl Acad Sci U S A. 2004;101 Suppl 2:14677–82.
O'Neil SE, Heinrich TK, Hales BJ, et al. The chitinase allergens Der p 15 and Der p 18 from Dermatophagoides pteronyssinus. Clin Exp Allergy. 2006;36:831–9.
Pauli G, Larsen TH, Rak S, et al. Efficacy of recombinant birch pollen vaccine for the treatment of birch-allergic rhinoconjunctivitis. J Allergy Clin Immunol. 2008;122:951–60.
Platts-Mills TA, Rakes G, Heymann PW. The relevance of allergen exposure to the development of asthma in childhood. J Allergy Clin Immunol. 2000;105:S503–8.
Reese G, Ayuso R, Lehrer SB. Tropomyosin: an invertebrate pan-allergen. Int Arch Allergy Immunol. 1999;119:247–58.
Satinover SM, Reefer AJ, Pomes A, et al. Specific IgE and IgG antibody-binding patterns to recombinant cockroach allergens. J Allergy Clin Immunol. 2005;115:803–9.
Schmitz R, Ellert U, Kalcklosch M, et al. Patterns of sensitization to inhalant and food allergens - findings from the German Health Interview and Examination Survey for Children and Adolescents. Int Arch Allergy Immunol. 2013;162:263–70.
Smith AM, Chapman MD. Reduction in IgE binding to allergen variants generated by site-directed mutagenesis: contribution of disulfide bonds to the antigenic structure of the major house dust mite allergen Der p 2. Mol Immunol. 1996;33:399–405.
Stewart GA, Ward LD, Simpson RJ, et al. The group III allergen from the house dust mite Dermatophagoides pteronyssinus is a trypsin-like enzyme. Immunology. 1992;75:29–35.
Sun G, Stacey MA, Schmidt M, et al. Interaction of mite allergens Der p3 and Der p9 with protease-activated receptor-2 expressed by lung epithelial cells. J Immunol. 2001;167:1014–21.
Sunyer J, Jarvis D, Pekkanen J, et al. Geographic variations in the effect of atopy on asthma in the European Community Respiratory Health Study. J Allergy Clin Immunol. 2004;114:1033–9.
Takai T, Yokota T, Yasue M, et al. Engineering of the major house dust mite allergen Der f 2 for allergen-specific immunotherapy. Nat Biotechnol. 1997;15:754–8.
Takai T, Mori A, Yuuki T, et al. Non-anaphylactic combination of partially deleted fragments of the major house dust mite allergen Der f 2 for allergen-specific immunotherapy. Mol Immunol. 1999;36:1055–65.

Takai T, Hatanaka H, Ichikawa S, et al. Effects of double mutation at two distant IgE-binding sites in the three-dimensional structure of the major house dust mite allergen Der f 2 on IgE-binding and histamine-releasing activity. Biosci Biotechnol Biochem. 2001;65:1601–9.
Thomas WR. Hierarchy and molecular properties of house dust mite allergens. Allergol Int Off J Japanese Soc Allergol. 2015;64:304–11.
Thomas WR, Smith WA, Hales BJ, et al. Characterization and immunobiology of house dust mite allergens. Int Arch Allergy Immunol. 2002;129:1–18.
Thomas WR, Hales BJ, Smith WA. Structural biology of allergens. Curr Allergy Asthma Rep. 2005;5:388–93.
Tovey ER, Chapman MD, Platts-Mills TA. Mite faeces are a major source of house dust allergens. Nature. 1981;289:592–3.
Trompette A, Divanovic S, Visintin A, et al. Allergenicity resulting from functional mimicry of a Toll-like receptor complex protein. Nature. 2009;457:585–8.
Tsai LC, Chao PL, Shen HD, et al. Isolation and characterization of a novel 98-kd Dermatophagoides farinae mite allergen. J Allergy Clin Immunol. 1998;102:295–303.
Van Hage-Hamsten M, Johansson SG, Hoglund S, et al. Storage mite allergy is common in a farming population. Clin Allergy. 1985;15:555–64.
Van Hage-Hamsten M, Johansson SG, Johansson E, et al. Lack of allergenic cross-reactivity between storage mites and Dermatophagoides pteronyssinus. Clin Allergy. 1987;17:23–31.
Voorhorst R, Spieksma-Boezeman MI, Spieksma FT. Is a mite (Dermatophagoides Sp.) the producer of the house-dust allergen? Allerg Asthma (Leipz). 1964;10:329–34.
Wahn U, Lau S, Bergmann R, et al. Indoor allergen exposure is a risk factor for sensitization during the first three years of life. J Allergy Clin Immunol. 1997;99:763–9.
Walton SF, Slender A, Pizutto S, et al. Analysis of IgE binding patterns to house dust mite allergens in scabies-endemic communities: insights for both diseases. Clin Exp Allergy. 2016;46:508.
Wan H, Winton HL, Soeller C, et al. Der p 1 facilitates transepithelial allergen delivery by disruption of tight junctions. J Clin Invest. 1999;104:123–33.
Weghofer M, Dall'antonia Y, Grote M, et al. Characterization of Der p 21, a new important allergen derived from the gut of house dust mites. Allergy. 2008a;63:758–67.
Weghofer M, Thomas WR, Kronqvist M, et al. Variability of IgE reactivity profiles among European mite allergic patients. Eur J Clin Invest. 2008b;38:959–65.
Weghofer M, Grote M, Resch Y, et al. Identification of Der p 23, a peritrophin-like protein, as a new major Dermatophagoides pteronyssinus allergen associated with the peritrophic matrix of mite fecal pellets. J Immunol. 2013;190:3059–67.
Wraith DG, Cunnington AM, Seymour WM. The role and allergenic importance of storage mites in house dust and other environments. Clin Allergy. 1979;9:545–61.
Yasueda H, Mita H, Akiyama K, et al. Allergens from Dermatophagoides mites with chymotryptic activity. Clin Exp Allergy. 1993;23:384–90.

Cockroach, Tick, Storage Mite, and Other Arthropod Allergies: Molecular Aspects 23

C. Hilger, A. Kuehn, M. Raulf, A. Pomés, and T. Jakob

23.1 Introduction

Arthropods form an extensive phylum of the animal kingdom, comprising widely varying members such as insects, arachnids, chitin-exoskeleton animals (e.g., crabs, shrimp, and lobsters), and centipedes (◉ Fig. 23.1). The molecular-based diagnoses of the common house dust mite allergy and the hymenoptera venom allergy are discussed in ▶ Chaps. 16 and 19. The present chapter deals with rarer allergies to specific members of the arthropod kingdom. The extracts available for diagnostic purposes, as well as the currently known individual allergens, are presented, and their potential application in allergy diagnostics is discussed.

The present chapter is based on, and modified from, an article by the authors published in 2014 in *Allergo Journal International* (Hilger C, Kuehn A, Raulf M, Jakob T: Cockroach, tick, storage mite and other arthropod allergies: Where do we stand with molecular allergy diagnostics? Allergo J Int 2014; 23: 172–178).
The authors gratefully thank Dr. Steve Love, PhD, Laguna Niguel, CA, USA, for reading the manuscript and editorial assistance with the English translation.

C. Hilger, PhD (✉) • A. Kuehn, PhD, Prof.
Allergology – Immunology – Inflammation Research Unit, Department of Infection and Immunity, Luxembourg Institute of Health, Esch-sur-Alzette, Luxembourg
e-mail: christiane.hilger@lih.lu; annette.kuehn@lih.lu; https://www.lih.lu/

M. Raulf, PhD
Center Allergology/Immunology, Institute for Prevention and Occupational Medicine of the German Social Accident Insurance, Institute of the Ruhr-Universität Bochum, Bochum, Germany
e-mail: raulf@ipa-dguv.de

A. Pomés, PhD
Basic Research Department, Indoor Biotechnologies, Inc, Charlottesville, VA, USA
e-mail: apomes@inbio.com

T. Jakob, MD, Prof.
Department of Dermatology and Allergology, University Medical Center Giessen (UKGM), Justus-Liebig-University, Giessen, Germany
e-mail: thilo.jakob@derma.med.uni-giessen.de

J. Kleine-Tebbe, T. Jakob (eds.), *Molecular Allergy Diagnostics*,
DOI 10.1007/978-3-319-42499-6_23

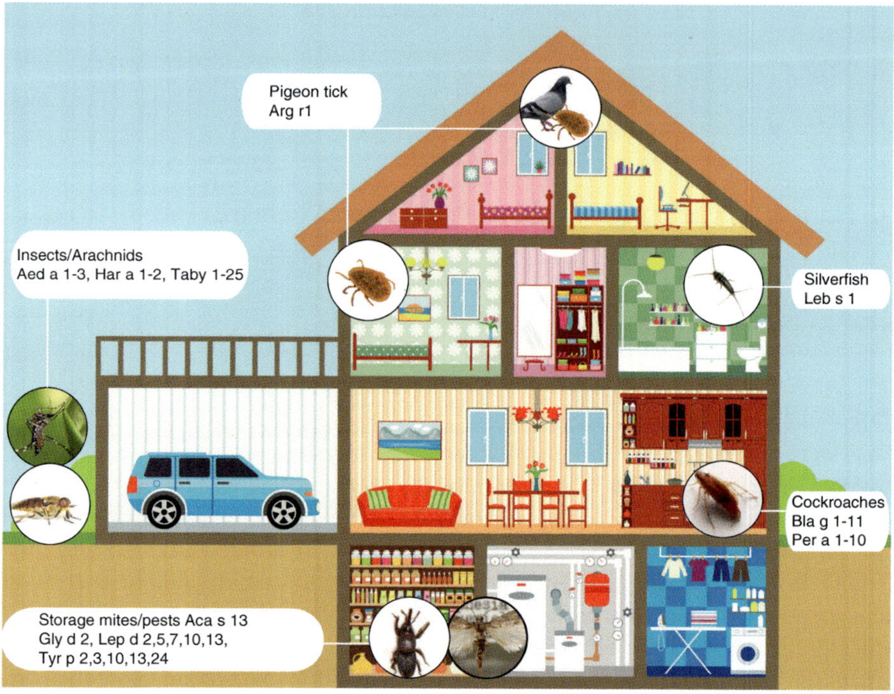
Pigeon tick
Arg r1
Insects/Arachnids
Aed a 1-3, Har a 1-2, Taby 1-25
Silverfish
Leb s 1
Cockroaches
Bla g 1-11
Per a 1-10
Storage mites/pests Aca s 13
Gly d 2, Lep d 2,5,7,10,13,
Tyr p 2,3,10,13,24

Fig. 23.1 Preferred habitats of various allergy-triggering arthropods in the house and garden, as well as their characterized allergens (© [M] mylisa/fotolia.com)

23.2 Cockroach Allergy

23.2.1 Exposure and Distribution

The cockroach order (Blattodea) comprises more than 4,600 species distributed worldwide. Most cockroaches are nocturnal and indigenous primarily to the tropics and subtropics. The domestic cockroaches best investigated as allergen sources include the German cockroach (*Blattella germanica*), which dominates in the USA in terms of numbers, as well as the American cockroach (*Periplaneta americana*) and the oriental cockroach (*Blatta orientalis*), which are common in South American and Asian countries. By infesting containers transported either by ship or air, the *Periplaneta fuliginosa* cockroach, which was originally indigenous only to Japan, Southeast Asia, and the Southern United States, has spread worldwide.

The frequency of cockroach allergies depends to a great extent on the level of exposure to cockroach allergens (Pomés and Arruda 2013). Allergen exposure in urban areas is as a whole significantly higher than in suburban areas, where, nevertheless, these allergens are found in up to 30 % of US households (Cohn et al. 2006; Matsui et al. 2003).

23.2.2 Allergen Identification

The official allergen database from the World Health Organization and International Union of Immunological Societies (WHO/IUIS) (www.allergen.org) includes German and American cockroach allergens from up to 12 different groups according to their molecular features and physiological functions (Pomés and Arruda 2013) (◉ Table 23.1). These allergens have been identified in feces, eggs, and exoskeletons. Homologous, possibly cross-reactive allergens have been described in other cockroach species.

Table 23.1 Single allergens of the German and American cockroaches identified according to the WHO/IUIS Allergen Nomenclature Sub-committee

Allergen	Name	Molecular weight (kDa)
Blattella germanica[a, c–f] (German cockroach)	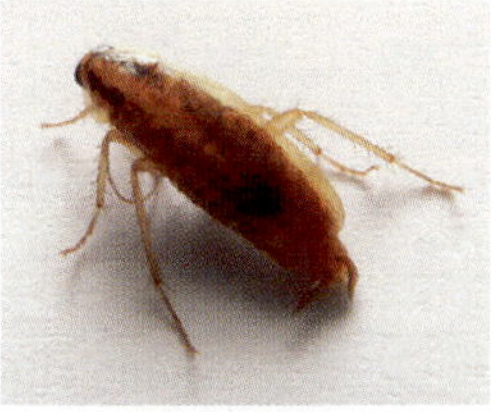	
Bla g 1[b]	Midgut microvilli protein homolog	25–90
Bla g 2[b]	Aspartic protease	36
Bla g 3	Hemocyanin	78.9
Bla g 4	Calycin	21
Bla g 5[b]	Glutathione S-transferase	23
Bla g 6	Troponin C	17
Bla g 7[b]	Tropomyosin	33
Bla g 8	Myosin light chain	–
Bla g 11	α-Amylase	57
Periplaneta americana[a, c, d] (American cockroach)	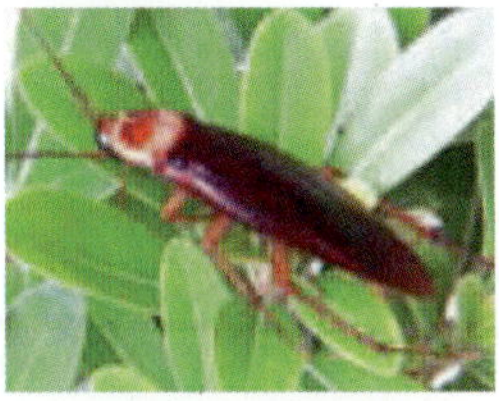	
Per a 1	Midgut microvilli protein homolog	25–45
Per a 2	Aspartic protease-like	42
Per a 3	Arylphorin/hemocyanin	46–79
Per a 6	Troponin C	17
Per a 7	Tropomyosin	33
Per a 9	Arginine kinase	43
Per a 10	Serine protease	28

(continued)

Table 23.1 (continued)

Allergen	Name	Molecular weight (kDa)
Per a 11	α-Amylase	55
Per a 12	Chitinase	45

[a]ImmunoCAP®, Phadia/ThermoScientific and Siemens Healthcare, Freiburg, Germany
[b]ImmunoCAP® ISAC, Phadia/ThermoScientific and Siemens Healthcare, Freiburg, Germany
[c]3gAllergy™/Immulite, Siemens Healthcare, Eschborn, Germany
[d]ALLERG-O-LIQ®, Dr Fooke Laboratorien GmbH, Neuss, Germany
[e]Allergozyme®, Omega Diagnostics, Reinbek, Germany
[f]Allercoat™, EuroImmun, Lübeck, Germany

23.2.3 Function and Structure

Some cockroach allergens are proteins associated with the digestive tract and presumably contribute to digestion, e.g., Bla g 1/Per a 1 (midgut proteins), Per a 9 (arginine kinase), Per a 10 (serine protease), and Bla g 11 (α-amylase) (Pomés et al 1998; Jeong et al. 2013; Suazo et al. 2009: Sudha et al. 2008; Yu et al. 2003). The basic structural unit of Bla g 1 has been determined and forms a spherical capsule with a large cavity that contains lipids (Mueller et al. 2013). This structure facilitated the standardization of assays in absolute units for the assessment of environmental allergen exposure.

Other cockroach allergens are involved in muscle contraction. These include Bla g 6/Per a 6 (troponin C), Bla g 7/Per a 7 (tropomyosin), and Bla g 8 (myosin light chain) (Hindley et al. 2006; Jeong et al. 2004). Bla g 6 and Per a 6 belong to the family of EF-hand proteins. They bind calcium ions via α-helices made up of 12 amino acids. Bla g 7 and Per a 7 are tropomyosins, consisting of two intertwined helical molecules. Myosin light chains are small, calcium-binding subunits of the high-molecular-weight myosin complex, which are associated with the heavy chains in a helical configuration (Messer and Kendrick-Jones 1988).

The biological function of the cockroach allergen Bla g 2 has not yet been elucidated. Analysis of the crystal structure demonstrated that the molecule is an inactive aspartic protease that preserves the typical fold of this group of enzymes (Wünschmann et al. 2005). Five disulfide bridges, as well as a binding site for the cofactor zinc, contribute to the stability of this allergen (Gustchina et al. 2005; Li et al. 2008).

The allergens Bla g 3 and Per a 3 are hemocyanins, the arthropod homolog of hemoglobins, responsible for oxygen transport (Mindykowski et al. 2010). Oxygen binding in hexameric cockroach proteins is coordinated via one copper ion per monomer.

The cockroach-specific protein, Bla g 4, belongs to the lipocalin family, which includes important inhalant allergens from dog (Can f 1, Can f 2), cat (Fel d 4), horse (Equ c 1, Equ c 2), and cow (Bos d 2, Bos d 5) (Hilger et al. 2012). Bla g 4 appears to be involved in reproduction as a transport molecule for low-molecular-weight hydrophobic compounds (Fan et al. 2005). Analysis of the crystal structure showed that it has a fold typical for lipocalins: a funnel-shaped structure that is closed off with a lid-like molecule following ligand binding (Tan et al. 2009).

As a glutathione S-transferase, the allergen Bla g 5 is biologically active and thought to be involved in metabolic detoxification processes (Arruda et al. 1997). IgE cross-reactivity was found between Bla g 5 and a GST homolog from glutathione S-transferase of *Wuchereria bancrofti*, a major lymphatic filarial pathogen of humans, despite a low amino acid identity between both proteins (30 %). This low degree of cross-reactivity was attributed to a similar N-terminal linear epitope (Santiago et al. 2012). Recently, the structures of Bla g 5, the homologs Der p 8 and Blo t 8 from mites, and the Ascaris allergen Asc s 13 were determined and compared. A low similarity at the level of the molecular surface explains the low cross-reactivity observed among these allergens in patients from temperate areas (Mueller et al. 2015).

23.2.4 Relevance and Sensitization Frequency

Cockroach allergen sensitization is one of the greatest risk factors for high asthma-related morbidity among the low-income population in the USA, with the greatest prevalence in densely populated inner city housing (Gruchalla et al. 2005). Sensitization rates in Europe are generally far lower (Raulf et al. 2014). A study by Hirsch et al. (2000) found that only 4.2 % of approximately 3000 children studied in Dresden, Germany, had specific IgE (>0.7 kU/l) to the German cockroach (*Blattella germanica*), although the prevalence of sensitization among asthmatic children was 6.1 %. Most cockroach-sensitized children in this study were also sensitized to other allergens. Also, in a study carried out at several European centers, where skin tests were performed using various indoor and outdoor allergens in over 3,000 patients, an overall prevalence of sensitization of 8.9 % was found to *Blattella germanica*; the rate was 12 % in German patients (Heinzerling et al. 2009).

The prevalence of specific IgE antibodies to single cockroach allergens varies significantly, a phenomenon that appears to depend on regional exposure (Barbosa et al. 2013; Sohn and Kim 2012). The major allergens are found in the protein groups 1–5 (Bla g 1–5). Since group-1 and group-2 cockroach allergens (Bla g 1 and Bla g 2) are released into the environment, they serve well as markers for the assessment of cockroach allergen exposure (Pomés and Arruda 2013).

23.2.5 Cross-Reactive Allergens

Homologous allergens from different cockroach species, e.g., Bla g 1 and Per a 1, exhibit high but variable cross-reactivity. The tropomyosins, Bla g 7 and Per a 7, as well as arginine kinase (Per a 9), are quite similar to the homologous allergens of other arthropods (>80 % identity). The clinical significance of IgE cross-reactivity between tropomyosins and arginine kinases of cockroaches, chitin-skeleton arthropods, and house dust mites has not yet been fully elucidated (Binder et al. 2001; Wang et al. 2011).

23.3 Storage Mite Allergy

23.3.1 Exposure and Distribution

Storage mites, microscopic arachnids, which feed on plant and animal matter, are typical storage (pertaining to their feeding on stored foodstuffs) pests. Depending on the species, they are found in grain and animal feed, including hay, as well as in straw. The storage mites most commonly found in Europe include *Lepidoglyphus destructor*, the flour mite *Acarus siro*, *Glycyphagus domesticus*, and the mold mite *Tyrophagus putrescentiae*. The latter has a predilection for foods containing protein and fat, such as ham or cheese. All species thrive at temperatures of 20–30 °C and at a relative humidity of >65 % (Fernández-Caldas et al. 2007; Franz et al. 1997; vanHage-Hamsten and Johansson 1998).

23.3.2 Allergen Identification

The groups of allergens listed in the allergen database are shown in ◉ Table 23.2 and include the panallergen tropomyosin (Lep d 10, Try p 10). However, with an IgE prevalence around 13 %, tropomyosin is a minor allergen. Allergens have been identified in carcasses as well as in feces. The major allergen belongs to group 2 (Lep d 2, Tyr p 2, and Gly d 2) and has been found in mite intestine; its function, however, is unknown.

23.3.3 Relevance

Airborne storage mite allergies frequently affect mainly farmers and individuals working in the animal-feed industry. Symptoms include allergic rhinitis and, eventually, bronchial asthma. Isolated cases of oral dust mite allergy have been described. Severe allergic symptoms occurred following the ingestion of flour-based foods baked using contaminated ingredients (Sánchez-Borges et al. 2013). These reports related to contamination with storage mites as well as with house dust mites.

23.3.4 Cross-Reactive Allergens

Although there is strong serological cross-reactivity between extracts from different species of storage mites (flour, stored food, mold), there is little IgE cross-reactivity between house dust and storage mites.

Table 23.2 Single allergens of storage mites identified according to the WHO/IUIS Allergen Nomenclature Sub-committee

Allergen	Name	Molecular weight (kDa)
Acarus siro[a, c–f] (Flour mite)		
Aca s 13	Fatty acid-binding protein	15
Glycophagus domesticus[a, c–f] (House mite)	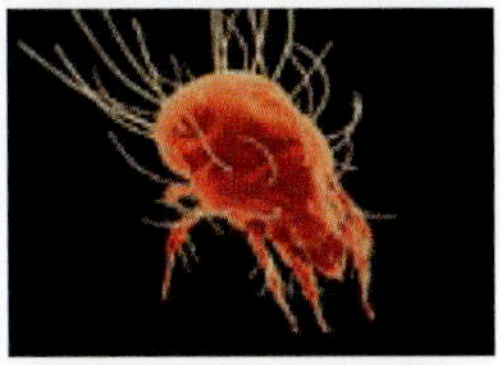	
Gly d 2		15
Lepidoglyphus destructor[a, c–f] (Storage mite)		
Lep d 2[b]	NPC2 family	16
Lep d 5		
Lep d 7		
Lep d 10	Tropomyosin	
Lep d 13	Fatty acid-binding protein	
Tyrophagus putrescentiae[a, c–f] (Mold mite)		
Tyr p 2	NPC2 family	16
Tyr p 3	Trypsin	26
Tyr p 10	Tropomyosin	
Tyr p 13	Fatty acid-binding protein	15
Tyr p 34	Troponin C	18

Diagnostic assays providing (molecular) allergens from the indicated source:
[a]ImmunoCAP®, Phadia/ThermoScientific and Siemens Healthcare, Freiburg, Germany
[b]ImmunoCAP® ISAC, Phadia/ThermoScientific and Siemens Healthcare, Freiburg, Germany
[c]3gAllergy™/Immulite, Siemens Healthcare, Eschborn, Germany
[d]ALLERG-O-LIQ®, Dr Fooke Laboratorien GmbH, Neuss, Germany
[e]Allergozyme®, Omega Diagnostics, Reinbek, Germany
[f]Allercoat™, EuroImmun, Lübeck, Germany

Co-sensitizations appear to be common. Group-2 allergens, in particular (Lep d 2 and Gly d 2), exhibit high sequence identity. The tropomyosin from storage mites (Lep d 10) has a high degree of identity with Der f 10 and Der p 10 in house dust mites, supporting the known cross-reactivity.

23.4 Tick Allergy

23.4.1 Exposure and Distribution

Cases of anaphylactic reactions to pigeon ticks have been consistently reported in recent years, most notably in France, Poland, and Italy but also in Germany

(Hilger et al. 2005; Kleine-Tebbe et al. 2006). The pigeon tick (*Argas reflexus*), which belongs to the soft tick family, is a temporary ectoparasite of wild pigeons in Southern and Central Europe. It feeds primarily nocturnally on blood from its host and seeks refuge in wall crevices and wood cracks during the day. If the pigeon does not return to its nest, the tick will seek new hosts by invading homes, where it infests humans. Adult ticks can be dormant for several years without food and are extremely challenging to combat. In addition to the severe anaphylactic reactions described in the literature, there are also many instances of mild local reactions. A study carried out in Leipzig found an 8 % rate of severe systemic reactions and a 99 % rate of local reactions in subjects with pigeon tick bites (Kleine-Tebbe et al. 2006).

In addition to pigeon ticks, isolated cases of classic immediate-type reactions have been described following bites from the common wood tick (*Ixodes ricinus*), the Australian paralysis tick (*Ixodes holocyclus*), and the brown dog tick (*Rhipicephalus sanguineus*), which is found primarily in Southern Europe. Such cases involve an IgE-mediated reaction to protein in tick saliva.

A specific form of allergy, the delayed red meat allergy, is also associated with tick bites. This allergy involves IgE sensitization to a sugar epitope, galactose-α-1.3-galactose, which is believed to be triggered by tick bites (Commins et al. 2011). While in the USA the American Lone Star tick (*Amblyomma americanum*) and in Australia the Australian paralysis tick (*Ixodes holocyclus*) are discussed as allergy triggers, the wood tick (*Ixodes ricinus*) and Dermacentor ticks (*Dermacentor*) are associated with sensitization to galactose-α-1.3-galactose in Europe (Steinke et al. 2015).

23.4.2 Allergen Identification

Like the cockroach allergen Bla g 4, the major allergen Arg r 1 from the pigeon tick belongs to the lipocalin family. Arg r 1 is a histamine-binding salivary protein. The crystal structure has been determined in complex with its ligand histamine (PDB code 2X45). The overall structure is that of a lipocalin. However, cross-reactivity within this group of proteins is most likely low or absent, since the structure (as well as the amino acid sequence) of the tick protein differs significantly from other allergenic lipocalins.

Galactose-α-1.3-galactose, the tick allergen epitope relevant in delayed red meat allergy, is a significant component of bovine thyroglobulin. Galactose-α-1.3-galactose in bovine thyroglobulin is available for the diagnosis of galactose-α-1.3-galactose sensitization in the ImmunoCAP system.

23.5 Allergies to Other Arthropods

Rarely, a variety of other arachnids and insects can cause allergies (Raulf et al. 2015) (◉ Table 23.3). Individuals who work in barns or stables, where spiders are found in abundance, can experience allergic reactions to the spiders themselves as well as to their cobwebs. Salivary proteins from mosquitoes and horseflies cause

Table 23.3 Single allergens from other arthropods identified according to the IUIS Allergen Nomenclature Sub-committee

Allergen	Name	Molecular weight (kDa)
Aedes aegypti (yellow fever mosquito), *Aedes* spp., *Culex pipiens* (common house mosquito)[a, c–f]	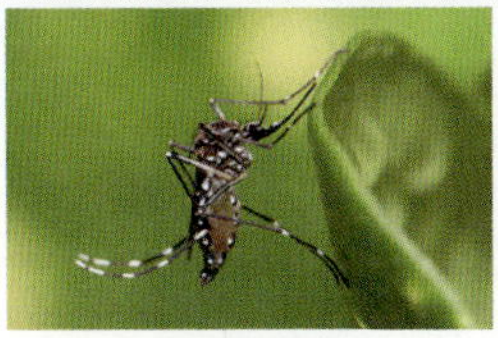	
Aed a 1	Apyrase	68
Aed a 2	Salivary D7 protein	37
Aed a 3	Undefined 30 kDa salivary protein	30
Aed a 4	α-Glucosidase	67
Aed a 5	Sarcoplasmic Ca+(EF-hand)-binding protein	
Aed a 6	Porin 3	
Aed a 7		
Aed a 8	Heat shock cognate protein-70	
Aed a 10	Tropomyosin	32
Aed a 11	Lysosomal aspartic protease	
Argas reflexus[e] (Pigeon tick)	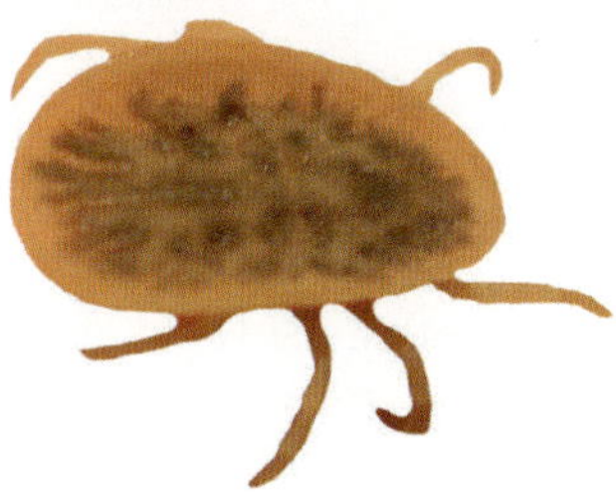	
Arg r 1	Lipocalin	17
Chironomus thummi thummi[a, c–f] (Red chironomid larvae)	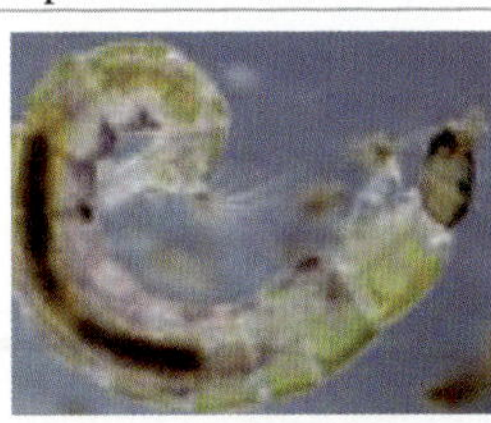	
Chi t 1	Hemoglobin component III/IV	16
Chi t 2	Hemoglobin component I/IA	16
Chi t 3	Hemoglobin component II-β, VI, VIII, IX	16
Chi t 4	Hemoglobin component IIIA	16
Chi t 9	Hemoglobin component X	16

(continued)

Table 23.3 (continued)

Allergen	Name	Molecular weight (kDa)
Harmonia axyridis (Ladybug)	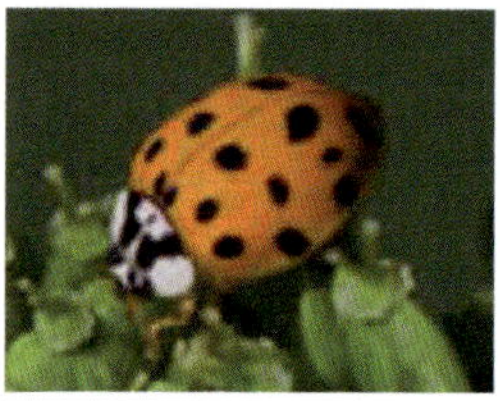	
Har a 1		10
Har a 2	Aldehyde dehydrogenase	55
Lepisma saccharina (Silverfish)	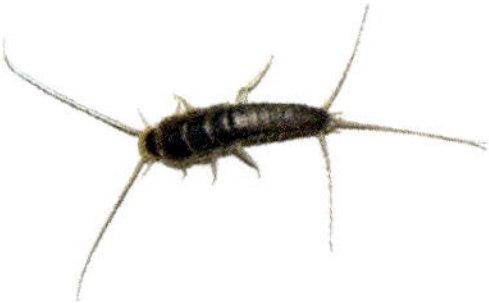	
Lep s 1	Tropomyosin	36
Tabanus yao, *Tabanus* spp.[a, c–f] (Horsefly)	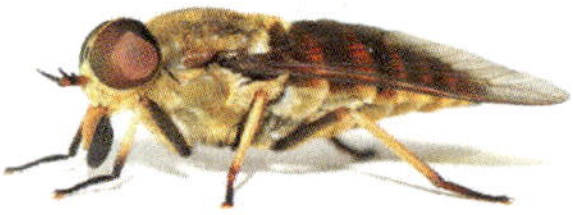	
Tab y 1	Apyrase	70
Tab y 2	Hyaluronidase	35
Tab y 5	Antigen 5-related protein	26

[a]ImmunoCAP®, Phadia/ThermoScientific and Siemens Healthcare, Freiburg, Germany
[b]ImmunoCAP® ISAC, Phadia/ThermoScientific and Siemens Healthcare, Freiburg, Germany
[c]3gAllergy™/Immulite, Siemens Healthcare, Eschborn, Germany
[d]ALLERG-O-LIQ®, Dr Fooke Laboratorien GmbH, Neuss, Germany
[e]Allergozyme®, Omega Diagnostics, Reinbek, Germany
[f]Allercoat™, EuroImmun, Lübeck, Germany

strong local allergic reactions of varying severity and, more rarely, systemic reactions (Ma et al. 2011; Simons and Peng 2001). Other insects can cause allergies in areas of the world that they infest (silkworm, pharaoh ant, Indian meal moth, pine processionary, caddisflies, etc.) (Pomés 2014).

To date, ten allergens from the *Aedes aegypti* mosquito are listed in the WHO/IUIS Allergen Database, including Aed a 1, an apyrase (68 kDa), Aed a 2 (37 kDa), and Aed a 3 (30 kDa), of as yet unknown function, tropomyosin Aed a 10 (32 kDa), and lysosomal aspartic protease (Aed a 11) (Simons and Peng 2001) (◉ Table 23.3).

Three major allergens have been identified to date from the horsefly (*Tabanus spp.*): Tab y 1, an apyrase; Tab y 2, a hyaluronidase; and Tab y 5, an antigen-5 protein (Ma et al. 2011). The last two show cross-reactivity with hyaluronidase and antigen 5 of the Vespidae family (An et al. 2012) and offer an explanation for presumed cross-reactions between wasp venom and horsefly saliva.

Table 23.4 Available storage pest extracts

Species name	Common English name
Ephestia kuehniella[a, c, e] 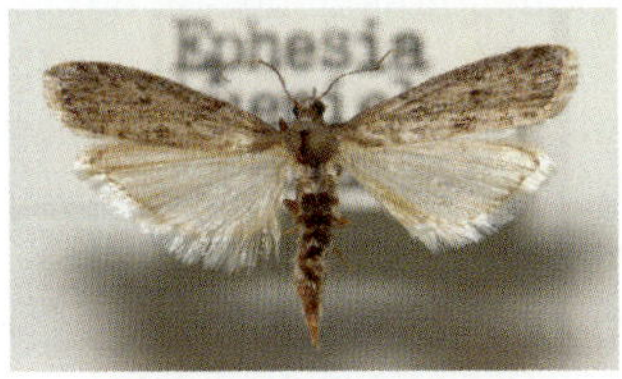	Mediterranean flour moth
Sitophilus granarius[a, e] 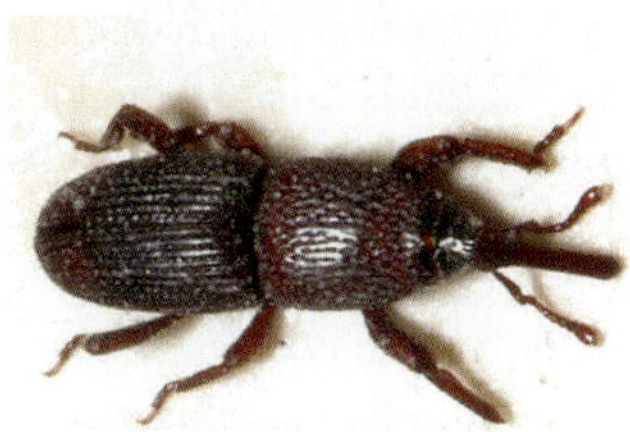	Wheat weevil
Tenebrio molitor[a] 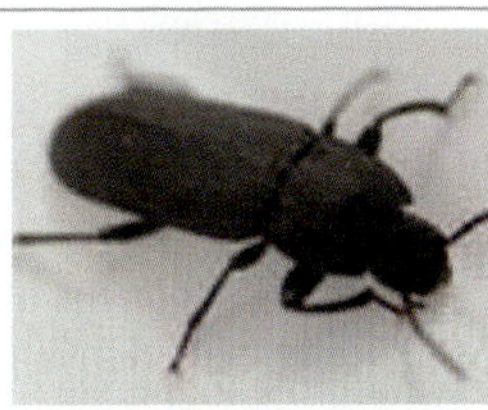	Mealworm beetle
Tribolium confusum[a, d–f] 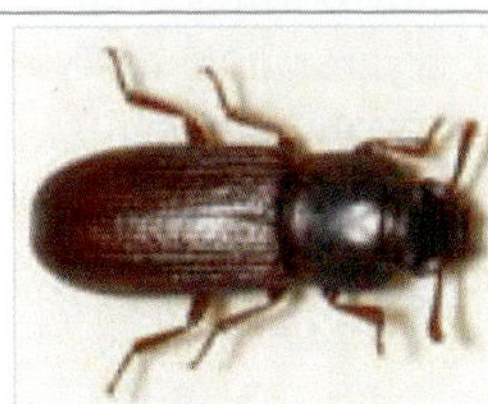	Confused flour beetle
Trogoderma angustum[a, e, f] 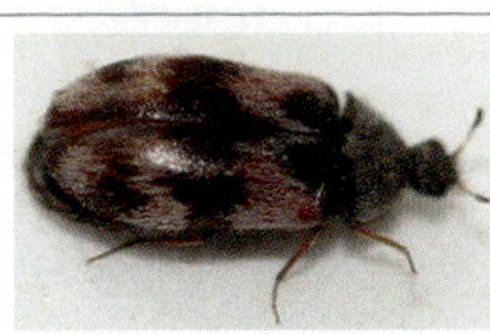	Berlin beetle

[a]ImmunoCAP®, Phadia/ThermoScientific and Siemens Healthcare, Freiburg, Germany
[b]ImmunoCAP® ISAC, Phadia/ThermoScientific and Siemens Healthcare, Freiburg, Germany
[c]3gAllergy™/Immulite, Siemens Healthcare, Eschborn, Germany
[d]ALLERG-O-LIQ®, Dr Fooke Laboratorien GmbH, Neuss, Germany
[e]Allergozyme®, Omega Diagnostics, Reinbek, Germany
[f]Allercoat™, EuroImmun, Lübeck, Germany

The red chironomid midge larvae (*Chironomus thummi thummi*) are popular as fishing bait and are known to trigger allergic respiratory symptoms in individuals working in fish food manufacture and in hobby-related aquarists (Baur and Liebers 1992). Their various hemoglobin components are recorded in the WHO/IUIS database as allergens Chi t 1–9.

The silverfish (*Lepisma saccharina*) is found primarily in kitchens, bathrooms, and cellars. In the case of high levels of infestation, allergens may be present in house dust. The tropomyosin Lep s 1 is the only known allergen to date. It exhibits cross-reactivity with tropomyosin of other arthropods, such as the house dust mite, the cockroach, and the shrimp (Barletta et al. 2005).

The multicolored Asian ladybug (*Harmonia axyridis*) was introduced in the USA between 1916 and 1990 to control aphids. Since then, ladybugs produce infestations, as they swarm out and invade houses and other buildings in their hundreds in order to hibernate. They have become a new and significant source of seasonal indoor allergens in the USA (Nakazawa et al. 2007). Extract-based diagnosis of ladybug allergy showed high cross-reactivity with cockroach extract (Nakazawa et al. 2007). Two major allergens have been identified to date: Har a 1 (10 kDa), a protein believed to be specific for ladybug sensitization, and Har a 2 (55 kDa), a protein related to the aldehyde dehydrogenase of the red flour beetle (Nakazawa et al. 2007).

Storage pests, such as the wheat weevil (*Sitophilus granarius*), the rice weevil (Kleine-Tebbe et al. 1992), the mealworm beetle (*Tenebrio molitor*), the confused flour beetle (*Tribolium confusum*), the Berlin beetle (*Trogoderma angustum*) (Kleine-Tebbe et al. 1983), and the Mediterranean flour moth (*Ephestia kuehniella*), have also been described as allergen sources (◉ Table 23.4). Since these storage pests are found primarily in stored grain, occupational groups such as farmers, bakers, millers, and grain storage workers are particularly affected and, depending on the duration of exposure, can develop allergic rhinitis and, eventually, bronchial asthma (Raulf et al. 2014). It has not been possible as yet to include any IgE-binding proteins from these sources in the WHO/IUIS allergen database.

23.6 Diagnostics and the Added Benefit of Molecular-Based Diagnosis

Routine diagnosis of the rarer allergies to arthropods is accomplished by means of skin testing or specific IgE antibody detection using extracts. At present, extracts from three cockroach species (*Periplaneta americana*, *Blatella germanica*, and *Blatta orientalis*), four storage mite species (*Lepidoglyphus destructor*, *Acarus siro*, *Glycyphagus domesticus*, and *Tyrophagus putrescentiae*), and a number of storage pests (*Sitophilus granarius*, *Tribolium confusum*, *Trogoderma angustum*, and *Ephestia kuehniella*) are available from a variety of manufacturers for in vitro diagnostic purposes. *Argas reflexus* extract from the pigeon tick is available only from Omega Diagnostics, Reinbeck, Germany. However, a clinical history can provide a strong indication of pigeon tick allergy: nighttime tick bite, typically during the warm months and in the vicinity of pigeon breeding sites. Allergen components

(Lep d 2, Bla g 1, Bla g 2, Bla g 5, and Bla g 7) are only available as yet in the ISAC test system (Thermo Scientific), but not in the ImmunoCAP system.

One advantage of molecular-based diagnostics (Matricardi et al. 2016) is that it employs standardized reagents, because both the protein and allergen content in commercial extracts vary, as previously demonstrated for cockroach extracts (Patterson and Slater 2002). The use of extracts also bears the risk of cross-reactivity with related arthropod species (Raulf et al. 2014). Since the IgE-binding profiles of patients vary not only on an individual but also on a geographic basis, the goal should be to make as complete a range of standardized allergens as possible available for diagnostic purposes (Barbosa et al. 2013; Matricardi et al. 2016).

23.7 Treatment and Diagnostic Outlook

Preparations for specific immunotherapy are currently available for storage mite allergy only in Germany. Studies on subcutaneous and sublingual immunotherapy of cockroach allergy are currently underway in the USA (Wood et al. 2014), and the results are promising.

Given that a variety of arthropod allergens (e.g., cockroach, tick, and storage mite) are already well characterized and for the most part available as recombinant molecules, the way has been paved for the development of IgE-based diagnostic tests using individual allergen components.

Conclusions

Although not well standardized, the available extracts permit IgE-based diagnosis of allergies to cockroaches, storage mites, and storage pests. A future broadening of IgE-based diagnostics with individual allergens would be beneficial.

An important goal for further developments in molecular testing systems should be the use of marker allergens for the unequivocal detection of sensitization and differentiation from cross-reactions. Marker allergens for tick sensitization, such as Arg r 1 from the pigeon tick, could be used to exclude pigeon tick allergy in cases of unexplained anaphylaxis.

References

An S, Chen L, Wei JF, et al. Purification and characterization of two new allergens from the venom of *Vespa magnifica*. PLoS One. 2012;7:e31920.

Arruda LK, Vailes LD, Platts-Mills TA, et al. Induction of IgE antibody responses by glutathione S-transferase from the German cockroach (*Blattella germanica*). J Biol Chem. 1997;272:20907–12.

Barbosa MC, Santos AB, Ferriani VP, et al. Efficacy of recombinant allergens for diagnosis of cockroach allergy in patients with asthma and/or rhinitis. Int Arch Allergy Immunol. 2013;161:213–9.

Barletta B, Butteroni C, Puggioni EM, et al. Immunological characterization of a recombinant tropomyosin from a new indoor source, *Lepisma saccharina*. Clin Exp Allergy. 2005;35:483–9.
Baur X, Liebers V. Insect hemoglobins (Chi tI) of the diptera family Chironomidae are relevant environmental, occupational, and hobby-related allergens. Int Arch Occup Environ Health. 1992;64:185–8.
Binder M, Mahler V, Hayek B, et al. Molecular and immunological characterization of arginine kinase from the Indianmeal moth, *Plodia interpunctella*, a novel cross-reactive invertebrate pan-allergen. J Immunol. 2001;167:5470–7.
Cohn RD, Arbes Jr SJ, Jaramillo R, et al. National prevalence and exposure risk for cockroach allergen in U.S. households. Environ Health Perspect. 2006;114:522–6.
Commins SP, James HR, Kelly LA, et al. The relevance of tick bites to the production of IgE antibodies to the mammalian oligosaccharide galactose-α-1,3-galactose. J Allergy Clin Immunol. 2011;127:1286–93.
Fan Y, Gore JC, Redding KO, Vailes LD, Chapman MD, Schal C. Tissue localization and regulation by juvenile hormone of human allergen Bla g 4 from the German cockroach, Blattella germanica (L.). Insect Mol Biol. 2005;14:45–53.
Fernández-Caldas E, Iraola V, Carnés J. Molecular and biochemical properties of storage mites (except Blomia species). Protein Pept Lett. 2007;14:954–9.
Franz JT, Masuch G, Müsken H, et al. Mite fauna of German farms. Allergy. 1997;52:1233–7.
Gruchalla RS, Pongracic J, Plaut M, et al. Inner City Asthma Study: relationships among sensitivity, allergen exposure, and asthma morbidity. J Allergy Clin Immunol. 2005;115:478–85.
Gustchina A, Li M, Wünschmann S, et al. Crystal structure of cockroach allergen Bla g 2, an unusual zinc binding aspartic protease with a novel mode of self-inhibition. J Mol Biol. 2005;348:433–44.
Heinzerling LM, Burbach GJ, Edenharter G, et al. GA(2)LEN skin test study I: GA(2)LEN harmonization of skin prick testing: novel sensitization patterns for inhalant allergens in Europe. Allergy. 2009;64:1498–506.
Hilger C, Bessot JC, Hutt N, et al. IgE-mediated anaphylaxis caused by bites of the pigeon tick *Argas reflexus*: cloning and expression of the major allergen Arg r 1. J Allergy Clin Immunol. 2005;115:617–22.
Hilger C, Kuehn A, Hentges F. Animal lipocalin allergens. Curr Allergy Asthma Rep. 2012;12:438–47.
Hindley J, Wünschmann S, Satinover SM, et al. Bla g 6: a troponin C allergen from *Blattella germanica* with IgE binding calcium dependence. J Allergy Clin Immunol. 2006;117:1389–95.
Hirsch T, Stappenbeck C, Neumeister V, et al. Exposure and allergic sensitization to cockroach allergen in East Germany. Clin Exp Allergy. 2000;30:529–37.
Jeong KY, Lee J, Lee IY, et al. Analysis of amino acid sequence variations and immunoglobulin E-binding epitopes of German cockroach tropomyosin. Clin Diagn Lab Immunol. 2004;11:874–8.
Jeong KY, Kim CR, Park J, et al. Identification of novel allergenic components from German cockroach fecal extract by a proteomic approach. Int Arch Allergy Immunol. 2013; 161:315–24.
Kleine-Tebbe J, Wahl R, Maasch HJ, et al. Histamine release studies in patients with positive Trogoderma-RAST. In: Serafin U, Errigo E, editors. Proceedings of the XII Congress of the European Academy of Allergology and Clinical Immunology (EAACI) Rome 1983. Firenze: O.I.C. Medical Press; 1983.
Kleine-Tebbe J, Jeep S, Josties C, Meysel U, O'Connor A, Kunkel G. IgE-mediated inhalant allergy in inhabitants of a building infested by the rice weevil (*Sitophilus oryzae*). Ann Allergy. 1992;69:497–504.
Kleine-Tebbe J, Heinatz A, Gräser I, et al. Bites of the European pigeon tick (*Argas reflexus*): risk of IgE-mediated sensitizations and anaphylactic reactions. J Allergy Clin Immunol. 2006;117:190–5.
Li M, Gustchina A, Alexandratos J, et al. Crystal structure of a dimerized cockroach allergen Bla g 2 complexed with a monoclonal antibody. J Biol Chem. 2008;283:22806–14.

Ma D, Li Y, Dong J, et al. Purification and characterization of two new allergens from the salivary glands of the horsefly, Tabanusyao. Allergy. 2011;66:101–9.
Matricardi PM, Kleine-Tebbe J, Hoffmann HJ, et al. EAACI molecular allergology user's guide. Pediatr Allergy Immunol. 2016;27(suppl23):1–250.
Matsui EC, Wood RA, Rand C, et al. Cockroach allergen exposure and sensitization in suburban middle-class children with asthma. J Allergy Clin Immunol. 2003;112:87–92.
Messer NG, Kendrick-Jones J. Molecular cloning and sequencing of the chicken smooth muscle myosin regulatory light chain. FEBS Lett. 1988;234:49–52.
Mindykowski B, Jaenicke E, Tenzer S, et al. Cockroach allergens Per a 3 are oligomers. Dev Comp Immunol. 2010;34:722–33.
Mueller GA, Pedersen LC, Lih FB, et al. The novel structure of the cockroach allergen Bla g 1 has implications for allergenicity and exposure assessment. J Allergy Clin Immunol. 2013;132:1420–6.
Mueller GA, Pedersen LC, Glesner J, et al. Analysis of glutathione S-transferase allergen cross-reactivity in a North American population: relevance for molecular diagnosis. J Allergy Clin Immunol. 2015;136:1369–77.
Nakazawa T, Satinover SM, Naccara L, et al. Asian ladybugs (Harmonia axyridis): a new seasonal indoor allergen. J Allergy Clin Immunol. 2007;119:421–7.
Patterson ML, Slater JE. Characterization and comparison of commercially available German and American cockroach allergen extracts. Clin Exp Allergy. 2002;32:721–7.
Pomés A. Cockroach and other inhalant insect allergens. In: Lockey RF, Ledford DK, editors. Allergens and allergen immunotherapy: subcutaneous, sublingual, and oral. 5th ed. New York: CRC Press/Taylor & Francis Group; 2014. p. 203–15.
Pomés A, Arruda LK. Investigating cockroach allergens: aiming to improve diagnosis and treatment of cockroach allergic patients. Methods. 2013;66:75–85.
Pomés A, Melén E, Vailes LD, et al. Novel allergen structures with tandem amino acid repeats derived from German and American cockroach. J Biol Chem. 1998;273:30801–7.
Raulf M, Bergmann KC, Kull S, Sander I, Hilger C, Brüning T, Jappe U, Müsken H, Sperl A, Vrtala S, Zahradnik E, Klimek L. Mites and other indoor allergens - from exposure to sensitization and treatment. Allergo J Int. 2015;24:68-80.
Raulf M, Sander I, Gonnissen D, et al. Schaben und Co. Die Rolle von Gesundheitsschädlingen als Allergenquelle. Bundesgesundheitsbl. 2014;57:585–92.
Sánchez-Borges M, SuárezChacón R, Capriles-Hulett A, et al. Anaphylaxis from ingestion of mites: pancake anaphylaxis. J Allergy Clin Immunol. 2013;131:31–5.
Santiago HC, LeeVan E, Bennuru S, et al. Molecular mimicry between cockroach and helminth glutathione S-transferases promotes cross-reactivity and cross-sensitization. J Allergy Clin Immunol. 2012;130:248–56.
Simons FE, Peng Z. Mosquito allergy: recombinant mosquito salivary antigens for new diagnostic tests. Int Arch Allergy Immunol. 2001;124:403–5.
Sohn MH, Kim KE. The cockroach and allergic diseases. Allergy Asthma Immunol Res. 2012;4:264–9.
Steinke JW, Platts-Mills TA, Commins SP. The alpha-gal story: lessons learned from connecting the dots. J Allergy Clin Immunol. 2015;135:589–96.
Suazo A, Gore C, Schal C. RNA interference-mediated knock-down of Bla g 1 in the German cockroach, *Blattella germanica* L., implicates this allergen-encoding gene in digestion and nutrient absorption. Insect Mol Biol. 2009;18:727–36.
Sudha VT, Arora N, Gaur SN, et al. Identification of a serine protease as a major allergen (Per a 10) of *Periplaneta americana*. Allergy. 2008;63:768–76.
Tan YW, Chan SL, Ong TC, et al. Structures of two major allergens, Bla g 4 and Per a 4, from cockroaches and their IgE binding epitopes. J Biol Chem. 2009;284:3148–57.
vanHage-Hamsten M, Johansson E. Clinical and immunologic aspects of storage mite allergy. Allergy. 1998;53:49–53.

Wang J, Calatroni A, Visness CM, et al. Correlation of specific IgE to shrimp with cockroach and dust mite exposure and sensitization in an inner-city population. J Allergy Clin Immunol. 2011;128:834–7.

Wood RA, Togias A, Wildfire J, et al. Development of cockroach immunotherapy by the Inner-City Asthma Consortium. J Allergy Clin Immunol. 2014;133:846–52.

Wünschmann S, Gustchina A, Chapman MD, et al. Cockroach allergen Bla g 2: an unusual aspartic proteinase. J Allergy Clin Immunol. 2005;116:140–5.

Yu CJ, Lin YF, Chiang BL, et al. Proteomics and immunological analysis of a novel shrimp allergen, Pen m 2. J Immunol. 2003;170:445–53.

Mold Allergens and Their Importance in Molecular Allergy Diagnosis

24

S. Kespohl and M. Raulf

24.1 Background

The aim of the present chapter is to give a comprehensive overview of the molecular allergy diagnosis for mold species based on the WHO/IUIS allergen database. In addition to providing information on the health risks posed by different fungal species, prominent mold allergen families are presented according to their biochemical function and in terms of the resulting probabilities of cross-reactions with fungi, as well as with other organisms. Moreover, the commercial availability and clinical relevance of recombinant single mold allergens are described.

This chapter is based on an article by Sabine Kespohl and Monika Raulf: "Mould allergens: Where do we stand with molecular allergy diagnostics?", published in *Allergo Journal International* (2014; 23: 120–125), which has been updated and extended for this book chapter.

The authors gratefully thank Emeritus Professor Robert K. Bush, MD (Madison, WI, USA), and Dr. Steve Love, PhD (Laguna Niguel, CA, USA), for reading the manuscript, for their helpful suggestions, and for their editorial assistance with the English translation.

S. Kespohl, PhD (✉)
Institute for Prevention and Occupational Medicine of the German Social Accident Insurance, Institute of the Ruhr-Universität Bochum (IPA), Bochum, Germany
e-mail: kespohl@ipa-dguv.de

M. Raulf, PhD, Prof.
Center Allergology/Immunology, Institute for Prevention and Occupational Medicine of the German Social Accident Insurance, Institute of the Ruhr-Universität Bochum, Bochum, Germany
e-mail: raulf@ipa-dguv.de

J. Kleine-Tebbe, T. Jakob (eds.), *Molecular Allergy Diagnostics*,
DOI 10.1007/978-3-319-42499-6_24

24.2 Classification of Fungal Allergens

Out of more than 100,000 known fungal species, approximately 400 organisms are listed as potential and/or identified sources for allergy at ▶ www.allergome.org. The WHO/IUIS allergen database is currently compiled from 111 fungal allergens originating from 29 fungal species (www.allergen.org).

Phylogenetically, mold species belong to the sac fungi (*Ascomycota*) or *Zygomycota*; however, pileated mushrooms (*Basidiomycota*) can also induce IgE-mediated allergies. Known fungal species that induce allergies are shown in ⊙ Fig. 24.1.

Among *Ascomycota,* 86 single allergens originating from ten fungal genera are currently categorized according to the WHO/IUIS criteria. Twenty-three allergens from five fungal genera have been identified among *Basidiomycota* (⊙ Fig. 24.1). Of these, ten single allergens belong to *Malassezia sympodialis* and three to *Malassezia furfur*. Among *Zygomycota*, two single allergens are currently listed in the WHO/IUIS database, and these come from *Rhizopus orycae*.

Medical mycologists differentiate fungal species independently of their systematic taxonomy, into dermatophytes, yeasts, and molds:

- *Dermatophytes* include the clinically relevant fungal species *Microsporum, Trichophyton*, and *Epidermatophyton*.
- Among yeasts, the genera *Candida* (noted as of controversial relevance) and *Malassezia* are relevant for clinical allergology.
- The term *mold* includes all fungal species of *Ascomycota* (excluding *Trichophyton* and *Candida*), plus *Rhizopus orycea* from *Zygomycota* (⊙ Fig. 24.2).

24.3 Mold Exposure and Health Risks

Several species of fungi are part of our natural environment and our daily life. While mushrooms grow and stay mostly on solid ground, releasing only mature spores into the air, mold and yeast fragments and/or spores are small enough to become airborne. As a result, mold exposure can occur almost anywhere. About 200 varieties of fungi are found in both indoor and outdoor air in Europe. The frequency and concentration of different types of mold in the atmosphere vary seasonally, especially for *Alternaria,* where the highest exposures occur during May to August in Southern Europe and July to September in Northern Europe (Canova et al. 2013). Exposure to *Aspergillus, Cladosporium*, and *Penicillium* is generally higher in autumn. A measure of the total amount of spores in ambient air (colony-forming units [cfu]/m^3; indoor as well as outdoor), indicated that, on average, spores from *Cladosporium* were usually present at a level that was eight times higher than the number of spores measured for *Alternaria* and *Aspergillus*, and four times more than *Penicillium* (de Ana et al. 2006). In general, no significant difference was found between the numbers of indoor versus outdoor spores, with the exception of *Alternaria*, where a clear outdoor bias was shown.

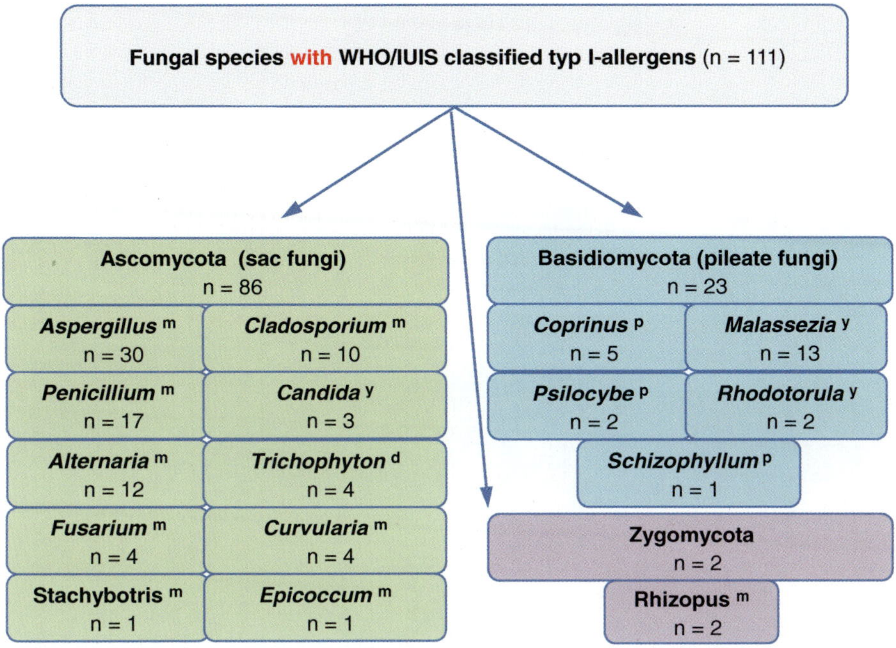

Fig. 24.1 Fungal species with World Health Organization/International Union of Immunological Societies (WHO/IUIS)-classified type-I allergens ([d] dermatophyte, [y] yeast, [m] mold, [p] (pileate-) fungi/mushroom. n: number of identified fungal allergens); adapted from www.allergen.org, 03.11.2015

Health risks posed by mold exposure include infectious diseases (especially in immunocompromised patients), odor nuisance from volatile organic compounds (VOCs), irritative and/or toxic effects such as organic dust toxic syndrome (ODTS) and mucous membrane irritation syndrome (MMIS), as well as sensitization and allergic symptoms. Nevertheless, although several thousand mold spores can be measured in standard airborne samples, the rates of sensitization to either indoor (e.g., *Aspergillus*, *Penicillium*) or outdoor molds (e.g., *Cladosporium*, *Alternaria*) are below 5 % (according to Haftenberger et al. 2013; Heinzerling et al. 2009; Schmitz et al. 2013; and Sennekamp et al. 2015). In other words, molds appear not to be the dominant allergen source in the majority of subjects with sensitization to environmental allergens. In some instances of very high mold exposure (e.g., after thunderstorms), high levels of fungal spores in the atmosphere are associated with an increased number and/or exacerbation of asthma attacks.

A different situation in regard to mold sensitization prevalence is seen among allergic or asthmatic subjects (Crameri et al. 2014). Here, rates are considerably higher than in the general population. A brief overview of mold sensitization summarized from different studies is given in ⊙ Table 24.1.

The data presented in ⊙ Table 24.1 include data for groups of subjects varying in age and status of clinically relevant allergy and testing procedures (e.g. skin prick testing versus specific IgE determination). In the general population, although rates

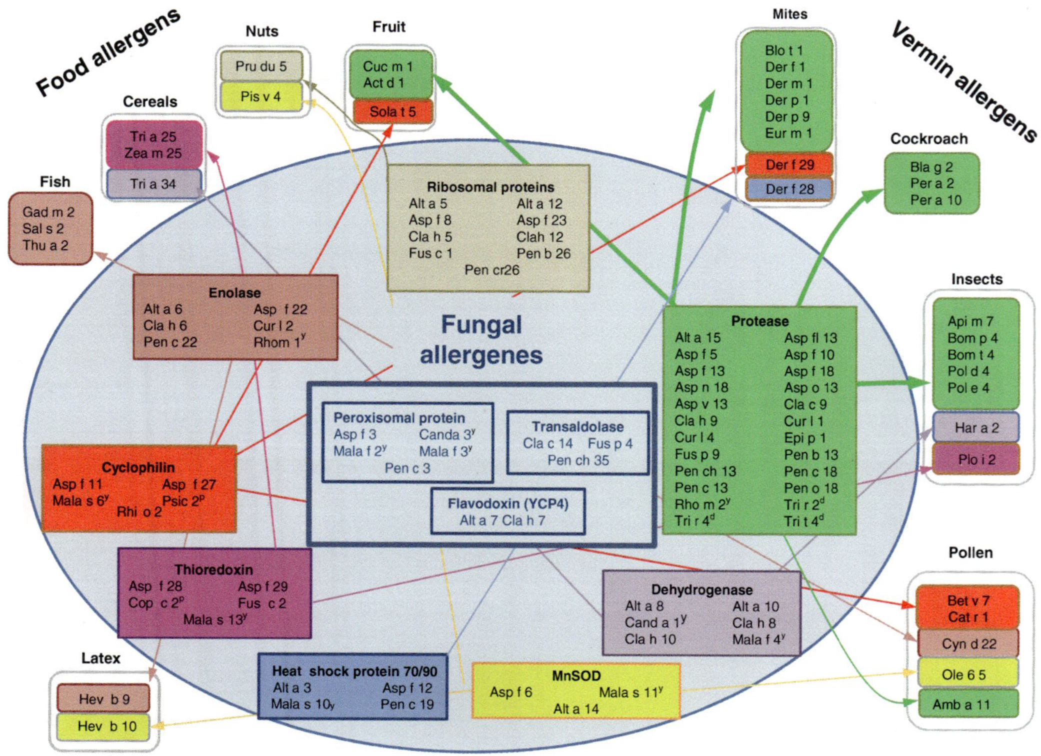

Fig. 24.2 Prominent mold allergen families with established/potential cross-reactions to other allergens. Mold allergen families (colored or clear boxes) on the blue background are known cross-reactive allergens in fungi. Outside the blue background are homologs/cross-reactive allergens in non-fungal organisms. To date, three protein families – peroxisomal protein, transaldolase, and flavodoxin (clear boxes on the blue background) – have been exclusively identified in fungi. *y* Yeast, *d* dermatophyte, *p* pileated mushroom

Table 24.1 Prevalence of mold sensitization among different groups

Molds	General population [%]	Patient group with allergic symptoms [%]	Asthmatic group [%]
Alternaria	13 % (Arbes et al. 2005); 3–4 % (Haftenberger et al. 2013); 2–13 % (Salo et al. 2014); 5 % (Szewzyk et al. 2011)	10 % (D'Amato et al. 1997); 8–10 % (Heinzerling et al. 2009); 3 % (Toppila-Salmi et al. 2015)	22 % (O'Driscoll et al. 2009); 6 % (Toppila-Salmi et al. 2015)
Aspergillus	2–3 % (Haftenberger et al. 2013); 3–10 % (Salo et al. 2014); 3 % (Szewzyk et al. 2011)	4–5 % (Heinzerling et al. 2009); 3 % (Toppila-Salmi et al. 2015)	33–44 % (Maturu and Agarwal 2015); 45 % (O'Driscoll et al. 2009); 11 % (Toppila-Salmi et al. 2015)
Cladosporium	8 % (Gent et al. 2012); 1–2 % (Haftenberger et al. 2013); 2 % (Szewzyk et al. 2011);	5 % (D'Amato et al. 1997); 4–6 % (Heinzerling et al. 2009); 2 % (Toppila-Salmi et al. 2015)	24 % (O'Driscoll et al. 2009); 4 % (Toppila-Salmi et al. 2015)
Penicillium	8 % (Gent et al. 2012); 5 % (Szewzyk et al. 2011)	–	29 % (O'Driscoll et al. 2009)

of mold sensitization are lower than rates of sensitization to other environmental allergens, subjects with asthma displayed high sensitization rates to different mold species. In particular, *Aspergillus* species seemed to be particularly important in subjects with severe asthma with fungal sensitization (SAFS) (O'Driscoll et al. 2009). Other studies have shown *Alternaria alternata* to be involved in the development and severity of asthma and allergic rhinitis (reviewed by Fukutomi and Taniguchi; 2015).

As well as IgE-based type-I allergic reactions to molds (mostly allergic rhinoconjunctivitis and SAFS), other types of allergy are also known.

Severe symptoms observed in ABPA are based on a mixed form of type-I and type-III allergic reactions, and occasionally type-IV allergy. ABPA is usually caused by the colonization of *Aspergillus fumigatus* in pulmonary tissue. This colonization is possible because *Aspergillus fumigatus*. is thermo-tolerant, and thus is capable of growing at human body temperature. Furthermore, its small spore size enables its passage to the terminal airways (Fukutomi and Taniguchi 2015), where spores can germinate. Other mold species with comparable growing conditions and small spore size are also potential sources of mycoses that can result in allergic bronchopulmonary mycoses (ABPM). Patients suffering from ABPM are often immunodeficient, a condition that is also present in approximately 1–2 % of asthma patients and 2–15 % of patients with cystic fibrosis (Agarwal 2009). Increased levels of specific IgE (sIgE; especially against the single Asp f allergen pattern) and sIgG against *Aspergillus fumigatus* are typically found on serological analysis and should be considered in the diagnosis of ABPM.

Another mold-induced disease that occurs in terminal lung tissue is hypersensitivity pneumonitis (HP) or extrinsic allergic alveolitis (EAA). In contrast to classical type-I allergic reactions, HP does not involve sIgE, but involves sIgG (type-III allergy), which induces immune reactions by antigen-IgG-complexes as well as by cellular components, depending on the status of the disease (acute versus chronic). Therefore, the determination of sIgG levels is a useful tool in the diagnosis of HP (Sennekamp et al. 2015).

To find the optimal therapy for patients with severe bronchial diseases such as asthma, it is important to know whether these patients also suffer from mold invasion, so as to decide whether antifungal medication can be helpful (Knutsen et al. 2012).

Monitoring mold exposure in chronically damp houses or workplaces is generally conducted by measuring vital mold fragments (colony-forming units; cfu) in airborne samples, dust, surface samples, or material samples. In general, culturing methods are only able to determine viable fungal spores that can grow under given culture conditions; however, these spores are not representative of all fungal fragments.

Viable spores, as well as non-viable spores and other mold fragments, contain allergens and are potential sensitizers. Consequently, if mold allergen monitoring considers only viable spores (cfu), the actual mold allergen load would be inaccurate.

To improve mold allergen monitoring, it would be necessary to assess mold allergen content directly in the collected samples using standardized test systems against single mold allergens, such as Alt a 1 from *Alternaria alternata* or Asp f 1 from *Aspergillus fumigatus.* Aeroallergen exposure assessment requires suitable strategies for monitoring exposure; that is, the use of sensitive and validated test systems. Immunoassays based on monoclonal or polyclonal antibodies are recommended for mold allergen quantification (Raulf et al. 2014). For a few mold species, quantification tools based on polyclonal antibodies against crude mold extracts are available (Sander et al. 2012). A comprehensive overview of mold exposure has been conducted by Eduard (2009) and is recommended reading.

24.4 Mold Allergens Belong to Various Protein Families, Most Often with Enzymatic Function in the Organism

Currently, 111 fungal allergens are listed in the official IUIS database (www.allergen.org). Of these, 81 are derived from mold species (*Ascomycota,* excluding yeast and dermatophytes and *Zygomycota*). A further 30 allergens have been identified among *Basidiomycota* (pileated mushrooms), yeasts ([y]), and dermatophytes ([d]). Fungal allergens can be distinguished from typical allergen families, such as those originating from pollen, food, or animals. The most prominent fungal allergen families are:

- Proteases ($n=24$: 20 mold, 1 yeast[(y)], 3 dermatophyte[(d)])
- Ribosomal proteins ($n=9$: all mold)
- Enolases ($n=6$: 5 mold, 1 yeast[(y)])
- Dehydrogenases ($n=6$: 4 mold, 2 yeast[(y)])
- Thioredoxins ($n=5$: 3 mold, 1 yeast[(y)], 1 mushroom[(p)])
- Heat shock proteins (HSP 70/90) ($n=4$: 3 mold, 1 yeast[(y)])

- Peroxisomal membrane proteins ($n=5$: 2 mold, 3 yeast[(y)])
- Manganese-dependent superoxide dismutases (MnSOD) ($n=3$: 2 mold, 1 yeast[(y)])
- Cyclophilins ($n=5$: 3 mold [including one *Rhizopus* allergen from *Zygomycota*], 1 yeast[(y)], 1 mushroom[(p)])
- Transaldolases ($n=3$: all mold)
- Flavodoxins (YCP4) ($n=2$: both mold).

Based on conserved protein regions, the biochemical functions of these allergens, in addition to their potential cross-reactions with other fungal and non-fungal allergens, were observed or postulated, as shown in ⦿ Fig. 24.2.

24.4.1 Proteases

More than 50 % (24 of 41) of the WHO/IUIS-classified allergen proteases can be found in molds. Of these 24 mold proteases, 21 (88 %) are serine proteases and represent the most characteristic mold allergen family. Unfortunately, none of these mold proteases are available yet for diagnostic purposes. Cross-reactions were described for alkaline, as well as for vacuolar, serine proteases among. Aspergillus and Penicillium Species (group 13 and 18 allergens of Asp f, Asp fl, penicillium (Pen) b, Pen c, Pen ch, and Pen o) on the basis of positive sIgE in 20–80 % of mold-sensitized subjects (Simon-Nobbe et al. 2008).

24.4.2 Ribosomal Proteins

Nine of the ten ribosomal proteins (90 %) identified as allergens occur in mold species. The ribosomal proteins are located in the cytoplasm and, together with rRNA, build the 60S-subunit of the ribosomes. Cross-reactive structures exist and are most probably based on sequence homology (Achatz et al. 1995; Mayer et al. 1999). A sensitization prevalence of 35 % to ribosomal mold allergens Fus c 1 was found in *Fusarium*-allergic subjects (Simon-Nobbe et al. 2008).

24.4.3 Enolases

The enolase protein family comprises 11 allergens, of which 5 were identified in mold, 1 in yeast, 3 in fish, and 2 in plants. Cross-reactions are described among enolase, Alt a 6, Cla h 6 , and Hev b 9 (Wagner et al. 2000), as well as among Asp f 22 and Pen c 22 (Lai et al. 2002). A sensitization prevalence of 20–30 % to enolases was detected of in mold-sensitized subjects (Simon-Nobbe et al. 2008).

24.4.4 Dehydrogenases

Four of the eight allergens classified as dehydrogenases (which oxidize proteins by transferring a anion to reductive moieties such as (NAD) nicotinamide adenine dinucleotide or (FAD) flavin adenine dinucleotide), are found in molds. Here, cross-reactivity between Cla h 8 and Alt a 8 has been shown (Schneider et al. 2006). The rate of sensitization against mold dehydrogenases among mold-sensitized subjects was 40–50 % (Simon-Nobbe et al. 2008).

24.4.5 Thioredoxins

Thioredoxins are small proteins consisting of about 100 amino acids. They are redox proteins that support the reduction of other proteins and are therefore essential in many biochemical processes in animal and plant cells. Three of the eight characterized thioredoxins are derived from molds. About 50 % of patients allergic to *Fusarium* had specific IgE against thioredoxin Fus c 2 (Simon-Nobbe et al. 2008).

24.4.6 Heat Shock Proteins

Heat shock proteins (HSP 70/90) or their molecular chaperones facilitate protein folding and stabilize secondary protein structure in all organisms. Prominent representatives of IgE-binding chaperones are Alt a 3 and Pen c 19 (HSP-70), with 41 % sensitization prevalence for Pen c 19 and 5 % for recombinant Alt a 3 in mold-sensitized subjects (Simon-Nobbe et al. 2008).

24.4.7 Peroxisomal Membrane Proteins

To date, five peroxisomal membrane proteins have been described as allergens in fungi, two in mold and three in yeast. In particular, mold allergen Asp f 3 demonstrated high sIgE-binding rates, of 32–100 %, in *Aspergillus*-sensitized subjects (Simon-Nobbe et al. 2008).

24.4.8 MnSODs

Three fungal allergens are MnSODs. Cross-reactivity was confirmed in sIgE-inhibition studies between the two mold allergens, Asp f 6 and Alt a 14. Rates of sensitization were between 63% and 70 % in the investigated patient groups (ABPA and cystic fibrosis; Simon-Nobbe et al. 2008).

24.4.9 Flavodoxins

Flavodoxins and flavodoxin-like proteins (YCP4-homologs) are gene-regulatory proteins that are expressed in the late phases of mold and yeast development. Among molds, Alt a 7 and Cla h 7 display flavodoxin properties, but with only minor sIgE-binding potency of 7–22 % in mold-sensitized patients (Simon-Nobbe et al. 2008).

24.4.10 Cyclophilins

Cyclophilins, also known as peptidyl-prolyl isomerases, are located in the cell cytoplasm and have been identified as allergens in mold and pollen. Mold Asp f 11 was ascertained as the major allergen in *Aspergillus*-sensitized subjects (90 % sensitization rate); in patients with atopic dermatitis, Mala a 6 sensitization rates ranged from 21% to 25 % (Simon-Nobbe et al. 2008).

Manganese superoxide dismutase allergens (Asp f 6, Mala s 11, latex Hevea (Hev) b 10 and Pis v 4, a food allergen from pistachio) were analyzed with respect to cross-reactivity based on homologous peptide sequences. The results indicated high peptide sequence concordance within plant allergens (83 % identity between pistachio Pis v 4 and latex Hev b 10) and fungal allergens (56 % identity between mold Asp f 6 and yeast Mala s 11). Further studies are necessary to determine whether homology could be an indicator of polysensitization to fungal and plant material.

24.5 Commercially Available Single Allergens Originating from Mold

Thirty to forty mold extracts for skin testing or serological testing of IgE-mediated allergy are currently available (data from Germany), but standardization is still a challenge. Comparison of mold test solutions from different manufacturers showed heterogeneous protein content, despite supposedly identical allergen sources (Kespohl et al. 2013). This might be one reason for the discrepancy between skin test results and serological IgE measurements.

The concordance between skin tests and serological tests can be less than 30 % depending on the mold species (O'Driscoll et al. 2009). A current study (Kespohl et al. 2016) showed that the antigen content of skin prick test solutions was positively associated with the concordant skin prick test, as well as with sIgE.

Although numerous fungal allergens have been identified, only eight single mold allergens from three mold genera are actually available for molecular diagnosis. These eight allergens cover the species *Alternaria alternata*, *Aspergillus fumigatus*, and *Cladosporium herbarum* (⦿ Table 24.2). Additionally, two other mold proteins are available. The first is Asp o 21, an alpha-amylase from *Aspergillus niger,* used as an enzyme in commercial bakery; this protein is a useful tool for studying occupational allergy in bakers. The other single mold component is mitogillin from *Aspergillus restrictus* (believed to be Asp r 1), which is not yet registered in the WHO/IUIS database.

- **rAlt a 1** is available in different test systems (ImmunoCAP and ISAC Allergen Chip; both from Thermo Scientific, Phadia AB, Uppsala, Sweden). Up to 98 % of IgE-mediated sensitizations to *Alternaria* can be detected by testing rAlt a 1, which makes this single allergen valuable for the standardization of test extracts

Table 24.2 Commercially available single mold allergens for specific immunoglobulin (Ig)E diagnosis

Allergen	Mold species	Test system	Allergen family
Recombinant (r)Alt a 1	*Alternaria alternata*	ImmunoCAP, ImmunoCAP ISAC	Protein without known function
rAlt a 6	*Alternaria alternata*	ImmunoCAP ISAC	Enolase
rAsp f 1	*Aspergillus fumigatus*	ImmunoCAP, ImmunoCAP ISAC	Mitogillin
rAsp f 2	*Aspergillus fumigatus*	ImmunoCAP	Fibrinogen binding protein
rAsp f 3	*Aspergillus fumigatus*	ImmunoCAP, ImmunoCAP ISAC	Peroxisomal protein
rAsp f 4	*Aspergillus fumigatus*	ImmunoCAP	Protein without known function
rAsp f 6	*Aspergillus fumigatus*	ImmunoCAP, ImmunoCAP ISAC	Manganese-dependent superoxide dismutases (MnSOD)
rCla h 8	*Cladosporium herbarum*	ImmunoCAP ISAC	Dehydrogenase
Native (n)Asp o 21 [a]	*Aspergillus oryzae*	ImmunoCAP, IMMULITE	α-Amylase
nAsp r 1 [b]	(*Aspergillus restrictus*)	IMMULITE	Mitogillin

[a]Baking enzyme: not a typical test allergen for mold sensitization
[b]Not WHO/IUIS-listed

(Simon-Nobbe et al. 2008). Alt a 1 is an acidic glycoprotein without known biochemical function and is expressed in *Alternaria* cell cultures, but not before 21–30 days in culture. The unique protein structure, a butterfly-like dimer, was exclusively found among mold proteins (Chruszcz et al. 2012). Alt a 1 homologs have been identified in Pleosporaceae genera: *Biopolaris*, *Curvularia, Pithomyces, Stemphylium, Ulocladium, Spondylocladium, Crivellia, Embellisia, Nimbya,* and *Sinomyces* (www.allergome.org). However, Alt a 1 homologs have not yet been detected in mold genera such as *Aspergillus, Penicillium,* or *Cladosporium.*

- **rAlt a 6** (enolase) can be tested only on an ImmunoCAP ISAC Allergen Chip. Alt a 6 is a minor allergen in *Alternaria alternata*-sensitized patients, with sensitization rates of 15–22 % in this cohort (Unger et al. 1999). Enolases have also been described as allergens in other mold species, such as *Cladosporium*, *Aspergilus,* and *Penicillium*, as well as in fish food (Gadus (Gad) m 2, Salmo (Sal) s 2, Thinnies (Thu) a 2) and natural rubber latex (Hev b 9). Based on the known sequence homology, cross-reactions between these allergens are likely. To date, IgE-cross-reactions for rHev b 9, rAlt a 6, and rCla h 6 have been shown by inhibition studies (Simon-Nobbe et al. 2008).
- rAsp f 1, 2, 3, 4, and 6 are available as single allergens in the ImmunoCAP system, and rAsp f 1, 3, and 6 are available on the ImmunoCAP ISAC Allergen Chip. A typical major allergen, comparable to Alt a 1 in *Alternaria*, is missing in *Aspergillus fumigatus,* as well as in all other mold species. Nevertheless, molecular allergy diagnosis with recombinant *A. fumigatus* single allergens (rAsp f) is

a valuable tool in the documentation of ABPA (Kurup et al. 2000). In the serum of patients with clinically verified ABPA, sIgE to rAsp f 2, rAsp f 4, and rAsp f 6 was frequently found. This single allergen pattern was significant in patients with ABPA compared with patterns in asthmatics or mold-sensitized patients. In contrast, the single allergens rAsp f 1 and rAsp f 3 were detected in ABPA patients, as well as in asthmatics and mold-sensitized patients. To discriminate between ABPA and allergic asthma, only the combination of rAsp f 2+rAsp f 4+rAsp f 6 seems to be definitive, whereas sensitization to rAsp f 1 and/or rAsp f 3 was not definitive for allergic asthma. Serologically positive results for recombinant Asp f single allergens can be observed in, for example, patients with cystic fibrosis or other chronic lung diseases.
- rCla h 8 (dehydrogenase) is obtainable only on the ImmunoCAP ISAC Allergen Chip. The sensitization prevalence to Cla h 8 is about 57 % among *Cladosporium herbarum*-sensitized subjects (Simon-Nobbe et al. 2008). Cross-reactions to other mold dehydrogenases were described for Alt a 8 from *Alternaria alternata* (Simon-Nobbe et al. 2008). Further potential (based on peptide sequence homology), but unproven cross-reactions can be expected for the dehydrogenase Har a 2 from Asian lady bugs (*Harmonia axyridis*) and for Tri a 34 from wheat flour (*Tritium aestivum*).

The two commercially available single-allergen components, nAsp o 21 and nAsp r 1, are not frequently used for the molecular diagnosis of mold sensitization (as noted above).

- nAsp o 21 is an α-amylase offered by the 3 g Allergy IMMULITE System (Siemens Healthcare Diagnostics, Tarrytown, NY, USA) and by the ImmunoCAP system. Asp o 21 is most relevant in subjects with baker's asthma due to occupational exposure to baking enzymes, but is not relevant in mold-sensitized subjects. Therefore, nAsp o 21 is generally included in the baker's asthma allergen panel.
- nAsp r 1, a mitogillin, is supplied by the 3 g Allergy IMMULITE System. The mitogillin protein family has sequential homology to ribonucleases from totally unrelated species such as birch pollen Betula (Bet) v 1, but also to Asp f1. There are, as yet, no published data on sensitization rates to nAsp r 1.

24.5.1 Specific IgG Tests

Specific IgG testing against mold antigens; for example, to verify HP, can be conducted only with crude mold extracts. Standardized assessment criteria, such as defined cut-off values, are currently being developed.

24.6 Outlook

There is a high demand for the improvement of mold allergy diagnosis using single allergen components (Matricardi et al. 2016), especially specific mold marker allergens. Mold serine proteases, such as Asp f 13 and Cla h 9, as well as single allergens from the ribosomal protein family; for example, Alt a 5/Cla h 5 and Alt a 12/Cla h 12, would be good candidates.

Crude mold extracts must be standardized to ensure accuracy in mold allergy diagnosis. This applies to skin and serological test extracts, as well as to solutions used for for immunotherapy. One improvement in this regard would be a defined allergen content in test solutions. However, the opposite of standardization can actually be observed. Formalities of the European Union (EU) directive 2001/83/EC, article 1(4b), defined test allergen solutions as pharmaceutical products; in other words, allergen test solutions need the same approval procedure as pharmaceutical products, making their development very work- and cost-intensive. As a result, less relevant allergen solutions, such as mold solutions, have been continuously disappearing from the panel of commercially available test solutions, thereby reducing the variety of available mold allergens. Future improvements in this regard are urgently needed to solve this problem on behalf of inadequately diagnosed and treated patients.

24.7 Conclusions for Routine Clinical Practice

Component resolved diagnosis for mold allergy based on single allergens is actually only applicable for the species *Alternaria alternata* and *Aspergillus fumigatus*, and in part for *Cladosporium herbarum*. Sensitization testing for other species must still be conducted with crude extracts.

References

Achatz G, Oberkofler H, Lechenauer E, Simon B, Unger A, Kandler D, Ebner C, Prillinger H, Kraft D, Breitenbach M. Molecular cloning of major and minor allergens of Alternaria alternata and Cladosporium herbarum. Mol Immunol. 1995;32:213–27.

Agarwal R. Allergic bronchopulmonary aspergillosis. Chest. 2009;135:805–26.

Arbes Jr SJ, Gergen PJ, Elliott L, Zeldin DC. Prevalences of positive skin test responses to 10 common allergens in the UA population: results from the third National Health and Nutrition Examination Survey. J Allergy ClinImmunol. 2005;116:377–83.

Canova C, Anto JM, Heinrich J, Anton JM, Leynaert B, Smith M, Kuenzli N, Zock JP, Janson C, Cerveri I, de Marco R, Toren K, Gislason T, Nowak D, Pin I, Wjst M, Manfreda J, Svanes C, Crane J, Abramson M, Burr M, Burney P, Jarvis D. The influence of sensitisation to pollens and moulds on seasonal variations in asthma attacks. Eur Respir J. 2013;42:935–45.

Chruszcz M, Chapman MD, Osinski T, Solberg R, Demas M, Porebski PJ, Majorek KA, Pomés A, Minor W. Alternaria alternata allergen Alt a 1: a unique β-barrel protein dimer found exclusively in fungi. J Allergy ClinImmunol. 2012;130:241–7.

Crameri R, Garbani M, Rhyner C, Huitema C. Fungi: the neglected allergenic sources. Allergy. 2014;69:176–85.

D'Amato G, Chatzigeorgiou G, Corsico R, Gioulekas D, Jäger L, Jäger S, Kontou-Fili K, Kouridakis S, Liccardi G, Meriggi A, Palma-Carlos A, Palma-Carlos ML, Pagan Aleman A, Parmiani S, Puccinelli P, Russo M, Spieksma FT, Torricelli R, Wüthrich B. Evaluation of the prevalence of skin prick test positivity to Alternaria and Cladosporium in patients with suspected respiratory allergy. A European multicenter study promoted by the Subcommittee on

Aerobiology and Environmental Aspects of Inhalant Allergens of the European Academy of Allergology and Clinical Immunology. Allergy. 1997;52:711–6.

de Ana SG, Torres-Rodríguez JM, Ramírez EA, García SM, Belmonte-Soler J. Seasonal distribution of Alternaria, Aspergillus, Cladosporium and Penicillium species isolated in homes of fungal allergic patients. J Investig Allergol Clin. 2006;16:357–63.

Eduard W. Fungal spores: a critical review of the toxicological and epidemiological evidence as a basis for occupational exposure limit setting. Crit Rev Toxicol. 2009;39:799–864.

Fukutomi Y, Taniguchi M. Sensitization to fungal allergens: resolved and unresolved issues. Allergol Int. 2015;64:321–31.

Gent JF, Kezik JM, Hill ME, Tsai E, Li DW, Leaderer BP. Household mold and dust allergens: exposure, sensitization and childhood asthma morbidity. Environ Res. 2012;118:86–93.

Haftenberger M, Laußmann D, Ellert U, Kalcklösch M, Langen U, Schlaud M, Schmitz R, Thamm M. Prävalenz von Sensibilisierungen gegen Inhalations- und Nahrungsmittelallergene – Ergebnisse der Studie zur Gesundheit Erwachsener in Deutschland (DEGS1). Bundesgesundheitsblatt. 2013;56:687–97.

Heinzerling LM, Burbach GJ, Edenharter G, Bachert C, Bindslev-Jensen C, Bonini S, Bousquet J, Bousquet-Rouanet L, Bousquet PJ, Bresciani M, Bruno A, Burney P, Canonica GW, Darsow U, Demoly P, Durham S, Fokkens WJ, Giavi S, Gjomarkaj M, Gramiccioni C, Haahtela T, Kowalski ML, Magyar P, Muraközi G, Orosz M, Papadopoulos NG, Röhnelt C, Stingl G, Todo-Bom A, von Mutius E, Wiesner A, Wöhrl S, Zuberbier T. GA(2)LEN skin test study I: GA(2)LEN harmonization of skin prick testing: novel sensitization patterns for inhalant allergens in Europe. Allergy. 2009;64:1498–506.

Kespohl S, Maryska S, Zahradnik E, Sander I, Brüning T, Raulf-Heimsoth M. Biochemical and immunological analysis of mould skin prick test solution: current status of standardization. Clin Exp Allergy. 2013;43:1286–96.

Kespohl S, Maryska S, Bünger J, Hagemeyer O, Jakob T, Joest M, Knecht R, Koschel D, Kotschy-Lang N, Merget R, Mülleneisen NK, Rabe U, Röseler S, Sander I, Stollewerk D, Straube H, Ulmer HM, van Kampen V, Walusiak-Skorupa J, Wiszniewska M, Wurpts G, Brüning T, Raulf M. How to diagnose mould allergy? Comparison of skin prick tests with specific IgE results. Clin Exp Allergy. 2016;46:981–91.

Knutsen AP, Bush RK, Demain JG, Denning DW, Dixit A, Fairs A, Greenberger PA, Kariuki B, Kita H, Kurup VP, Moss RB, Niven RM, Pashley CH, Slavin RG, Vijay HM, Wardlaw AJ. Fungi and allergic lower respiratory tract diseases. J Allergy Clin Immunol. 2012;129:280–91.

Kurup VP, Banerjee B, Hemmann S, Greenberger PA, Blaser K, Crameri R. Selected recombinant Aspergillus fumigatus allergens bind specifically to IgE in ABPA. Clin Exp Allergy. 2000;30:988–93.

Lai HY, Tam MF, Tang RB, Chou H, Chang CY, Tsai JJ, Shen HD. cDNA cloning and immunological characterization of a newly identified enolase allergen from Penicillium citrinum and Aspergillus fumigatus. Int Arch Allergy Immunol. 2002;121:181–90.

Matricardi PM, Kleine-Tebbe J, Hoffmann HJ, Valenta R, Hilger C, Hofmaier S, Aalberse RC, Agache I, Asero R, Ballmer-Weber B, Barber D, Beyer K, Biedermann T, Biló MB, Blank S, Bohle B, Bosshard PP, Breiteneder H, Brough HA, Caraballo L, Caubet JC, Crameri R, Davies JM, Douladiris N, Ebisawa M, Eigenmann PA, Fernandez-Rivas M, Ferreira F, Gadermaier G, Glatz M, Hamilton RG, Hawranek T, Hellings P, Hoffmann-Sommergruber K, Jakob T, Jappe U, Jutel M, Kamath SD, Knol EF, Korosec P, Kuehn A, Lack G, Lopata AL, Mäkelä M, Morisset M, Niederberger V, Nowak-Wezgrzyn AH, Papadopoulos NG, Pastorello EA, Pauli G, Platts-Mills T, Posa D, Poulsen LK, Raulf M, Sastre J, Scala E, Schmid JM, Schmid-Grendelmeier P, van Hage M, van Ree R, Vieths S, Weber R, Wickman M, Muraro A, Ollert M. EAACI molecular allergology user's guide. Pediatr Allergy Immunol. 2016;27(suppl23):1–250.

Maturu VN, Agarwal R. Prevalence of Aspergillus sensitization and allergic bronchopulmonary aspergillosis in cystic fibrosis: systematic review and meta-analysis. Clin Exp Allergy. 2015;45:1765–78.

Mayer C, Appenzeller U, Seelbach H, Achatz G, Oberkofler H, Breitenbach M, Blaser K, Crameri R. Humoral and cell-mediated autoimmune reactions to human acidic ribosomal P2 protein in individuals sensitized to Aspergillus fumigatus P2 protein. J Exp Med. 1999;189:1507–12.

O'Driscoll BR, Powell G, Chew F, Niven RM, Miles JF, Vyas A, Denning DW. Comparison of skin prick tests with specific serum immunoglobulin E in the diagnosis of fungal sensitization in patients with severe asthma. Clin Exp Allergy. 2009;39:1677–83.

Raulf M, Buters J, Chapman M, Cecchi L, de Blay F, Doekes G, Eduard W, Heederik D, Jeebhay MF, Kespohl S, Krop E, Moscato G, Pala G, Quirce S, Sander I, Schlünssen V, Sigsgaard T, Walusiak-Skorupa J, Wiszniewska M, Wouters IM, Annesi-Maesano I. Monitoring of occupational and environmental aeroallergens-- EAACI Position Paper. Concerted action of the EAACI IG Occupational Allergy and Aerobiology & Air Pollution. Allergy. 2014;69:1280–99.

Salo PM, Arbes Jr SJ, Jaramillo R, Calatroni A, Weir CH, Sever ML, Hoppin JA, Rose KM, Liu AH, Gergen PJ, Mitchell HE, Zeldin DC. Prevalence of allergic sensitization in the United States: results from the National Health and Nutrition Examination Survey (NHANES) 2005–2006. Allergy Clin Immunol. 2014;134:350–9.

Sander I, Zahradnik E, van Kampen V, Kespohl S, Stubel H, Fischer G, Brüning T, Bünger J, Raulf-Heimsoth M. Development and application of mold antigen-specific enzyme-linked immunosorbent assays (ELISA) to quantify airborne antigen exposure. J Toxicol Environ Health. 2012;75:1185–93.

Schmitz R, Ellert U, Kalcklösch M, Dahm S, Thamm M. Patterns of sensitization to inhalant and food allergens – findings from the German Health Interview and Examination Survey for Children and Adolescents. Int Arch Allergy Immunol. 2013;162:263–70.

Schneider PB, Denk U, Breitenbach M, Richter K, Schmid-Grendelmeier P, Nobbe S, Himly M, Mari A, Ebner C, Simon-Nobbe B. Alternaria alternata NADP-dependent mannitol dehydrogenase is an important fungal allergen. Clin Exp Allergy. 2006;36:1513–24.

Sennekamp J, Lehmann E, Joest M. Berufsbedingte exogen-allergische Alveolitis. ASU. 2015;50:38–52.

Simon-Nobbe B, Denk U, Pöll V, Rid R, Breitenbach M. The spectrum of fungal allergy. Int Arch Allergy Immunol. 2008;145:58–86.

Szewzyk R, Becker K, Hünken A, Pick-Fuß H, Kolossa-Gehring M. Kinder-Umwelt-Survey (KUS) 2003/06 Sensibilisierung gegenüber Innenraumschimmelpilzen. Schriftreihe Umwelt & Gesundheit im Auftrag des Umweltbundesamt; 2011.

Toppila-Salmi S, Huhtala H, Karjalainen J, Renkonen R, Mäkelä MJ, Wang DY, Pekkanen J. Sensitization pattern affects the asthma risk in Finnish adult population. Allergy. 2015;70:1112–20.

Unger A, Stöger P, Simon-Nobbe B, Susani M, Crameri R, Ebner C, Hintner H, Breitenbach M. Clinical testing of recombinant allergens of the mold Alternaria alternata. Int Arch Allergy Immunol. 1999;118:220–1.

Wagner S, Breiteneder H, Simon-Nobbe B, Susani M, Krebitz M, Niggemann B, Brehler R, Scheiner O, Hoffmann-Sommergruber K. Hev b 9, an enolase and a new cross-reactive allergen from Hevea latex and molds. Purification, characterization, cloning and expression. Eur J Biochem. 2000;267:7006–14.

Latex Allergens: Source of Sensitization and Single Allergens

25

M. Raulf and H.-P. Rihs

25.1 Introduction

Allergy to natural rubber latex (NRL) is a phenomenon of the late twentieth century, arising primarily because of elevated hygiene standards in medicine with regard to transmissible infectious diseases (especially AIDS). These increased standards led to a significant increase in the use of NRL products, especially powdered NRL gloves, in healthcare facilities (Raulf 2014). Besides healthcare workers (HCWs), patients with a history of multiple interventions, especially children with spina bifida, are at a high risk of developing NRL allergy. Consequently, due to the tremendous health and economic implications of NRL allergy, NRL became one of the most investigated allergen sources. Cross-reactivity with food products ('latex fruit syndrome') and non-food plants increased the problem. Therefore, tremendous efforts were made to identify the source and inducer of NRL allergy, and to develop appropriate diagnostic tools, which continue to be improved and updated. NRL proteins are 'model allergens' as they optimally illustrate the application and benefit of how recombinant single allergens improve *in-vitro*-immunoglobulin (Ig)E diagnosis by the addition of relevant but labile single allergens to the whole natural extract. Results obtained from basic research on the allergenicity of latex proteins have stimulated numerous preventive measures.

For example, NRL and NRL-containing dust were classified as airway and skin sensitizers, and the introduction of powder-free, latex-poor gloves decreased the high frequency of latex allergy in risk populations such as healthcare workers (Allmers

M. Raulf, PhD, Prof. (✉)
Center Allergology/Immunology, Institute for Prevention and Occupational Medicine of the German Social Accident Insurance, Institute of the Ruhr-Universität Bochum, Bochum, Germany
e-mail: raulf@ipa-dguv.de

H.-P. Rihs, PhD
Institute for Prevention and Occupational Medicine of the German Social Accident Insurance, Institute of the Ruhr-University Bochum (IPA), Bochum, Germany
e-mail: rihs@ipa-dguv.de

J. Kleine-Tebbe, T. Jakob (eds.), *Molecular Allergy Diagnostics*,
DOI 10.1007/978-3-319-42499-6_25

et al. 2002) and patients with spina bifida (Levy et al. 1999; Niggemann 2010; Cremer et al. 1998). Data from Germany have demonstrated the effectiveness of primary prevention measures by showing a clear association between the introduction of powder-free gloves with low protein levels and the decline in the number of suspected cases of occupational NRL allergies on a nationwide scale (Allmers et al. 2002).

25.2 Source of Proteins and Denomination of Allergens

Latex – the milky sap of the rubber tree *Hevea brasiliensis*, is synthesized by specialized laticifer cells and secreted from damaged tree bark, or from incisions made in the bark for latex collection. In about 1770 in England, dried latex was given the name "rubber", as it was found to be well suited to "rub out" pencil marks. In German, the term "Kautschuk" – which originated from the Native American word for "weeping tree – caoutchouc", was established. The main constituent of latex is the polymeric hydrocarbon, 1,4 cis-polyisoprene. Only 2% of the fresh weight of Hevea latex is made up of proteins that are heterogeneously distributed in the latex sap (Yeang et al. 2002). These proteins are involved in the biosynthesis of the polyisoprene associated with the coagulation of latex and in the defense of the plant against various diseases. More than 240 polypeptides were detected in latex by two-dimensional electrophoresis, and 60 IgE-binding structures were identified (Posch et al. 1997). To date, 26 NRL allergens, including isoforms and variants with molecular weight between 4.7 and 60 kDa, have been listed by the World Health Organization/International Union of Immunological Societies (WHO/IUIS) Allergen Nomenclature Sub-Committee, as Hev b 1–15 (www.allergen.org) (Raulf-Heimsoth and Rihs 2011) (◉ Table 25.1).

25.3 Function of NRL Allergens

In 1993, the first NRL allergen, "rubber elongation factor" (REF),was identified by Czuppon et al. (1993) and was listed and denominated as Hev b 1 according to the rules of the WHO/IUIS Allergen Nomenclature Sub-Committee. Today, most of the NRL allergens are available in recombinant form.

Hev b 1 (14.6 kDa) is a latex-specific, particle-bound protein involved in the synthesis of polyisoprene, the basic matrix of latex, without any relevant homology to other plant proteins. It was characterized on the B- and T-cell epitope level (Raulf-Heimsoth et al. 1998).

Hev b 2 is a glycosylated basic β-1,3-glucanase (34 kDa) belonging to the defense PR-3 protein family (PR; pathogenesis-related), and is synthesized by the plants as a control strategy against microbial attack. Hev b 2 is not commercially available as a recombinant protein.

Hev b 3 (23 kDa), like Hev b 1, belongs to the particle-bound allergens (small rubber particle protein) and was first described by Alenius et al. (1993) as a latex sensitizer.

Hev b 4 (53–55 kDa) is a lecithinase homolog of minor relevance (Bernstein et al. 2003).

Table. 25.1 Characterized latex allergens of the rubber tree *Hevea brasiliensis* – biochemical and clinical properties

	Latex allergens*[a]	Molecular weight [kDa]	Protein name, biological function or physiological role
Major allergens	Hev b 1*[b]	14	Rubber elongation factor (REF)
	Hev b 3*[b]	24	Small rubber particle proteins
	Hev b 5*[b, c]	16	Acidic structural proteins
	Hev b 6.01*[c]***	20	Prohevein (precursor of hevein Hev b 6.02)
Minor allergens	Hev b 2*[d]	34	β-1,3-glucanase
	Hev b 4	53-55	Lecithinase homolog
	Hev b 7	42	Patatin-like protein (esterase) from latex-B- and C-serum
	Hev b 8	15	Profilin (actin-binding protein)
	Hev b 9	51	Enolase
	Hev b 10	26	Manganese superoxide dismutase (MnSOD)
	Hev b 11	30	Class I chitinase
	Hev b 12	9	Non-specific lipid transfer protein type 1 (nsLTP1)
	Hev b 13*[d]	42	Esterase
	Hev b 14	30	Hevamine
	Hev b 15	7.5	Serine protease inhibitor

□ recombinant form available and suitable for the diagnosis; *italic* and **bold**: for clarification of cross-reactivity applicable

[a]IUIS (International Union of Immunological Societies) nomenclature (www.allergen.org, October 2015)

[b]Major allergens for spina bifida patients

[c]Major allergens for healthcare workers

[d]Relevance under discussion

Hev b 5 is detectable in latex C-serum and represents an acidic (pH 3.5), heat-stable 16-kDa protein, rich in glutamic acid, as well as in proline residues. Its physiological function is unknown. Native Hev b 5 was characterized by Akasawa et al. (1996), whereas the first recombinant Hev b 5 (rHev b 5) was described by Slater et al. (1996). Hev b 5 has multiple isoforms.

Hev b 6 or Hev b 6.01 (prohevein) represents the 20-kDa precursor protein of hevein and belongs to the class I chitinases. It harbors two allergenic components, the N-terminal hevein (Hev b 6.02) and the C-terminal Hev b 6.03. The maturing process of the mRNA is necessary for the development of a mature prohevein. A post-translational cleavage precedes the formation of two further proteins – the 4.7-kDa Hev b 6.02 and the 14-kDa C-terminal domain Hev b 6.03. All three allergens exist in the plant, with the ratio between Hev b 6.01 and Hev b 6.03 being about 30:1 (Yeang et al. 2002). In the Hev b 6.01 molecule, the regions responsible for IgE-binding and those for inducing T-cell proliferation responses are located in different parts of the protein. Hev b 6.03 is a better inducer of proliferation and contains HLA-DR4-binding motifs, whereas the Hev b 6.02 domain is responsible for IgE-binding and is the important allergenic part, carrying discontinuous B-cell epitopes (Raulf-Heimsoth et al. 2004a). A comparison of the different sequences showed that hevein has similarities with known plant PR-proteins (Broekaert et al. 1990), including a structure homologous to lectins and endochitinases, which exist in fruits.

Hev b 7 is a 42-kDa patatin-like protein with sequence homology to patatins from *Solanaceae*, such as tomato and potato (Kostyal et al. 1998; Schmidt et al. 2002; Seppala et al. 2000). Isoforms of Hev b 7 with post-translational modifications are present in latex C-serum, as well as in the bottom (B) fraction of the latex sap.

Hev b 8 is a 15-kDa latex profilin and belongs to a group of panallergens that are widespread in plants. It could be responsible for cross-reactivity with fruits or pollen (Vallier et al. 1995).

Separation of latex proteins by two-dimensional electrophoresis and immunoblotting with sera from latex-allergic patients, followed by microsequencing of the IgE-binding spots, enabled the identification of **Hev b 9**, a 51-kDa enolase, and Hev b 10, a 26-kDa manganese-superoxide dismutase (Posch et al. 1997). *In-vitro* cross-reactivity of Hev b 9 with enolases from fungi of the genera *Cladosporium* and *Alternaria* has been shown, but the clinical significance of these results is debatable (Wagner et al. 2000). **Hev b 10** displays homology with enzymes of the same family (Mn-superoxide dismutase) that is present in *Aspergillus* (Rihs et al. 2001).

Hev b 11 is a 30-kDa class I chitinase with a hevein domain, but the cross-reactivity to Hev b 6.02 is low (Posch et al. 1999).

Additional latex allergens include the following proteins: Hev b 12, a non-specific lipid transfer protein (Beezhold et al. 2003; Rihs et al. 2006; Faber et al. 2015), a Mediterranean plant panallergen that is included in the defense protein group; Hev b 13, a latex esterase (42 kDa) found in B-serum; Hev b 14 (hevamine, 39 kDa), a bifunctional enzyme with lysozyme and chitinase activity (Jekel et al. 1991) and Hev b 15, a serine protease inhibitor, with molecular weight of 7.5 kDa, which belongs to the PR-6 family (Rihs et al. 2015).

25.4 Importance of the Major Allergens

Currently, sufficient evidence exists suggesting that various risk groups are sensitized by different NRL allergens (Rihs et al. 2015). It is also quite obvious that the mode of contact with the allergenic proteins is of enormous importance for the development of sensitization. HCWs can become sensitized to airborne latex allergens that are adsorbed to the powder in the gloves they or their co-workers wear, whereas patients with, for example, spina bifida or multiple surgeries, become sensitized through the direct contact of latex-containing devices with their body fluids and mucosa. Whereas Hev b 5, Hev b 6.01 (especially the hevein domain Hev b 6.02), and Hev b 2 have been recognized as major allergens in HCWs, patients with spina bifida have predominantly IgE-reactivity to Hev b 1, Hev b 3, and Hev b 5.

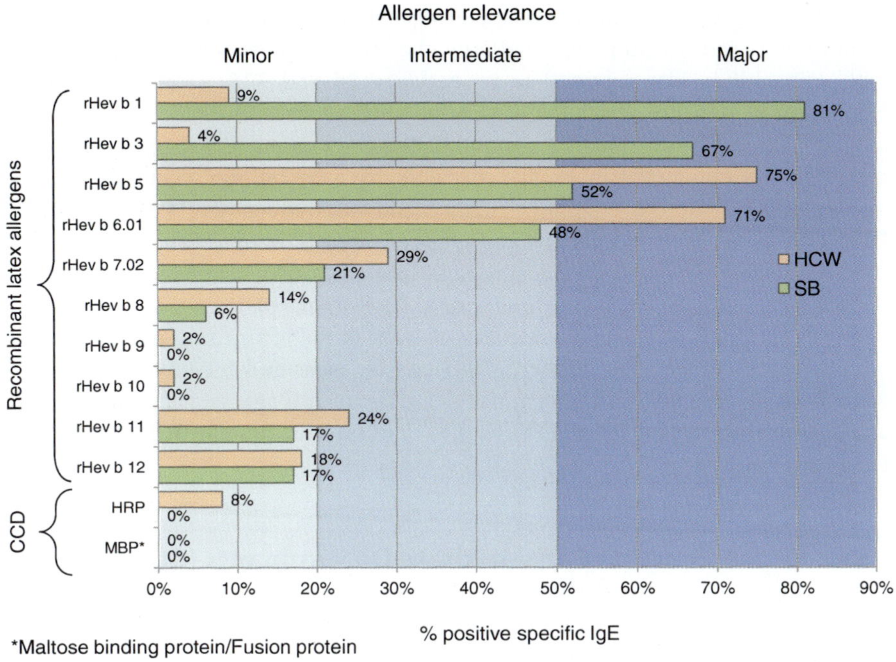

Fig. 25.1 Specific latex sensitization profile of 31 patients with spina bifida and 104 healthcare workers with clinically relevant latex allergy, according to data in Raulf-Heimsoth et al. (2007a)

All other allergens are of minor relevance, but may help to complete and elucidate the diagnostic picture in specific cases (◉ Fig. 25.1).

25.5 Dissemination of Latex Allergy

Many theories have been proposed to explain the sudden increase in the number of persons affected by latex allergy that began in the 1980s and extended into the 1990s (Raulf 2014; Ownby 2002). One factor was the improved hygiene standards in medicine with respect to transmissible infectious diseases (especially AIDS), whereby the number of NRL products, especially NRL gloves, increased.

Before the initiation of primary NRL prophylactic measures – such as the introduction in hospitals of powder-free gloves with reduced protein levels, and the introduction of latex-free surgeries for spina bifida patients – HCWs, children with spina bifida, and people with a history of multiple surgeries were all at a high risk of developing NRL allergy. In addition, high risks were also described for non-HCWs who might be exposed to latex; for example, hairdressers, cleaners, and food-service workers, as well as workers in industrial rubber companies or people with food allergies and atopy.

Depending on the definition of the groups studied and the methods for assessment of latex sensitization and/or allergy, the observed prevalence among children with spina bifida was reported to be between 25 and 72 % (Konz et al. 1995; Bernardini et al. 1999; Yassin et al. 1992), whereas the prevalence among HCWs ranged between 0 and 30 % (Yassin et al. 1994; Garabrant and Schweitzer 2002). A meta-analysis conducted in France revealed that latex allergy occurred at a frequency of 1.37 % in the general population and at a frequency of 4.32 % in HCWs (Bousquet et al. 2006; Caballero and Quirce 2015). The introduction of powder-free, latex-poor gloves decreased the high frequency of latex allergy in high-risk populations, such as HCWs (Allmers et al. 2002) and patients with spina bifida (Levy et al. 1999; Niggemann 2010). However, in polysensitized allergic patients without latex contact, latex-specific IgE can be measured based on IgE against cross-reactive carbohydrate determinants (CCDs) or IgE against panallergens, such as latex profilin (Hev b 8) or non-specific lipid transfer protein (Rihs et al. 2006; Faber et al. 2015).

25.6 Cross-Reactive Carbohydrate Determinants (CCDs)

Latex proteins include glycoproteins (CCDs) with potential cross-reactivity, but with carbohydrate determinants of low clinical relevance. Determination of specific IgE against CCDs is highly recommended, especially in people with unexpected specific IgE antibodies against latex, such as the two following groups:

- In patients allergic to pollen or Hymenoptera venom (Jappe et al. 2006) without clinical symptoms induced by latex
- In patients sensitized to plant food listed in the 'latex-fruit-syndrome', but who have no clinical symptoms.

25.7 Latex-Food Syndrome

About 30–50 % of latex-allergic patients have allergic symptoms to plant-derived foods, especially fresh fruits (Radauer et al. 2011). This association was called latex-fruit syndrome (review in Blanco (2003); Wagner and Breiteneder (2002)) and is a growing problem due to the large amounts of available fruits. The fruits most commonly involved are avocado, banana, chestnut, and kiwi. In contrast to primary food allergens that are heat stable and resistant to degradation or proteolytic digestion, allergens involved in the latex-fruit-syndrome are usually heat-labile proteins, which are easily degradable. The number of patients suffering from latex-fruit syndrome is greater than the number of patients who are allergic to these associated fresh foods and fruits and who are not latex-allergic. Importantly, only a few of these sensitizations are clinically relevant. In addition, it is also possible that aeroallergens, e.g., components of *Ficus benjamina*, *Euphorbia pulcherrima*, or grass/

weed pollen show cross-reactivity to latex, although no taxonomic relationships exist between *Hevea brasiliensis* and these plants. Several latex allergens, such as Hev b 2 (Barre et al. 2009), Hev b 6.02 (Posch et al. 1999; Chen et al. 1998; Raulf-Heimsoth et al. 2002), Hev b 7 (Schmidt et al. 2002), Hev b 8 (Raulf-Heimsoth et al. 2007b), and Hev b 12 (◉ Fig. 25.2) (Beezhold et al. 2003), have been considered to be responsible for the latex-fruit cross-reactivity.

Using recombinant latex allergens, several cross-reactions could be identified as potential causes of the latex-fruit syndrome:

Hev b 8 (latex profilin) for latex and chestnut (Raulf-Heimsoth et al. 2007b)
Hev b 6.01/Hev b 6.02 for latex and acerola (Raulf-Heimsoth et al. 2002)
Hev b 12 (latex-non-specific lipid transfer protein type) for latex and previous peach allergy, mainly in Mediterranean countries (Rihs et al. 2006; Faber et al. 2015)

On the other hand, there are latex-allergic patients without latex-associated fruit allergy, although Hev b 6.02 or chitinases with hevein domains have been recognized as major allergens (◉ Fig 25.2).

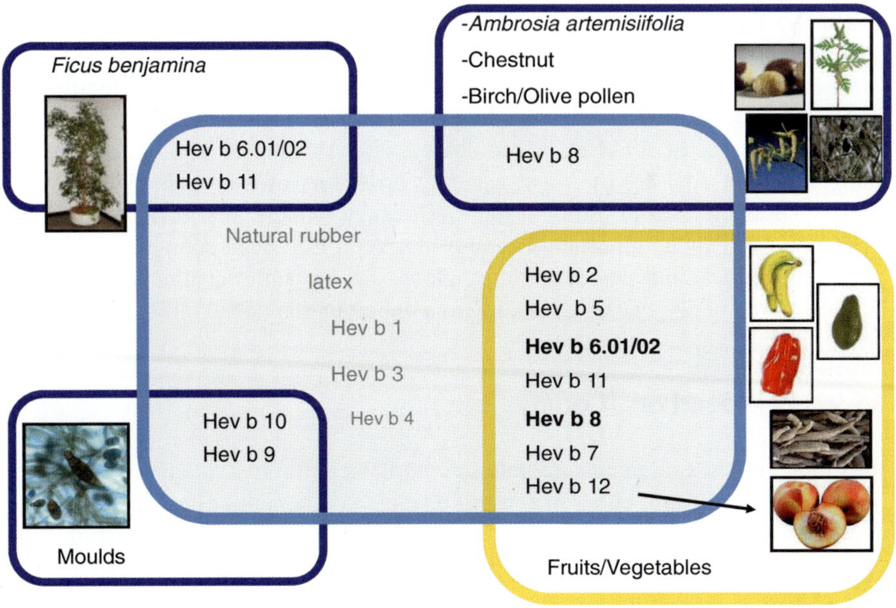

Fig. 25.2 Molecular basis of cross-reactivity between natural rubber latex and other (mostly plant) allergen sources, according to Raulf-Heimsoth and Rihs (2011) and Raulf (2016), with modifications

25.8 Diagnosis with Single Latex Allergens

Since the first synthesis of the recombinant latex allergen Hev b 1 (Yeang et al. 1996; Rihs et al. 2000), more than a dozen latex allergens have been synthesized successfully in recombinant form in *Escherichia coli*. Because post-translational modifications have, in general, no influence on the IgE reactivity of the recombinant latex allergens, most have proved successful in actual *in vitro*-diagnostics. One exception is rHev b 2, which exhibits dramatically reduced allergenic potential in comparison with its natural counterpart nHev b 2. Of note, the missing glycosylation of rHev b 2 does not seem to be the main cause of the reduced IgE reactivity (Yeang et al. 2002; Raulf-Heimsoth et al. 2004b). Another exception is Hev b 13 (rHev b 13), a second latex allergen that is not suitable for *in vitro*-diagnostics. All other recombinant latex allergens are appropriate for use in IgE assays and most are commercially available for single tests (ImmunoCAP; ThermoFisher Scientific, Freiburg, Germany), as well as for multiplex specific-IgE screening platforms (ImmunoCAP ISAC; Thermo Fisher Scientific).

In summary, with the application of single recombinant latex allergens it is possible to detect a specific latex allergy and to exclude CCD-specific IgE when using the diagnostic algorithm shown in ◉ Fig. 25.3. Nevertheless, we should be aware that it is difficult to achieve higher diagnostic sensitivity with single latex allergens compared with the 'spiked' natural latex extract. In the latter case, an increased sensitivity of the IgE *in-vitro* assay for latex allergy was achieved by adding recombinant Hev b 5 allergen to the natural latex (Raulf-Heimsoth et al. 2007a; Chen et al. 2000; Lundberg et al. 2001), with the result that sera which previously tested negative were now positive with the 'spiked' latex extract (ThermoFisher Scientific k82 with rHev b 5). A current study (Vandenplast et al. 2016) has demonstrated that high levels of IgE specific for rHev b 5 combined with rHev b 6.01 or 6.02 (determined using ImmunoCAP) are the most accurate predictors of a bronchial response to NRL, showing better diagnostic efficiency than the NRL-(k82)-sIgE ImmunoCAP. This is important, because in several European countries, NRL skin prick test extracts and powdered latex gloves for bronchial challenge test are no longer commercially available, leading to a deficit in diagnostic tools.

25.9 Perspectives (Conclusions)

Recombinant latex allergens are able to complement the individual patient's diagnostic armamentarium, either in form of a single component or together with other allergens on a microarray chip. Therefore, from the currently available studies the following conclusions can be drawn and implemented in day-to-day practice:

1. The addition of a relevant single latex recombinant allergen (rHev b 5) to the natural latex extract provides a significant improvement for *in-vitro*-IgE diagnosis.

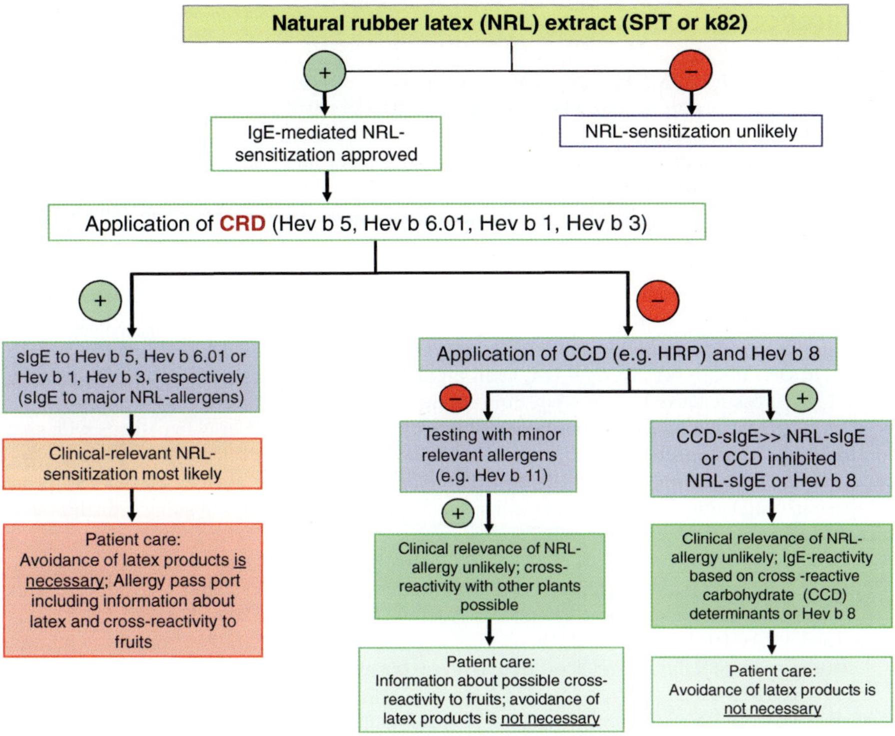

Fig.25.3 Diagnostic algorithm for suspicion of latex allergy or suspicion of polysensitization in patients with positive specific IgE to latex, according to Rauf-Heimsoth and Rihs (2011) and Raulf (2016), with modifications

2. Depending on their exposure, latex-allergic individuals are sensitized to the following major allergens:

   (a) Healthcare workers: Hev b 5, Hev b 6.01/6.02, and Hev b 2
   (b) Spina bifida patients: Hev b 1, Hev b 3, and Hev b 5

3. In polysensitized individuals with specific IgE to latex extract but without any corresponding symptoms, the cause for exhibiting IgE reactivity is usually based on CCDs.
4. A panel of specific recombinant latex allergens facilitates the definition of a specific sensitization profile. For example, rHev b 6.01/6.02, rHev b 8, and rHev b 12 represent potential markers that clarify a possible cross-reactivity in the context of the 'latex-fruit syndrome'.
5. With respect to the sensitivity of the IgE assays, the improved natural latex extract 'spiked' with recombinant rHev b 5 is more sensitive than assays using the available panel of recombinant latex allergens.
6. The most reliable tool for predicting bronchial reactivity to NRL is a combination of the levels of specific IgE antibodies against the recombinant allergen components Hev b 5 with Hev b 6.01 or 6.02 (Vandenplast et al. 2016).

References

Akasawa A, Hsieh LS, Martin BM, et al. A novel acidic allergen, Hev b 5, in latex. Purification, cloning and characterization. J Biol Chem. 1996;271:25389–93.

Alenius H, Palosuo T, Kelly K, et al. IgE reactivity to 14-kD and 27-kD natural rubber proteins in latex-allergic children with spina bifida and other congenital anomalies. Int Arch Allergy Immunol. 1993;102:61–6.

Allmers H, Schmengler J, Skudlik C. Primary prevention of natural rubber latex allergy in the German health care system through education and intervention. J Allergy Clin Immunol. 2002;110:318–23.

Barre A, Culerrier R, Granier C, et al. Mapping of IgE-binding epitopes on the major latex allergen Hev b 2 and the cross-reacting 1,3 beta-glucanase fruit allergens as a molecular basis for the latex-fruit syndrome. Mol Immunol. 2009;46:1595–604.

Beezhold DH, Hickey VL, Kostyal DA, et al. Lipid transfer protein from *Hevea brasiliensis* (Hev b 12), a cross-reactive latex protein. Ann Allergy Asthma Immunol. 2003;90:439–45.

Bernardini R, Novembre E, Lombardi E, et al. Risk factors for latex allergy in patients with spina bifida and latex sensitization. Clin Exp Allergy. 1999;29:681–6.

Bernstein DI, Biagini RE, Karnani R, et al. In vivo sensitization to purified Hevea brasiliensis proteins in health care workers sensitized to natural rubber latex. J Allergy Clin Immunol. 2003;111:610–6.

Blanco C. Latex-fruit syndrome. Curr Allergy Asthma Rep. 2003;3:47–53.

Bousquet J, Flahault A, Vandenplas O, et al. Natural rubber latex allergy among health care workers: a systematic review of the evidence. J Allergy Clin Immunol. 2006;118:447–54.

Broekaert I, Lee HI, Kush A, et al. Wound-induced accumulation of mRNA containing a hevein sequence in laticifers of rubber tree (Hevea brasiliensis). Proc Natl Acad Sci U S A. 1990;87:7633–7.

Caballero ML, Quirce S. Identification and practical management of latex allergy in occupational settings. Expert Rev Clin Immunol. 2015;11:977–92.

Chen Z, Posch A, Cremer R, et al. Identification of hevein (Hev b 6.02) in Hevea latex as a major cross-reacting allergen with avocado fruit in patients with latex allergy. J Allergy Clin Immunol. 1998;102:476–81.

Chen Z, Rihs HP, Slater JE, Paupore EJ, Schneider EM, Baur X. The absence of Hev b 5 in capture antigen may cause false-negative results in serologic assays for latex-specific IgE antibodies. J Allergy Clin Immunol. 2000;105:S8.

Cremer R, Kleine-Diepenbruck U, Hoppe A, et al. Latex allergy in spina bifida patients – prevention by primary prophylaxis. Allergy. 1998;3:709–11.

Czuppon AB, Chen Z, Rennert S, et al. The rubber elongation factor of rubber trees (*Hevea brasiliensis*) is the major allergen in latex. J Allergy Clin Immunol. 1993;92:690–7.

Faber MA, Sabato V, Bridts CH, et al. Clinical relevance of the Hevea brasiliensis lipid transfer protein Hev b 12. J Allergy Clin Immunol. 2015;135:1645–8.

Garabrant DH, Schweitzer S. Epidemiology of latex sensitization and allergies in health care workers. J Allergy Clin Immunol. 2002;110:S82–95.

Jappe U, Raulf-Heimsoth M, Hoffmann M, et al. In vitro hymenoptera venom allergy diagnosis: improved by screening for cross-reactive carbohydrate determinants and reciprocal inhibition. Allergy. 2006;61:1220–9.

Jekel PA, Bernard J, Hartmann H, et al. The primary structure of hevamine, an enzyme with lysozyme/chitinase activity from Hevea brasiliensis latex. Eur J Biochem. 1991;200:123–30.

Konz KR, Chia JK, Kurup VP, et al. Comparison of latex hypersensitivity among patients with neurologic defects. J Allergy Clin Immunol. 1995;95:950–4.

Kostyal DA, Hickey VL, Noti JD, et al. Cloning and characterization of a latex allergen (Hev b 7): homology to patatin, a plant PLA2. Clin Exp Immunol. 1998;112:355–62.

Levy D, Allouache S, Chabane MH, et al. Powder-free protein-poor rubber latex gloves and latex sensitization. JAMA. 1999;281:988.

Lundberg M, Chen Z, Rihs HP, Wrangsjö K. Recombinant spiked allergen extract. Allergy. 2001;56:794–5.
Niggemann B. IgE-mediated latex allergy – an exciting and instructive piece of allergy history. Pediatr Allergy Immunol. 2010;21:997–1001.
Ownby DR. A history of latex allergy. J Allergy Clin Immunol. 2002;110:S27–32.
Posch A, Chen Z, Wheeler C, et al. Characterization and identification of latex allergens by two-dimensional electrophoresis and protein microsequencing. J Allergy Clin Immunol. 1997;99:385–95.
Posch A, Wheeler CH, Chen Z, et al. Class I endochitinase containing a hevein domain is the causative allergen in latex-associated avocado allergy. Clin Exp Allergy. 1999;29:667–72.
Radauer C, Adhami F, Fürtler I, et al. Latex-allergic patients sensitized to the major allergen hevein and hevein-like domains of class I chitinases show no increased frequency of latex-associated plant food allergy. Mol Immunol. 2011;48:600–9.
Raulf M. The latex story. In: Bergmann K-C, Ring J, editors. History of allergy. Chem immunol allergy, vol. 100. Basel: Karger; 2014.
Raulf M: "Latex Allergy (B22)" published in: Matricardi PM, Kleine-Tebbe J, Hoffmann HJ, Valenta R, Hilger C, Hofmaier S, Aalberse RC, Agache I, Asero R, Ballmer-Weber B, Barber D, Beyer K, Biedermann T, Biló MB, Blank S, Bohle B, Bosshard PP, Breiteneder H, Brough HA, Caraballo L, Caubet JC, Crameri R, Davies JM, Douladiris N, Ebisawa M, Eigenmann PA, Fernandez-Rivas M, Ferreira F, Gadermaier G, Glatz M, Hamilton RG, Hawranek T, Hellings P, Hoffmann-Sommergruber K, Jakob T, Jappe U, Jutel M, Kamath SD, Knol EF, Korosec P, Kuehn A, Lack G, Lopata AL, Mäkelä M, Morisset M, Niederberger V, Nowak-Wezgrzyn AH, Papadopoulos NG, Pastorello EA, Pauli G, Platts-Mills T, Posa D, Poulsen LK, Raulf M, Sastre J, Scala E, Schmid JM, Schmid- Grendelmeier P, van Hage M, van Ree R, Vieths S, Weber R, Wickman M, Muraro A, Ollert M. EAACI molecular allergology user's guide. Pediatr Allergy Immunol. 2016;27(suppl23):1–250.
Raulf-Heimsoth M, Rihs H-P. Latexallergene: Sensibilisierungsquellen und Einzelallergenprofile erkennen. Allergo J. 2011;20:241–3.
Raulf-Heimsoth M, Chen Z, Rihs HP, et al. Analysis of T-cell reactive regions and HLA-DR4 binding motifs on the latex allergen Hev b 1 (rubber elongation factor). Clin Exp Allergy. 1998;28:339–48.
Raulf-Heimsoth M, Stark R, Sander I, et al. Anaphylactic reaction to apple juice containing acerola: cross-reactivity to latex due to prohevein. J Allergy Clin Immunol. 2002;109:715–6.
Raulf-Heimsoth M, Rozynek P, Brüning T, et al. Characterization of B- and T-cell responses and HLA-DR4 binding motifs of the latex allergen Hev b 6.01 (prohevein) and its post-transcriptionally formed proteins Hev b 6.02 and Hev b 6.03. Allergy. 2004;59:724–33.
Raulf-Heimsoth M, Rozynek P, Sander I, Brüning T, Rihs HP. Naturlatexallergie: molekulare Grundlagen und Kreuzreaktivitäten. Allergo J. 2004;13:328–36.
Raulf-Heimsoth M, Rihs HP, Rozynek P, et al. Quantitative analysis of IgE reactivity profiles in patients allergic or sensitized to natural rubber latex (Hevea brasiliensis). Clin Exp Allergy. 2007;37:1657–67.
Raulf-Heimsoth M, Kespohl S, Crespo JF, et al. Natural rubber latex and chestnut allergy: cross-reactivity or co-sensitization? Allergy. 2007;62:1277–81.
Rihs HP, Chen Z, Schumacher S, Rozynek P, Cremer R, Lundberg M, Raulf-Heimsoth M, Petersen A, Baur X. Recombinant Hev b 1: Large-scale production and immunological characterization. Clin Exp Allergy. 2000;30:1285–92.
Rihs HP, Chen Z, Rozynek P, et al. Allergenicity of rHev b 10 (manganese-superoxide dismutase). Allergy. 2001;56:85–6.
Rihs HP, Ruëff F, Lundberg M, et al. Relevance of the recombinant lipid transfer protein of Hevea brasiliensis: IgE-binding reactivity in fruit-allergic adults. Ann Allergy Asthma Immunol. 2006;97:643–9.
Rihs HP, Sander I, Heimann H, et al. The new latex allergen Hev b 15: IgE-binding properties of a recombinant serine protease inhibitor. J Investig Allergol Clin Immunol. 2015;25:160–2.

Schmidt MH, Raulf-Heimsoth M, Posch A. Evaluation of patatin as a major cross-reactive allergen in latex-induced potato allergy. Ann Allergy Asthma Immunol. 2002;89:613–8.

Seppala U, Palosuo T, Seppala U, et al. IgE reactivity to patatin-like latex allergen, Hev b 7, and to patatin of potato tuber, Sol t 1, in adults and children allergic to natural rubber latex. Allergy. 2000;55:266–73.

Slater JE, Vedvick T, Arthur-Smith A, et al. Identification, cloning, and sequence of a major allergen (Hev b 5) from natural rubber latex (*Hevea brasiliensis*). J Biol Chem. 1996;271:25394–9.

Vallier P, Balland S, Harf R, et al. Identification of profilin as an IgE-binding component in latex from Hevea brasiliensis: clinical implications. Clin Exp Allergy. 1995;25:332–9.

Vandenplast O, Froidure A, Meurer U, Rihs HP, Rifflart C, Soetaert S, Jamart J, Pilette C, Raulf M. The role of allergen components for the diagnosis of latex-induced occupational asthma. Allergy. 2016;71:840–9.

Wagner S, Breiteneder H. The latex-fruit syndrome. Biochem Soc Trans. 2002;30:935–40.

Wagner S, Breiteneder H, Simon-Nobbe B, et al. Hev b 9, an enolase and a new cross-reactive allergen from hevea latex and molds. Purification, characterization, cloning and expression. Eur J Biochem. 2000;267:7006–14.

Yassin MS, Sanyurah S, Lierl MB, et al. Evaluation of latex allergy in patients with meningomyelocele. Ann Allergy. 1992;69:207–11.

Yassin MS, Lierl MB, Fischer TJ, et al. Latex allergy in hospital employees. Ann Allergy. 1994;72:245–9.

Yeang HY, Cheong KF, Sunderasan E, Hamzah S, Chew NP, Hamid S, Hamilton RG, Cardosa MJ. The 14.6 kD rubber elongation factor (Hev b 1) and 24 kD (Hev b 3) rubber particle proteins are recognized by IgE from patients with spina bifida and latex allergy. J Allergy Clin Immunol. 1996;98:628–39.

Yeang HY, Arif SA, Yusof F, et al. Allergenic proteins of natural rubber latex. Methods. 2002;27:32–45.

Part IV

Designer Allergens, Hypoallergens and Fusion Allergens

Recombinant Allergens in Specific Immunotherapy

26

A. Nandy, P.S. Creticos, and D. Häfner

26.1 Introduction

Extract-based allergen-specific immunotherapy (AIT) has long been established as an effective treatment method for a wide variety of type-1 allergies including seasonal allergic rhinitis/conjunctivitis, perennial allergic rhinitis/conjunctivitis, allergic asthma, and venom sensitivity. Unmodified or chemically modified extracts with reduced immunoglobulin-E (IgE) reactivity, i.e., allergoids that can be used at higher doses, are finding application.

Since extracts are natural products, their allergen contents can differ from one another according to raw material and extraction method. As a result, extract standardization is realistically limited to only total IgE-binding activity and quantification of the most relevant major allergen. Moreover, extracts are largely made up of components that can be considered unnecessary or even counterproductive for effective AIT. These include minor allergens in low concentrations, nonallergenic

The present chapter is based on, and modified from, an article by the authors published in 2015 in *Allergo Journal International* (Nandy A, Häfner D, Klysner S: Recombinant allergens for specific immunotherapy: Current concepts and developments. Allergo J Int 2015; 24:143–151).

A. Nandy, PhD (✉)
Business Unit Allergy, Research & Development,
Allergopharma GmbH and Co. KG, Reinbek, Germany
e-mail: andreas.nandy@allergopharma.com

P.S. Creticos, MD, Prof.
Johns Hopkins University School of Medicine, Division of Allergy and Clinical Immunology, Baltimore, MD, USA

Creticos Research Group, LLC, Crownsville, MD, USA

D. Häfner, PhD
Allergopharma GmbH and Co. KG, Reinbek, Germany

J. Kleine-Tebbe, T. Jakob (eds.), *Molecular Allergy Diagnostics*,
DOI 10.1007/978-3-319-42499-6_26

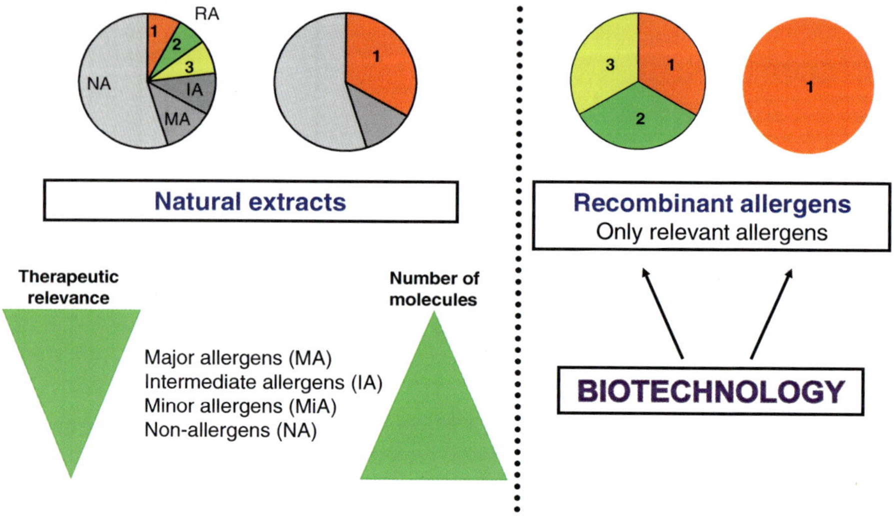

Fig. 26.1 Natural extracts are made up of a mixture of relevant allergens, intermediary allergens, minor allergens, and a large quantity of undefined nonallergenic materials (e.g., proteins, sugars, lipids). Genetically engineered allergens, in contrast, comprise only those components relevant to treatment, can be precisely standardized, and can be reproduced to consistent quality. According to the concept of major allergens, preparations for recombinant treatment are made up of a cocktail of relevant allergens (e.g., grasses, house dust mites) or can be obtained as a monopreparation in cases where only one relevant major allergen is available (e.g., birch, cat, ragweed)

proteins, lipids, sugar, or other components that have not been further characterized (◉ Fig. 26.1). In contrast, genetically engineered allergens can be characterized extensively and can be produced in a reproducible manner to a quality that meets the regulatory requirements for pharmaceutical products (Cromwell et al. 2011).

26.2 Advantages and Opportunities Posed by Recombinant Allergens for Allergen-Specific Immunotherapy

26.2.1 Recombinant Allergens for Specific Immunotherapy: Why?

Recombinant production of allergens makes it possible to precisely select those allergens that have been identified as relevant for the allergy and for AIT. Only these allergens are then produced in a highly pure form and administered to allergic patients in a therapeutic formulation (◉ Fig. 26.1). Standardization is performed by means of absolute protein quantification. Whereas the composition of allergens in natural extracts can vary depending on the raw material, i.e., individual allergens may be underrepresented or lacking altogether, allergens in recombinant preparations can be combined using precisely defined parameters (e.g., concentration, mixture ratios, etc.). Similarly, it is possible to avoid adverse side effects, for instance, due to proteases in extracts, as well as contamination, e.g., by lipopolysaccharides

(LPS). Potential new sensitizations due to low levels of extract components are unlikely with recombinant allergens (Jutel et al. 2005).

26.2.2 The Challenge: Selecting the Relevant Allergens

One of the main challenges in the development of AIT with recombinant allergens lies in correctly selecting those allergens relevant to treatment success.

While the frequency of sensitization to an allergen, i.e., the percentage of allergy sufferers sensitized to this allergen, is considered a guide to selection on the one hand, the level of specific IgE to a single allergen in total IgE to the allergen source is, on the other, an important criterion when estimating relevance of this allergen.

For some allergen sources, such as birch or cat, there is only one relevant major allergen (Bet v 1 from birch; Fel d 1 from cat): considerably more than 90% of allergy sufferers are sensitized to these allergens, and specific IgE accounts for the major part of total IgE. In such cases, monopreparations are sufficient and have already been tested in clinical trials (◉ Table 26.1). In the case of other allergen sources, combinations of various allergens, so-called cocktails, are required in the majority of these patients to cover most allergen-specific IgE. Cocktails comprising four allergens (Phl p 1, Phl p 2, Phl p 5, and Phl p 6) have been clinically tested for the treatment of grass pollen allergy (◉ Table 26.1). One preparation contained the two isoallergens, Phl p 5.01 and Phl p 5.02, from the allergen Phl p 5, which differ in their primary sequence at approximately 35% of amino acid positions (Jutel et al. 2005). The major allergen of ragweed, Amb a 1, also has five isoallergens with around 60–88% sequence identity (Radauer et al. 2014). In addition to IgE cross-reactivity, it is important here to take as broad a coverage of T-cell epitopes as possible into account when selecting isoallergens.

While allergens in extracts are present as a mixture of isoallergens and isoforms, which are subject to geographic differences in composition in terms of both quality and quantity, the concept of recombinant allergens focuses on one or a few sequences that contain the important and relevant epitopes (T-cell and/or B-cell epitopes, depending on the strategy). Due to high sequence homology and the associated cross-reactivity of the epitopes, one can expect a variety of species to be covered (e.g., Pooideae grass species, early bloomers such as birch, alder, hazel, or the mite species *Dermatophagoides pteronyssinus* and *D. farinae*). However, appropriate preliminary immunological investigations need to be carried out to confirm this in order to identify the most important sequences. Selecting the epitopes relevant to treatment success represents an additional challenge for treatment strategies not based on the use of complete molecules, but which depend solely on the use of pure epitopes.

Table 26.1 Clinical studies on recombinantly produced active allergenic substances

Active substances	Study design	Phase	References[a]
Birch pollen allergy			
Bet v 1 trimer Bet v 1 fragments (hypoallergenic)	SCIT DBPC	II	Niederberger et al. (2004) Purohit et al. (2008)
Bet v 1 (hypoallergenic) Birch pollen extract (native)	SCIT Open	II	NCT00266526
Bet v 1 (native) nBet v 1 (native) Birch pollen extract (native)	SCIT DBPC	II	NCT00410930 Pauli et al. (2008)
Bet v 1 (hypoallergenic)	SCIT DBPC	III	NCT00309062 Narkus et al. (2008)
Bet v 1 (hypoallergenic)	SCIT DBPC	III	NCT00554983
Bet v 1 (hypoallergenic)	SCIT	II	NCT00841516
Bet v 1 (hypoallergenic)	SCIT DRF	II	NCT01490411
Bet v 1 (native)	SLIT	I	NCT00889460 Winther et al. (2009)
Bet v 1 (native)	SLIT DRF	I	NCT00396149 Winther et al. (2009)
Bet v 1 (native)	SLIT DBPC		NCT00901914
Grass pollen allergy			
Phl p 1, 2, 5.01, 5.02, 6	SCIT DBPC	II	Jutel et al. (2005)
Phl p 1, 2, 5.01, 5.02, 6	SCIT DBPC DRF	II	NCT00666341 Klimek et al. (2012)
Phl p 1, 2, 5.01, 5.02, 6	SCIT DBPC	III	NCT00309036
Phl p 1, 2, 5.01, 5.02, 6	SCIT DBPC	III	NCT00671268
Phl p 1, 2, 5.01, 5.02, 6	SCIT DBPC	III	NCT01353755
BM32 (Phl p 1, 2, 5, 6 IgE epitopes)	SCIT DBPC DRF	IIa	NCT01445002
BM32 (Phl p 1, 2, 5, 6 IgE epitopes)	SCIT DBPC	IIb	NCT01538979
Cat allergy			
Fel d 1-MAT	ILIT		Senti et al. (2009)
Peanut allergy			
EMP123 (Ara h 1, 2, 3 modified)	Rectal		NCT00850668
Fish allergy			
Cyp c 1 (hypoallergenic)	SCIT DBPC	I/II	NCT02017626

DBPC double-blind placebo controlled, *DRF* dose-*response* finding, *IDIT* intradermal immunotherapy, *ILIT* intralymphatic immunotherapy, *SCIT* subcutaneous immunotherapy, *SLIT* sublingual immunotherapy

[a]NCT number: Studies listed under www.clinicaltrials.gov

26.2.3 Various Treatment Strategies Using Recombinant Allergens

Expectations in terms of novel innovative products in AIT, particularly in recombinant strategies, are high. The desired goal is to achieve better efficacy, as well as even greater safety and patient-friendly use, e.g., shorter treatment times and fewer administrations, compared with preparations already available.

The majority of clinical studies performed with recombinant allergens to date have been based on identifying relevant allergens in order to obtain the most representative picture of the extract as possible. As part of this process, the form of administration compared with extract-based preparations was virtually unmodified. Thus, SCIT preparations are made up of either a mixture of five grass pollen allergens or, in the case of birch pollen allergy, of the major birch pollen allergen Bet v 1 in native form or, alternatively, as a "Bet v 1 allergenoid" (hypoallergenic variant) (◉ Fig. 26.2). These preparations were each administered in aluminum hydroxide-absorbed form. Dose escalation protocols and treatment duration were guided by experience of treatment with unmodified extracts or chemically modified, hypoallergenic allergoids.

Clinical trials with alternate routes of immunization – sublingual (as opposed to subcutaneous) administration and local injection of allergen into regional lymph nodes (intralymphatic immunotherapy) – have also been performed. The sublingual studies have focused on native Bet v 1, incorporating one major isotype of birch

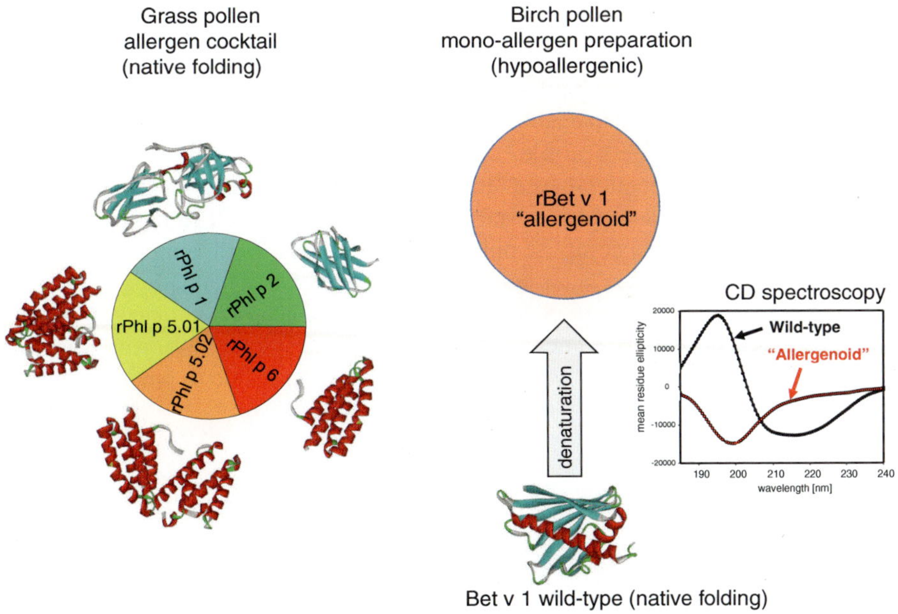

Fig. 26.2 The vast majority of clinical experience has been gained with a grass pollen allergen cocktail (single allergens in their native fold in equimolar composition) and a hypoallergenic birch pollen mono-allergen preparation. Circular dichroism (*CD*) spectra (*right*) show the loss of secondary structural elements (β-pleated sheet, α-helix) in the allergenoid. IgE binding is reduced by the modified surface structure (Adapted from Kahlert et al. 2008)

pollen (Winther et al. 2009). This method is believed to be more convenient for the patient since the patient can administer the treatment at home. However, the amount of allergen product needed is higher as compared to AIT, and the efficacy of SLIT seems to be slightly inferior indirectly compared to AIT (Durham and Penagos 2016).

A different administration strategy, intralymphatic immunotherapy, has been pursued with Fel d 1, the major cat allergenic moiety. Initial dosing studies provided confirmatory findings that injection of allergen directly into the target organ (inguinal lymph nodes) would enable a more efficient uptake of allergen – both lowering the dose requirement (μg of allergen) and the frequency of injections (Senti et al. 2012). The investigational construct incorporated the modified recombinant allergen of the major cat allergen protein (rFel d 1) fused to a translocator peptide trans-activating transcription factor (TAT) and to part of the human invariate chain (Ii) to generate a modular antigen transporter (MAT) vaccine that targeted the major histocompatibility complex (MHC) class II pathway for antigen presentation (Senti et al. 2012).

Additional concepts include fusion or coupling with molecules, such as antibodies or sugar structures, which directly bind specific receptors of desired target cells of the immune system (e.g., dendritic cells) in order to facilitate uptake. Furthermore, recombinant allergens can be fused with substances that have an adjuvant effect, with a goal of redirecting the untoward immune response to that of immunologic balance (i.e., restoring a Th2/Th1 balance), e.g., coupling with immunostimulatory oligonucleotides [non-methylated cytosine phosphatidyl guanine (CpG) DNA] or cystatin. Likewise, there is interest in evaluating the salutatory effects of coadministration with vitamin D3 and probiotics.

Moreover, hypoallergenic variants of recombinant allergens that show reduced IgE reactivity have been generated (allergenoids). These recombinant molecules can be considered as the biotechnical equivalent of allergoids (hypoallergenic extracts) and are intended to enable the use of higher therapeutic doses while retaining an undiminished safety profile.

Finally, there are peptide-based strategies that involve the use of long overlapping peptides with reduced IgE reactivity and preserved T-cell reactivity (Spertini et al. 2014) or those that comprise only IgE epitopes. The T-cell epitopes necessary for immunogenicity in the latter approach are derived from a nonallergenic carrier molecule (hepatitis B virus preS domain) (Marth et al. 2014).

The approaches described here address the immune system in varying ways and are based on differing modes of action. It is not as yet possible to predict which of these strategies will ultimately prove to be the most effective.

26.3 Clinical Experience with Recombinant Allergens

26.3.1 Regulatory Requirements

Recombinant allergens are approved as biotechnological products by the European Medicines Agency (EMA) through a centralized process. As with extract-based preparations, their production must comply with the rules of good manufacturing practice (GMP) (European Commission 2010). Safety and efficacy need to be shown in clinical trials. ◉ Figure 26.3 provides an overview of the production process for a recombinant allergen, from research and development to production.

◉ Table 26.1 offers an overview of clinical studies with recombinant allergens. Toxicological and stability studies precede clinical trials. Guidelines on the quality of recombinant allergens (European Medicines European Medicines and Committee for Medicinal Products for Human Use 2008) include physicochemical investigations to characterize their structure and verify their identity and purity. Product-related impurities, such as by-products, aggregates, or modifications (e.g., deamidation, oxidation), need to be investigated in the same way as process-related impurities, such as host cell protein and DNA, medium components, and microbial contamination. Recombinant proteins also require immunological characterization.

26.3.2 Studies with Unmodified Recombinant Allergens

The characteristics of unmodified recombinant allergens are comparable with natural allergens in terms of structure (native fold) and IgE reactivity. Recombinant allergens produced in bacterial cells, however, lack the sugar content that can

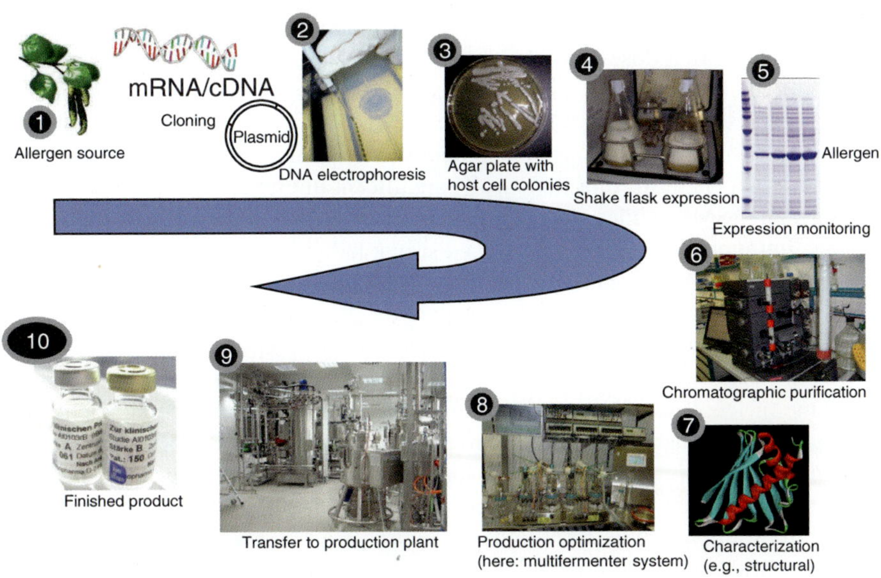

Fig. 26.3 Simplified representation of the production process for recombinant allergens. mRNA is isolated from the allergen source, e.g., pollen (*1*), and complementary DNA (*cDNA*) is produced and cloned in an expression plasmid (*2*). Host cells (e.g., *Escherichia coli* or yeast) are transformed with the plasmid (*3*), isolated, and cultured in fluid culture medium (*4*); they then express the heterologous allergen protein (*5*). Following chromatographic separation to remove host cell components (*6*), the pure protein is extensively characterized physicochemically and immunologically (*7*). Production processes are developed, optimized (*8*), and upscaled (*9*) for selected proteins that are candidates for therapy. Material for toxicological investigations and clinical tests (*10*) is produced in its final formulation under conditions that comply with GMP conditions, which correspond to the production process of the subsequent preparation for market release

occur in some natural allergens as an IgE cross-reactive carbohydrate component (e.g., Phl p 1). However, this has no effect on IgE binding, T-cell reactivity, or the immunogenicity of the molecule (Cromwell et al. 2006; Jutel et al. 2005; Suck et al. 2006).

An aluminum hydroxide-adsorbed cocktail comprising the five most important allergens of Timothy grass (*Phleum pratense*; ◉ Fig. 26.2) was tested in a double-blind, placebo-controlled phase-II trial on grass pollen allergy (Jutel et al. 2005). The study included 62 patients with grass pollen allergy and rhinoconjunctivitis with or without asthma. Patients were treated preseasonally with a subcutaneous maintenance dose of 40 **μ**g (equimolar dose of the five allergens: 10 μg Phl p 1, 10 μg Phl p 5.01, 10 μg Phl p 5.02, 5 μg Phl p 2, and 5 μg Phl p 6). The initial dose contained 0.02 μg total protein. The dose was increased to 0.16 μg in the second injection and then doubled at subsequent injections to a maximum of 40 μg total protein (0.8 mL).Using the symptom medication score (SMS) as the primary endpoint, efficacy was shown in the form of a significant improvement of 39% compared with placebo. The recombinant cocktail components showed high immunogenicity, which was expressed as the ability to induce high specific IgG_1 and in particular IgG_4 levels. Four patients in the verum group were not sensitized to Phl p 5. Moreover, no new sensitizations to Ph1 p 5 occurred following treatment. This method's safety profile is described as very good, as was confirmed in a dose-finding study with maximum maintenance doses of 120 μg (Klimek et al. 2012).

However, the promising results of these early studies could not be confirmed in subsequent double-blind, placebo-controlled multinational phase-III trials (◉ Table 26.1) in terms of a statistically significant improvement in symptom medication score (SMS) under natural geographical conditions compared with placebo, despite immunological parameters (e.g., strong induction of specific IgG_4) showing a distinct effect (Allergopharma, publication in preparation). An important aspect in the evaluation of results is the dependence of clinical data on external influences (pollen count), which account for a marked improvement in SMS in the placebo group in years with low pollen counts. In order to minimize these effects on the outcome of lengthy and expensive clinical studies, a number of manufacturers of allergen immunotherapeutic agents are currently working on establishing the use of pollen exposure chambers and their approval for the collection of data that could serve as the primary endpoint for approval trials.

A further approach using recombinant birch allergens has been investigated in a double-blind, placebo-controlled phase-II study. The study compared the subcutaneous administration of birch pollen extract ($n=29$), purified natural (n) Bet v 1 ($n=29$), and recombinant (r) Bet v 1 ($n=32$) with placebo ($n=35$) (Pauli et al. 2008). The three preparations were adsorbed on aluminum hydroxide, administered preseasonally, and each contained 15 μg Bet v 1 in the maximum maintenance dose. The rhinoconjunctivitis symptom score improved by 48.0% (extract), 58.3% (nBet v 1), and 64.2% (rBet v 1) during the first pollen season following treatment, while the medication score improved by 69.9% (extract),

63.5% (nBet v 1), and 64.2% (rBet v 1). If one takes the number of patients into consideration, the three preparations showed comparable efficacy. What is also remarkable is that three patients in the extract group developed new sensitizations to the birch pollen minor allergen Bet v 2, while the IgE value rose in one patient that was already sensitized to Bet v 2. In the nBet v 1 and rBet v 1 groups, no new sensitizations to Bet v 2 or increases in IgE were observed in two patients that were already sensitized to Bet v 2.

Further studies with recombinant Bet v 1 administered sublingually in tablet form have been published as abstracts (Rak et al. 2010; Winther et al. 2009). The safety profile at 12.5, 25, and 50 μg Bet v 1 was described *as "very good,"* particularly at the two lower concentrations. Clinical efficacy, as measured by patient-reported symptom scores, showed ~25% improvement compared with placebo-treated subjects.

26.3.3 Studies with Hypoallergenic Recombinant Allergenoids

A number of strategies to generate hypoallergenic variants (allergenoids) from IgE-reactive native folded allergens, i.e., allergens that are structurally equivalent to naturally occurring allergens, have been described. This concept is based on experience with allergoids, chemically modified hypoallergenic extracts, which, due to the reduction of IgE-mediated side effects, can be administered in AIT at higher doses with an undiminished safety profile. This can be achieved, e.g., by means of point mutations in IgE epitopes, deletion of IgE-binding areas, sequence reorganization (allergen "shuffling"), or disulfide-bond elimination via cysteine mutations.

Most clinical experience has been gained with hypoallergenic variants of the birch pollen allergen Bet v 1. This Bet v 1 allergoid was unfolded by chemical denaturing, such that the existing secondary structure elements (α-helical regions and β-pleated sheet structures) were eliminated (◉ Fig. 26.2), thereby significantly reducing IgE binding as a result of the loss of IgE conformational epitopes (◉ Fig. 26.4). Since T-cell epitopes are not conformation-dependent, T-cell reactivity was conserved (Kahlert et al. 2008). An open randomized controlled proof-of-concept comparative study on an unmodified birch extract (Novo-Helisen Depot, Allergopharma) investigated efficacy and safety. The Bet v 1 content of native Bet v 1 in the extract was 20 μg in the maintenance dose, while that in the hypoallergenic recombinant Bet v 1 was 80 μg; moreover, the hypoallergenic preparation was faster in terms of dose escalation. After the first year of preseasonal treatment, the combined SMS dropped to 5.9 with the recombinant preparation and to 12.4 with the extract, as compared to 14.7 in the reference group (Narkus et al. 2008). A further improvement in SMS values of 3.00 (recombinant Bet v 1) and 2.93 (extract) was observed in the second year (Kettner et al. 2007a, b). Both the extract and the hypoallergenic recombinant Bet v 1 variants induced comparable specific IgG_1 and IgG_4 responses to birch pollen extract (Klimek et al. 2015). This study yielded

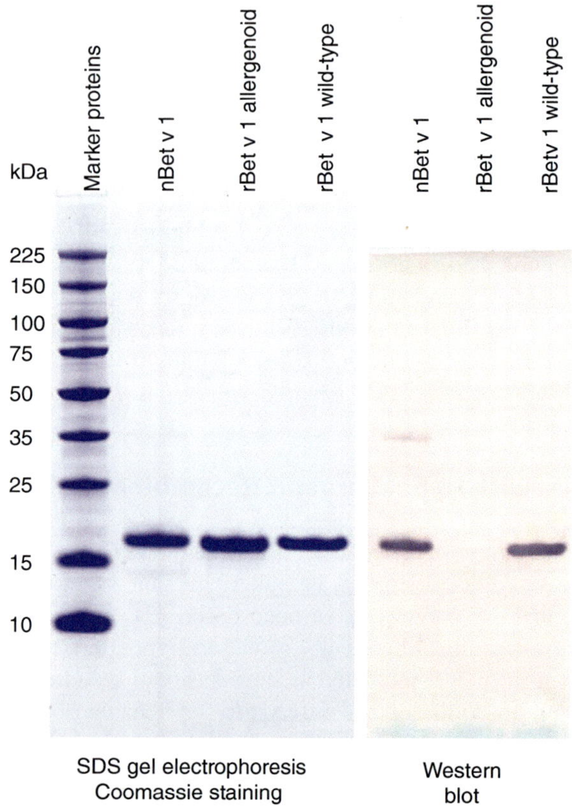

Fig. 26.4 The natural (*n*) Bet v 1 derived from a pollen extract, the recombinant (*r*) allergenoid, and the wild-type recombinant with native fold all behave in the same manner in sodium dodecyl sulfate (*SDS*) gel electrophoresis. Once the proteins have been transferred to a membrane (Western blot) and incubated with pooled serum from individuals with birch allergy, IgE binding can be detected. The correctly folded wild-type nBet v 1 and rBet v 1 show IgE binding. For the unfolded rBet v 1 allergenoid, in contrast, IgE binding can no longer be detected (Modified from Kahlert et al. (2008) with kind permission)

important conclusions for AIT with both recombinant and hypoallergenic preparations:

1. A single molecule can replace a complete extract in the case of birch pollen allergy treatment.
2. One isoform of the allergen is sufficient.
3. In the first year of therapy, treatment with a hypoallergenic recombinant allergenoid was superior to treatment with an unmodified extract.
4. The hypoallergenic concept (treatment with allergoids) was investigated and confirmed using a recombinant allergenoid.

Furthermore, a dose-finding study showed Bet v 1 allergenoids to be tolerated up to a dose of 320 μg, whereby the optimal dose for efficacy was 80 μg in the maintenance dose (Meyer et al. 2012).

A double-blind, placebo-controlled study on 226 patients with allergic rhinitis with or without asthma also demonstrated the efficacy of the recombinant preparation (Kettner et al. 2007a, b); moreover, the therapeutic effect was maintained at 2 years following completion of treatment (Hansen et al. 2011). However, further development of this preparation was ceased, since it was not deemed to offer greater value compared with commercially available hypoallergenic extract-based allergoid preparations (according to information from the company Allergopharma).

The results of further clinical trials with hypoallergenic recombinant allergens for food allergies are expected soon. Parvalbumin (Cyp c 1), the major allergen of the carp, has been produced as a hypoallergenic variant by four mutations in the calcium-binding site (Swoboda et al. 2007). Initial clinical phase-I/phase-II studies are currently underway.

26.3.4 Studies Involving Alternative Concepts

Fel d 1 is described as the most relevant major allergen in cat allergy. An immunotherapeutic approach currently in clinical phase-II trials is based on recombinant Fel d 1, fused to a translocation domain for more effective uptake by antigen-presenting cells and a truncated invariant chain for improved presentation of MHC class-II molecules (Senti et al. 2009). This construct, molecular antigen transporter (MAT)-Fel d 1, was administered in the form of intralymphatic immunotherapy (ILIT). Since the preparation is administered directly to the target organ, a lower dose is required. This method's safety profile is described as very good. Moreover, the clinical study yielded promising results, with tolerance induced after only three injections of 1.3 and 10 μg MAT-Fel d 1 (Senti et al. 2012).

Besides the goal to identify and utilize specific synthetic peptide sequences based on MHC class II binding in conjunction with T-cell proliferation assays and histamine release against an allergen (e.g., cat), another interesting approach involves that of producing overlapping peptides, in which the entire amino acid sequence of the allergen is included in order to "cover" all T-cell epitopes (Pellaton et al. 2013, Fallrath et al. 2003). A clinical trial with a significantly reduced treatment period was carried out with a preparation of three aluminum hydroxide-adsorbed synthetic overlapping fragments of the birch major allergen Bet v 1 (Spertini et al. 2014). Dosing was performed at 15 min intervals on the first day, followed by four further injections. The induction of IgG_4 antibodies and an increase in interleukin (IL)-10 production were measured immunologically. Efficacy was demonstrated by a 30% (50 μg preparation) and 19% (100 μg preparation) improvement in the rhinoconjunctivitis symptom and medication score (RSMS) through the birch pollen season. Both treatment regimens were also associated with similar improvements in QOL scores. A similar approach by Purohit et al. (2008) with two recombinant Bet v 1 fragments produced modifications of immunological parameters, yet no significant improvements in SMS.

Valenta and his collaborators have recently focused on the development of a recombinant B-cell epitope vaccine. With their recombinant methodology, linear peptides are fused to a carrier molecule and expressed as a fusion protein that has the capability to induce allergen-specific IgG against the IgE epitopes, thereby blocking the binding of IgE. In an initial study, exclusively B-cell epitopes were selected from four grass pollen allergens, Phl p 1, Phl p 2, Phl p 5, and Phl p 6, and fused to a carrier protein, hepatitis B preS (Marth et al. 2014). The aim with this approach is to induce therapeutically effective blocking IgG antibodies, while avoiding specific T-cell-mediated reactions. This preparation (BM32), which was injected subcutaneously four times annually, was evaluated with a study design that employed skin test provocation to assess preliminary safety and efficacy of the product (Niederberger et al. 2015). A double-blind, placebo-controlled phase-II trial on efficacy is currently underway (NCT01538979). Further work being undertaken includes a new Phase II (BM32) grass study utilizing an environmental chamber exposure model to optimize dose regimens for subsequent field trials.

26.4 Molecular Diagnosis for Molecular Treatment?

An attractive vision for the future of molecular allergology is individualized, component-based treatment selected for the individual on the basis of component-resolved diagnosis (Valenta et al. 1999). The appropriate treatment for each sensitization pattern of not only one allergen source but rather as a mixture of allergens from different allergen sources appears to be the ideal treatment form, tailored in a targeted manner to the individual patient. However, since each new mixture represents a new product from a regulatory perspective and therefore requires marketing authorization and its own clinical trials, this approach is not feasible under the current regulatory requirements.

Conclusions

1. The proof of concept for the efficacy and safety of recombinant allergens in AIT has been demonstrated. A single allergen (Bet v 1) can replace an extract for the treatment of birch pollen allergy.
2. The hypoallergenic concept has been confirmed by the clinical efficacy of a recombinant hypoallergenic Bet v 1 monopreparation.
3. The envisaged advantages of recombinant allergens compared with established extract-based preparations have not as yet been demonstrated in clinical trials.
4. New concepts based on recombinant immunotherapeutic agents are currently undergoing research and development and have the potential to significantly improve AIT in the future.

References

Cromwell O, Fiebig H, Suck R, et al. Strategies for recombinant allergen vaccines and fruitful results from first clinical trials. Immunol Allergy Clin North Am. 2006;26:261–81.

Cromwell O, Häfner D, Nandy A. Recombinant allergens for specific immunotherapy. J Allergy Clin Immunol. 2011;127:865–72.

Durham SR, Penagos M. Sublingual or subcutaneous immunotherapy for allergic rhinitis? J Allergy Clin Immunol. 2016;137:339–49.

European Commission, editor. EudraLex: the rules governing medicinal products in the European Union, Volume 4: EU guidelines for good manufacturing practice for medicinal products for human and veterinary use, annex 2, manufacture of biological active substances and medicinal products for human use. 2010.

European Medicines Agency, Committee for Medicinal Products for Human Use.Guideline on Allergen Products: production and quality issues; note for guidance on specifications: test procedures and acceptance criteria for biotechnological/biological products CPMP/ICH/365/96 [Q6B]. 2008.

Fallrath JM, Kettner A, Dufour N, et al. Allergen-specific T-cell tolerance induction with allergen-derived long synthetic peptides: Results of a phase I trial. J Allergy Clin Immunol. 2003;111:854–56.

Hansen S, Mußler S, Meyer H, et al. First long-term efficacy data of subcutaneous specific immunotherapy with a recombinant birch pollen product. Allergy. 2011;66:62.

Jutel M, Jaeger L, Suck R, et al. Allergen-specific immunotherapy with recombinant grass pollen allergens. J Allergy Clin Immunol. 2005;116:608–13.

Kahlert H, Suck R, Weber B, et al. Characterization of a hypoallergenic recombinant Bet v 1 variant as a candidate for allergen-specific immunotherapy. Int Arch Allergy Immunol. 2008;145:193–206.

Kettner J, Meyer H, Narkus A, et al. Specific immunotherapy with recombinant birch pollen allergen rBet v 1-FV is clinically efficacious—results of a phase III study [abstract]. Allergy. 2007a;62:33.

Kettner J, Meyer H, Cromwell O, et al. Specific immunotherapy with recombinant birch pollen allergen Bet v 1-FV. Results of 2 years treatment (Phase II Trial) [Abstract]. Allergy. 2007b;62:262.

Klimek L, Schendzielorz P, Pinol R, et al. Specific subcutaneous immunotherapy with recombinant grass pollen allergens: first randomized dose-ranging safety study. Clin Exp Allergy. 2012;42:936–45.

Klimek L, Bachert C, Lukat KF, et al. Allergy immunotherapy with a hypoallergenic recombinant birch pollen allergen rBet v 1-FV in a randomized controlled trial. Clin Transl Allergy. 2015;5:28.

Marth K, Focke-Tejkl M, Lupinek C, et al. Allergen peptides, recombinant allergens and hypoallergens for allergen-specific immunotherapy. Curr Treat Options Allergy. 2014;1:91–106.

Meyer W, Narkus A, Salapatek A, et al. Efficacy and safety of four dose regimes of a hypoallergenic recombinant birch pollen major allergen (rBet v 1-FV) in birch pollen allergic patients studied in an environmental exposure chamber [Abstract]. Allergy. 2012;67:89.

Narkus A, Kniest F, Menzel A et al. Clinical trials with recombinant allergens—three perspectives: industry. Arbeiten aus dem Paul-Ehrlich-Institut, 12th International Paul-Ehrlich-Seminar, Bad Homburg. Chmielorz, Wiesbaden; 2008. p. 270–8.

Niederberger V, Horak F, Vrtala S, et al. Vaccination with genetically engineered allergens prevents progression of allergic disease. Proc Nat Acad Sci USA. 2004;101 Suppl 2:14677–82.

Niederberger V, Marth K, Eckl-Dorna J, et al. Skin test evaluation of a novel peptide carrier-based vaccine, BM32, in grass pollen-allergic patients. J Allergy Clin Immunol. 2015;136:1101–3.

Pauli G, Larsen TH, Rak S, et al. Efficacy of recombinant birch pollen vaccine for the treatment of birch-allergic rhinoconjunctivitis. J Allergy Clin Immunol. 2008;122:951–60.

Pellaton C, Perrin Y, Boudousquie C, et al. Novel birch pollen specific immunotherapy formulation based on contiguous overlapping peptides. Clin Transl Allergy. 2013;3:17.
Purohit A, Niederberger V, Kronquist M, et al. Clinical effects of immunotherapy with genetically modified recombinant birch pollen Bet v 1 derivatives. Clin Exp Allergy. 2008;38:1514–25.
Radauer C, Nandy A, Ferreira F, et al. Update of the WHO/IUIS Allergen Nomenclature Database based on analysis of allergen sequences. Allergy. 2014;69:413–9.
Rak S, De Blay F, Worm M, et al. Efficacy and safety of recombinant Bet v 1 (rBet v 1) tablets in sublingual immunotherapy [abstract]. Allergy. 2010;65 Suppl 65:4.
Senti G, Kuster D, Martinez-Gomez J, et al. Intralymphatic allergen specific immunotherapy using modified recombinant allergen targeting the MHC class II pathway: a double-blind placebo-controlled clinical trial in cat dander allergic patients [abstract]. Allergy. 2009;64 Suppl 90:74.
Senti G, Crameri R, Kuster D, et al. Intralymphatic immunotherapy for cat allergy induces tolerance after only 3 injections. J Allergy Clin Immunol. 2012;129:1290–6.
Suck R, Kamionka T, Schaffer B, et al. Bacterially expressed and optimized recombinant Phl p 1 is immunobiochemically equivalent to natural Phl p 1. Biochim Biophy Acta. 2006; 1764:1701–9.
Spertini F, Perrin Y, Audran R, et al. Safety and immunogenicity of immunotherapy with Bet v 1-derived contiguous overlapping peptides. J Allergy Clin Immunol. 2014;134:239–40.
Swoboda I, Bugajska-Schretter A, Linhart B, et al. A recombinant hypoallergenic parvalbumin mutant for immunotherapy of IgE-mediated fish allergy. J Immunol. 2007;178:6290–6.
Valenta R, Lidholm J, Niederberger V, et al. The recombinant allergen-based concept of component-resolved diagnostics and immunotherapy (CRD and CRIT). Clin Exp Allergy. 1999; 29:896–904.
Winther L, Poulsen LK, Robin B, et al. Safety and tolerability of recombinant Bet v 1 (rBet v 1) tablets in sublingual immunotherapy SLIT [abstract]. J Allergy Clin Immunol. 2009; 123(Suppl):S215.

Definition and Design of Hypoallergenic Foods

27

V. Mahler and R.E. Goodman

Abbreviations

DBPCFC	Double-blind placebo-controlled food challenge
dsRNA	Double-stranded RNA
EAST	Enzyme allergosorbent test
EFSA	European Food Safety Authority
ELISA	Enzyme-linked immunosorbent assay
GenTG	Deutsches Gentechnikgesetz German Genetic Engineering Act
GM	Genetically modified
GMO	Genetically modified organisms
HA	Hypoallergenic
HPLC	High-performance liquid chromatography
hpRNA	Hairpin RNA
IgE	Immunoglobulin E
LOAEL	Lowest observed adverse effect level
LTP	Lipid transfer protein
mRNA	Messenger RNA
nsLTP	Nonspecific lipid transfer protein

This contribution is based on a publication by the first author that appeared in the *Allergo Journal International* in 2015 (Mahler V. Definition and design of hypoallergenic foods. Allergo J Int 2015;24: 244–55), which has been updated and expanded as a chapter for this book.

V. Mahler, MD, Prof. (✉)
Department of Dermatology, University Hospital Erlangen, Friedrich-Alexander-University Erlangen-Nuremberg, Erlangen, Germany

Allergology, Paul-Ehrlich Institute, Federal Institute for Vaccines and Biomedicines, D-63225 Langen, Germany
e-mail: vera.mahler@uk-erlangen.de; vera.mahler@fau.de; vera.mahler@pei.de

R.E. Goodman, PhD, Prof.
Department of Food Science & Technology, University of Nebraska, Lincoln, NE, USA

J. Kleine-Tebbe, T. Jakob (eds.), *Molecular Allergy Diagnostics*,
DOI 10.1007/978-3-319-42499-6_27

NTWG	New Techniques Working Group
PR-10	Pathogenesis-related protein family 10
PTGS	Posttranscriptional gene silencing
RNA	Ribonucleic acid
RNAi	RNA interference
RNase	Ribonuclease
RT-PCR	Reverse transcriptase-polymerase chain reaction
siRNA	Short interfering RNA
SIT	Specific immunotherapy
TALEN	Transcription activator-like effector nucleases
TILLING	Targeting induced local lesions in genomes
UDP	Uridine diphosphate
WT	Wild type
ZKBS	German Central Commission for Biological Safety (*Zentrale Kommission für die Biologische Sicherheit*)

27.1 Introduction

In addition to nuts, legumes, fish, and crustacean shellfish, the most common food allergies in adults in industrialized countries are to fruits and vegetables (Ballmer-Weber and Hoffmann-Sommergruber 2014; Sicherer 2011). A number of recent studies have used molecular methods for the diagnosis of fruit and vegetable allergy and identified a few allergen families as the likely cause of cross-reactivity as reviewed in 2014 (Ballmer-Weber and Hoffmann-Sommergruber 2014). Different allergens in plant foods are recognized with varying frequency by food allergy sufferers (Asero et al. 2008). Regional differences exist in this regard (Hoffmann-Sommergruber et al. 2015; Palacín et al. 2012; Schmidt-Andersen et al. 2011). Epidemiologically important allergens (proteins) are often considered to be those recognized by IgE of more than 50% of the population *allergic to a source*, and these are referred to as *major allergens* (Chapman 2008). However, in some cases, the most commonly bound protein is a pan-allergen (e.g., profilin) that may or may not be associated with clinical elicitation, and the term major might be more accurately described as most commonly bound by IgE using sera from clinically diagnosed allergic subjects (Asero et al. 2015).

The severity of an allergic reaction to an allergen is determined on an individual consumer and allergen basis influenced by the amount and specificity of IgE, number of epitopes bound by the subjects' IgE, as well as very diverse and variable environmental factors that may augment the response (e.g., infection, physical exertion, psychological stressors, hormonal influences, cold, heat, alcohol consumption, drug use) and by the dose and structural characteristics of the respective allergen (Hauser et al. 2012; Hompes et al. 2010; Kleine-Tebbe et al. 2010; Petersen and Scheurer 2011; Radauer et al. 2012). Heat-stable and acid and pepsin-resistant allergens generally cause more severe reactions compared with heat- and gastric acid and pepsin-labile allergens (Hauser et al. 2012; Kleine-Tebbe et al. 2010; Petersen and Scheurer 2011; Radauer et al. 2012; Asero et al. 2000).

The only generally recognized effective treatment for food allergy to date is the consistent avoidance of the relevant allergenic food. However, vigilant avoidance can also be associated with a significant reduction in quality of life (Beyer 2007; Taylor and Hefle 2001).

A number of research groups are evaluating the potential efficacy of reducing the expression of specific proteins in allergenic species of plants as a way to reduce risks for allergic consumers.

Hypoallergenic foods—in which immunodominant immunoglobulin E (IgE)-binding allergens are lacking or markedly reduced—could contribute to primary and secondary prevention in terms of reducing new sensitizations and cross-reactivity. But in addition, they may serve the purpose of avoiding elicitation of reactions in already-sensitized food allergy sufferers.

This article discusses the current state of the science with regard to the definition and design of hypoallergenic foods. Perspectives and challenges are highlighted.

27.2 Definition of Hypoallergenic Foods

Foods intended for consumption by food-allergic individuals should be hypoallergenic, i.e., have significantly reduced in vivo capacity to elicit an allergic sufferer's reaction compared with naturally occurring foods (Muraro et al. 2004).

However, the term hypoallergenicity—although frequently used in conjunction with foods—is not precisely defined. Foods defined as hypoallergenic to date have primarily been restricted to cow's milk formulations that are modified to reduce the concentration of intact or substantial fragments of allergenic proteins to peptides or amino acids below the size that can cross-link IgE on FcεRI receptors on mast cells and basophils or reducing T-cell activation. The products labeled hypoallergenic (HA) infant formulas have been treated using food processing techniques (enzymatic protein hydrolysis, heat treatment, and/or ultrafiltration), with the aim of destroying or inactivating IgE-binding and T-cell epitopes (Beyer 2007; Fritsché 2009). For each new product, the success of allergenicity reduction in these hypoallergenic formulations needs to be verified in the preclinical setting as well as in clinical use by in vitro and in vivo methods (Beyer 2007; Muraro et al. 2004; Fritsché 2009; American Academy of Pediatrics Committee on Nutrition 2000). The practical definition of hypoallergenic requires that at least 90 % of children with proven cow's milk allergy tolerate these formulations in double-blind, placebo-controlled food challenge (DBPCFC) (Beyer 2007; Muraro et al. 2004; Chung and Reed 2014). The possibilities and limitations of food processing techniques to reduce allergens in raw foods by means of physical and chemical methods during processing are discussed elsewhere (Taylor and Hefle 2001; Chung and Reed 2014).

Beyond process of allergenic animal products, some attention has been focused on allergenic plant ingredients in foods in recent years (Ballmer-Weber and Hoffmann-Sommergruber 2014; Radauer and Breiteneder 2007). New molecular biological approaches to reducing the IgE binding of food allergens in unprocessed foods have become the focus of several researchers using various techniques to "silence" the production of proteins by insertion of modified DNA that expresses interfering RNA for the reduction of specific allergens, using newer gene-editing techniques to remove the allergenic genes (Gallo and Sayre 2009; Hebert et al. 2008; Song et al. 2015).

27.3 Design and Evaluation of Hypoallergenic Foods

Using various gene silencing methods, it has been possible to successfully achieve reduced or blocked expression of genes that code for particular food allergens in rice, soybean, apple, tomato, carrot, and peanut as models of allergen sources (Gallo and Sayre 2009).

Model allergens—due either to their common prevalence or to the severity of allergic manifestations they cause—are the focus of scientific interest in terms of the design of hypoallergenic foods in the current proof-of-concept investigations. Knowledge gained through initial trials to eliminate certain model allergens or reduce the IgE-binding capacity of these proteins in plant-based foods may open the door for development of the multigene-targeted silencing strategies needed for the possible long-term sustainable production of hypoallergenic foods in which all epidemiologically relevant allergens have been simultaneously eliminated.

A number of steps are required to confirm the presumed hypoallergenicity of allergen-reduced foods (Herman et al. 2003):

- Sustained production of the food with reduced allergen expression
- Verification of the postulated hypoallergenicity verified by in vitro testing using SDS-PAGE immunoblotting or ELISA assays demonstrating low IgE binding
- In vivo testing in animal models
- Skin prick testing with extracts from the hypoallergenic food in sensitized patients
- Open oral food challenge in patients with known allergy to the relevant food

It is essential that transgenic allergen-reduced plants are monitored to evaluate the entire protein profile for simultaneous upregulation of other known or new allergens and, additionally, to ensure equivalence in terms of the agronomic characteristics of crop species (Gallo and Sayre 2009; Goodman et al. 2008).

There are recommendations, decision trees, and legal requirements [Regulation (EC) No 1829/2003 of the European Parliament and of the Council of 22 September 2003 on genetically modified food and feed] for the risk assessment of genetically modified (GM) foods that need to be taken into account if commercial marketing of the product is intended as discussed briefly here.

A scientific opinion issued by the European Food Safety Authority (EFSA) summarizes the amended, wholistic recommendations on risk assessment strategies for:

1. Proteins that are newly expressed in the plant (most are intended to increase the agronomic performance potential, pest resistance, herbicide tolerance, or nutritional value of a plant-based food)

2. GM foods including the hypoallergenic foods produced using RNA interference (RNAi) are mentioned as follows (EFSA Panel on Genetically Modified Organisms (GMO Panel) 2010):
    - Each modified (GM) protein must be evaluated by a computer search for existing sequence identity matches, with a conservative sequence alignment to known allergens set as the minimal requirement. Sequence identities greater than 35 % to a known allergen over a length of at least 80 amino acids are considered the threshold of concern.
    - Where IgE-binding tests are considered necessary (e.g., in the case of existing sequence homology if the source of the gene is a known allergenic source), sera from individuals allergic to the source, but not pooled sera, should be used to evaluate potential IgE binding.
    - A pepsin resistance test is also performed under fixed laboratory conditions (Ofori-Anti et al. 2008); other in vitro digestibility tests that imitate physiological conditions in humans may provide useful information for the risk assessment.
    - If the recipient plant of a newly introduced gene is known to be allergenic (e.g., peanut, wheat), it is recommended that the known endogenous allergens are included in the compositional analysis of the GM plant and its appropriate non-modified counterparts in order to compare allergenicity. A hypoallergenic GM variety would have to be demonstrated to have markedly lower concentrations of known allergenic proteins under food labeling laws in many countries in order to be marketed as such.

The EFSA recommendations are in line with the Codex Alimentarius (Codex Alimentarius Commission 2003; Ladics 2008) and pursue a weight-of-evidence approach, whereby all abovementioned areas need to be evaluated (Goodman et al. 2008).

27.4 Methods of Gene Silencing to Produce Hypoallergenic Foods

While new methods of gene editing including CRISPR/Cas9 and TALONs are being used to silence specific genes in plants, so far there are no publications demonstrating removal of allergens from a food crop using these new methods. However, various posttranscriptional gene silencing (PTGS) methods (Fagard and Vaucheret 2000) have been used with varying degrees of success in proof-of-concept studies on obtaining hypoallergenic foods in different plant models (◉ Table 27.1) (Gallo and Sayre 2009; Scheuer and Sonnewald 2009):

- *Posttranscriptional gene silencing by sense transgenes (co-suppression):* Introducing a transcribable gene that is identical to the target gene (sense transgene) can downregulate expression of the homologous endogenous gene.

Table 27.1 Overview of the posttranscriptional gene silencing methods used in the design of hypoallergenic foods

Method	Silencing of	Allergen source	References
Co-suppression	Gly m Bd 30K	Soybean	Herman et al. (2003)
Antisense gene silencing	14- to 16-kDa allergens (α-amylase/trypsin inhibitor)	Rice	Tada et al. (1996)
RNAi silencing (chimeric RNAi construct)	Simultaneously: 14- to 16-kDa allergens (α-amylase/trypsin inhibitor) and 33-kDa allergen (β-glyoxalase)	Rice	Wakasa et al. (2011)
RNAi silencing	Mal d 1 (PR-10 protein)	Apple	Gilissen et al. (2005)
RNAi silencing	Sola l 1 (profilin)	Tomato	Le et al. (2006a)
RNAi silencing	β-1,2-Xylosyltransferase enzyme (→ alteration of the IgE epitope of Sola l 2)	Tomato	Paulus et al. (2011)
RNAi silencing	Sola l 3 (nsLTP)	Tomato	Le et al. (2006b)
RNAi silencing (chimeric RNAi construct)	Simultaneously: Sola l 4 (PR-10 protein, TSI-1) and chitinase B and osmotin-like protein	Tomato	Paulus (2012)
RNAi silencing (chimeric RNAi construct)	Simultaneously: polygalacturonase 2A and pectinesterase	Tomato	Paulus (2012)
RNAi silencing and co-expression	Sola l 1 (profilin) Simultaneously: co-expression of yeast profilin	Tomato	Le et al. (2010)
RNAi silencing	Dau c 1.01 (PR-10 protein)	Carrot	Peters et al. (2011)
RNAi silencing	Dau c 1.02 (PR-10 protein)	Carrot	Peters et al. (2011)
RNAi silencing	Ara h 2.02	Peanut	Dodo et al. (2008)
RNAi silencing	Simultaneously: Ara h 2.01 and Ara h 2.02, as well as simultaneously reduced expression of Ara h 6	Peanut	Chu et al. (2008)

IgE immunoglobulin E, *nsLTP* nonspecific lipid transfer protein, *RNAi* RNA interference

Co-suppression is based on endogenous and transgenic ribonucleic acid (RNA) degradation following their common transcription (Herman et al. 2003). More efficient reductions have been achieved using transgenes designed specifically to produce either full-length or partial sequence antisense RNA copies of the gene that is intended to be reduced as described below.

- *Posttranscriptional gene silencing by antisense transgenes:* The antisense strategy involves introducing a complementary antisense gene (antisense transgene) in the plant cell. The antisense gene's messenger RNA (mRNA) binds to endogenous mRNA as a matching counterpart and blocks translation of the protein. The resulting double-stranded RNA (dsRNA) can either block translation or leads to degradation of the translatable mRNA. These RNA interference (RNAi) methods, which have been applied with increasing success in plants in recent years, involve a sequence-specific gene silencing mechanism triggered by the introduction of double-stranded RNA and which causes degradation of the plant's own mRNA (Nusrat et al. 2010). RNAi can be successfully induced in plants using a dsRNA construct in the form of a hairpin (hairpin RNA, hpRNA) (Wesley et al. 2001; Smith et al. 2000). An appropriate DNA construct that codes for a specific sequence in sense and antisense orientation—separated by an intron—is introduced into the cell by transformation. The abovementioned sequence-specific dsRNA constructs are formed through DNA-dependent synthesis; due to the intron, they form a hairpin structure. These dsRNA molecules are recognized by a ribonuclease (RNase/Dicer) and cleaved into smaller fragments of 21–23 nucleotides, which are referred to as short interfering RNA (siRNA). These siRNA are then integrated into a riboprotein complex (RNA-induced silencing complex), where they mediate translational repression of protein synthesis or cleavage of the target mRNA (◉ Fig. 27.1) (Zhang and Hua 2004).

27.5 Allergen Reduction Achieved in Allergen Source Models of Plant-Based Foods

27.5.1 Rice (*Oryza sativa*)

Antisense gene silencing was first used to suppress allergen gene expression in maturing rice seeds (Tada et al. 1996). The prevalence of type 1 sensitization (antigen-specific IgE-mediated immediate hypersensitivity) to rice in population-based studies of adults (aged 22–44 years) in 13 countries (11 European countries, the USA, and Australia) is reportedly between 0.3 % in Iceland and 4.9 % in the USA (Burney et al. 2010), while the highest prevalence within Europe is found in Italy at 3.6 % (Burney et al. 2010). The prevalence of IgE-mediated rice allergy in atopic subjects has been reported to be as high as 10 % in Japan (Wakasa et al. 2011). However, the actual prevalence of proven food allergy to rice is much lower (Trcka et al. 2012). The majority of studies demonstrating IgE binding to rice proteins have used sera from subjects with asthma or dermatitis and without symptoms of food allergy due to consumption of rice.

Two rice allergens are listed in the official allergen database of the World Health Organization (WHO) and International Union of Immunological Societies (IUIS) Allergen Nomenclature Subcommittee (2014) the major rice pollen allergen Ory s 1, a beta-expansin (35 kDa), and Ory s 12, a profilin A with a molecular weight of 14 kDa (contained in pollen and seed). Other potential food allergens from rice that

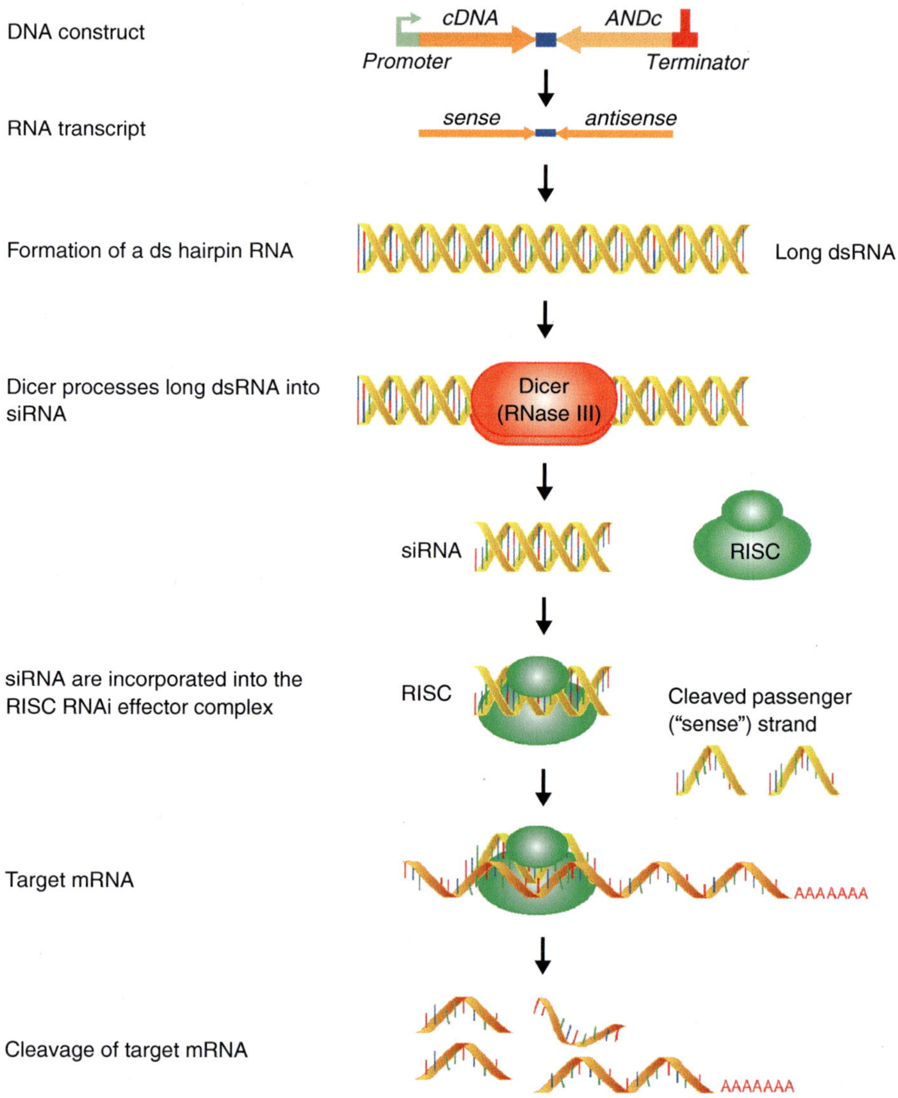

Fig. 27.1 Mechanism of RNAi silencing using dsRNA. *dsRNA* double-strand RNA, *RNAi* RNA interference

have not yet fulfilled IUIS criteria have been described in rice (Trcka et al. 2012; Allergome et al. 2014), including α-amylase/trypsin inhibitors (14–16 kDa), α-globulin (26 kDa), and β-glyoxalase I (33 kDa), which are considered major allergens based on IgE recognition by serum IgE from allergy patients (Wakasa et al. 2011) and a 56 kDa glycoportein which seems to be responsible for anaphylaxis after consumption of rice in a German patient. Whereas 14- to 16-kDa allergens represent a multigene family with >80 % nucleotide sequence identity, the 26-kDa and 33-kDa allergen both are based on single-copy genes (Wakasa et al. 2011).

Antisense gene silencing was used to suppress gene expression of the 14- to 16-kDa allergens (α-amylase/trypsin inhibitors) in maturing rice seeds (Tada et al. 1996).

Immunoblotting and RNA blot analysis of seeds from the transgenic rice plants using allergen-specific monoclonal antibodies and a sequence-specific antisense RNA probe showed that both the mRNA and the protein content of the allergens were significantly lower compared with wild-type rice and remained so in a stable manner for several generations (Tada et al. 1996). However, it was not possible to achieve complete suppression, explained in part by poor sequence homology between the antisense constructs used and the various members of the multigene family that encode for the 14- to 16-kDa allergens (Tada et al. 1996).

Whereas antisense gene silencing reduced the 14- to 16-kDa allergen content to only 20 % of that in wild type, a recent multi-target approach involving dsRNA interference using transformation of a type of rice (Koshihikari)—in which the 26-kDa allergen (α-globulin) was already lacking due to mutation breeding—was able to achieve the simultaneous inhibition of 14- to 16-kDa allergens (α-amylase-trypsin inhibitors) and the 33-kDa allergen (β-glyoxalase). Simultaneous inhibition of the three allergens in the transgenic plants reduced IgE-binding capacity by up to 90 %. Data to assess allergenicity based on the basophil histamine release test or skin testing in rice allergic patients are still lacking. No effect on the rice seed phenotype was observed (Wakasa et al. 2011).

27.5.2 Soybean (*Glycine max*)

The prevalence of type 1 sensitization to soy in a population-based study of adults (aged 20–44 years) in the 13 countries mentioned above is between 0.0 % in Iceland and 4.7 % in the USA (overall average for all countries, 2.1 %; overall average for all countries excluding birch pollen-sensitized subjects, 1.4 % (Burney et al. 2010). The highest prevalence within Europe was found in Italy at 3.6 %.

In addition to the eight soybean food allergens currently included in the WHO/IUIS list (Gly m 1–8) (International Union of Immunological Societies (IUIS) Allergen Nomenclature Sub-Committee 2014), other food allergens have been described, including the allergen Gly m Bd 30K, also known as P34 (cysteine protease) present in the 7S-globulin fraction, which is frequently recognized by sera from soy-sensitized patients as sole allergen (Ogawa et al. 1991).

Although it was not possible to silence the immunodominant Gly m Bd 30K allergen using mutagenesis and conventional breeding, transgene-induced gene silencing (co-suppression) was able to achieve a complete knockdown of the Gly m Bd 30K gene, resulting in the full elimination of Gly m Bd 30K-specific binding in immunoblotting analysis with patient sera. No morphological or reproductive differences between transgenic and wild-type plants were seen (Herman et al. 2003).

The authors concluded that combined suppression of the Gly m Bd 30K allergen and other major soybean allergens is necessary in order to obtain a hypoallergenic soybean that is tolerated not only by the abovementioned group of Gly-m-Bd30K-monosensitized allergy patients (Herman et al. 2003). Others have shown that major seed storage proteins, three beta-conglycinins (Gly m 5.0101, 5.0201, and 5.0301) as well as five glycinins (Gly m 6.0101–6.0501), are major food allergens in soybean and comprise a major portion of the proteins in seeds (Holzhauser et al. 2009).

27.5.3 Apple (*Malus domestica*)

RNAi as a method of posttranscriptional gene silencing was first used in apple plants as an allergen source model to inhibit the expression of Mal d 1, the major apple allergen (Hoffmann-Sommergruber et al. 2015; Gilissen et al. 2005). Mal d 1 occurs in 30 different isoforms and exhibits marked cross-reactivity with the major birch allergen, Bet v 1 (Hoffmann-Sommergruber et al. 2015; Gilissen et al. 2005; Krath et al. 2009). Mal d 1 and Bet v 1 share 64.5 % amino acid sequence identity (Krath et al. 2009). At least 18 genes for Mal d 1 have been identified in the apple genome (Gilissen et al. 2005). Mal d 1 is found in the fruit as well as in the leaves.

In addition to Mal d 1, Mal d 2 [thaumatin-like protein, a pathogenesis-related (PR) protein belonging to the PR-5 family], Mal d 3 [nonspecific lipid transfer protein 1 (nsLTP1) belonging to the PR-14 family], and Mal d 4 (profilin) are listed as food allergens in apple in the official WHO/IUIS database (Hoffmann-Sommergruber et al. 2015). Approximately 70 % of birch pollen-allergic individuals suffer from allergic symptoms, predominantly oral allergy syndrome to ingestion of apple due to the homology between Bet v 1 and Mal d 1, both of which belong to the PR-10 family (Gilissen et al. 2005). The prevalence of sensitization to apple in a population-based study of young adults (aged 20–44 years) in 13 European countries was between 0.0 % in Iceland and 10.3 % in Germany (overall average for all countries, 4.2 %; overall average for all countries excluding birch pollen-sensitized subjects, 2.0 %) (Burney et al. 2010).

RNAi proved to be a suitable method to simultaneously inhibit the expression of all genes belonging to the PR-10 gene family (Hebert et al. 2008). As part of the SAFE project, plantlets of the apple cultivar "Elstar" were transformed with a construct that contained a Mal d 1-specific inverted repeat sequence and coded for an intron-spliced hairpin RNA (Hoffmann-Sommergruber et al. 2015; Gilissen et al. 2005). Gene silencing is based on the sequence-specific degradation of endogenous mRNA, which undergoes enzymatic degradation via RNA interference with double-stranded hairpin RNA (Gilissen et al. 2006).

The resulting reduction in Mal d 1 protein expression could be shown in extracts of the transformed plant using IgE immunoblotting with a serum pool from patients. The leaves of the transformed plants exhibited significantly lower skin test reactivity compared with wild type in skin prick testing on patients with birch pollen and apple allergy (Gilissen et al. 2005). In a follow-up project, GM plants were grafted onto wild-type rootstock and cultivated under greenhouse conditions (Krath et al. 2009): eight of the 10 plants showed significant silencing (up to 10,000 fold) in Mal d 1 gene expression, and these levels remained stable over a period of more than 3 years (Krath et al. 2009). Due, in all likelihood, to in vitro culture or genetic modification, some of the GM Elstar trees showed altered morphology, involving darker, more serrated leaves and slower growth compared with other GM plants (Krath et al. 2009). One of the disadvantages of apple as a model allergen source is its latency period of several years between transformation and fruit-bearing, which explains why allergenicity studies have been carried out on leaves from GM plants.

Recently, food challenges with apples derived from the gene silenced genetically modified apple lines, expressing extensively downregulated mRNA levels for Mal d 1.02 and other Mal d 1 genes compared to wild-type Elstar, proved to induce significantly less intense symptoms in apple-allergic individuals (Dubois et al. 2015).

27.5.4 Tomato (*Solanum lycopersicum*, Formerly: *Lycopersicon esculentum*)

The prevalence of type 1 sensitization to tomato in a population-based study of adults (aged 20–44 years) in the 13 countries mentioned above was 0.8 % in Iceland and 5.6 % in Germany (overall average for all countries, 3.3 %; overall average for all countries not including birch pollen sensitized subjects, 2.3 %) (Burney et al. 2010).

Five tomato allergens [Sola l 1 (profilin), Sola l 2 (β-fructofuranosidase, synonym: invertase), Sola l 3 (nsLTP 2), Sola l 4 (PR-10, Bet v 1 family member, TSI-1), Sola l 5 (cyclophilin)] have been included in the official WHO/IUIS allergen nomenclature list. The tomato allergens Sola l 1–3 are given in the literature under their former allergen names (Lyc e 1–3). As a result of an update of the botanical nomenclature (new: *Solanum lycopersicum*, formerly: *Lycopersicon esculentum*), allergen names were also updated in the recent review of the WHO/IUIS Allergen Nomenclature Database (Radauer et al. 2014).

Approximately 32 % of food-allergic (Willerroider et al. 2003) and 22 % of tomato-allergic individuals are sensitized to tomato profilin Sola l 1 (Westphal et al. 2003), 17 % to Sola l 2 (invertase) (Westphal et al. 2004), and 35 % of Spanish patients with fruit allergy to Sola l 3 (nsLTP), whereas sensitization to Sola l 3 (nsLTP), which is resistant to heat and pepsin action and can cause severe allergic symptoms, is a rarity in tomato-allergic patients in Germany (Foetisch et al. 2001). Sola l 4 (PR-10 protein), on the other hand, was recognized by 76 % of German patients with tomato and birch pollen allergy (Wangorsch et al. 2014). With an amino acid identity of over 40 % and similar protein structure, there is considerable cross-reactivity between the two PR-10 proteins, Sola l 4 and Bet v 1 (Wangorsch et al. 2014). Furthermore, numerous other putative tomato allergens have been described (Bässler et al. 2009; Kondo et al. 2001; López-Matas et al. 2011; Welter et al. 2013a, b).

Most tomato-allergic individuals are polysensitized to several tomato fruit allergens; according to own investigations in a German collective, the proportion of monosensitized patients that recognize only a single tomato allergen is just under 5 %, whereas 15 % of tomato-allergic individuals in an Italian collective were monosensitized to nsLTP (Sola l 3) (Le et al. 2006a; Pravettoni et al. 2009).

Varying environmental conditions (e.g., climate factors, aridity, tomato plant infections) result in varying levels of gene expression of individual proteins in the tomato plant and its fruit (Welter et al. 2013b; Plant et al. 1991), which can be relevant in terms of successful gene silencing. The advantages of the tomato as a model allergen plant include its short (approximately 2–3 months) generation time and latency period between successful transformation and the bearing of initial fruit with reduced allergenicity, a known genome, as well as the existence of various—both glycosylated and non-glycosylated—tomato allergens that can be used as models to gain insight into gene silencing in different allergens.

Three tomato allergens have been suppressed by RNAi silencing (Le et al. 2006a, b; Paulus et al. 2011). It was possible to confirm reduced or absent IgE reactivity of allergen-reduced tomatoes in subsequent daughter generations, suggesting that RNAi silencing remains stable over several generations. No compensatory expression of other endogenous tomato allergens was detected.

Sola l 1 (profilin) and Sola l 3 (nsLTP), which each occur in two isoforms, were successfully silenced in transgenic plants by using constitutive expression of specially conceived constructs of allergen-specific hairpin RNA (Le et al. 2006a, b). Successful silencing of both profilin genes (Le et al. 2006a) and both LTP genes (Le et al. 2006b), as well as the resulting reduction in allergenicity of the GM plants and their tomato fruit, was confirmed:

- On an RNA level (Northern blot)
- On a protein level (Western blot with profilin or LTP-specific rabbit antiserum and IgE immunoblotting with sera from tomato-allergic patients (Le et al. 2006a; Lorenz et al. 2006) or basophil histamine release (Le et al. 2006b)
- In skin tests on patients (Le et al. 2006a; Lorenz et al. 2006)

A number of transgenic plant lines yielded red tomatoes with a tenfold reduced Sola l 1 content compared with wild-type plants (Le et al. 2006a). LTP could no longer be detected in Sola l 3-silenced transgenic tomatoes using Northern or Western blot assays. Ten- to 100-fold higher protein extract levels were required for Sola l 3-silenced transgenic tomato fruits to trigger basophil histamine release; IgE

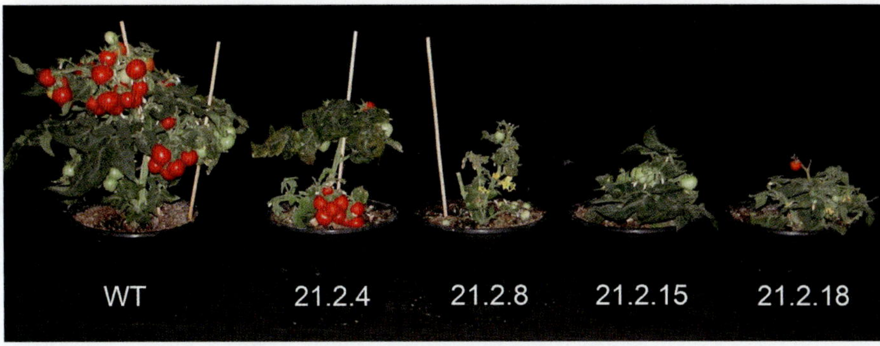

Fig. 27.2 Sola l 1 (profilin-)silenced transgenic tomato plants (lines 21.2.4, 21.2.8, 21.2.15, and 21.2.18) compared with the wild-type (*WT*) Micro-Tom variety (Figure courtesy of Dr. Kathrin Paulus and Prof. Uwe Sonnewald, Department of Biochemistry, Friedrich-Alexander University Erlangen-Nürnberg, Germany)

immunoblotting assays with sera from tomato-allergic subjects, as well as skin prick testing in tomato-allergic subjects, exhibited significantly reduced IgE binding and reduced skin test reactivity (Le et al. 2006b).

A different approach was chosen in terms of reducing the allergenicity of Sola l 2 (invertase): it could be shown that the IgE-binding epitope in the tomato allergen, Sola l 2, contains a β-1,2-linked xylose. In plants, the transfer of xylose from uridine phosphate (UDP) xylose to the core mannose of N-glycans is mediated by the enzyme β-1,2-xylosyltransferase. By silencing this enzyme via RNAi, it was possible to obtain GM tomatoes that contained undiminished concentrations of Sola l 2, but without the β-1,2-linked xylose sugar residue. As a result the allergen's ability to bind IgE in vitro and in vivo was completely lost demonstrating that the IgE was targeting a cross-reactive carbohydrate determinant (CCD) (Paulus et al. 2011).

Although it was possible to achieve Sola l 3 reduction via RNAi and hypoallergenic Sola l 2 in the tomato plant and fruit via RNAi silencing of β-1,2-xylosyltransferase without morphological changes (Le et al. 2006b; Paulus et al. 2011), markedly diminished growth and reduced fruit setting were observed in Sola l 1-silenced plants (Le et al. 2006a) (◉ Fig. 27.2), suggesting that profilin and its function are of physiological relevance in the regulation of the plant's cytoskeleton.

It was possible to compensate for this deficiency via simultaneous RNAi silencing of endogenous tomato profilin (Sola l 1) and co-expression of hypoallergenic yeast (*Saccharomyces cerevisiae*) profilin (◉ Fig. 27.3) (Le et al. 2010): phenotype and growth behavior could be virtually normalized in Sola l 1-silenced transgenic plants (with a residual content of Sola l 1<5 %) when complemented with yeast profilin. The production of green biomass in these plants was 77 % that of wild type (compared with noncomplemented Sola l 1-silenced transgenic plants: 44 % that of wild type) (Le et al. 2010).

Amino acid identity between the tomato allergen, Sola l 1, and yeast profilin, which has not as yet been described as an allergen, is a mere 32.6 % and is not

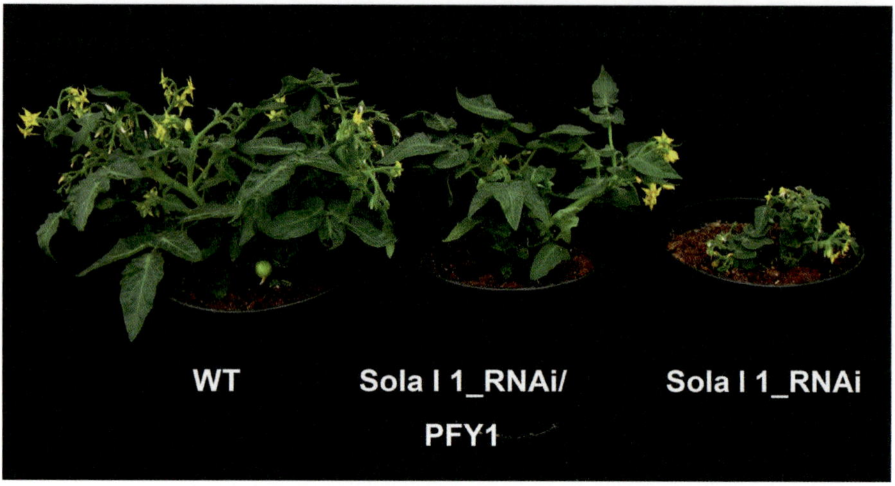

Fig. 27.3 Limitations of the Sola l 1-silenced plant, Sola l 1_RNAi, in terms of biomass development were compensated for by simultaneous Sola l 1-silencing and co-expression of hypoallergenic yeast profilin (PFY1) in the transgenic plant, Sola l 1_RNAi/PFY1. By comparison: wild-type (WT) Micro-Tom variety (Figure courtesy of Dr. Kathrin Paulus and Prof. Uwe Sonnewald, Department of Biochemistry, Friedrich-Alexander University Erlangen-Nürnberg, Germany)

associated with clinically manifest cross-reactivity (Le et al. 2010). The allergenicity of Sola l 1-silenced tomatoes is not increased by the co-expression of yeast profilin (as demonstrated with the basophil histamine release test and prick-to-prick test using native fruit pulp in tomato-allergic subjects) (Le et al. 2010).

Since most tomato-allergic individuals are polysensitized to several tomato allergens, simultaneous silencing of several allergens appears necessary in order to obtain a hypoallergenic tomato fruit that is generally tolerated. In a proof-of-concept study for gene suppression of several target genes (multi-target silencing), a number of chimeric RNAi constructs were generated, e.g., to simultaneously silence Sola l 4 and two putative tomato allergens (chitinase B and osmotin-like protein from tomato) (Paulus 2012). These were stably transformed in the "Micro-Tom" tomato variety. The green fruits of selected RNAi lines exhibited a reduction in the three target genes, while others exhibited a reduction in only two target genes or overexpression of individual target genes as a result of the silencing construct (Paulus 2012). The allergenic potential of this multi-target silencing in tomatoes is the subject of current research.

27.5.5 Carrot (*Daucus carota*)

The prevalence of sensitization to carrot in a population-based study of adults (aged 20–44 years) in 13 countries was between 0.0 % in Iceland and 7.7 % in Germany (overall average for all countries, 3.6 %; overall average for all countries excluding birch pollen-sensitized subjects, 2.0 %) (Burney et al. 2010). Three allergens have been included in the IUIS database to date: Dau c 1 (PR-10, Bet v 1 family member), Dau c 4 (profilin), and Dau c 5 (isoflavone reductase-like protein). Other carrot allergens (LTP and cyclophilin) have been described (Allergome et al. 2014).

It was possible to generate Dau c 1-silenced carrots using RNAi (Peters et al. 2011). The successful silencing of the genes that code for the two isoforms, Dau c 1.01 and Dau c 1.02, by stably expressed Dau c 1.01- and Dau c 1.02-specific hairpin RNA was confirmed in separate plant lines by means of quantitative reverse transcriptase-polymerase chain reaction (RT-PCR) and, on the protein level, by means of immunoblotting with allergen-specific monoclonal antibodies in different plant lines. No attempts have been made to simultaneous RNAi silence both isoforms in the same plant line. IgE immunoblotting with patient sera showed reduced IgE binding to extracts of the Dau c 1.01-silenced carrots compared with wild type; however, reduced IgE binding to extracts of the Dau c 1.02-silenced carrots was not demonstrated via IgE immunoblotting. A reduction in average wheal diameter of 21–50 % compared with wild-type carrots was observed in skin prick tests on carrot-allergic subjects (Peters et al. 2011). A third isoform (Dau c 1.03) was recently identified, but no attempt has been made to silence that gene with RNAi. Coincidental suppression of Dau c 1.03 transcription in the Dau c 1.01- and Dau c 1.02-silenced transgenic carrot roots was ruled out, which may explain why the IgE-binding capacity of the transgenic carrots was preserved.

Physical injury (cutting of the carrot root, i.e., abiotic stress) and infection (biotic stress) caused increased transcription of isoform Dau c 1.03, both in the wild-type and in the transgenic carrot root (Wangorsch et al. 2012). Knowing about the existence of isoforms and their different expression behaviors is of particular importance in the design of RNAi constructs with regard to successful simultaneous RNAi silencing, since even very small quantities, depending on the individual sensitization profile of the carrot-allergic patient (0.55–34.46 μg cumulative dose of Dau c 1.01, Dau c 1.02, and Dau c 4), may be sufficient to trigger allergic symptoms (Foetisch et al. 2013).

A limitation of using carrot as a model plant for allergen modification in root crops lies in the fact that the latency period between transformation and obtaining a testable food (carrot root) is twice as long as that of tomato.

27.5.6 Peanut (*Arachis hypogaea*)

The prevalence of sensitization to peanut in a population-based study of adults (aged 20–44 years) in 13 countries was between 0.8 % in Norway and 9.3 % in the USA (overall average for all countries, 2.6 %; overall average for all countries not including birch pollen sensitized subjects, 1.8 %). The highest prevalence in European countries was seen in Germany at 4.2 % (Burney et al. 2010). According to current data from the German anaphylaxis register, peanut is the most common food-related trigger of anaphylaxis in childhood (Worm et al. 2014). The WHO/IUIS allergen database includes 12 food allergens in peanut: Ara h 1 (vicillin,7S globulin), Ara h 2 (2S albumin), Ara h 3 (11S globulin, glycinin), Ara h 5 (profilin), Ara h 6 (2S albumin), Ara h 7 (2S albumin), Ara h 8 (PR-10, Bet-v-1 homolog), Ara h 9 (nsLTP), Ara h 10 (16-kDa oleosin), Ara h 11 (14-kDa oleosin), Ara h 12 (defensin), and Ara h 13 (defensin).

Ara h 2 is a heat-stable storage protein belonging to the prolamin family that is recognized by more than 90 % of peanut food-allergic individuals and has been the focus of RNAi silencing. Two homologous genes (ara h 2.01 and ara h 2.02) encode for the two isoforms, Ara h 2.01 and Ara h 2.02 (Dodo et al. 2008).

Successful transformation using an Ara h 2.02 RNAi construct—based on a genomic clone—resulted in Ara h 2-silenced transgenic plants. The percentage of Ara h 2 in the total protein content was between 2.87 % and 6.24 % based on animal antibody detection enzyme-linked immunosorbent assays (ELISA) of raw peanut extracts selected from transgenic plants, compared with 27.73 % in wild-type peanuts. Western blot detection of Ara h 2 in the GM peanut using specific monoclonal antibodies was negative. Indirect ELISA tests using patient sera showed a significant reduction in IgE binding to the extracts of selected transgenic peanuts compared with wild type. However, the protein profiles of extracts from some transgenic peanuts were overall altered in the protein gel. The number of mature pods (between two and 32 from transgenic plants compared with 25 on average from wild-type plants) varied considerably (Dodo et al. 2008).

Transformation with another RNAi construct targeting Ara h 2.01 generated plant lines in which expression of both Ara h 2.01 and Ara h 2.02 was silenced and expression of Ara h 6—another 2S albumin that shares 63 % sequence homology with Ara h 2 and is encoded by three genes—was reduced (Chu et al. 2008). One of the plant lines showed complete silencing of Ara h 2 and Ara h 6 in Western blot analysis with chicken-anti-Ara h 2 and anti-Ara h 6 antibodies, as well as a lack of IgE binding using sera from three peanut-allergic human donors. Although the trypsin inhibitory effect of Ara h 2 was missing in transgenic plants, they did not exhibit greater susceptibility to infections by *Aspergillus flavus*. However, mass spectroscopy showed some plant lines to have greater expression of other allergens (Stevenson et al. 2009).

27.6 Acceptance of Hypoallergenic GM Foods Among Consumers

Cultivation rules and bans as well as the reluctance of many consumers to purchase GM foods are recurring subjects in the lay press which predominantly deals with gene-modified crops that are tolerant to herbicides or resistant to particular insect pests. Some voices claim such products only benefit farmers or big agribusiness companies. However, the development of GM hypoallergenic foods discussed above represents products that could provide an immediate benefit for the consumer (Gallo and Sayre 2009).

A questionnaire-based pilot study investigated consumer acceptance of GM hypoallergenic foods among food-allergic subjects in three allergy departments in Austria, the Netherlands, and Spain (20 subjects per department) (Miles et al. 2005). Overall, 83 % of respondents (95 % in Spain, 85 % in the Netherlands, and 70 % in Austria) expressed an interest in the availability of hypoallergenic foods. The majority (89 %) cited a vested interest in such foods as they are currently food allergic and hope to one day to be able to eat foods without fear of an allergic reaction. Price, taste, and safety were given as three further factors that would influence consumer behavior. On average 77 % of respondents (85 % of Spanish respondents, 80 % of Dutch respondents, and 55 % of Austrian) accepted the use of GM methods used to produce hypoallergenic foods and stated they would buy such. Given the choice between GM technology and conventional cultivation, 27 % (30 % of Spanish, 30 % of Dutch, and 20 % of Austrian respondents) expressed no preference for either, while 67 % (65 % of Spanish, 55 % of Dutch, and 80 % of Austrian respondents) stated a preference for conventional cultivation (Miles et al. 2005). Although the small number of respondents makes a conclusive assessment impossible, it is striking that about 75 % of the food-allergic subjects questioned stated that they would purchase GM foods—an indication of the burden caused by avoidance of the relevant foods. The study also highlighted regional/national differences.

27.7 Additional Benefits of Molecular Diagnostics

Using molecular diagnosis in allergy, it is possible to identify allergens that are epidemiologically relevant to food allergy sufferers and which represent suitable target structures in the plant and plant foods for specific allergen reduction strategies. These may vary according to the geographical location (Schmidt-Andersen et al. 2011).

27.8 Treatment and Recommendations

The hypoallergenic foods discussed above are all undergoing testing at the proof-of-concept stage.

Thus, besides the strict avoidance of food or foods containing allergenic components to which food-allergic individuals have developed allergic symptoms, current food allergy treatment options comprise symptomatic, drug-based approaches to suppress allergic symptoms (e.g., H1 receptor antagonists). These will not be discussed in greater detail here. With regard to the management of IgE-mediated food allergies and current treatment recommendations, the reader is referred to the revised guidelines (Muraro et al. 2014; Worm et al. 2015).

Providing patients with emergency medication as a preventive measure is particularly important in the case of previous severe reactions. The "Anaphylaxis" guidelines provide information on the recognition and treatment of anaphylactic reactions (Muraro et al. 2014; Ring et al. 2014). Suffice it to say here that prompt administration of adrenaline is the treatment of first choice in anaphylaxis (Worm et al. 2014).

27.9 Perspectives

The commercial marketing of hypoallergenic foods is not foreseeable at the present time (Chung and Reed 2014). Even the complete silencing of individual allergens achieved to date does not automatically result in the complete loss of allergenicity, since most food-allergic individuals are sensitized to more than one allergen in the same food. Thus, multi-target knockdown approaches aimed at simultaneously silencing several allergens in a food are required and currently the subject of early feasibility studies (Wakasa et al. 2011; Paulus 2012; Chu et al. 2008). Demonstration of stable reduction or elimination of the biologically relevant allergens will need to be demonstrated, and the products will have to meet other safety tests and evaluation before marketing of any hypoallergenic GM product can take place (Goodman et al. 2008; Scheurer and Sonnewald 2009). In vivo investigations of allergenic activity to date have mainly been evaluated by skin prick testing in patients with some of the reviewed hypoallergenic foods; except for apple (Dubois et al. 2015), oral food challenges are lacking. Allergen-resolved threshold doses (LOAEL, lowest observed adverse effect level), i.e., doses below which sensitized patients are not expected to develop allergic symptoms (Foetisch et al. 2013), have been identified for only a few food allergens. Thus, it is not possible at present to conclusively assess whether the 100-fold allergen reduction *in planta* achieved by RNAi silencing is sufficient to enable allergic individuals to consume relevant foods free from symptoms. Although investigations to date demonstrate the stable transformation and expression of RNAi constructs over generations, further investigations are required to establish their stability under extreme climatic conditions and in the case of plant infections. Further scientific investigations are underway to resolve these questions.

Food-specific allergy vaccines to treat food allergies using specific immunotherapy (SIT) are currently only available within the context of clinical trials (Chung and Reed 2014). Anaphylactic side effects (sometimes severe) have been observed in attempts at SIT with food extracts (Pons et al. 2005). Stable allergen extracts that are standardized in terms of their relevant allergen content have not as yet received market authorization nor are they commercially available.

Targeted mutagenesis has been used to generate hypoallergenic mutants of food allergens as recombinant proteins [e.g., hypoallergenic mutants of Pru av 1 (cherry) (Neudecker et al. 2003; Wiche et al. 2005), Ara h 2 (peanut) (King et al. 2005), Ara h 6 (Hazebrouck et al. 2012), Mal d 1 (apple) (Hoffmann-Sommergruber et al. 2015; Bolhaar et al. 2005)].

IgE immunoblotting or immunoblotting and enzyme allergosorbent test (EAST) inhibition confirmed significantly reduced in vitro IgE-binding capacity in these mutated proteins. The modulation of IgE-binding sites by targeted mutagenesis represents a promising approach to obtaining hypoallergenic proteins, the use of which appears conceivable in the midterm in SIT as a treatment measure for tertiary prevention in existing type 1 allergy (Wiche et al. 2005; Hazebrouck et al. 2012; Bolhaar et al. 2005). In contrast, the design of hypoallergenic foods is following a global approach to allergy prevention which, in addition to avoiding allergic symptoms in existing sensitization, also aims primarily at preventing the development of de novo sensitizations to allergenic foods (Gallo and Sayre 2009).

Due to the current controversy surrounding GM foods, new techniques in crop cultivation have become of interest [e.g., targeting induced local lesions in genomes (TILLING) and transcription activator-like effector nucleases (TALEN)], which, according to a report by the New Techniques Working Group (NTWG), involve molecular biological methods classified in Europe as belonging to conventional cultivation. A position statement of the German Central Commission for Biological Safety (*Zentrale Kommission für die Biologische Sicherheit*)—formulated on the basis of assessments made on a European level—classifies these new techniques according to European Directives and the German Genetic Engineering Act (*Gentechnikgesetz*, GenTG) in terms of whether they give rise to genetically modified organisms within the meaning of EU Directives 2001/18/EG and 2009/41/EG or not (Lebensmittelsicherheit & Zentrale Kommission für die Biologische Sicherheit (ZKBS) 2012).

The TILLING method, for example, combines the standard breeding technique of ethyl methanesulfonate mutagenesis with a screening procedure based on the detection of mismatch hybridization using high-performance liquid chromatography (HPLC), which enables the simultaneous investigation of numerous potential mutants (McCallum et al. 2000). TALEN bind to a target site in the genome in a sequence-specific manner and induce a double-strand break, which permits, e.g., mutation or deletion (Morbitzer et al. 2010).

These new methods of conventional breeding appear to make it possible to obtain, e.g., null mutants with partially similar, stable characteristics, as in the proof-of-concept studies with GM methods, pointing to novel non-GM strategies to produce hypoallergenic foods.

Conclusions

Food allergies in adulthood are most commonly to plant foods (nuts, legumes, fruits, and vegetables). Eliminating relevant allergens in the plant itself represents a new approach to allergen avoidance for the primary, secondary, and tertiary prevention of food allergies.

At present, the development of hypoallergenic foods is largely still at the preclinical experimental stage using GM techniques. Proof-of-concept studies have successfully established strategies to stably silence or reduce allergen expression in plant-based foods. Only profilin silencing exhibited serious limitations in terms of growth and fruit setting in tomato plants; this, however, could be compensated for by simultaneously complementing plants with a hypoallergenic yeast profilin.

Multi-target strategies to simultaneously silence several allergens are the subject of current investigations.

Based on the findings of these proof-of-concept studies, producing allergen-reduced foods is technically feasible. However, in the eventuality that their acceptance proves problematic, it would appear reasonable, in terms of the further development of hypoallergenic foods, to examine the option of reproducing the results obtained with allergen-silenced transgenic plants discussed above using modern breeding methods.

However, a major obstacle remains before the dream of having hypoallergenic foods for common consumption becomes a reality: in order to protect food-allergic consumers, it will be necessary to develop systems that control the entire food supply chain in order to guarantee that a food (e.g., peanut butter) labeled as a hypoallergenic will indeed be safe for consumers with severe peanut allergy. That requires fail-safe controls from seed production through farming, harvest, wholesale markets, food production facilities, packaging, and labeling of foods. Controls and quality checks will need to be developed that will prevent comingling of wild-type, fully allergenic varieties of crop materials with hypoallergenic materials and foods. At present it is not possible to guarantee perfect control of allergenic food sources to prevent comingling and allergen cross-contact in our complex food supply system in spite of great improvements in allergen detection, quality control plans, strict labeling, and regulatory processes.

References

Allergome, The Platform of Allergen Knowledge, editor. www.allergome.org/script/search_step1.php?clear=1. accessed 30 Nov 2014.

American Academy of Pediatrics Committee on Nutrition, editor. Clinical testing of hypoallergenic formulas. Pediatrics. 2000;106:346–9.

Asero R, Mistrello G, Roncarolo D, de Vries SC, Gautier MF, Ciurana CL, et al. Lipid-transfer protein: a pan-allergen in plant-derived foods that is highly resistant to pepsin digestion. Int Arch Allergy Immunol. 2000;122:20–32.

Asero R, Jimeno L, Barber D. Component-resolved diagnosis of plant food allergy by SPT. Eur Ann Allergy Clin Immunol. 2008;40:115–21.

Asero R, Tripodi S, Dondi A, et al. Prevalence and clinical relevance of IgE sensitization to profilin in childhood: a multicenter study. Int Arch Allergy Immunol. 2015;168:25–31.

Ballmer-Weber BK, Hoffmann-Sommergruber K. Update: molecular diagnostics of allergies to vegetables and fruits. Allergo J Int. 2014;23:24–34.

Bässler OY, Weiss J, Wienkoop S, Lehmann K, Scheler C, Dölle S, et al. Evidence for novel tomato seed allergens: IgE-reactive legumin and vicilin proteins identified by multidimensional protein fractionation-mass spectrometry and in silico epitope modeling. J Proteome Res. 2009;8:1111–22.

Beyer K. Hypoallergenicity: a principle for the treatment of food allergy. In: Cooke RJ, Vandenplas Y, Wahn U, editors. Nutrition support for infants and children at risk. 59th Nestlé Nutrition Workshop, Pediatric Program, Berlin 2006. Basel: Karger; 2007. p. 37–47.

Bolhaar ST, Zuidmeer L, Ma Y, Ferreira F, Bruijnzeel-Koomen CA, Hoffmann-Sommergruber K, et al. A mutant of the major apple allergen, Mal d 1, demonstrating hypo-allergenicity in the target organ by double-blind placebo-controlled food challenge. Clin Exp Allergy. 2005;35:1638–44.

Bundesamt für Verbraucherschutz und Lebensmittelsicherheit, Zentrale Kommission für die Biologische Sicherheit (ZKBS), editors. Stellungnahme der ZKBS zu neuen Techniken für die Pflanzenzüchtung. Az.: 402.45310.0104; Juni 2012. www.keine-gentechnik.de/fileadmin/pics/Informationsdienst/ZKBS_Neue_Techniken_Pflanzenzuechtung_D_2012.pdf.

Burney P, Summers C, Chinn S, Hooper R, van Ree R, Lidholm J. Prevalence and distribution of sensitization to foods in the European Community Respiratory Health Survey: a EuroPrevall analysis. Allergy. 2010;65:1182–8.

Chapman MD. Allergen nomenclature. In: Lockey RF, Ledford DK, editors. Allergens and allergen immunotherapy. 4th ed. New York: Informa Healthcare; 2008. p. 47–58.

Chu Y, Faustinelli P, Ramos ML, Hajduch M, Stevenson S, Thelen JJ, et al. Reduction of IgE binding and nonpromotion of Aspergillus flavus fungal growth by simultaneously silencing Ara h 2 and Ara h 6 in peanut. J Agric Food Chem. 2008;56:11225–33.

Chung SY, Reed S. Reducing food allergy: is there promise for food applications? Curr Pharm Des. 2014;20:924–30.

Codex Alimentarius Commission. Alinorm 03/34: Joint FAO/WHO Food Standard Programme, 25th Session, Rome; 2003. Appendix III, Guideline for the conduct of food safety assessment of foods derived from recombinant-DNA plants; Appendix IV, Annex on the assessment of possible allergenicity, p. 47–60.

Dodo HW, Konan KN, Chen FC, Egnin M, Viquez OM. Alleviating peanut allergy using genetic engineering: the silencing of the immunodominant allergen Ara h 2 leads to its significant reduction and a decrease in peanut allergenicity. Plant Biotechnol J. 2008;6:135–45.

Dubois AE, Pagliarani G, Brouwer RM, Kollen BJ, Dragsted LO, Eriksen FD, Callesen O, Gilissen LJ, Krens FA, Visser RG, Smulders MJ, Vlieg-Boerstra BJ, Flokstra-de Blok BJ, van de Weg WE. First successful reduction of clinical allergenicity of food by genetic modification: Mal d 1-silenced apples cause fewer allergy symptoms than the wild-type cultivar. Allergy. 2015;70:1406–12.

EFSA Panel on Genetically Modified Organisms (GMO Panel), editor. Scientific opinion on the assessment of allergenicity of GM plants and microorganisms and derived food and feed. EFSA J. 2010;8:1700.

Fagard M, Vaucheret H. (Trans)gene silencing in plants: how many mechanisms? Annu Rev Plant Physiol Plant Mol Biol. 2000;51:167–94.

Foetisch K, Son AY, Altmann F, Aulepp H, Conti A, Haustein D, Vieths S. Tomato (Lycopersicon esculentum) allergens in pollen-allergic patients. Eur Food Res Technol. 2001;213:259–66.

Foetisch K, Scheurer S, Vieths S, Hanschmann KM, Lidholm J, Mahler V. Identification of allergen-resolved threshold doses of carrot (Daucus carota) by means of oral challenge and ELISA. J Allergy Clin Immunol. 2013;131:1711–3.

Fritsché R. Utility of animal models for evaluating hypoallergenicity. Mol Nutr Food Res. 2009;53:979–83.

Gallo M, Sayre R. Removing allergens and reducing toxins from food crops. Curr Opin Biotechnol. 2009;20:191–6.

Gilissen LJWJ, Bolhaar STHP, Matos CI, Rouwendal GJA, Boone MJ, Krens FA, et al. Silencing the major apple allergen Mal d 1 by using the RNA interference approach. J Allergy Clin Immunol. 2005;115:364–9.

Gilissen LJWJ, Bolhaar STHP, Knulst AC, Zuidmeeri L, van Ree R, Gao ZS, et al. Production of hypoallergenic plant foods by selection, breeding and genetic modification. In: Gilissen LJEJ, Wichers HJ, Savelkoul HFJ, Bogers RJ, editors. Allergy matters: new approaches to allergy prevention and management. Heidelberg: Springer; 2006. p. 95–105.

Goodman RE, Vieths S, Sampson HA, Hill D, Ebisawa M, Taylor SL, van Ree R. Allergenicity assessment of genetically modified crops – what makes sense? Nat Biotechnol. 2008;26:73–81.

Hauser M, Wallner M, Ferreira F, Mahler V, Kleine-Tebbe J. Das Konzept der Pollen-Panallergene: Profiline und Polcalcine. Allergo J. 2012;21:291–3.

Hazebrouck S, Guillon B, Drumare MF, Paty E, Wal JM, Bernard H. Trypsin resistance of the major peanut allergen Ara h 6 and allergenicity of the digestion products are abolished after selective disruption of disulfide bonds. Mol Nutr Food Res. 2012;56:548–57.

Hebert CG, Valdes JJ, Bentley WE. Beyond silencing engineering applications of RNA interference and antisense technology for altering cellular phenotype. Curr Opin Biotechnol. 2008;19:500–5.

Herman EM, Helm RM, Jung R, Kinney AJ. Genetic modification removes an immunodominant allergen from soybean. Plant Physiol. 2003;132:36–43.

Hoffmann-Sommergruber K, SAFE Consortium, editors. The SAFE project: 'plant food allergies: field to table strategies for reducing their incidence in Europe' an EC-funded study. Allergy. 2015;60:436–42.

Holzhauser T, Wackermann O, Ballmer-Weber BK, Bindslev-Jensen C, Scibilia J, Perono-Garoffo L, Utsumi S, Pousen KL, Vieths S. Soybean (Glycine max) allergy in Europe: Gly m 5 (beta-conglycinin) and Gly m 6 (glycinin) are potential diagnostic markers for severe allergic reactions to soy. J Allergy Clin Immunol. 2009;123:452–8.

Hompes S, Scherer K, Köhli A, Rueff F, Mahler V, Lange L, et al. Nahrungsmittel-Anaphylaxie: Daten aus dem Anaphylaxie-Register. Allergo J. 2010;19:234–42.

International Union of Immunological Societies (IUIS) Allergen Nomenclature Sub-Committee, editor. Allergen nomenclature. 2014. www.allergen.org/index.php. Zugegriffen 30 Nov 2014.

King N, Helm R, Stanley JS, Vieths S, Lüttkopf D, Hatahet L, et al. Allergenic characteristics of a modified peanut allergen. Mol Nutr Food Res. 2005;49:963–71.

Kleine-Tebbe J, Ballmer-Weber B, Breiteneder H, Vieths S. Bet v 1 und Homologe – Verursacher der Baumpollenallergie und birkenpollenassoziierter Kreuzreaktionen. Allergo J. 2010; 19:462–3.

Kondo Y, Urisu A, Tokuda R. Identification and characterization of the allergens in the tomato fruit by immunoblotting. Int Arch Allergy Immunol. 2001;126:294–9.

Krath BN, Eriksen FD, Pedersen BH, Gilissen LJWJ, van der Weg WE, Dragsted LO. Development of hypo-allergenic apples: silencing of the major allergen Mal d 1 gene in 'Elstar' apple and the effect of grafting. J Hortic Sci Biotechnol. 2009;ISAFRUIT Special Issue:52–7.

Ladics GS. Current codex guidelines for assessment of potential protein allergenicity. Food Chem Toxicol. 2008;46 Suppl 10:S20–3.

Le LQ, Mahler V, Lorenz Y, Scheurer S, Biemelt S, Vieths S, Sonnewald U. Reduced allergenicity of tomato fruits harvested from Lyc e 1-silenced transgenic tomato plants. J Allergy Clin Immunol. 2006a;118:1176–83.

Le LQ, Lorenz Y, Scheurer S, Fotisch K, Enrique E, Bartra J, et al. Design of tomato fruits with reduced allergenicity by dsRNAi-mediated inhibition of ns-LTP (Lyc e 3) expression. Plant Biotechnol J. 2006b;4:231–42.

Le LQ, Mahler V, Scheurer S, Foetisch K, Braun Y, Weigand D. Yeast profilin complements profilin deficiency in transgenic tomato fruits and allows development of hypoallergenic tomato fruits. FASEB J. 2010;24:4939–47.

López-Matas MÁ, Larramendi CH, Ferrer A, Huertas AJ, Pagán JA, García-Abujeta JL, et al. Identification and quantification of tomato allergens: in vitro characterization of six different varieties. Ann Allergy Asthma Immunol. 2011;106:230–8.

Lorenz Y, Enrique E, Lequynh L, Fötisch K, Retzek M, Biemelt S, et al. Skin prick tests reveal stable and heritable reduction of allergenic potency of gene-silenced tomato fruits. J Allergy Clin Immunol. 2006;118:711–8.

McCallum CM, Comai L, Greene EA, Henikoff S. Targeting induced local lesions in genomes (TILLING) for plant functional genomics. Plant Physiol. 2000;123:439–42.

Miles S, Bolhaar S, Gonzalez-Mancebo E, Hafner C, Hoffmann-Sommergruber K, Fernandez-Rivas M, Knulst A. Attitudes towards low allergen food in food allergic consumers. Nutr Food Sci. 2005;35:220–8.

Morbitzer R, Römer P, Boch J, Lahaye T. Regulation of selected genome loci using de novo-engineered transcription activator-like effector (TALE)-type transcription factors. Proc Natl Acad Sci U S A. 2010;107:21617–22.

Muraro A, Dreborg S, Halken S, Høst A, Niggemann B, Aalberse R, et al. Dietary prevention of allergic diseases in infants and small children. Part I: immunologic background and criteria for hypoallergenicity. Pediatr Allergy Immunol. 2004;15:103–11.

Muraro A, Werfel T, Hoffmann-Sommergruber K, Roberts G, Beyer K, Bindslev-Jensen C, et al. EAACI food allergy and anaphylaxis guidelines: diagnosis and management of food allergy. Allergy. 2014;69:1008–25.

Neudecker P, Lehmann K, Nerkamp J, Haase T, Wangorsch A, Fötisch K, et al. Mutational epitope analysis of Pru av 1 and Api g 1, the major allergens of cherry (Prunus avium) and celery (Apium graveolens): correlating IgE reactivity with three-dimensional structure. Biochem J. 2003;376(Pt 1):97–107.

Nusrat A, Datta SK, Datta K. RNA interference in designing transgenic crops. GM Crops. 2010;1:207–13.

Ofori-Anti AO, Ariyarathna H, Chen L, Lee HL, Pramod SN, Goodman RE. Establishing objective detection limits for the pepsin digestion assay used in the assessment of genetically modified foods. Regul Toxicol Pharmacol. 2008;52(2):94–103.

Ogawa T, Bando N, Tsuji H, Okajima H, Nishikawa K, Sasaoka K. Investigation of the IgE-binding proteins in soybeans by immunoblotting with the sera of the soybean-sensitive patients with atopic dermatitis. J Nutr Sci Vitaminol. 1991;37:555–65.

Palacín A, Gómez-Casado C, Rivas LA, Aguirre J, Tordesillas L, Bartra J, et al. Graph based study of allergen cross-reactivity of plant lipid transfer proteins (LTPs) using microarray in a multi-center study. PLoS One. 2012;7:e50799.

Paulus KE. Molekulare Ansätze zur Reduktion des allergenen Potenzials von Tomatenfrüchten. Dissertation an der Naturwissenschaftlichen Fakultät der Friedrich-Alexander-Universität Erlangen-Nürnberg; 2012.

Paulus KE, Mahler V, Pabst M, Kogel KH, Altmann F, Sonnewald U. Silencing β1,2-xylosyltransferase in transgenic tomato fruits reveals xylose as constitutive component of Ige-binding epitopes. Front Plant Sci. 2011;2:42.

Peters S, Imani J, Mahler V, Foetisch K, Kaul S, Paulus KE, et al. Dau c 1.01 and Dau c 1.02-silenced transgenic carrot plants show reduced allergenicity to patients with carrot allergy. Transgenic Res. 2011;20:547–56.

Petersen A, Scheurer S. Stabile pflanzliche Nahrungsmittelallergene: lipid-transfer-proteine. Allergo J. 2011;20:384–6.

Plant AL, Cohen A, Moses MS, Bray EA. Nucleotide sequence and spatial expression pattern of a drought- and abscisic acid-induced gene of tomato. Plant Physiol. 1991;97:900–6.

Pons L, Palmer K, Burks W. Towards immunotherapy for peanut allergy. Curr Opin Allergy Clin Immunol. 2005;5:558–62.

Pravettoni V, Primavesi L, Farioli L, Brenna OV, Pompei C, Conti A, et al. Tomato allergy: detection of IgE-binding lipid transfer proteins in tomato derivatives and in fresh tomato peel, pulp, and seeds. J Agric Food Chem. 2009;57:10749–54.

Radauer C, Breiteneder H. Evolutionary biology of plant food allergens. J Allergy Clin Immunol. 2007;120:518–25.

Radauer C, Kleine-Tebbe J, Beyer K. Stabile pflanzliche Nahrungsmittelallergene: Speicherproteine. Allergo J. 2012;21:155–8.

Radauer C, Nandy A, Ferreira F, Goodman RE, Larsen JN, Lidholm J, et al. Update of the WHO/IUIS Allergen Nomenclature Database based on analysis of allergen sequences. Allergy. 2014;69:413–9.

Ring J, Beyer K, Biedermann T, Bircher A, Duda D, Fischer J, et al. Akuttherapie und Management der Anaphylaxie. Allergo J Int. 2014;23:96–112.

Scheurer S, Sonnewald S. Genetic engineering of plant food with reduced allergenicity. Front Biosci. 2009;14:59–71.

Schmidt-Andersen MB, Hall S, Dragsted LO. Identification of European allergy patterns to the allergen families PR-10, LTP, and profilin from Rosaceae fruits. Clin Rev Allergy Immunol. 2011;41:4–19.

Sicherer SH. Epidemiology of food allergy. J Allergy Clin Immunol. 2011;127:594–602.

Smith NA, Singh SP, Wang MB, Stoutjesdijk PA, Green AG, Waterhouse PM. Total silencing by intron-spliced hairpin RNAs. Nature. 2000;407:319–20.

Song Y, Cui C, Zhu H, Li Q, Zhao F, Jin Y. Expression, purification and characterization of zinc-finger nucleases to knockout the goat beta-lactoglobulin gene. Protein Expr Purif. 2015;112:1–7.

Stevenson SE, Chu Y, Ozias-Akins P, Thelen JJ. Validation of gelfree, label-free quantitative proteomics approaches: applications for seed allergen profiling. J Proteomics. 2009;72:555–66.

Tada Y, Nakase M, Adachi T, Nakamura R, Shimada H, Takahashi M, et al. Reduction of 14–16 kDa allergenic proteins in transgenic rice plants by antisense gene. FEBS Lett. 1996;391:341–5.

Taylor SL, Hefle SL. Food allergies and other food sensitivities. A publication of the Institute of Food Technologists' Expert Panel on Food Safety and Nutrition. Food Technol. 2001;55:68–83.

Trcka J, Schad SG, Scheurer S, Conti A, Vieths S, Gross G, Trautmann A. Rice-induced anaphylaxis: IgE-mediated allergy against a 56-kDa glycoprotein. Int Arch Allergy Immunol. 2012;158:9–17.

Wakasa Y, Hirano K, Urisu A, Matsuda T, Takaiwa F. Generation of transgenic rice lines with reduced contents of multiple potential allergens using a null mutant in combination with an RNA silencing method. Plant Cell Physiol. 2011;52:2190–9.

Wangorsch A, Weigand D, Peters S, Mahler V, Fötisch K, Reuter A, et al. Identification of a Dau c PRPlike protein (Dau c 1.03) as a new allergenic isoform in carrots (cultivar Rodelika). Clin Exp Allergy. 2012;42:156–66.

Wangorsch A, Jamin A, Foetisch K, Malczyk A, Reuter A, Vierecke S, et al. Identification of Sola l 4 as Bet v 1 homologous pathogenesis related-10 allergen in tomato fruits. Mol Nutr Food Res. 2014;59:582–92.

Welter S, Lehmann K, Dölle S, Schwarz D, Weckwerth W, Scheler C, et al. Identification of putative new tomato allergens and differential interaction with IgEs of tomato allergic subjects. Clin Exp Allergy. 2013a;43:1419–27.

Welter S, Dölle S, Lehmann K, Schwarz D, Weckwerth W, Worm M, Franken P. Pepino mosaic virus infection of tomato affects allergen expression, but not the allergenic potential of fruits. PLoS One. 2013b;8:e65116.

Wesley SV, Helliwell CA, Smith NA, Wang MB, Rouse DT, Liu Q, et al. Construct design for efficient, effective and high-throughput gene silencing in plants. Plant J. 2001;27:581–90.

Westphal S, Kolarich D, Foetisch K, Lauer I, Altmann F, Conti A, et al. Molecular characterization and allergenic activity of Lyc e 2 (beta-fructofuranosidase), a glycosylated allergen of tomato. Eur J Biochem. 2003;270:1327–37.

Westphal S, Kempf W, Foetisch K, Retzek M, Vieths S, Scheurer S. Tomato profilin Lyc e 1: IgE cross-reactivity and allergenic potency. Allergy. 2004;59:526–32.

Wiche R, Gubesch M, König H, Fötisch K, Hoffmann A, Wangorsch A, et al. Molecular basis of pollen-related food allergy: Identification of a second cross-reactive IgE epitope on Pru av 1, the major cherry allergen. Biochem J. 2005;385:319–27.

Willerroider M, Fuchs H, Ballmer-Weber BK, Focke M, Susani M, Thalhamer J, et al. Cloning and molecular and immunological characterisation of two new food allergens, Cap a 2 and Lyc e 1, profilins from bell pepper (Capsicum annuum) and tomato (Lycopersicon esculentum). Int Arch Allergy Immunol. 2003;131:245–55.

Worm M, Eckermann O, Dölle S, Aberer W, Beyer K, Hawranek T, et al. Auslöser und Therapie der Anaphylaxie: Auswertung von mehr als 4000 Fällen aus Deutschland, Österreich und der Schweiz. Dtsch Arztebl Int. 2014;111:367–75.

Worm M, Reese I, Ballmer-Weber B, et al. Guidelines on the management of IgE-mediated food allergies: S2k-Guidelines of the German Society for Allergology and Clinical Immunology (DGAKI) in collaboration with other German Medical Societies including the Association of the Scientific Medical Societies in Germany (AWMF). Allergo J Int. 2015;24:256–293.
Zhang J, Hua ZC. Targeted gene silencing by small interfering RNA-based knock-down technology. Curr Pharm Biotechnol. 2004;5:1–7.

Index

J. Kleine-Tebbe, T. Jakob (eds.), *Molecular Allergy Diagnostics*,
DOI 10.1007/978-3-319-42499-6

D

J

K

L

M

N

O

U

V

W

Printed by Printforce, the Netherlands